To my husband,
Robert,
and my son,
Michael,
who support me in all
my professional
and personal endeavors

Contributors

Tiffany Kay Bennett, RNC-OB, MS-NL
RN Senior Manager
Labor, Delivery, and Triage
Banner Thunderbird Medical Center
Glendale, Arizona

Teresa K. Buchda RNC-OB, MS-NL
RN Director, Women and Infant Services
Banner Thunderbird Medical Center
Glendale, Arizona

Deborah L. Davis, PhD
Developmental Psychologist and Writer
    Author of *Empty Cradle, Broken Heart*
Denver, Colorado
Tulsa, Oklahoma

Suzanne Helzer, RNC-OB, LCCE
Bereavement Services/RTS Program
    Coordinator
Banner Desert Medical Center
Mesa, Arizona

Terance L. Kranz, RNC-OB, MSN
Clinical Education Specialist
Banner Del E. Webb Medical Center
Sun City West, Arizona

Karen M. Marshall, RNC–OB, MSN, CNS
Clinical Nurse Specialist
Banner Thunderbird Medical Center
Glendale, Arizona

Barbara Oxley, NMD, RN, BSN, IBCLC
Director
Bethany Ranch Health Clinic
Phoenix, Arizona

Sheryl Parfitt, MSN, RNC
Clinical Educator, Obstetrics
Scottsdale Heathcare
Scottsdale, Arizona

Mary L. Sciuto, RN, MS
RN-Clinical Education Specialist
Banner Good Samaritan Medical Center
Phoenix, Arizona

Christina Tussey, MSN, CNS, RNC-OB, RNC-MN
Women and Infants Clinical Nurse
    Specialist
Banner Good Samaritan Medical Center
Phoenix, Arizona

Amy Warengo, RN, MS-NL
RN Senior Manager
Antepartum and Maternal Fetal
    Medicine Center
Banner Thunderbird Medical Center
Glendale, Arizona

Preface

Today's technologic advances make it possible to offer the woman and her family, who are experiencing a high risk pregnancy and delivery, a good chance for a positive outcome. The evidence-based practice nursing and medical literature were the primary resources used in the writing of this manual such as the Cochrane Reviews, a database of systematic reviews, and evidence-based clinical guidelines such as Agency for Healthcare Research and Quality (AHRQ), National Guideline Clearinghouse (NGC), Institute for Clinical Systems Improvement (ICSI), and Society of Obstetricians and Gynaecologists of Canada (SOGC) as well as references from professional organizations such as AWHONN and ACOG. As nurses, nurse practitioners, and nurse-midwives, we each have a responsibility to keep our practices up-to-date and evidence-based. Nurses play a key role in ensuring that women and their fetuses receive the best possible care. Perinatal nurses in all obstetric facilities must know about screening for risk factors, they must provide preventive management using effective alternative and complementary therapies, and appropriately intervene when complications develop. Unfortunately, many women do not receive adequate prenatal care and enter the health care system only after complications occur. Because these women seek assistance from various types of facilities, nurses who practice in clinics, emergency rooms, and primary care settings must also be alert to perinatal complications and be prepared to provide immediate stabilizing care in ambulatory or other inpatient care settings.

Manual of High Risk Pregnancy & Delivery is designed as a practical reference manual to provide comprehensive information in a concise, portable, and accessible format. Clearly written text and numerous tables and boxes enhance comprehension and facilitate easy retrieval of information. The nursing process serves as the organizational framework for discussions of both preventive and emergent care for a wide range of topics. Nursing interventions are grounded in evidence-based practice recommendations.

The coverage of common medical and obstetric problems experienced during childbearing are presented in a layout style that includes incidence, etiology, physiology, pathophysiology, as well as the usual, expected, and intensive care management protocols for advanced nurse practitioners. Management and intervention protocols are addressed with emphases on ambulatory care prevention and inpatient high-risk care with critical care protocols, as appropriate. Psychosocial implications and family considerations are incorporated throughout. A unique, contributed chapter discusses and emphasizes how advance practice nurses can access relevant alternative and complementary therapies, which are evidence-based for high risk pregnancy and delivery care.

It is my conviction that with thorough, knowledgeable, and evidence-based care of the mother and fetus, neonatal morbidity and mortality can be considerably decreased, and complications for the mother can be lessened. It is my intent and hope that this text will enable health care professionals to provide optimal care for mother, fetus, and family from ambulatory, preventive, inpatient, and critical care arenas through the early postpartum period.

Elizabeth Stepp Gilbert

Contents

UNIT I PHYSIOLOGIC CONSIDERATIONS, ASSESSMENTS, AND INTEGRATIVE THERAPIES

1. Physiologic and Nutritional Adaptations to Pregnancy, 1
2. General Nursing Assessment of the High Risk Expectant Family, 25
3. Assessment of Fetal Well-Being, 43
4. Perinatal Screening, Diagnoses, and Fetal Therapies, 88
5. Integrative Therapies in Pregnancy and Childbirth, 107

UNIT II PSYCHOLOGIC IMPLICATIONS OF A HIGH RISK PREGNANCY

6. Psychologic Adaptations, 128
7. Perinatal Death and Bereavement Care, 149

UNIT III ETHICAL DILEMMAS AND LEGAL CONSIDERATIONS IN PERINATAL NURSING

8. Ethical Decision Making, 170
9. Legal Issues and Risk Management, 181

UNIT IV HEALTH DISORDERS COMPLICATING PREGNANCY

10. Diabetes, 200
11. Cardiac Disease, 243
12. Renal Disease, 258
13. Autoimmune Rheumatic Diseases, 271
14. Venous Thromboembolic Disease, 282
15. Pulmonary Disease and Respiratory Distress, 289

UNIT V COMPLICATIONS IN PREGNANCY

16. Spontaneous Abortion, 311
17. Ectopic Pregnancy, 331
18. Gestational Trophoblastic Disease, 351
19. Placental Abnormalities, 364
20. Disseminated Intravascular Coagulation, 395
21. Hemolytic Incompatibility, 402

22. Hypertensive Disorders, 416

23. Preterm Labor and Multiple Gestation, 460

24. Premature Rupture of Membranes, 488

25. Trauma, 500

UNIT VI TERATOGENS AND SOCIAL ISSUES COMPLICATING PREGNANCY

26. Sexually and Nonsexually Transmitted Genitourinary Infections, 519

27. Substance Abuse, 558

UNIT VII ALTERATIONS IN THE MECHANISM OF LABOR

28. Labor Stimulation, 582

29. Dysfunctional Labor, 610

30. Prolonged Pregnancy, 660

Index, 671

1

Physiologic and Nutritional Adaptations to Pregnancy

T he foundation of high risk pregnancy management is based on careful, thorough physiologic and nutritional assessments. The nurse caring for the high risk expectant mother must have a thorough understanding of the anatomic and physiologic changes that occur in a pregnant woman's body to be able to recognize normal as well as abnormal responses.

ADAPTATIONS

Cardiovascular

The most dramatic changes during pregnancy involve the cardiovascular system. These changes are anatomic and hemodynamic. The following normal hemodynamic changes occur during pregnancy:

- *Hypervolemia.* Blood volume increases 48%, leading to such auscultatory changes as S_1 splitting, auditory S_3 by 20 weeks of gestation, systolic murmur, and, occasionally, a transient diastolic murmur.
- *Hemodilution.* Plasma volume increases approximately 50%, whereas red blood cell volume increases only 20%, causing hemodilution. This leads to a lower colloid osmotic pressure (COP), which is the force that holds fluid in the capillaries. The opposing force, capillary hydrostatic pressure measured as pulmonary capillary wedge pressure (PCWP), which moves fluid out of the capillaries into the interstitial space, remains the same. COP is dependent on the plasma concentration of colloids, plasma proteins such as albumin, and to a lesser extent, globulin and fibrinogen. Because the hemodilution of the plasma colloids causes the COP to decrease while there is no change in the PCWP, there is a tendency to develop dependent edema. During a pregnancy coupled with a high risk condition that further decreases the COP or increases the PCWP, the risk for pulmonary edema is greater.

- *Hyperdynamic state.* Cardiac output increases 40% by 36 to 38 weeks of gestation (cardiac output = heart rate × stroke volume). Both stroke volume and heart rate increase 20% by this point in gestation.
- *Low resistance.* Normally, systemic vascular resistance decreases 20%, and pulmonary vascular resistance decreases 35% related to progesterone, local prostaglandins such as prostacyclin, and nitric oxide. This lowered systemic vascular resistance usually causes the baseline blood pressure to decrease at the end of the first trimester and throughout the second trimester and to return to the nonpregnancy baseline during the third trimester.
- Anatomically, the heart is displaced upward and to the left throughout pregnancy, changing the location of the point of maximum impulse (PMI) from the fifth intercostal space (ICS) to approximately the fourth ICS and moving it more lateral to the midclavicular line. This results in electrocardiogram changes such as a left axis deviation of the QRS complex, a nonspecific S-T segment, and an abnormal T wave.

Respiratory

The normal respiratory changes follow:

- *Thoracic breathing.* During pregnancy, the mother changes from being an abdominal breather to being a thoracic breather. This is because the diaphragm raises 4 to 7 cm and the ribs flare, increasing the anterior to posterior diameter.
- *Improved oxygen delivery.* Oxygen consumption increases by 20% to meet fetal growth and development needs and increased maternal growth and basal metabolism. Oxygen consumption further increases during labor, and it is higher during pregnancy with multiples.
- *Hyperventilation.* Maternal tidal volume (volume of air that is exchanged with each breath) increases 40% related to progesterone. Maternal functional residual capacity (volume of air that remains in the lung on expiration) decreases 25%. The result is increased depth of respirations because there is increased oxygenated air mixed with a smaller amount of carbon deoxygenated air. For high risk management, note that hyperventilation lowers oxygen reserve and that hypoxia can develop more rapidly in a high risk condition. This can enhance induction of and recovery from general anesthesia.
- *Compensatory respiratory alkalosis.* Because of the hyperventilation effect of pregnancy, the arterial oxygen tension is increased (normal Po_2, 100 to 108 mm Hg) and the arterial carbon dioxide tension is reduced (normal Pco_2, 27 to 32 mm Hg) because the excess CO_2 is exhaled, decreasing carbonic acid. Maternal serum bicarbonate decreases (normal, 18 to 22 mEq/L) to maintain the maternal acid-base balance. Therefore the normal arterial blood gases of pregnancy reflect the state of chronic compensatory respiratory alkalosis. Women with high risk pregnancies can develop respiratory and metabolic acidosis rapidly.

Hematologic

The normal hematologic changes during pregnancy follow:

- *Hypercoagulation.* During pregnancy, the equilibrium for coagulation-fibrinolysis is skewed toward coagulation. Plasma fibrinogen rises throughout pregnancy.

The fibrinogen clotting factors are increased, and the fibrinolytic activity is suppressed because there is a decrease in circulatory plasminogen activators. Platelet count either remains normal or is reduced insignificantly.

- *Leukocytosis, especially neutrophils.* White blood cells, or leukocytes, are primarily responsible for fighting infections. Leukocytes are either granulocytes or nongranulocytes. When infection occurs, granulocytes increase and nongranulocytes migrate to inflammatory areas by way of the circulatory system. During pregnancy, the number of neutrophils that are granulocytes increases. This increase is stimulated by estrogen and plasma cortisol.

Renal

The normal renal changes follow:

- *Hypervolemia.* Increased blood volume circulates through the kidneys. Renal blood flow constitutes about one fifth of the cardiac output; therefore it is increased 50% to 80%. The entire plasma volume is filtered about 60 times per day.
- *Hyperdynamics.* Substances to be retained by the body are first filtered and then reabsorbed in the tubules. Substances to be excreted are added to the fluid and flow to the distal portion of the tubules. During pregnancy, larger quantities are filtered in the glomerulus because of the greater capillary pressures associated with the increased blood flow; the glomerular filtration rate increases about 50%. Glucose, nitrogenous waste products of metabolism, and bicarbonate are therefore excreted in the urine in greater quantities. In turn, blood levels of nitrogenous waste products decrease. During pregnancy, normal laboratory values indicating renal function must be adjusted. A blood urea nitrogen level higher than 12 mg/dl is abnormal even though it is within the nonpregnant normal range. Serum creatinine levels higher than 0.8 mg/dl are considered abnormal for pregnancy. Creatinine clearance levels are normally elevated (110 to 160 ml/min) during pregnancy.
- *Physiologic hydroureter and hydronephrosis.* As the gravid uterus displaces other organs in the abdomen, it causes a physiologic hydroureter and hydronephrosis. It is usually more pronounced on the right side than on the left. The dilation of the ureters is further facilitated by estrogen. During pregnancy, the bladder has decreased tone because of hormonal influences. This factor and the distended ureters cause the pregnant woman to be more vulnerable to urinary tract infections. The increased glucose excretion into the urine also promotes bacterial growth.

Gastrointestinal

The predominant gastrointestinal change is hypotonic. A hypotonic gastrointestinal tract leads to decreased gastric motility and a prolonged stomach-emptying time, resulting primarily from the anatomic shifting of abdominal contents. Constipation is frequently a problem during pregnancy.

The gallbladder is influenced by estrogen and becomes hypotonic. This causes an increased concentration of bile. An increased incidence of gallstones can result. Acute cholecystitis can lead to the second most common nonobstetric surgical condition of pregnancy, following appendicitis. Intrahepatic cholestasis of pregnancy, the most common liver disorder unique to pregnancy, is the result of retained bile in the liver. Pruritus is the predominant presenting factor.

For high risk management, it is important to note that giving an order for nothing by mouth before surgery does not necessarily mean an empty stomach. Gastric pH is normally more acid during pregnancy because of the hypertonic states of the gastrointestinal system. Therefore there is an increased risk for aspiration of high acidic gastric content in the event of general anesthesia.

Metabolic

The predominant metabolic change during pregnancy is hyperinsulinemia, causing a diabetogenic state. This is related to the increased insulin resistance caused by the placental hormone and lactogen and by prolactin, cortisol, and glucagon.

DEVELOPMENT OF THE MATERNAL-FETAL UNIT

Knowledge of the growth and development of the maternal-fetal unit provides a basis for care of the mother or fetus at risk for disease or for treatment of pregnancy complications. This knowledge provides a basis for early detection of maternal or fetal problems, enabling more serious complications to be prevented.

Embryo

During the luteal phase of the menstrual cycle, cervical mucus becomes receptive to spermatozoa. Ejaculation of sperm into the vagina is aided by mucoid receptivity, which allows rapid migration of spermatozoa through the cervix, into the uterine cavity, and into the fallopian tube.

Active spermatozoa can reach the outer portion of the fallopian tube within 75 minutes. The sperm and ovum meet in the distal portion of the fallopian tube. Fertilization occurs when the sperm penetrates the vitelline membrane of the ovum. Cell division begins, forming a small cell mass called the *morula*.

The morula passes through the fallopian tube by way of tubal peristalsis and ciliary propulsion. The outer cell layer of the morula secretes a fluid that pools in a segmentation cavity. Now the cell mass is called a *blastocyst*.

The blastocyst takes approximately 6 to 7 days to form. Implantation takes place at the blastocyst stage, usually occurring high in the uterine fundus. At this time, the outer cells on the blastocyst are called *trophoblasts*.

The trophoblasts then invade the endometrium. It is thought that the reason the trophoblast cells are not treated as foreign and rejected by the mother is because there is an exchange of fetal and maternal cytoplasmic and nuclear material from the trophoblastic cells. This exchange allows the maternal immunologic system to tolerate the fetus as a part of the body rather than as foreign to it.

Progesterone from the corpus luteum provides stored nutritive substances in the endometrium, called the *decidua*. The trophoblasts secrete proteolytic and cytolytic enzymes, permitting them to destroy vessels, glands, and stroma in the endometrium.

Placenta

The trophoblasts proliferate rapidly after implantation, and three layers of cells appear. These send out fingerlike projections called *villi*. The outer layer of cells (syncytiotrophoblast), the inner layer (cytotrophoblast), and the dividing layer of thin connective tissue (mesotrophoblast), are formed within these fingerlike projections. The mesotrophoblast forms the support for the villi and fetal vascular tissue. The syncytial cells then synthesize proteins, glucose, and hormones for use by the embryo.

After 2 or 3 weeks, the chorion begins to develop within the villi. While the chorion is developing, the amnion and its cavity are forming. Two cavities form in the embryonic pole. The ventral cavity is the yolk sac. The dorsal cavity becomes the amniotic cavity. As the chorion enlarges, it forces the formation of the body stalk, the allantois, the blood vessels, and the beginning of the umbilical cord.

The decidua basalis, the layer beneath the embryoblast tissue, comes into contact with the villi, which then multiply rapidly. During villi multiplication, the decidua basalis is called the *chorion frondosum.*

By 14 weeks, the chorion frondosum organizes into the discrete organ called the *placenta.* The placenta has segments, called *cotyledons,* which are connected by vascular channels to the umbilical cord. The placental surface is exposed to the maternal blood in the intervillous space and thins to a single layer of cells called the *placental membrane.* The exposure of fetal blood to maternal blood across this membrane provides for fetal oxygenation, nutrition, and excretion of fetal wastes. The two umbilical arteries carry CO_2 and other waste from the fetus to the mother. The vein carries nutrition and oxygen to the fetus.

Transfer of O_2, CO_2, nutrition, and waste depends on molecular size. Smaller molecules, such as O_2, CO_2, electrolytes, and water, transfer by simple diffusion, moving passively from the side of greater to the side of lesser molecular concentration. Their transfer largely depends on the adequacy of uterine blood flow into the intervillous space.

A more complex process called *facilitated diffusion* selectively transfers larger molecules, such as glucose. This process occurs against a large concentration gradient and requires a carrier system. Energy expenditure can also provide for selective transfer. Facilitated diffusion and selective transfer depend primarily on placental surface area and thickness for their diffusion.

In addition to simple and complex diffusion, the placenta also adopts an endocrine function. Early in pregnancy, it assumes responsibility for maintenance of the pregnancy. The principal hormones produced by the placenta are estrogen, progesterone, human chorionic gonadotropin, and human placental lactogen.

Amniotic Fluid

Origin

Initially, the amnion fetal membrane primarily produces the amniotic fluid by actively transporting solute and passively transporting water from maternal serum to the amniotic fluid space. As the fetus develops, the amnion fetal membrane makes a significant contribution by excreting urine into the amniotic fluid.

Functions

Amniotic fluid is normally swallowed by the fetus and absorbed in the gastrointestinal tract. If there are abnormalities of the fetal gastrointestinal tract or renal system, neurotube defects, or ruptured membranes, amniotic fluid may be excessive, deficient, or absent. Sufficient amounts of amniotic fluid provide a buoyant medium, which does the following:

- Permits symmetric growth and development
- Prevents adherence of the amnion to embryo or fetal parts
- Cushions the fetus against jolts by distributing impacts the mother may receive
- Helps control the fetal body temperature by maintaining a relatively constant temperature
- Enables the fetus to flex, extend, and move freely, thus aiding musculoskeletal development
- Provides fetal nutritional development
- Allows the umbilical cord to be relatively free of compression

Fetus

The first trimester is a period of tremendous growth and organogenesis from an embryo into a fetus. By the end of the second week, the three embryologic germ layers develop to form body organs and systems. The formation of these layers is called *gastrulation.*

The ectoderm gives rise to the skin, hair, and nails; the epithelium of the internal and external ear, nasal cavity, mouth, and anus; the nervous system tissues; and the glands. The mesoderm forms the connective tissue, blood vessels, lymphatic tissue, kidneys, pleura, peritoneum, pericardium, muscles, and skeleton. The endoderm forms the respiratory tract, bladder, liver, pancreas, and digestive tract.

By 6 weeks, a single-chamber heart is functioning and lung buds appear, as do a rudimentary kidney and gut. By the end of the first trimester, the heart has compartmentalized into four chambers; the lungs have bronchi; the gut, liver, pancreas, and spleen have developed; and the gender can be distinguished.

During the second trimester, facial features become defined. Fine body hair, called *lanugo*, appears, and vernix is produced to protect fetal skin. Meconium begins to appear in the gut. Maturation of organs allows some immature functioning.

In the third trimester, the fetus rapidly gains weight and the final maturation of the organs for extrauterine life occurs. Subcutaneous fat deposits appear, and the body has a rounded appearance.

Assessing fetal well-being has become sophisticated. In addition to estimating fetal well-being by examining maternal well-being, it can be estimated biochemically by using laboratory studies and physically by observing fetal heart activity on the fetal monitor and by visualizing the fetus using ultrasound techniques.

EXERCISE AND BEDREST

For healthy women with a normal pregnancy, exercise is safe and promotes the health and well-being of the mother and fetus (Talmadge, Kravitz, and Robergs, 2000; ACOG, 2002; NICE, 2008). Exercise has been shown to improve a woman's fitness and comfort during pregnancy, decrease the risk for gestational diabetes and hypertension, reduce the risk of cesarean delivery (Bungum, 2000; ICSI, 2008), and enhance her postpartum recovery because muscle loss and excessive fat gain are minimized.

In general, the following exercise guidelines are recommended by the American College of Obstetricians and Gynecologists (ACOG, 2002) for healthy pregnant women:

- Moderate exercise for 30 minutes or more is recommended throughout pregnancy. The exercise heart rate is the same as for a nonpregnant woman. That rate is 60% to 80% of the maximum heart rate (200 minus age). Although the fetal heart rate increases similarly, no negative effects have been shown (ACOG, 2002).
- Exercise is modified based on maternal symptoms such as shortness of breath, lightheadedness, and nausea.
- Exercise is stopped when the woman is fatigued, and she must never exercise to exhaustion.
- No exercise is performed in a supine position after the third month. Exercise positions must be modified by inserting support under the head, neck, and shoulders and by tilting the abdomen to the left.
- Breathing must be regular at all times during exercise. The Valsalva maneuver is to be avoided.
- Caloric intake should be adequate to meet the demands of both the pregnancy and the exercise. The pregnant woman who exercises regularly needs about 300 additional calories.
- Prevent dehydration by frequently drinking fluids.
- Movements are to be smooth at all times. Jerky, bouncy motions must be avoided to prevent injury.
- Avoid long periods of motionless standing because this position decreases cardiac output.
- Avoid contact sports, scuba diving, and exertion at high altitudes.

Women with a preexisting medical condition involving the heart, kidney, lungs, or thyroid should be referred to a specialist for appropriate, individualized exercise plans. Contraindications to exercise are listed in the following (ACOG, 2002):

- Incompetent cervix or cerclage
- Intrauterine growth-restricted fetus
- Preeclampsia
- Preterm premature rupture of membranes
- History of preterm labor or current preterm labor symptoms, indicating high risk for preterm labor
- Persistent second or third trimester bleeding
- Multiple gestation

In the event the pregnancy becomes high risk, restricting activity to varying degrees or prescribing bedrest is frequently part of the management plan. It is estimated that nearly 20% of all women who deliver each year in the United States were prescribed bedrest by their physicians for some period during their pregnancy after 20 weeks of gestation (Maloni and Kutil, 2000; Sprague, 2004). The benefits of this liberal use of bedrest during pregnancy are under review. There is conclusive evidence of adverse physical and psychosocial effects in both women and their families when compliance with bedrest was reported.

Negative physical effects of bedrest include the following (Maloni and others, 1993; Maloni and Kutil, 2000; Maloni, 2002; Sprague, 2004):

- Skeletal muscle atrophy within 6 hours, with greatest progression of atrophy in 3 to 7 days
- Muscle volume loss of more than 25% to 30% in 5 weeks
- Weight loss despite reduced activities and controlled calorie intake
- Plasma and blood volume decrease by approximately 7% of body weight
- Increased blood coagulation
- Heartburn and reflux
- Decreased cardiac output and stroke volume
- Glucose intolerance and insulin resistance
- Prolonged postpartum physical recovery, including symptoms of muscular and cardiovascular deconditioning

Negative psychosocial effects of bedrest on pregnant women and their families include the following (Maloni and others, 1993; Maloni and Kutil, 2000; Maloni and others, 2001):

- Increased stress, family and marital
- Specific increased concerns about family status, emotional changes, health, and body image
- Loss of financial support
- Disruption of routine

Except in the high risk conditions that are serious enough to be life threatening to the mother or fetus, the benefits of bedrest are not evidence based. High risk conditions that do require bedrest include serious kidney, hypertension, and heart disease and placental abnormalities such as abruptio placentae or placenta previa (Schroeder, 1998). Because studies of newborns do not show improved outcomes and some studies suggest deleterious physical and psychosocial effects with antenatal home or hospital bedrest, we must reevaluate the frequent recommendations for these expensive measures. This is especially true for otherwise healthy women who experience preterm labor or who are pregnant with multiples (Crowther and Dodd, 2005).

The nurse's focus should be one of preventive counseling, thereby decreasing the development or severity of the high risk condition that predisposes that woman to bedrest. Furthermore, nurses can be advocates of evidence-based practice to promote changes in the prescription of bedrest (Sprague, 2004). If bedrest becomes necessary—that is, it is related to a life-threatening risk—then the nurse should implement care to decrease the physical effects of bedrest with isometric exercises. The isometric exercises listed in Box 1-1 can help prevent some of these problems for women who must have long-term bedrest or severely curtailed exercise. These exercises are not aerobic, but they do maintain conditioning and provide a sense of physical well-being. A support group or a referral to the national bedrest support group Sidelines can reduce the psychosocial stress of bedrest. See the Sidelines web site (*http://www.sidelines.org*).

Box 1-1   Isometric Exercises for Pregnant Women on Therapeutic Bedrest

Kegel Exercise
- Lying on your back at a left tilt or sitting up, tighten your pelvic floor muscles (as if stopping and starting your urine). Hold for three counts and then relax.

Abdominal Breathing
- Lying on your back at a left tilt with knees bent, breathe in deeply, letting your abdominal wall rise. Exhale slowly through your mouth as you tighten your stomach muscles.

Bridging
- Lying on your back at a left tilt with knees bent, raise your hips off the bed while keeping your shoulders down (see figure below).

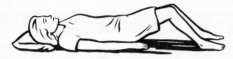

Curl-Ups
- Lying on your back at a left tilt with knees bent, put your hands on your stomach. Lift your head and shoulders up (tuck your chin). Keep small of your back against the bed (see figure below).

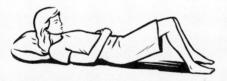

Leg Sliding
- Lying on your back at a left tilt with knees bent, slide your legs out slowly, straightening your knees. Keep small of your back flat against the bed. Slowly pull both knees back up (see figure below).

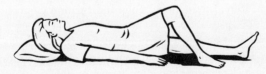

Modified Leg Raises
- Lying on your back at a left tilt with one knee bent, bend opposite knee up toward your chest. Then straighten leg by kicking it up toward the ceiling and lower it to bed. Repeat with first bent knee.

Abduction
- Lying on your back at a left tilt with knees bent, let your knees come apart and then squeeze them back together.

Continued

Box 1-1	Isometric Exercises for Pregnant Women on Therapeutic Bedrest—cont'd

Ankle Circles
- Pump ankles up and down. Circle the foot first in one direction, then in the other while resting your right ankle on left knee. Repeat with left ankle on right knee.

Arm Lifts
- Exhale deeply through your nose as you lift one arm up to the side over your head. The sides of your chest should expand. Exhale as you bring your arm down. Repeat with opposite arm.

ANTEPARTUM NUTRITION

Nutrition plays a significant role in fetal well-being and in the prevention and treatment of a high risk pregnancy. To give adequate counseling, the nurse caring for high risk patients must know about nutrition needs, modifications, and risks for potential deficiencies. Utilize the new U.S. Department of Agriculture (USDA, 2005) food guide pyramid (*http://www.mypyramid.gov*) and the Department of Health and Human Services (HHS) and USDA Dietary Guidelines for Americans, 2005 (*http://www. healthierus.gov/dietaryguidelines*).

Nutrient Needs

Adequate nutrients are critical for cell growth to take place during pregnancy. A 25% deficit in needed calories and protein can interfere with the synthesis of DNA. The cells that are undergoing rapid division at the time of insult are the ones most damaged (Reifsnider and Gill, 2000).

During the first 2 months of pregnancy, a deficit in adequate nutrients can have teratogenic effects or cause a spontaneous abortion. After the second month, a nutritional deficit can impede fetal growth, causing a small-for-gestational-age infant or a small-brain-growth infant (Kretchmer and Zimmermann, 1997). These infants may, as a consequence, have limited stature, intellect, and future health (Kretchmer and Zimmermann, 1997; International Food Information Council Foundation and March of Dimes [2003]).

After 24 weeks of gestation, a nutritional deficit is associated with significantly increased preterm delivery and decreased fetal stores of nutrients, especially calcium, magnesium, and iron (Kretchmer and Zimmermann, 1997).

Cell division occurs by two processes: (1) hyperplasia, or an increase in cell number, and (2) hypertrophy, or an increase in the size of the cell. If the insult occurs during hyperplastic cell division, the number of cells will be permanently reduced. This can cause mental retardation, even in developed countries, where nutritional concerns are frequently overlooked.

Protein: Body's Basic Building Blocks

Protein, 70 g daily or about 1 g/kg per day (Institute of Medicine, 2002; Trumbo and others, 2002), is very important to support the increased embryonic-fetal cellular growth, promote the increased maternal blood volume, and possibly facilitate the prevention of preeclampsia. To prevent the development of anemia, pregnant women also require an adequate intake of iron, folic acid, and vitamins B_6 and B_{12}.

Carbohydrates: Provide Energy

Carbohydrate needs are individualized based on the woman's recommended weight gain and her level of exercise. However, the Institute of Medicine (2002) recommends an average intake of 175 g per day.

Fat: Promotes Proper Central Nervous System Development

Essential fatty acids such as linoleic (omega 6) and alpha-linolenic (omega 3) acids are important for tissue formation, especially the neuron system and the eyes. Food sources include egg yolks, green leafy vegetables, cold water fatty fish, and oils such as canola, flaxseed, soybean, corn, or safflower. The intake of these essential fatty acids should be increased slightly for the singleton pregnancy and even more for the multifetal pregnancy (Monti, 2003).

Iron

Iron deficiency anemia is a serious condition during pregnancy and has been associated with preterm labor, decreased fetal iron stores resulting in anemia during the first year of life, and increased risk for hypertension in adulthood (Hindmarsh and others, 2000; Reifsnider and Gill, 2000; Strong, 2005). To prevent iron deficiency during pregnancy, women need 27 mg of iron per day but should not exceed 45 mg daily (Institute of Medicine, 2001; ODS and NIH, 2005). Foods high in iron include meats and plant foods such as legumes, dried fruits, whole grains, and green leafy vegetables. Iron from plants (non-heme iron) is less well absorbed by the body, but absorption can be improved by eating these foods along with a food high in vitamin C. Caffeinated beverages should be avoided or consumed between meals because they interfere with iron absorption.

All pregnant women on their first prenatal visit should be screened for iron deficiency anemia. It is estimated that in the United States 12% of pregnant women are iron deficient (Cogswell and others, 2003). The initial screen usually is best made by the hemoglobin, hematocrit, and serum ferritin values. The serum ferritin value reflects iron reserves. A ferritin value lower than 12 mcg/dl in the presence of a low hemoglobin value (11.0 g/dl in the first trimester, 10.5 g/dl in the second, and 11 g/dl in the third) indicates iron deficiency anemia. Then 60 to 120 mg of iron per day is usually prescribed in divided doses to increase absorption (CDC, 1998; Kaiser and Allen, 2002). Excessive iron levels can lower zinc absorption and increase the risk for free radicals and oxidative damage resulting possibly in cardiac disease (Strong, 2005).

Prophylactic iron supplementation can be given selectively or routinely. Very little information is available on pregnancy outcome with its use according to a Cochrane Review (Peña-Rosas, 2006). Currently, the CDC, IOM, and ACOG recommend iron supplementation use during pregnancy starting after the first prenatal visit (Lee, 2004; Cox and Phelan, 2008). When prophylactic iron supplementation is used, 30 mg of ferrous iron in the form of ferrous gluconate, 300 mg daily, or ferrous sulfate, 150 mg daily, is given. For best absorption, instruct the woman to take the supplemental iron between meals. Ascorbic acid does not increase absorption of iron supplements in ferrous form.

Folate

Folic acid, one of the most important vitamins during pregnancy, is intimately involved in all DNA synthesis and functions as a coenzyme in amino acid metabolism. Therefore this vitamin is essential to all cell division such as the fetus, placenta, and maternal red blood cell synthesis, and protein synthesis. Folic acid deficiency has been associated with an increased occurrence of neural tube defects (AAP, 1999; ACOG, 2003; Moos and others, 2008). The ACOG (2003) recommended that all women of childbearing age capable of becoming pregnant consume 400 mcg of folic acid daily. Folic acid is commonly found in dark green leafy vegetables, citrus fruits, eggs, legumes, and whole grains. In January 1998, the U.S. Food and Drug Administration (FDA) established rules under which specified grain products are fortified with approximately 140 mcg of folic acid.

During pregnancy the RDA for folic acid increases to 600 mcg/day (IOM, 1998; Cox and Phelan, 2008). Therefore if the woman is eating at least five servings of fruits and vegetables and includes whole or fortified grains in her diet, supplementation is not necessary. If the diet is inadequate or if the patient is at risk for folic acid deficiency because of cigarette smoking or drug or alcohol abuse, a folic acid supplement is recommended (Reifsnider and Gill, 2000). If the mother has a personal obstetric history of a major central nervous system anomaly, such as a neural tube defect, a 4 mg/day dosage of folate is recommended. The woman should start taking the folate before conception and continue through the first three gestational months (International Food Information Council Foundation and March of Dimes, 2003; ICSI, 2008).

Zinc

Zinc is an essential mineral for normal growth and development, DNA synthesis, and immune function. During pregnancy, the diet should contain between 11 and 12 mg of zinc each day (IOM, 2001). Zinc is commonly found in nuts, meats, whole grains, legumes, and dairy products.

Sodium

Restricted sodium intake, as well as excessive intake, can cause problems during pregnancy. Restricted sodium intake can interfere with adequate maternal blood volume increase. Excessive sodium intake can increase the sensitivity of the blood vessel wall to angiotensin, causing vasoconstriction. Thus an average sodium intake of 1.5 to 2.3 g/day is considered therapeutic during pregnancy (IOM, 2004; Duley, Henderson-Smart, and Meher, 2005).

Calcium

According to the new dietary reference values, the pregnant woman needs 1000 mg of calcium and the pregnant adolescent needs 1300 mg/day (Trumbo and others, 2002). Intakes greater than 2500 mg/day are associated with increased incidence of kidney stones. Supplemental calcium has been shown to reduce the risk of preeclampsia in women with low dietary intake in pregnant women at risk of a hypertensive disorder according to a Cochrane Review (Hofmeyr, Atallah, and Duley, 2006).

Vitamin A

The current recommendation for vitamin A is 2500 IU per day. It is a fat-soluble vitamin and is stored in the body. More than 10,000 IU per day may be teratogenic (van den Broek and others, 2002; Gardiner and others, 2008).

Vitamin D

Another lipid-soluble vitamin, vitamin D, promotes calcium absorption and bone mineralization. A deficiency in vitamin D in pregnant women and infants has been noted in a number of studies in recent years (Thacher and others, 2006; Bodnar and others, 2007; Dawodu and others, 2007; Dijkstra and others, 2007; McCullough, 2007; Ward and others, 2007). The current recommended daily consumption is 400 to 800 IU daily with some sun exposure (Gardiner and others, 2008; NICE, 2008).

Fluids

Hofmeyr and Gülmezoglu (2002) indicated that oral hydration is important for amniotic fluid volume. In the presence of oligohydramnios, oral fluids appear to increase the amniotic fluid volume by increasing maternal plasma volume, thereby improving uteroplacental blood flow. Decreased fluids also increase the risk for uterine irritability and urinary tract infections. The amount of fluid is unique to each individual, but the dietary reference intake (DRI) for water during pregnancy is 3 L/day (IOM, 2004).

Assessment

To determine whether the pregnant woman is obtaining adequate nutrition and to prevent nutrition-related complications, the nurse must conduct an ongoing assessment. To assess the nutritional needs and status of the pregnant woman, her pattern of weight gain, prepregnancy body mass index (BMI), daily activities, and dietary intake should be evaluated throughout the pregnancy. The formation of fatty and lean body tissues is important. These act as a reserve for energy that the fetus can draw on during the last part of pregnancy and provide a source of energy during labor and delivery and lactation.

Prepregnancy Weight Status: Underweight or Overweight

Underweight is defined as a BMI of less than 19.8 kg/m². A prepregnancy underweight status increases the risk of complications during pregnancy, such as increased risk of a birth defect such as gastroschisis, small-for-gestational age, intrauterine growth restriction, and preterm birth (Cox and Phelan, 2008; Gardiner and others, 2008). Frequently these patients have some type of eating disorder such as anorexia nervosa or bulimia nervosa. Eating disorders are associated with not only nutritional alterations but also metabolic, endocrine, and psychologic changes that can cause infertility and if conceiving can have potentially negative effects on fetal development as well.

Obesity is defined as a BMI of 30 kg/m^2 or greater. Prepregnancy obesity is associated with less optimal reproductive outcomes for the fetus, increasing the risk of congenital anomalies such as neural tube defects (King, 2006; Gardiner and others, 2008), macrosomia (King, 2006), stillbirth, childhood obesity (Gale and others, 2007), and metabolic syndrome as an adult (Cox and Phelan, 2008). The risks to the pregnant mother are gestational diabetes, hypertensive disorders, deep vein thrombosis, labor dystocia, shoulder dystocia, increased cesarean rate, and postpartum complications such as aspiration with general anesthesia, hemorrhage, infections, and depression (Chu and others, 2008; Cox and Phelan, 2008; Gardiner and others, 2008; Guelinckx, Devlieger, Beckers, and Vansant, 2008; Moos and others, 2008). Following bariatric surgery, the pregnant patient is at greater risk of vitamin B$_{12}$, vitamin D, folate, iron, and calcium deficiencies (ACOG, 2005). These patients require individualized nutrient supplementation such as multivitamins, calcium, and iron to maximize the health of mother and fetus (Guelinckx and others, 2008). Their risk of complications is less than for the obese patient but they still have an increased risk of gestational diabetes, preeclampsia, cesarean delivery, and anemia (Maggard and others, 2008). The most common risks for the fetus following maternal bariatric surgery is premature delivery, low birth weight, macrosomia, and perinatal mortality (Maggard and others, 2008).

Weight Gain for Singleton Pregnancy

An average weight gain during a normal singleton pregnancy (Table 1-1) is between 25 and 35 pounds, according to the U.S. Department of Health and Human Services, Healthy People 2010 document (USDHHS, 2000) and the Institute of Medicine (IOM, 2009). During the first 2 months, a 2- to 4-pound weight gain is considered average, with a gain of about 1 pound per week during the remainder of the pregnancy. Differences in fat deposition and water retention, as well as in body frame, influence the amount and rate of gain fluid. Low gestational weight gain increases the risk of preterm birth, small-for-gestational age and increased risk of cesarean birth (AHRQ and USDHHS, 2008).

According to the Food and Nutrition Board of the National Academy of Science (USDHHS, 2000; IOM, 2009), a woman whose BMI is below 18.5 should gain more than the average (28 to 40 pounds) to offset the increased risk for fetal mortality and maternal complications of pregnancy. During the first 2 months, the woman

Table 1-1   Weight Gain During Pregnancy: IOM Recommendations

Weight Before Pregnancy	Recommended Weight Gain During Pregnancy (Pounds)
Underweight (BMI <18.5)	28–40
Normal weight (BMI 18.5–24.9)	25–35
Moderate overweight (BMI 25.0–29.9)	15–25
Severe overweight (BMI >29.9)	11–20

Adapted from Institute of Medicine (IOM): Weight gain during pregnancy: reexamining the guidelines, Washington D.C., 2009, National Academies Press.

should gain the pounds that she is underweight, with a gain of 1 pound or more per week during the remainder of the pregnancy.

A woman whose prepregnancy weight is BMI 25.0 to 29.9 needs to gain less than average (15 to 25 pounds). She needs to gain only a couple of pounds during the first trimester and then approximately 0.5 to 0.7 pounds per week for the remainder of the pregnancy.

If she is more than 135% of standard weight (BMI >29), a gain of approximately 11 to 20 pounds is recommended in the U.S. Department of Health and Human Services, *Healthy People 2010* document (USDHHS, 2000), and by the Institute of Medicine (IOM, 2009). However, because of the increased risk for macrosomia related to a prepregnancy maternal overweight state (above 135% of standard weight for height), some health care providers recommend for these women a nutritious diet that maintains their prepregnancy weight instead of a weight gain. Weight loss is never appropriate during pregnancy (AHRQ and USDHHS, 2008).

Even if the pregnant patient begins pregnancy at an ideal weight, high gestational weight gain increases complications. There is moderate to strong evidence for high birth weight, large for gestational age infant and increased postpartum weight retention (AHRQ and USDHHS, 2008).

Weight Gain in Multifetal Pregnancy

In multifetal pregnancies, early weight gain is important, with a recommended gain of 1.5 pounds per week in the second and third trimesters (Brown and Carlson, 2000). In a twin pregnancy, a weight gain of 37 to 54 pounds has been associated with improved outcomes (Brown and Carlson, 2000; IOM, 2009). In triple gestation, a weight gain of 50 pounds improves outcome (IFICF and MOD, 2003). Just as in a singleton gestation, underweight women should gain at the high end, 1.75 to 2.0 pounds per week, and overweight women should gain somewhat less (Table 1-2).

Food Groups

To ensure that the body receives the needed additional nutrients, a pregnant woman is encouraged to select nutrient-rich foods using the guide to daily food choices. She should select servings from each of the food groups: protein, grains, milk and milk products, fruits, and vegetables (Table 1-3). Fried foods and calorie-laden foods that are void of nutrients should be avoided. These foods increase the number of calories but do not supply the body with any nutrients. Thus they promote an abnormal weight gain. In addition, social habits such as drinking alcohol, smoking cigarettes, and abusing drugs, if continued during pregnancy, interfere with adequate absorption and intake of various nutrients (see Chapter 27).

According to the Institute of Medicine (1990), women with multifetal pregnancy should eat a healthy diet (Table 1-4). In addition, they should receive a supplement that contains the following (Brown and Carlson, 2000):

- Iron: 30 mg
- Zinc: 15 mg
- Copper: 2 mg
- Calcium: 250 mg
- Vitamin B_6: 2 mg

Table 1-2   Dietary Requirements for Pregnancy*

Because we are interested in helping you, through good nutrition, to produce a healthy baby and experience an optimally healthy pregnancy, some of these guidelines may need to be adjusted for your usual weight, pregnancy complications, and food preferences or religious or other dietary habits. This is intended as a guideline. The recommendations will be discussed with you, your questions will be answered, and any specific modifications you require will be made with you.

Nutrients	Nonpregnant	Singleton	Twins	Triplets	Quadruplets
Proteins, fats, calories, and carbohydrates per day	2200	2500	3500	4000	4500
Recommended weight gain before 24 weeks		½ lb/wk	1 lb/wk	1½ lb/wk	2 lb/wk
Recommended weight gain after 24 weeks		1 lb/wk	2 lb/wk	2½ lb/wk	3 lb/wk
Optimal total weight gain		25–30 lb	40–50 lb	50–60 lb	65–80 lb
Average length of gestation		40 wk	36 wk	32 wk	30 wk

*Gaining the recommended amount of weight from recommended nutrients can help prevent some preterm and premature labor and extremely premature deliveries.

Table 1-3   Guide to Daily Food Choices

Food Groups	Adolescents (Under 17 yr)	Adults (Over 18 yr)
Protein	6 oz	6 oz
Grains	6–11 servings	6–11 servings

Fruits and vegetables
  1 Yellow fruit or vegetable
  1 Vitamin C fruit or vegetable
  1 Green leafy vegetable
	5–9 servings	5–9 servings

Dairy	5 servings	4 servings
Fats and sweets	Cautious use	Cautious use

- Folate: 300 mcg
- Vitamin C: 50 mg
- Vitamin D: 5 mcg or 200 international units

Referrals

When obvious deficiencies cannot be met using a balanced meal plan, arrange a consultation with a registered dietitian. Cultural or religious practices can also influence and complicate nutritional intake. Careful planning in these situations may allow for

Table 1-4 Menu Guidelines

Food Group	Serving Size	Singleton	Twins	Triplets	Quadruplets
Dairy	8 oz milk 8 oz cottage cheese 8 oz ice cream 1 oz hard cheese 1 cup yogurt*	6 servings per day	8 servings per day	10 servings per day	12 servings per day
Meats, fish, poultry	1 oz	6 servings per day	10 servings per day	10 servings per day	12 servings per day
Eggs	1	1 per day	2 per day	2 per day	2 per day
Vegetables	½ cup cooked or 1 cup fresh	4 per day	5 per day	6 per day	6 per day
Fruits	½ cup or 1 cup fresh	4 per day	7 per day	8 per day	8 per day
Grains and breads	1 oz; ½ cup cooked or 1 slice	8 per day	10 per day	12 per day	12 per day
Fats, oils, and nuts	1 T oil 1 pat butter 1 oz nuts	5 per day	6 per day	7 per day	8 per day

Fats and oils are heroes, not villains, for expectant moms.
Stock cupboards, refrigerator, and freezer with the basics.
Do not disparage fast foods.
Practice on-the-job snacking savvy.
Eat right, on the job and at home.

Adapted from Luke B, Johnson T, Petrie R: *Clinical maternal-fetal nutrition*, Boston, 1993, Little, Brown.
*Contains two times the calcium, ounce-per-ounce, compared with other dairy servings listed.

alternative food selections that provide adequate nutrition while still meeting cultural and religious practices. Financial aid agencies, such as the Special Supplementary Food Program for Women, Infants, and Children (WIC), can be used if income is inadequate to purchase healthful foods.

Hyperphenylalaninemia

Women with phenylketonuria (PKU) are put on a dietary phenylalanine restriction before conception and throughout pregnancy (AAP, 2001; Dunlop and others, 2008). According to the National Institutes of Health (2000) and the American College of Obstetricians and Gynecologists (2001), levels of the amino acid phenylalanine (Phe) are recommended to be below 6 mg/dl for at least 3 months before conception. This decreases the risk for PKU-related teratogenic effects of high levels of phenylalanine. The dietary modification normally excludes all high-protein foods such as meat, milk, eggs, and nuts as well as wheat products. Throughout pregnancy, the Phe levels are monitored at least once but preferably twice a week. The recommended level is 2 to 6 mg/dl during pregnancy (National Institutes of Health, 2000; Dunlop and others, 2008).

Hyperemesis Gravidarum

Hyperemesis is a condition characterized by severe nausea and vomiting with weight loss and dehydration. It may be seen more frequently in patients with hydatidiform mole, advanced diabetes, anorexia nervosa or bulimia, or gastrointestinal diseases such as peptic ulcers. Many explanations have been postulated in the literature, including the following:

- High levels of human chorionic gonadotropin
- High levels of estrogen
- Increased glucose drain on maternal metabolism
- Family history (genetics)
- Psychogenic factors

To date, these explanations have not proved to be causes because these same factors are present in women without hyperemesis and in women who have mild early pregnancy nausea with or without vomiting.

One major nutritional concern with severe nausea and vomiting is the vitamin B complex and protein deficiency. Various therapies have been tried. Therapies that correlate with supportive therapy seem to be the most effective (Box 1-2). The few women who experience intractable vomiting need close nutritional supervision. Therapy involves lifestyle changes and the following approach:

- Prevention—Multivitamin at time of conception (ACOG, 2004)
- Increased dietary sources of potassium and magnesium (Boxes 1-3 and 1-4)
- Ginger 1 g (Smith and others, 2004; Borrelli and others, 2005)
- Acupressure to stimulate the P6 acupuncture site (3 fingerwidths above the wrist on the anterior side) with a wristband-type, miniaturized, battery-operated transcutaneous electrical nerve stimulator called *ReliefBand* (Davis, 2004; NICE, 2008)
- Acupuncture at the P6 acupuncture point (Smith and others, 2002; NICE, 2008)

Box 1-2   Managing Morning Sickness

- Rest and eat a small amount of carbohydrates such as biscuits.
- Follow the salty and sweet approach—even so-called junk foods are okay.
- Eat frequently, at least every 2 to 3 hours. Separate liquids from solids and alternate every 2 to 3 hours.
- Eat protein after sweets.
- Be aware that foods normally liked may have no appeal at this time.
- Some find that dairy products stay down most easily.
- If you vomit even when your stomach is empty, try sucking on a popsicle.
- Try ginger tea. Peel and finely dice a knuckle-sized piece of ginger and place it in a mug of boiling water. Steep for 5 to 8 minutes and add brown sugar to taste.
- Try warm ginger ale (with sugar, not artificial sweetener).
- Try acupressure or antinausea wristbands advertised for motion sickness. When they are worn, they apply acupressure to point P6.
- In general, eat what sounds good, rather than trying to balance your meals. Nongreasy, dry, sweet, and salty may sound good to you.
- Turbo-boosters *(assist in adding calories fast)*

Sweet Success	Ensure
Instant Breakfast	ReSource
Boost	Sustacal-Plus
Sustacal	Ensure-Plus

Adapted from Jewell D, Young G: Interventions for nausea and vomiting in early pregnancy. *Cochrane Database of Syst Rev* 2003, Issue 4. Art. No.: CD000145; and Luke B, Eberlein T: *When you're expecting twins, triplets, and quads*, New York, 1999, Harper and Row.

Box 1-3   Foods Rich in Potassium

Fruits	Fruit Juices	Vegetables
Avocados	Apricot nectar	Broccoli
Bananas	Grapefruit juice	Cooked dry beans
Cantaloupes	Orange juice	Peanuts
Dates	Pineapple juice	Potatoes
Dried figs	Prune juice	Spinach
Prunes	Tomato juice	Dark yellow or orange
Raisins		squashes
Watermelons		Yams
Dried apricots		

- Pyridoxine (vitamin B_6) 25 mg every 8 hours with or without doxylamine; one half of a scored 25-mg tablet orally (ACOG, 2004). According to the Cochrane Review, pyridoxine may be the most effective in reducing the severity (Jewell and Young, 2003; NICE, 2008).
- Antiemetic pharmacologic management, including prochlorperazine (Compazine), trimethobenzamide (Tigan), or ondansetron (Zofran)

Box 1-4   Food Sources of Magnesium

Foods Rich in Magnesium	Foods Moderately Rich in Magnesium
Vegetables	*Fruits*
Spinach	Avocados
Swiss chard	*Vegetables*
Nuts and Seeds	Beans, including garbanzo, kidney,
Nuts	navy, pinto, or soy
Pumpkin seeds	Beet greens
Sunflower seeds	Broccoli
	Lima beans
	Tofu
	Cereals and Grains
	Cereal: bran or whole wheat
	Wheat germ
	Whole wheat bread or muffin
	Nuts and Seeds
	Peanuts
	Peanut butter

Table 1-5   Nutrient Composition of One Suggested Formula for Intravenous Supplementation

Nutrients	Pregnancy RDA	Actual Intake Using D_5 Lactated Ringer's Solution
Vitamin A (international units)	4000	3300
Vitamin B_{12} (mcg)	2.2	5
Vitamin C (mg)	70	100
Vitamin D (international units)	400	200
Vitamin E (international units)	15	10
Calcium (mg)	1200	80
Niacinamide (mg)	17	40
Potassium (mg)	2000	156
Magnesium (mg)	320	192
Thiamine (mg)	1.5	3.0
Riboflavin (mg)	1.6	3.6
Folic acid (mcg)	400	400
Sodium (mg)	500	3381
Biotin (mcg)	30–100	60
Pantothenic acid (mg)	447	15
Pyridoxine (mg)	2.2	14
Dextrose (kcal)	170	—
Chloride (mg)	750	5538

Data from Newman V, Fullerton J, Anderson P: Clinical advances in the management of severe nausea and vomiting during pregnancy, *J Obstet Gynecol Neonatal Nurs* 22(6):483–490, 1993.
RDA, Recommended daily allowance.

- Antihistamines such as diphenhydramine (Benadryl), meclizine (Antivert), or dimenhydrinate (Dramamine)
- Motility drugs that increase GI motility through the stomach, such as metoclopramide (Reglan)
- Intravenous formula for nutrients and supplementation as follows: add one multivitamin injection, 10 mg pyridoxine, and 2 g magnesium sulfate (192 elemental magnesium) to 1 L of lactated Ringer's solution; administered for 2 hours (Table 1-5)
- Enteral feeding

With any of these therapies or interventions, the goal is for the woman to obtain food, nutrients, vitamins, and protein from oral intake.

CONCLUSION

Knowledge of maternal physiology and the normal adaptations to pregnancy is essential in the management of high risk and complicated pregnancy. Nutrition and fitness play a significant role in fetal well-being and in prevention and treatment of a high risk pregnancy. The content in this chapter provides the foundation for optimal high risk pregnancy and delivery care.

BIBLIOGRAPHY
General
Cunningham F, and others: *Williams obstetrics*, ed 22, Norwalk, CT, 2005, Appleton and Lange.

Exercise and Bedrest
American College of Obstetricians and Gynecologists (ACOG) Committee on Obstetric Practice: ACOG Committee Opinion: Exercise during pregnancy and the postpartum period, Number *267*, *Int J Gynaecol Obstet* 77(1):79–81, 2002.

Bungum T, Peaslee D, Jackson A, and others: Exercise during pregnancy and type of delivery in nulliparae, *J Obstet Gynecol Neonatal Nurs* 29:258–264, 2000.

Crowther C, Dodd J: Multiple pregnancy. In James D, and others, editors: *High risk pregnancy: management options*, ed 3, Philadelphia, 2005, Saunders.

Heffernan A: Exercise and pregnancy in primary care, *Nurse Pract* 25(3):42, 2000.

Institute for Clinical Systems Improvement (ICSI): *Health care guidelines: routine prenatal care*, ed 12, Bloomington, MN, 2008, ICSI. Retrieved from http://www.icsi.org.

Maloni J: Astronauts and pregnancy bed rest, *AWHONN Lifelines* 6(4):319, 2002.

Maloni J, Brezinski-Tomasi J, Johnson L: Antepartum bed rest: effect upon the family, *J Obstet Gynecol Neonatal Nurs* 30(2):165–173, 2001.

Maloni J, Kutil RL: Antepartum support group for women hospitalized on bed rest, *MCN Am J Matern Child Nurs* 25(4):204–210, 2000.

Maloni J, and others: Physical and psychosocial side effects of antepartum hospital bed rest, *Nurs Res* 42(4):197–203, 1993.

National Institute for Health and Clinical Excellence (NICE): *Quick reference guide: Antenatal care for the healthy pregnant woman*, ed 2, London, 2008, RCOG Press. Retrieved from http://www.nice.org.uk/CG62.

Schroeder C: Bed rest in complicated pregnancy: a critical analysis, *MCN Am J Matern Child Nurs* 23(1):45–49, 1998.

Sprague A: The evolution of bed rest as a clinical intervention, *J Obstet Gynecol Neonatal Nurs* 33(5):542–549, 2004.

Talmadge A, Kravitz L, Robergs R: Exercise during pregnancy: research and application, *IDEA Health and Fitness Source* 18:28–35, 2000.

Nutrition

Agency for Healthcare Research and Quality (AHRQ) and U.S. Department of Health and Human Services (USDHHS): *Outcomes of maternal weight gain, Publication No. 08-E009*, Rockville, MD, 2008, AHRQ. Retrieved from http://www.ahrq.gov/clinic/tp/admattp.htm.

American Academy of Pediatrics (AAP) Committee on Genetics: Folic acid for the prevention of neural tube defects, *Pediatrics* 104(2 Pt 1):325–327, 1999.

American Academy of Pediatrics (AAP) Committee on Genetics: Maternal phenylketonuria, *Pediatrics* 107(2):427–428, 2001.

American College of Obstetricians and Gynecologists Committee on Genetics: Maternal phenylketonuria, *Int J Gynecol Obstet* 72:83–84, 2001.

American College of Obstetrics and Gynecology (ACOG): *Obesity in pregnancy, ACOG Committee Opinion*, No. 44, Washington, July, 2003, ACOG.

American College of Obstetrics and Gynecology (ACOG): *Neural tube defects, Practice Bulletin*, No. 315, *Obstet Gyncol* 206(3):671–675, 2005.

Bodnar L, Simhan H, Powers R, Frank M, and others: High prevalence of vitamin D insufficiency in black and white pregnant women residing in the northern United States and their neonates, *J Nutr* 137:447–452, 2007.

Brown J, Carlson M: Nutrition and multifetal pregnancy, *J Am Diet Assoc* 100(3):343–348, 2000.

Calhoun S: Focus on fluids: examining maternal hydration and amniotic fluid volume, *AWHONN Lifelines* 3(6):20–24, 2000.

Centers for Disease Control and Prevention (CDC) and others: Recommendations to prevent and control iron deficiency in the United States, *MMWR Morb Mortal Wkly Rep* 47:1–36, 1998.

Chu S, Bachman D, Callaghan W, and others: Association between obesity during pregnancy and increased use of health care, *N Engl J Med* 358(14):1444–1453, 2008.

Cogswell M, and others: Iron supplementation during pregnancy, anemia, and birth weight: a randomized controlled trial, *Am J Clin Nutr* 78(4):773–781, 2003.

Cox J, Phelan S: Nutrition during pregnancy, *Obstet Gynecol Clin North Am* 35:369–383, 2008.

Cunningham F, Leveno K, Bloom S, Hauth J, Rouse D, Spong C: *Williams obstetrics*, ed 23, New York, 2010, McGraw-Hill Medical.

Dawodu A, Wagner C: Mother-child vitamin D deficiency: an international perspective, *Arch Dis Child* 92:737–740, 2007.

Dijkstra S, van Beek A, Janssen J, de Vleeschouwer L, and others: High prevalence of vitamin D deficiency in newborn infants of high-risk mothers, *Arch Dis Child* 92:750–753, 2007.

Duley L, Henderson-Smart D, Meher S: Altered dietary salt for preventing pre-eclampsia, and its complications, *Cochrane Database Syst Rev* (Issue 4), Art. No.: CD005548, 2005.

Dunlop A, Jack B, Bottalico J, and others: The clinical content of preconception care: Women with chronic medical conditions, *Am J Obstet Gynecol* 199(6B):S310–S327, 2008.

Gale C, Javaid M, Robinson S, and others: Maternal size in pregnancy and body composition in children, *J Clin Endocrinol Metab* 92(10):3904–3911, 2007.

Gardiner P, Nelson L, Shellhaas C, Dunlop A, and others: The clinical content of preconception care: Nutrition and dietary supplements, *AJOG* 199(6B):S2345–S23356, 2008.

Guelinckx I, Devlieger R, Beckers K, Vansant G: Maternal obesity: Pregnancy complications, gestational weight gain and nutrition, *Obes Rev* 9(2):140–150, 2008.

Hindmarsh P, and others: Effect of early maternal iron stores on placental weight and structure, *Lancet* 356(9231):719–723, 2000.

Hofmeyr GJ, Atallah AN, Duley L: Calcium supplementation during pregnancy for preventing hypertensive disorders and related problems, *Cochrane Database Syst Rev* (Issue 3), Art. No.: CD001059, 2006.

Hofmeyr GJ, Gülmezoglu AM: Maternal hydration for increasing amniotic fluid volume in oligohydramnios and normal amniotic fluid volume, *Cochrane Database Syst Rev* (Issue 1), Art. No.: CD000134, 2002.

Institute of Medicine, Subcommittee for a Clinical Application Guide, Committee on Nutritional Status During Pregnancy and Lactation, Food and Nutrition Board: *Nutrition during pregnancy and lactation: an implementation guide*, Washington, DC, 1998, National Academy Press.

Institute of Medicine, Subcommittee on Nutritional Status and Weight Gain During Pregnancy: *Nutrition during pregnancy*, Washington, DC, 1990, National Academy Press. Retrieved from http://www.nal.usda.gov/fnic/etext/000105.html.

Institute of Medicine: *Dietary reference intake for energy, carbohydrate, fiber, fat, fatty acids, cholesterol, protein, and amino acids*, Washington, DC, 2002, National Academy of Science, Retrieved from http://www.nal.usda.gov/fnic/etext/000105.html.

Institute of Medicine: *Dietary reference intake for vitamin A, vitamin K, arsenic, boron, chromium, copper, iodine, iron, manganese, molybdenum, nickel, silicon, vanadium, and zinc*, Washington, DC, 2001, National Academy Press, Retrieved from http://www.nal.usda.gov/fnic/etext/000105.html.

Institute of Medicine: *Dietary reference intake for water, potassium, sodium, chloride, and sulfate*, Washington, DC, 2004, National Academy Press. Retrieved from http://www.nal.usda.gov/fnic/etext/000105.html.

Institute of Medicine: *Dietary reference intakes for calcium, phosphorus, magnesium, vitamin D and fluoride*, Washington, DC, 1997, National Academy Press. Retrieved from http://www.nal.usda.gov/fnic/etext/000105.html.

Institute of Medicine: *Dietary reference intakes for thiamin, riboflavin, niacin, vitamin B_6, folate, vitamin B_{12}, pantothenic acid, biotin, and choline*, Washington, DC, 1998, National Academy.

Institute of Medicine (IOM): *Weight gain during pregnancy: reexamining the guidelines*, Washington D.C, 2009, National Academies Press.

Institute for Clinical Systems Improvement (ICSI): *Health care guidelines: routine prenatal care*, ed 12, Bloomington, MN, 2008, ICSI. Retrieved from http://www.icsi.org

International Food Information Council Foundation (IFICF) and March of Dimes (MOD): *Healthy eating during pregnancy*, Washington, DC, 2003, IFIC Foundation. Retrieved from http://www.ific.org/publications/brochures/pregnancybroch.cfm.

Kaiser L, Allen L: Position of the American Dietetic Association: nutrition and lifestyle for a healthy pregnancy outcome, *J Am Diet Assoc* 102(10):1479–1497, 2002.

Kaiser L, Allen L: Position of the American Dietetic Association: Nutrition and lifestyle for a healthy pregnancy outcome, *J Am Diet Assoc* 108(3):553–561, 2008.

King J: Maternal obesity, metabolism, and pregnancy outcomes, *Ann Rev Nutr* 26:271–291, 2006.

Kretchmer N, Zimmermann M: *Developmental nutrition*, Boston, 1997, Allyn and Bacon.

Lee R: *Iron deficiency anemia*, IOM Food and Nutrition Board, Washington, DC, 2004. Retrieved from http://www.cdph.ca.gov/healthinfo/healthyliving/childfamily/documents/mo-agb-anemiairondefhandout.pdf.

Luke B: Nutrition in multiple gestations, *Clin Perinatol* 32(2):403–429, 2005.

Luke B, Eberlein T: *When you're expecting twins, triplets, quads*, New York, 1999, Harper and Row.

Maggard M, Yermilov I, Li Z, Maglione M, Newberry S, and others: Pregnancy and fertility following bariatric surgery: a systematic review, *JAMA* 300(19):2286–2296, 2008.

McCullough M: Vitamin D deficiency in pregnancy: bringing the issues to light, *J Nutr* 137:305–306, 2007.

Monti D: What's so "essential" about essential fatty acids in pregnancy?, *IJCE* 18:3, 2003.

Moos M, Dunlop A, Jack B, Nelson L, and others: Healthier women, healthier reproductive outcomes: Recommendations for the routine care of all women of reproductive age, *Am J Obstet Gynecol* 199(6B):S280–S289, 2008.

National Institute for Health and Clinical Excellence (NICE): *Quick reference guide: Antenatal care for the healthy pregnant woman*, ed 2, London, 2008, RCOG Press. Retrieved from http://www.nice.org.uk/guidance/index.jsp?CG62.

National Institutes of Health: *Phenylketonuria: screening and management, Consensus development conference statement*, October 16-18, 2000. Retrieved from http://www.consensus.nih.gov.

Newman V, Fullerton J, Anderson P: Clinical advances in the management of severe nausea and vomiting during pregnancy, *J Obstet Gynecol Neonatal Nurs* 22(6):483–490, 1993.

Office of Dietary Supplements (ODS) and National Institutes of Health (NIH): *Dietary supplement fact sheet*, Bethesda, Maryland, 2005. Retrieved from http://ods.od.nih.gov/factsheets/iron.asp

Peña-Rosas JP, Viteri FE: Effects of routine oral iron supplementation with or without folic acid for women during pregnancy, *Cochrane Database Syst Rev* (Issue 3), Art. No.: CD004736, 2006. Press. Retrieved from http://www.nal.usda.gov/fnic/etext/000105.html.

Reifsnider E, Gill S: Nutrition for the childbearing years, *J Obstet Gynecol Neonatal Nurs* 29(1):43–55, 2000.

Strong J: Anemia white blood cell disorders. In James D, and others, editors: *High risk pregnancy: management options,* ed 3, Philadelphia, 2005, Saunders.

Suitor C: *Maternal weight gain: a report of an expert work group,* Arlington, VA, 1997, National Center for Education in Maternal and Child Health. Retrieved from http://www.ncemch.org

Suitor C: Nutritional assessment of the pregnant woman, *Clin Obstet Gynecol* 37(3):501–514, 1994.

Thacher T, Fischer P, Strand M, Pettifor J: Nutritional rickets around the world: causes and future directions, *Ann Trop Paediatr* 26:1–16, 2006.

Trumbo P, Schlicker S, Yates A, and others: Dietary reference intakes for energy, carbohydrate, fiber, fat, fatty acids, cholesterol, protein, and amino acids, *J Am Diet Assoc* 102(11):1621–1630, 2002.

U.S. Department of Agriculture: *Dietary guidelines for Americans,* 2005. Retrieved from http://www. healthierus.gov/dietaryguidelines.

U.S. Department of Agriculture: *My Pyramid Food Guide,* 2005. Retrieved from http://www.mypyramid. gov.

U.S. Department of Health and Human Services: *Healthy People 2010: understanding and improving health,* Washington, DC, 2000, USDHHS. Retrieved from http://health.gov/healthypeople/ Document/tableofcontents.htm.

van den Broek N, Kulier R, Gülmezoglu AM, Villar J: Vitamin A supplementation during pregnancy, *Cochrane Database Syst Rev* (Issue 4), Art. No.: CD001996, 2002.

Ward L, Gaboury I, Ladhani M, Zlotkin S: Vitamin D-deficiency rickets among children in Canada, *CMAJ* 177:161–166, 2007.

Williams A: Vitamin D in pregnancy: An old problem still to be solved? *Arch Dis Child* 92:740–741, 2007.

Hyperemesis Gravidarum

American College of Obstetrics and Gynecology (ACOG): *Nausea and vomiting of pregnancy, Practice Bulletin,* No. 52, Washington, April, 2004, ACOG.

Borrelli F, Capasso G, Aviello M, Pittler M, Izzo A: Effectiveness and safety of ginger in the treatment of pregnancy-induced nausea and vomiting, *Obstet Gynecol* 105(4):849–856, 2005.

Davis M: Nausea and vomiting of pregnancy: an evidence-based review, *J Perinat Neonatal Nurs* 18(4):312–328, 2004.

Jewell D, Young G: Interventions for nausea and vomiting in early pregnancy, *Cochrane Database Syst Rev* (Issue 4), Art. No.: CD000145, 2003.

National Institute for Health and Clinical Excellence (NICE): *Quick reference guide: Antenatal care for the healthy pregnant woman,* ed 2, London, 2008, RCOG Press. Retrieved from http://www.nice.org.uk/ CG62.

Smith C, and others: Acupuncture to treat nausea and vomiting in early pregnancy: a randomized controlled trial, *Birth* 29(1):1–9, 2002.

Smith C, and others: A randomized controlled trial of ginger to treat nausea and vomiting in pregnancy, *Obstet Gynecol* 103(4):639–645, 2004.

2

General Nursing Assessment of the High Risk Expectant Family

A pregnancy becomes high risk when the mother or fetus has a significantly increased risk for disability (morbidity) or death (mortality). To achieve an optimal perinatal outcome, high risk factors must be recognized early so that appropriate and timely treatment can be implemented.

Nursing care for the family experiencing a high risk pregnancy focuses on the nurse's independent and collaborative roles. The independent role of the perinatal nurse is to diagnose and treat the expectant family's reactions or concerns about the potential risks inherent to this condition. This role is based on the American Nurses Association's (2003) definition of the unique role of the professional nurse:

Nursing is the protection, promotion, and optimization of health and abilities, prevention of illness and injury, alleviation of suffering through the diagnosis and treatment of human response, and advocacy in the care of individuals, families, communities, and populations.

The second and equally important role of the perinatal nurse is collaborative management of a high risk condition with other health team members in a way that facilitates health and healing. According to Carpenito-Moyet (2009), the nurse's collaborative role is to monitor the high risk condition and implement physician- and nurse-prescribed interventions to minimize fetal and maternal complications. These interventions should be evidence-based whenever evidence is available.

ANTEPARTUM NURSING ASSESSMENT

We have used the problem-solving process as the framework for patient care. To make appropriate nursing diagnoses, a comprehensive nursing database must be compiled. We chose Gordon's functional health patterns (1994) because they are relevant to all conceptual nursing models and they provide a systematic way to collect data to determine an individual's or a family's functioning response to a potential or actual threat to the optimal physical and emotional pregnancy outcome.

A prenatal assessment guide using the functional health patterns have been developed (Box 2-1). This tool can help health care providers assess the expectant mother and family in the acute care setting or home care in several ways:

- It provides a way to assess prenatal physical and emotional risks to make screening easier for a high risk complication.
- It assesses the patient's and family's reactions to hypothetical high risk conditions so that if one develops, it is easier to formulate a nursing strategy.
- It assesses the members of the support system, the resources, and the belief system of the family. This facilitates individualized care planning.
- It assesses the patient's and family's cultural beliefs and practices to enable creation of a patient care strategy that takes these important aspects into consideration. This facilitates optimal health outcomes.

ANTEPARTUM DIAGNOSTIC ASSESSMENT

Laboratory Studies

Initial laboratory studies provide baseline data about previous maternal disease, existing maternal disease, or predisposition to disease or complications during pregnancy. A typical prenatal profile includes several laboratory studies.

Complete Blood Cell Count

A complete blood cell count at the first prenatal visit provides information about leukocyte and erythrocyte levels and the plasma-to-volume ratio. It also supplies information about platelets and erythrocyte formation. If leukocyte levels are high, infection may be present and it can be treated early. Shifts in the granular and nongranular leukocyte counts can help determine whether viral or bacterial infections are present. If the erythrocyte count is low or hemoglobin and hematocrit levels are low, anemia may be a problem; it should be treated vigorously with nutritive and iron supplements. If the woman is of African or Mediterranean descent, further screening for sickle cell disease (thalassemia) may be needed.

All women should have repeat hemoglobin and hematocrit levels taken at 28 to 32 weeks. Although serum volume increases slightly more than the proportion of erythrocytes, anemia should not occur if red blood cells are normal before pregnancy and iron and folic acid intake are increased throughout pregnancy. True anemia of pregnancy is defined as a hemoglobin level lower than 11 g/dl in the first and third trimesters and lower than 10.5 g/dl in the second trimester.

Urine Culture

Urine culture and sensitivity for asymptomatic bacteriuria (ASB) is recommended on the first prenatal visit. If renal function is thought to be compromised, further evaluation may be needed to evaluate creatinine, protein, and uric acid in the urine and serum. If infection is present, treatment can be started before renal function is impaired and before the pregnancy is threatened by premature labor.

Text continued on p. 33.

Box 2-1   Functional Health Pattern Assessment for High Risk Pregnancy

Health Perception and Health Management Pattern (i.e., the perceived or actual prenatal risks)
Individual Assessment (Ask questions in all of the following areas)
- Demographic risks: geographic location, socioeconomic status, educational attainment, marital status, age, racial or ethnic group, occupational hazards, and blood type
- Behavioral characteristics
- Time prenatal care first sought
- Usage patterns and perception of effects on health of self and fetus of alcohol, tobacco, prescription and nonprescription drugs, illegal drugs, passive smoke, and sexual contact with an illegal drug user
- Health screening patterns, such as physical, dental, and eye examinations; Pap tests; and immunizations (especially rubella)
- Seat belt use
- Breast self-examination pattern
- Current medication use—over-the-counter and prescription
- Complementary and alternative therapy use, including herbal medications, acupuncture, massage therapy, and therapeutic touch
- Current general health (any of the following health problems?)
  - Known allergies
  - Anemia (severe)
  - Cardiac disease
  - Chronic hypertension
  - Chronic lung disease
  - Diabetes
  - Emotional problems
  - Metabolic disease, such as phenylketonuria
  - Phlebitis
  - Renal disease
  - Seizure disorder
  - Thyroid disease
  - Ulcers
- Medical history, including childhood diseases
  - Sexually transmitted diseases
  - Surgeries
  - Hereditary disorders
  - Multiple births
  - Diethylstilbestrol use
  - Premature birth
- Environmental or chemical exposure
  - Heavy metals
  - Organic solvents
  - Pollutants
- Radiation or x-ray exposure
- Viral infections such as cytomegalovirus, rubella, or toxoplasmosis
- Prenatal health care resources used or planned, such as childbirth education classes, support groups, social services, and community agencies

Continued

Box 2-1   Functional Health Pattern Assessment for High Risk Pregnancy—cont'd

- Expectations of the health care providers
- Birth plan
- Need for control

Family Assessment
- What is your family medical history? (Are there any health problems in your family? If yes, what?)
- Who in the family determines such things as what the family eats, when and how they exercise, or when to visit the doctor?
- What does your family do to stay healthy?
- What are your bathing and dental hygiene practices?

Community Assessment
- What, if anything, does the community do to help or hinder your attempts to be healthy?
- What, if anything, does the community do to help or hinder you in raising children?

Cultural Practice Assessment
- Do you plan to immunize your child?
- How often do you or your family get routine checkups?
- What is your belief about health care during pregnancy?

Nutritional-Metabolic Pattern
Individual Assessment
- What is a typical daily food and fluid intake? Eating times? Food likes and dislikes? Dieting patterns? Ways you like your meat cooked (rare)?
- What is your understanding as to the needed dietary changes, especially in folic acid and calcium intake, in (use the appropriate situation) normal pregnancy/high risk pregnancy/adolescent pregnancy/multiple gestation/lactation/postdelivery recovery?
- How is your appetite?
- What supplements do you use: iron, vitamins, and/or minerals?
- What food restrictions or cravings are you experiencing? Are you experiencing pica?
- What eating-related discomforts, such as nausea or vomiting, leg cramps, heartburn, or bleeding gums, are you experiencing?
- What is your nutritional status: height and weight, amount of weight gained or lost, condition of skin, teeth, hair, and nails?

Family Assessment
- Which family member makes the nutrition-related decisions?
- Is the cost of nutritional foods within your family's budget?

Community Assessment
- Are stores reasonably accessible to your family?
- Are any community resources such as WIC or food stamps needed?
- Is the water supply safe?

Cultural Practices Assessment
- Are there any cultural practices regarding foods or fluids that you and/or your family value?

Box 2-1 Functional Health Pattern Assessment for High Risk Pregnancy—cont'd

Elimination Pattern
Individual Assessment
- Urinary elimination pattern: Have you experienced changes or problems in urinating such as frequency, odor, or burning pain?
- Bowel elimination pattern: Have you experienced changes or problems such as flatulence, constipation, odor, or hemorrhoids?
- What remedies have you used?

Family Assessment
- What is the family's use of laxatives?
- Do you have an indoor cat? If so, who changes the litter box?

Pest Control and Garbage Disposal
Community Assessment
- What are the sanitation and disposal practices of the community?
- Are there any hazardous waste disposal plants near the community?
- How is the air quality?

Cultural Practices Assessment
- Are there any cultural practices in the area of elimination that you or your family value?
- When do you think a child should be toilet trained?

Activity and Exercise Pattern
Individual Assessment
- What is your usual pattern of exercise, activity, use of leisure time, and recreation?
- Do you plan to change this pattern during pregnancy/high risk condition/ postdelivery recovery in any way? Be specific.
- Are you experiencing any problems that interfere with the desired or expected pattern of activity?
- Since becoming pregnant, what has been your level of energy?
- Have you been experiencing any discomforts such as backache, round ligament pain, or varicosities?
- If a high risk condition develops and limited physical activity or bedrest becomes necessary: Do you understand the reason for the treatment?

Family Assessment
- What are the family's activity, leisure, and recreational patterns?
- Does the family have adequate transportation available?

Community Assessment
- What activities are available in the community for an expectant and new family?

Cultural Practices Assessment
- What activities or movements are prescribed during pregnancy or puerperium?
- What activities or movements are forbidden during pregnancy or puerperium, such as bathing or type of water used?

Continued

Box 2-1   Functional Health Pattern Assessment for High Risk Pregnancy—cont'd

Sleep-Rest Pattern
Individual Assessment
- What is your pattern of sleep, rest, and relaxation? Any problems? If so, what remedies are you using?
- Which position(s) do you sleep in?

Family Assessment
- What are the family's sleeping arrangements and plans for where the new baby will sleep?
- When do you believe a child should start sleeping through the night?

Community Assessment
- Do any community activities interfere with the family's sleep?

Cultural Practices Assessment
- How much sleep should the pregnant woman get?
- In what position should one sleep?

Cognitive-Perceptual Pattern
Individual Assessment
- Do you find it easy or difficult to communicate with family members or health care providers?
- Is there any information you would like to know about the following?
  - Reproduction
  - High risk condition you are at risk for
  - Screening methods to be ordered
  - Labor and delivery
  - Postdelivery recovery
- What are your perceptions of the needs of the fetus and infant? How do you propose to meet these needs?
- Do you know how to care for an infant? Do you have prior experience? Do you have a planned method of infant feeding?
- How do you learn best? (teaching method, strategies, preferred method, level of education, language spoken, readiness, and motivation)
- What are the nature and location of your pains and discomforts?
- Are your sensory modes or the prosthesis that you use adequate?

Family Assessment (Family's decision-making process and pattern of communication)
- Which family member decides whether to attend a childbirth education class?

Community Assessment
- If community resources are needed, such as a support group, are they available if a high risk condition develops?

Cultural Practices Assessment
- What educational goals do you have for yourself? For this child?
- How should a person respond to pain?

Self-Perception/Self-Concept Pattern
Individual Assessment
- How do you feel about yourself, your general mood, body image, sense of worth, sense of control over your life?

Box 2-1   Functional Health Pattern Assessment for High Risk Pregnancy—cont'd

- How do you feel about your life situation (use appropriate situation): health status, being pregnant, physical and emotional changes that you are experiencing, parenthood, pregnancy loss?
- How would you describe your childhood?

Family Assessment
- What is your significant other's response to the present life situation (choose the appropriate situation): the pregnancy, high risk condition, your physical and emotional changes, parenthood, pregnancy loss?
- How would the father-to-be describe his childhood?
- What are the family's feelings, in general?
- What is the response of the other family members, such as your other children, to the pregnancy?

Community Assessment
- What are the housing conditions where you live?
- What would you say is the overall feeling in your neighborhood?

Cultural Practices Assessment
- Are there any cultural practices where you live that will influence parenting?

Role-Relationship Pattern
Individual Assessment
- Do you feel loved and secure in your family relationship?
- What are your home responsibilities, child care, housework?
- What is your present or former occupation?
- How would you describe your work environment, commuting distance, hours at work, stress level, involvement in work activities such as lifting or standing, exposure to chemicals or infections?
- What are your hobbies?
- What is your perception of how pregnancy or a high risk condition will affect your responsibilities?
- Anticipatory guidance: What would you do if you had to be hospitalized for a few days? Who will take care of your home or other children while you are in the hospital to have your baby?
- What is your greatest concern?

Family Assessment
- Who is in your family? What are the living arrangements?
- What are the responsibilities of each family member in the home? At work? In the community?
- What are your significant other's and your perceptions of how parenthood will affect the future activities and plans of the family?

Community Assessment
- What referral services are needed, such as homemaker, child care, and financial assistance?

Cultural Practices Assessment
- What are the family's beliefs about the role of the father during pregnancy, during labor, and in child care?

Continued

Box 2-1   Functional Health Pattern Assessment for High Risk Pregnancy—cont'd

Sexuality and Reproductive Pattern
Individual Assessment
- Are your sexual relationships satisfying during this pregnancy?
- Are you experiencing any sexuality problems?
- How are you dealing with the modified or restricted sexual activity (if indicated because of a high risk condition)?
- Menstrual history: What was the length of your menstrual cycle and period? What was the date of your last normal menstrual period? What is the estimated date of delivery?
- Contraceptive history: What method of contraception did you use? Did you experience any problems? What do you know about alternative methods? What do you plan to use for future contraception?
- What is your obstetric history?
- Gravid/para (FPAL); dates of previous pregnancies
- Spontaneous abortions; induced abortions; ectopic pregnancy; abruptio placentae; placenta previa
- History of low-birth-weight or large-for-gestational-age infants
- History of multiple birth
- History of birth defects or intrauterine fetal death
- History of preterm birth
- History of labor dystocia/operative delivery/breech delivery
- Rh or ABO incompatibility
- High risk pregnancy complicated with gestational diabetes or preeclampsia
- Postpartum depression
- What is your current obstetric status?
- Prenatal care
- Multiple gestation
- Fetal presentation
- Bleeding
- Complications
- Fundal height; quickening; gestational age when first heard FHR (correlate with gestational age)
- Diagnostic tests such as hemoglobin, urinalysis, blood sugar (within normal limits)

Family Assessment
- What is your desired family size?
- What is your significant other's sexuality response to pregnancy? (sexual restrictions, if necessary)

Community Assessment
- What are your community's patterns of reproduction? (birth rates, teenage pregnancy rate, maternal and fetal mortality)
- Are you aware of the various prenatal care alternatives, family planning, abortion services, and adoption services available? (community resources)

Cultural Practices Assessment
- Are there any beliefs about sexual practices during pregnancy that you follow?

Box 2-1   Functional Health Pattern Assessment for High Risk Pregnancy—cont'd

- Where should delivery take place?
- What does the due date mean to you?

Coping and Stress-Tolerance Pattern
Individual Assessment
Perceived life stressors
- Is there anything in particular that is worrying you about yourself? Your significant other? Your baby?
- What do you think about childbirth, high risk condition, hospitalization?
- Have you had or are you anticipating any other major life changes during this pregnancy?
- How do you feel you are doing, adjusting to the role of parent? Have you had lifestyle changes?
- Have you ever been physically, emotionally, or sexually abused by someone?
- Have you ever been forced to participate in sexual activities?

Losses experienced
- Have you ever had an infant or a child who died?
- Have you had a recent death in your immediate family?
- Are you still grieving about the death?

Coping mechanisms used
- What do you do when you are upset?

Perception of support system
- Who comforts you when you have a problem?
- Who do you talk with about your pregnancy?
- Fill in the blanks. The baby's father is _____. Your mother is
_____.
- What can the nurses do to provide you with more comfort and security?

Family Assessment
- Is there anything in particular that is worrying your significant other? Your family?

Community Assessment
- Does the community where you live cause you added stress?
- Do you need any referral services? (social worker, community health nurse, mental health nurse, mental health referral, support group)

Cultural Practices Assessment
- Are there any religious practices that are important to you?
- Do you feel your faith in God is helpful to you? If so, how?
- Is prayer important to you?

ABO and Rho (D) Blood Typing

ABO and D (formally Rh) blood typing are important to know to prevent and treat erythroblastosis in the fetus. Repeat Rho (D) antibody testing at 28 weeks. If the mother is Rho (D) negative and unsensitized, Rho (D) immune globulin should be given at 28 weeks as well as within 72 hours postpartum.

Antibody Screen

Antibody screening should be done regardless of the D type because other hemolytic incompatibilities may be present. Clinically significant disease may develop because of various blood group antigens shown in the ABO, Rho (D), Duffy, and Kell systems. A mnemonic device to help remember the significance of various antibodies is "Duffy dies, Kell kills, and Lewis lives."

Rubella/Rubeola/Varicella Screen

A rubella, rubeola, and varicella screen provides information about immunity against these diseases. If titers indicate lack of immunity, the patient cannot be vaccinated with the MMR or varicella vaccine during pregnancy because these vaccines contain a live virus and could cause fetal anomalies. The patient should be instructed to avoid contact with people who could potentially infect her. Vaccination is recommended with the use of contraception at a minimum of 1 month postpartum for rubella and 3 months' postpartum for varicella.

Venereal Disease Research Laboratory (RPR or VDRL)

All mothers should receive a serologic test to screen for syphilis because the presence of this disease affects the treatment of the mother and the fetus for potential congenital syphilis caused by maternal infection. The prenatal health examination may be the first time the woman learns that she is infected. Treatment with antibiotics and follow-up serology must be undertaken.

Sexually Transmitted Infections

All patients 25 years or younger or at risk for sexually transmitted infections should be screened for venereal gonococcus and chlamydia at the first prenatal visit. All women should be screened for syphilis at the first prenatal visit (CDC, 2006) (see Chapter 26).

Hepatitis B Virus Screen

The Centers for Disease Control and Prevention and the American College of Obstetricians and Gynecologists (ACOG) recommend that all pregnant women be screened for hepatitis B surface antigen (HBsAg) at the initial prenatal visit (see Chapter 26).

Human Immunodeficiency Virus (HIV) Screening

HIV testing is routinely recommended. Pregnant women should be encouraged to undergo testing, and confidentiality of test results should be explained. If test results are positive, the woman can be treated with antiviral medications and combination drug therapies to prevent transmitting HIV to the fetus and lessen the likelihood of developing overt or worsening disease (see Chapter 26).

Glucose Test for Gestational Diabetes

All pregnant women, except those who are at low risk, should be screened between 24 and 28 weeks of gestation for gestational diabetes. All those who are at high risk for developing gestational diabetes should be screened at the first prenatal visit and again between 24 and 28 weeks of gestation (see Chapter 10).

Papanicolaou (Pap) Test

A Pap test should be done on all pregnant women at the time of their first prenatal visit if one was not done in the previous year. If third trimester bleeding develops, a Pap test can be repeated to rule out bleeding caused by carcinoma. Pregnancy may increase cervical cancerous growth because of hormonal influences. In the presence of cervical cancer, pregnancy might need to be terminated so that the mother may be treated.

Other diseases, such as *Monilia* and bacterial vaginitis infections, may be detected on the Pap test. These should be treated even if the woman is asymptomatic. Organism proliferation found on the Pap test may become significant enough to cause miscarriage or premature rupture of membranes if left untreated.

Purified Protein Derivative Test for Tuberculosis

A purified protein derivative (PPD) screen (Mantoux skin test) should be performed for all at-risk patients to identify any old infection or active disease.

Group B *Streptococcus* Screening

All pregnant women should be screened for group B-*streptococcus* between 35 and 37 weeks of gestation (CDC, 2002) (see Chapter 26).

Maternal Serum Markers Screen

Optimally, second trimester maternal serum markers or the quadruple marker screen—which includes unconjugated estriol, human chorionic gonadotropin (hCG) (the free beta subunit), inhibin-A, and alpha fetoprotein—should be measured between 14 and 22 weeks of gestation. Such serum markers may be measured to assess for developmental defects such as neurotube defects, ventral abdominal wall defects, and esophageal and duodenal atresia. These markers also detect such trisomies as Down syndrome and trisomy 18. There is a 5% false positive rate that produces anxiety for the expectant couple (Wald, Huttly, and Hackshaw, 2003).

First-trimester ultrasound nuchal translucency (NT) combined with hCG and pregnancy-associated plasma protein-A (PAPP-A) can be measured between 10 and 13 weeks to screen for Down syndrome, trisomy 18, or major heart defects but not spina bifida (ACOG, 2007). See Chapter 4 for greater detail regarding these screens.

Antepartum Ultrasound

Ultrasound has become commonplace in obstetric care. However, according to the Cochrane Review (Bricker and Neilson, 2000) and Phelan (2008), evidence exist that routine ultrasound in low risk women do not reduce perinatal morbidity and mortality or lower the rate of unnecessary interventions. They concluded that ultrasound should be performed only for specific indications in low risk pregnancies:

- To verify gestational age
- To evaluate fetal growth
- To diagnose fetal malformation
- To confirm cardiac activity
- To count fetuses
- To determine placenta location

- To diagnose uterine anomaly
- To rule out ectopic pregnancy, spontaneous abortion, hydatidiform mole, or fetal demise
- To determine fetal presentation
- As a special procedure adjunct for tests such as amniocentesis or chorionic villus sampling, biophysical profile, amniotic fluid index, and external version. However, if the family requests the test, it is reasonable to grant their request (ACOG, 2007).

ANTEPARTUM PHYSICAL ASSESSMENT

Ongoing assessment of a high risk pregnancy demands more frequent prenatal visits. An in-depth physical assessment should be done at each prenatal visit, along with an evaluation of complication-related parameters. Various parameters to evaluate follow.

Maternal Weight

See the section on nutrition (Chapter 1).

Fundus Height

Fundus height should be measured each visit after 20 weeks of gestation. It is measured in centimeters from the top of the symphysis pubis to the top of the fundus of the uterus. It is roughly equal in centimeters to the number of weeks of gestation. Thus at 28 weeks, fundal height would be expected to be 28 cm. Because care providers have varying techniques, it is important to use a consistent method and to know how each staff member takes this measurement. It is acceptable to find variations of 1 to 3 cm. Variations more than 3 cm should prompt further investigation of possible estimated date of delivery inaccuracies or growth abnormalities.

Blood Pressure

Blood pressure should be taken at each visit in the same arm and in the same position. The diastolic blood pressure normally drops 7 to 10 mm Hg during the first and second trimesters, followed by a return to nonpregnant baseline during the third trimester. A blood pressure of 140/90 or greater may warn of a hypertensive disorder of pregnancy and should be evaluated.

Physiologic/Pathologic Edema

Because edema has a low specificity and sensitivity in predicting the development of preeclampsia, the Institute for Clinical Systems Improvement (ICSI, 2008) recommended discontinuing routine evaluation for edema.

Urine Dipstick Test

Because a urine dipstick test gives unreliable protein and glucose readings, the ICSI (2008) recommended discontinuing its use as a diagnostic tool for pathologic conditions. Its value lies only in screening and then, if positive, in using it as diagnostic evaluation specific to the concern.

Fetal Heart Rate

Doppler readings begin at 10 to 12 weeks of gestation and continue at each visit. They enable the practitioner to auscultate the fetal heart rate (FHR). The technique for calculating heart rate is to listen for a full 60 seconds. The FHR is usually not detectable by fetoscope until 16 to 18 weeks. FHR documentation helps to confirm early dating and document fetal life.

Fetal Movement

After 18 weeks of gestation, the woman is asked about fetal movement. After 24 weeks, she is instructed to count movements at least once daily as a simple way of creating a dependable report of expected fetal well-being. See Chapter 3 for further discussion.

Risk Evaluation (ICSI, 2008)

The following assessments help evaluate fetal and maternal risks:
- Prescription and over-the-counter medication use
- Domestic violence screen (see Chapter 25)
- Personal or family history of psychiatric disease, including depression (see Chapter 6)
- Occupational hazards
- Genetic anomalies
- Preterm labor risk factors (see Chapter 23)
- Gestational diabetes risk factors (see Chapter 10)
- Modifiable infection risk factors: rubella/varicella immunity, tuberculosis, HIV, and other sexually transmitted diseases (see Chapter 26)
- Nutritional insufficiency (see Chapter 1)
- Substance use including alcohol, tobacco, and illicit drugs (see Chapter 27)

HIGH RISK FACTORS

Factors that significantly influence the pregnancy's outcome may be divided into categories.

Vaccination Risk

According to the CDC (2007) guidelines, inactivated vaccines are considered safe during pregnancy. Inactivated influenza is recommended for all women who will be pregnant during the influenza season. Hepatitis B, tetanus-diphtheria (Td), meningococcal, and rabies vaccines can be considered if otherwise indicated. All the live attenuated vaccines are contraindicated during pregnancy.

Genetic Risk

There is a 5% risk for a congenital abnormality and a 7% risk of developmental disability in the general population (ICSI, 2008; Rappaport, 2008). To determine the family's heritable risk, conduct a genetic risk assessment. A sample prenatal genetic risk assessment form can be found in the Institute for Clinical Systems Improvement (ICSI, 2008) Health Care Guidelines for Routine Prenatal Care (*http://www.icsi.org*).

Demographic Characteristics

Geographic Location

Factors such as altitude, unsafe soil conditions, environmental exposure to pollutants, and water contamination are indigenous to certain regions of the United States and should be considered.

Socioeconomic Status

Factors such as substandard living conditions, poor hygiene, inadequate nutritional status, limited income, and limited educational level are interrelated in adverse perinatal outcomes.

Educational Attainment

The risk for adverse prenatal outcome decreases as the length of education increases, probably related to the socioeconomic index, improved nutrition, and decreased substance use (Hays and others, 2000).

Marital Status

An unmarried mother or a mother from a broken marriage has twice the risk for an adverse perinatal outcome, which is usually related to a low birth weight and inadequate prenatal care (McIntosh, Roumayah, and Bottoms, 1995).

Maternal Age

The ideal childbearing age range is 20 to 34 years, with a slightly increased adverse perinatal outcome for mothers younger than 20 years and those older than 34 years (Cogswell and Yip, 1995).

Racial and Ethnic Origins

In different countries, the ethnic groups at risk vary. In the United States, African Americans are at increased risk (USDHHS, 2000). As reported in the *Healthy People 2010* report, overall maternal mortality was 5.1/100,000 in the United States in the year 2000 (USDHHS, 2000). For African-American women, maternal mortality was 20.3/100,000. The reasons for the disparity in maternal mortality are unclear, but suppositions include lack of access to or use of early prenatal care and differences in pregnancy-related morbidity. American Indians or Alaska natives have a 5.2/1000 risk for fetal alcohol syndrome, compared with a 0.4/1000 risk in the general population (USDHHS, 2000).

Occupational Hazards and Environmental Exposures

Because a broad range of adverse perinatal risks are related to various occupational health hazards, the perinatal nurse has an important role in screening women for work place hazards. The most common adverse work place conditions (Pompeii and others, 2005; ICSI, 2008) associated with increased preterm birth, low birth weight, and preeclampsia are:
- Work week longer than 36 hours or work day longer than 10 hours
- Standing for longer than 6 hours/shift

- Lifting more than 25 to 30 pounds
- Exposure to excessive noise or extreme heat or cold

The most common environmental exposures are outlined in Table 2-1. The risk to the growing fetus depends primarily on dose, timing of exposure, and maternal and fetal susceptibility. The greatest risk for a congenital abnormality occurs during embryogenesis (the first 60 days). However, brain development can be affected significantly between 8 and 15 weeks of gestation and even up through 25 weeks (Lidstrom, 1990). Exposure to environmental hazards later in pregnancy most frequently restricts fetal growth. The Organization of Teratology Information Specialists (OTIS) web site provides helpful fact sheets on common environmental fetal risks and ways to minimize the risk to the fetus (*http://www.otispregnancy.org/hm/inside.php?id=41*)

Behavioral Characteristics

Preconception and Prenatal Care

Preconception health status is significantly important in positively influencing pregnancy outcomes. Inadequate prenatal care has been linked to an increased risk of preterm delivery (Krueger and Scholl, 2000). Quality, rather than number of, prenatal visits that focus on improved patient education and patient responsibility of their own health and their family's health improves pregnancy outcome. Innovative approaches to prenatal care need to be considered. Group prenatal care is one innovative approach that has been shown to improve outcomes without additional cost (Ickovics and others, 2007).

Substance Abuse

Smoking is the cause of 20% to 30% of all low-birth-weight infants in the United States, related to intrauterine growth restriction (USDHHS, 2000). The uses of licit and illicit drugs increase the risk for spontaneous abortion, preterm delivery, and infectious diseases (USDHHS, 2000). See Chapter 27 for specific factors.

Nutritional Status

Inadequate or excessive nutritional intake are the two most significant factors influencing pregnancy outcome. A low prepregnancy weight and an inadequate pregnancy weight gain are important indicators of poor nutritional status. An inadequate pregnancy weight gain, especially during the second trimester, may negatively affect the maternal plasma value, reducing the transfer of nutrients to support appropriate growth (Cox and Phelan, 2008). On the other hand, prepregnancy obesity, defined as a body mass index (BMI) of 30 kg/m^3 or greater, is associated with less optimal reproductive outcomes and increase maternal complications (see Chapter 1).

Dental Hygiene

Periodontal disease may increase the risk or serve as a clinical marker for preterm birth, low birth weight, and preeclampsia (AAPD, 2007). This is probably because the endotoxins from the periodontal infection cause fetotoxic substances (Boggess, 2008).

Table 2-1   Environmental Exposures and Possible Reproductive Risk

Environmental Exposures	Possible Reproductive Risk
Chemical	
Mercury	Spontaneous abortion, low birth weight, cognitive impairment (McDiarmid, Gardiner, & Jack, 2008)
Lead: jewelry making, stained glass, paint removal, etc.	Spontaneous abortion, low birth weight, fetal death, impaired neurologic development, cognitive impairment, lymphangiomas, hemangiomas (McDiarmid, Gardiner, & Jack, 2008)
Passive smoking	Increase risk of attention deficit hyperactivity (ADHD) and conduct disorders related to overstimulation of the dopamine center of the fetal brain (Gatzke-Kopp & Beauchaine, 2007)
Pesticides, herbicides, and rodenticides	Decreased fertility, congenital anomalies (Keleher, 1991; McDiarmid, Gardiner, & Jack, 2008)
Anesthetic agents, cancer chemotherapeutic agents, use of oil based paints, paint-stripping agents that contain methylene chloride, jewelry making	Spontaneous abortion, congenital defect (ICSI, 2008; McDiarmid, Gardiner, & Jack, 2008)
Nail salon chemicals such as solvents, acrylates, and phthalates	Spontaneous abortion, congenital defects (OTIS, 2006; Ross, 2009)
Personal care products may contain chemicals that pose a risk	Various congenital defects (Ross, 2009)
Environmental	
BPA (Bisphenol A) exposure from canned food liners or water bottled in containers identified by the number 7	National Toxicology Program and the Center for the Evaluation of Risk to Human Reproduction found no direct evidence of risk to humans. Inconclusive animal studies indicated "some concern" regarding effects on the brain, behavior, and the prostate gland (NTP and CERHR, 2008)
Radiation, such as x-ray	Reduced fertility, childhood leukemia, and central nervous system congenital anomalies, especially microcephaly and mental retardation related to doses over 10 rads (Toppenberg, Hill, & Miller, 1999)
Biologic	
Contact in crowded places or with a group at higher risk, such as school children and the sick	If the woman contracts an infectious disease, congenital anomalies and premature rupture of membranes (Chamberlain, 1991)

Abuse and Violence

Domestic violence is a serious problem, and the risk increases during pregnancy (FVPF, 2005). Physical abuse during pregnancy increases the risk for abruptio placentae, preterm delivery, and low-birth-weight infants, possibly related to abdominal trauma and subsequent placental damage, infection from forced sex, or stress (Krug and others, 2002; ICSI, 2008). There is also an increased risk for child abuse once the baby is born (Lemmey and others, 2001).

Multiples

The incidence of multiple births continues to rise. There are associated physiologic and psychologic risks related to multiple births. Risk factors identified by Watson-Blasioli (2001) include:
- Preterm labor
- Pregnancy-induced hypertension (PIH)
- Fetal growth restriction and low birth weight
- Maternal anemia
- Discomfort
- Parental stress (related to health outcomes, pregnancy progress, and care issues)
- Child abuse
- Marital breakdown
- Substance abuse
- Postpartum depression

CONCLUSION

Meticulous, ongoing prenatal assessment is essential in order to achieve an optimal perinatal outcome. In a thorough nursing assessment, the nurse focuses on (1) health-promoting activities that can prevent complications, and (2) recognizing developing complications early, when treatment is most effective.

BIBLIOGRAPHY

American Academy of Pediatric Dentistry (AAPD): *Guidelines on oral health care for the pregnant adolescent*, Chicago, IL, 2007, American Academy of Pediatric Dentistry (AAPD).

American College of Obstetricians and Gynecologists (ACOG): *Screening for fetal chromosomal abnormalities, Practice Bulletin*, No. 77, Washington, DC, 2007, ACOG.

American Nurses Association: *Nursing's social policy statement*, ed 2, Kansas City, MO, 2003, ANA.

Boggess K: Maternal oral health in pregnancy, *Obstet Gynecol* 111:976–986, 2008.

Bricker L, Neilson JP: Routine Doppler ultrasound in pregnancy, *Cochrane Database Syst Rev* (Issue 2), Art. No.: CD001450, 2000.

Carpenito-Moyet L: *Nursing diagnosis: application to clinical practice*, ed 13, Philadelphia, 2009, Lippincott Williams & Wilkins.

Centers for Disease Control and Prevention (CDC): *Guidelines for vaccinating pregnant women*, Atlanta, GA, 2007, Centers for Disease Control and Prevention, Retrieved from http://www.cdc.gov/vaccines/pubs/downloads/b_preg_guide.pdf.

Centers for Disease Control and Prevention (CDC): Sexually transmitted disease treatment guidelines, *MMWR Morb Mortal Wkly Rep* 55, No. RR-11, 1–94, 2006. Retrieved from http://www.cdc.gov/std/treatment/.

Centers for Disease Control and Prevention: Prevention of perinatal group B streptococcal disease, *MMWR Morb Mortal Wkly Rep* 51:1–22, 2002.

Chamberlain G: ABCs of antenatal care: work in pregnancy, *BMJ* 302(6784):1070–1073, 1991.

Cogswell M, Yip R: The influence of fetal and maternal factors on the distribution of birthweight, *Semin Perinatol* 19(3):222–240, 1995.

Cox J, Phelan S: Nutrition during pregnancy, *Obstet Gynecol Clin North Am* 35:369–383, 2008.

Family Violence Prevention Fund's National Health Resource Center on Domestic Violence (FVPF): *Domestic violence risk measurement tool online*, San Francisco, 2005, FVPF. Retrieved from http://endabuse.org/programs/healthcare.

Gatzke-Kopp L, Beauchaine T: Direct and passive prenatal nicotine exposure and the development of externalizing psychopathology, *Child Psychiatry Human Development* 38:255–269, 2007.

Gordon M: *Nursing diagnosis: process and application*, ed 3, St Louis, 1994, Mosby.

Hays B, and others: Public health nursing data: building the knowledge base for high-risk prenatal clients, *MCN Am J Matern Child Nurs* 25(3):151–158, 2000.

Ickovics J, Kershaw T, Westdahl C, Magriples U, and others: Group prenatal care improves pregnancy outcomes at no additional cost, *Obstet Gynecol* 110(2):330–339, 2007.

Institute for Clinical Systems Improvement (ICSI): *Health care guideline: routine prenatal care*, Bloomington, Minn, 2008, ICSI. Retrieved from http://www.icsi.org.

Keleher K: Occupational health: how work environments can affect reproductive capacity and outcome, *Nurse Pract* 16(1):23–30, 1991.

Krueger P, Scholl T: Adequacy of prenatal care and pregnancy outcome, *JAOA* 100(8):485–492, 2000.

Krug E, Mercy J, Dahlberg L, Zwi A: The world report on violence and health, *Lancet* 360:1083–1088, 2002.

Lemmey D, and others: Intimate partner violence: mothers' perspectives of effects on their children, *MCN Am J Matern Child Nurs* 26(2):98–103, 2001.

Lidstrom I: Pregnant women in the workplace, *Semin Perinatol* 14(4):329–333, 1990.

March of Dimes (MOD): *Environmental risks and pregnancy*, White Plains, NY, 2005, March of Dimes Birth Defects Foundation. Retrieved from http://www.marchofdimes.com/printableArticles/14332_9146.asp?printable=true.

McDiarmid M, Gardiner P, Jack B: The clinical content of preconception care: environmental exposures, *Am J Obstet Gynecol* 199(6B):S357–S361, 2008.

McIntosh L, Roumayah N, Bottoms S: Perinatal outcome of broken marriage in the inner city, *Obstet Gynecol* 85(2):233–236, 1995.

National Toxicology Program (NTP) and Center for the Evaluation of Risk to Human Reproduction (CERHR): *Bisphenol A Safety Confirmed in Final National Toxicology Program Report*, Research. Triangle Park, NC, 2008. Retrieved from http://www.bisphenol-a.org/whatsNew/20080905.html.

Organization of Teratology Information Specialists (OTIS): *Can my pregnant patient keep her job at the nail salon*, 2006. Retrieved from http://www.otispregnancy.org/hm/.

Phelan S: Components and timing of prenatal care, *Obstet Gynecol Clin North Am* 35:339–353, 2008.

Pompeii L, Savitz D, Evenson K, and others: Physical exertion at work and the risk of preterm delivery and small for gestational age birth, *Obstet Gynceol* 106:1279–1288, 2005.

Rappaport V: Prenatal diagnosis and genetic screening: integration into prenatal care, *Obstet Gynecol Clin North Am* 35:3435–3458, 2008.

Ross K: Health effects of personal care products, *Nursing for Women's Health* 13(5):391–401, 2009.

Toppenberg K, Hill D, Miller D: Safety of radiographic imaging during pregnancy, *Am Fam Physician* 59(7):1813–1818, 1999.

U.S. Department of Health and Human Services (USDHHS): *Healthy People 2010: Understanding and improving health*, Washington, DC, 2000, USDHHS. Retrieved from http://www.healthypeople.gov/document.

Wald N, Huttly W, Hackshaw A: Antenatal screening for Down's syndrome with the quadruple test, *Lancet* 361(9360):835–836, 2003.

Watson-Blasioli J: Double-take: defining the need for specialized prenatal care for women expecting twins: a Canadian perspective, *AWHONN Lifelines* 5(2):34–42, 2001.

3

Assessment of Fetal Well-Being

etal surveillance is utilized to assess well-being. There are several modalities available to accomplish this task. During the antepartum period assessments may include the non-stress test (NST), contraction stress test (CST), amniotic fluid volume (AFV) assessment, biophysical profile (BPP), Modified BPP (includes an NST and AFV), Doppler velocimetry, and fetal movement counts. During the intrapartum period assessment is generally accomplished through the use of fetal monitoring by auscultation or application of the electronic fetal monitor. Our understanding of the limitations of fetal surveillance, as well as the benefits, has changed dramatically over the years and will continue to change as new technology and practices are supported. The body of evidence to support the use of technology into our practice continues to increase. The goal of these evidence based findings is to support improved patient outcomes.

PHYSIOLOGY AND PATHOPHYSIOLOGY OF FETAL OXYGENATION

Maternal Circulatory and Cardiovascular Adaptation

One of the most dramatic adaptations to pregnancy is the increase in maternal blood volume by 20% to 100% over prepregnant volume. Plasma increases plateau around 32 to 34 weeks of gestation. The number of red blood cells increases in response to the plasma volume. Both volume and blood cell increases are in response to cell proliferation and growth of the uterus, placenta, and fetus.

Under physiologically nonstressful conditions, the vascular system in the maternal pelvic region remains widely dilated. In the presence of stressors, it is capable of marked constriction and reduction of uteroplacental blood supply. The most common and easily preventable stressor is mechanical obstruction of the maternal inferior vena cava and aorta by the gravid uterus when in a supine position. Activation of the maternal autonomic nervous system (ANS), in response to other hemodynamic changes, may also trigger marked constriction of the pelvic vasculature, which is physiologically expendable to general maternal circulatory needs.

The usual state of the uterine vasculature is one of low resistance to blood flow. This occurs in part because of new vascularization of the uterus and in response to the systemic influence of estrogens, which increases overall vasodilation. It is now estimated that uterine blood flow increases from 50 ml/min in early pregnancy to 700 ml/min by term.

Because of vasodilation and increased volume, cardiac output (Stroke Volume × Heart Rate) is greater during pregnancy. The heart rate is generally 10 to 15 bpm faster than prepregnant rates, and stroke volume is increased by approximately 15% because of increased blood volume. The increase in cardiac output helps circulate more blood to the uterus during pregnancy.

UTEROPLACENTAL-FETAL EXCHANGE*

The placenta performs several major organ functions for the fetus. It acts as the following:

- Lung for respiratory functions of exchanging oxygen (O_2) and carbon dioxide (CO_2)
- Gastrointestinal tract for nutritive functions and exchange of waste products and electrolytes
- Skin for thermoregulation
- Kidney for renal functions of acid-base balance and electrolyte homeostasis
- Endocrine organ for production of hormones that promote placental perpetuation
- Barrier to maternal blood and bacteria

After implantation, the placenta begins to form the chorionic tissues. By 14 weeks, the placenta is a discrete organ with independent functions and purpose. It is at this point that segments of the placenta, called *cotyledons*, form and connect by vascular channels to the umbilical cord. The surface of the placenta then thins to a membranous, single layer of cells. Maternal blood and fetal blood, although not mixing, are exposed to one another across this membrane. By this exposure, fetal respiration, acid-base and electrolyte homeostasis, nutrition, and excretion take place. The space in which these functions take place is the intervillous space, which contains maternal blood. Therefore, the fetus totally depends on its mother for most homeostatic mechanisms.

Transfer and exchange of molecules occur in the intervillous space. Molecules enter through the epithelial cells on the surface of the villi and move through the villous stroma and into the fetal capillary vessels within the villi. Molecules pass back and forth between maternal and fetal tissues. Transport increases during gestation, caused by changes in the structure of the placenta, increased fetal and maternal blood flow, and fetal demands. Transfer may be modified by maternal nutritional status, exercise, and the effects of disease (i.e., diabetes, hypertension). Exchange processes are accomplished by means of simple or selective diffusion.

Simple (passive) diffusion is a relatively uncomplicated process responsible for the rapid exchange of small molecules, such as O_2, CO_2, water, electrolytes, creatinine, and uric acid, across the placental membrane. Simple diffusion also allows potentially harmful drugs—antibiotics, narcotics, barbiturates, and anesthetic agents, to name a few—to cross quickly to the fetus. Simple diffusion depends totally on the adequacy of uterine blood flow and the concentration gradient of the molecules.

---

*Blackburn, 2007; Meschia, 2009.

Facilitated diffusion is a complex process and therefore occurs more slowly than simple diffusion. It can occur against a concentration gradient by an energy-dependent process. Glucose, for instance, is transported in this manner from stores in the placenta.

Selective transfer can also be actively facilitated by specific enzyme systems. For example, through *active transport* amino acids and buffering substances are transferred using specific enzyme groups to facilitate the process. Selective transfer, by energy- or enzyme-dependent processes, depends on the sufficiency of the placental surface area and placental thickness rather than on uterine blood flow.

Because simple diffusion is faster (taking only minutes), O_2, CO_2, and water can be transported and exchanged rapidly to correct fetal hypoxia if uterine and umbilical blood flow and maternal O_2 are sufficient. On the other hand, the more complex processes of selective transfer, which take hours, cannot correct an acid-base imbalance from hypoxia.

Fetal Capabilities for Maintaining Health

The fetus has certain remarkable capabilities that enable it to withstand stressors. Fetal stressors may be caused by physiologic maternal adaptation failures, disease, or mechanical or physiologic obstruction of maternal blood flow through the uterus and into the intravillous space. The fetus is equipped with a high concentration of hemoglobin in plasma (60% hematocrit). Each hemoglobin molecule, because of its unique shape, can be supersaturated with O_2. This is fortunate and necessary because by the time maternal O_2 is transferred to the fetus, the O_2 partial pressure (Po_2) is at best 35 to 40 mm Hg. Compared with an adult Po_2 of 90 to 96 mm Hg, the fetal Po_2 would be inadequate were it not for different fetal hemoglobin. The low fetal Po_2 causes the diffusion gradient to facilitate O_2 delivery from mother to fetus (Meschia, 2009).

The fetal heart must be significantly hypoxic before myocardial depression occurs. It is only after fetal myocardial depression that significant fetal central nervous system (CNS) hypoxia occurs. Protection from myocardial hypoxia exists, in part, because of the well-supplied and unimpeded blood supply from the coronary vessels. Impulses travel through the heart, originating at the sinoatrial node and traveling across the atrioventricular junction, down the bundle branches, and out the Purkinje fibers in the ventricles. When myocardial depression occurs from hypoxia, cardiac arrhythmias may occur. The fetus can effectively compensate only by increasing FHR; it cannot increase output by changing cardiac output.

Function of Amniotic Fluid Related to Evaluation of Fetal Heart Rate

Early in gestation amniotic fluid is produced primarily by maternal blood. By week 11 of gestation the fetus contributes to the volume through urinary excretion. Amniotic fluid has a number of functions. It is a buoyant medium, allowing the umbilical cord to float and preventing it from becoming entrapped between the wall of the uterus and the fetal body, especially during contractions. This function is imperfect but, for the most part, effective.

When the amniotic fluid is filled with fetal meconium, the meconium promotes stiffening and loss of flexibility of the cord with extended exposure. This is one reason why it is dangerous for meconium to be passed before the baby is born.

PHYSIOLOGIC BASIS OF FETAL HEART RATE CONTROL

Central Nervous System Control

Regulation of the FHR originates in the fetal CNS. By week 10 of gestation, both the CNS and the cardiac system are developed enough to begin and maintain the FHR.

Sympathetic

Initially, the sympathetic portion of the rudimentary ANS is functionally active. The sympathetic branch is responsible for establishing and sustaining FHR. The normal rate throughout fetal life ranges from 110 to 160 bpm for most, tending toward the upper range of 150 to 160 in early fetal life and the middle to lower range of 110 to 140 by term. The sympathetic branch of the ANS supports acceleration of the FHR in response to various stimuli, as needed for fetal circulation, and supporting compensatory responses to physical insults.

Parasympathetic

Early in fetal life, the parasympathetic branch of the ANS begins to influence the FHR. The parasympathetic branch serves as an opposing force against the steady beat sustained by the dominant sympathetic branch. This opposition exerts a differing strength of opposing force on each beat. The effects of this opposing force are observed on the FHR as it gradually slows the intrinsic rate from early gestation through term gestation.

The opposition between the sympathetic and parasympathetic nervous systems results in visual fluctuations in the FHR over time referred to as variability. Beat-to-beat differences in the FHR have been referred to as *short-term* variability and cyclic fluctuations that occur over a minute have been referred to as *long-term* variability. There is no current evidence that the distinction between short- and long-term variability has any clinical significance. Because they are visually determined as a unit the National Institute of Child Health and Human Development (NICHD) do not recommend differentiating between the two (Cunningham, 2010).

FETAL HEART RATE MONITORING

Electronic Monitoring

Electronic fetal heart monitoring (EFM) provides a current and continuous observation of indirect, subjective information about fetal oxygenation at the time the monitoring is being done. Continuous or intermittent FHR tracings provide a convenient and reasonably predictable way of assessing fetal well-being. Of approximately 4 million live births in 2002, 85% were assessed with EFM in the United States (ACOG, 2009). It does not explain oxygenation in the past or predict the future oxygenation during fetal life in the same way we once expected. When EFM was introduced in the 1960s it was believed the continuous recording would prevent fetal deaths and decrease cerebral palsy. Thus the use of the fetal monitor was accepted despite the lack of evidence to support this practice.

U.S. health statistics from 2005 indicated that overall infant mortality (deaths per 1000 live births) was at 6.86 in 1000 births (MacDorman and Mathews, 2008). The United States was ranked 29th among industrialized nations based on available data in 2004 (MacDorman and Mathews, 2008).

In the United States, continuous EFM is routine in most hospital perinatal/maternity centers. Given the available data, ACOG (2009) stated that intermittent auscultation or EFM are acceptable options for a patient without complications. A Cochrane meta-analysis (Alfirevic, Devane, and Gyte, 2006) on EFM included a review of 12 trials that identified no difference in the perinatal death rates or incidence of cerebral palsy. Other data from the review of these 12 studies showed that neonatal seizures were decreased by half, but there was an increase in the number of cesarean births and operative deliveries.

Perinatal mortality has improved over the years, and EFM is one reason for the improvement. However, morbidity statistics have not improved, raising three main concerns regarding routine use of EFM (Thacker, Stroup, and Chang, 2001; ACOG, 2009):

- Effects of EFM on the incidence of cerebral palsy (CP)
- Effects of routine continuous EFM on cesarean birth rates
- Legal implications of FHR assessment (Mahlmeister, 2000)

Cerebral Palsy

The Centers for Disease Control and Prevention (CDC, 2006) estimates the rate of CP to be 3.6 per 1000 children. This rate has not decreased with the advent of the use of EFM. In fact, because more premature infants are surviving and because they have an associated increased risk for congenitally acquired neurologic damage, CP rates are unlikely to improve (Phelan and Kim, 2000; Freeman, Garite, and Nageotte, 2003). There is also some suggestion in the literature that CP actually may start with the development of an abnormal fetal brain (Phelan and Kim, 2000). A large percentage of asphyxial damage occurs before labor and thus would not benefit from electronic FHR monitoring-prompted interventions offered during labor (Freeman, 2002; Freeman, Garite, and Nageotte, 2003).

Cesarean Section

The most discussed risk of EFM is the rise of cesarean birth rates. In the United States, the current cesarean birth rate is 31.8% (Hamilton, Martin, and Ventura, 2009). One study examined the cesarean birth rate in more than 7000 births at a large Southwestern tertiary perinatal center in a more divided manner (Radin, Harmon, and Hanson, 1993). In this study, term primiparas, regardless of demographic data, physician practice, complications, induction, regional anesthesia, or stage of labor when admitted, had an 18% cesarean birth rate. Excluded from the study were those with multiple gestations, those with intrauterine fetal death, and those who were less than 35 weeks pregnant.

Three discrete groups of nurses were identified. The low cesarean birth rate group had a cesarean birth rate lower than 5%. The middle cesarean birth group had an overall 18% cesarean birth rate. The highest cesarean birth rate group had a rate as high as 35% to 49%. No significant differences existed in neonatal Apgar scores.

This study suggested that some nurses may manage technologic data from EFM to provide expert nursing care and manage patients with epidurals differently, whereas other nurses may use the data solely to report fetal assessment data to the physician to alter medical management. This study warrants further investigation of specific differences in the patient population, and nursing care practices, including designation of patient care assignments.

Legal Implications

In the care of the antepartum and intrapartum patient, accurate interpretation of FHR patterns is essential. One challenge that has been identified is the lack of consistent terminology and definitions in describing fetal heart patterns. Simpson (2004) identified this as a critical issue and recommended the need to select one set of definitions for fetal heart rate patterns and the need to communicate consistently to avoid confusion between health care providers.

In April 2008, the Eunice Kennedy Shriver National Institute of Child Health and Human Development (NICHD), the American College of Obstetricians and Gynecologists (ACOG), and the Society for Maternal-Fetal Medicine partnered to sponsor a workshop with three goals:

- To review and update FHR definitions
- To assess existing classification systems for interpreting specific FHR patterns
- To make recommendations for research priorities for EFM (Macones and others, 2008a,b)

The incorporation of these terms into practice has also been endorsed by the Association of Women's Health, Obstetric, and Neonatal Nurses (AWHONN, 2009).

Failures in communication have been identified as a contributor to birth injury litigation (Knox, Simpson, and Garite, 1999). McKeon, Cunningham, and Detty Oswaks (2008) suggest the need for effective communication as a strategy to improve patient safety. Working in complex work environments, health care providers can support prevention of adverse fetal outcomes through the use of a standardized "language." Incorporating standardized FHR definitions into practice will prevent failure to report fetal monitor strip information or pursue chain of command, failures related to intervention, those related to interpreting the fetal monitor tracing, and failures related to contacting the health care provider.

Intermittent Auscultation

Feinstein, Sprague, and Trepanier (2008) suggest that institutions develop protocols and policies to support the use of intermittent auscultation (IA). They identify the importance of listening to the FHR immediately after a contraction for at least 30 to 60 seconds. During that 30- to 60-second period of time the need to identify a baseline and the fetal response following the contraction must be assessed. Differentiating the maternal pulse from the FHR must also be accomplished. The nurse must place a finger on the woman's radial pulse as part of the assessment.

ACOG (2009) identified that although intermittent auscultation may not be appropriate for all pregnancies, it may be acceptable in the patient with no complications. When a woman requests IA during labor the care providers must collaborate. Areas to consider are the woman's perspectives, preferences, risk factors, staffing, practitioner's experiences, and institutional guidelines (Feinstein, Sprague, and Trepanier, 2008). Research in support of this technique will make IA a more desired option for certain identified populations.

With research findings supporting the use of both EFM and IA, it is apparent that perinatal nurses must understand how to use FHR monitoring. To do this, perinatal nurses must be fully acquainted with the following (Haggerty and Nuttall, 2000; Schmidt, 2000):

- Physiology and pathophysiology of fetal oxygenation
- Physiologic basis of FHR control
- Instrumentation and the application of external and internal fetal monitoring methods
- Baseline FHR, variability patterns, periodic rate changes, arrhythmias, and artifacts, which describe effects of maternal contractions on FHR control
- Nursing management related to EFM
- Skills and techniques for antepartum evaluation of fetal well-being through auscultation, EFM testing, and fetal movement counts
- Advanced methods of fetal evaluation, such as biophysical profile and Doppler flow studies

Instrumentation and Application of Fetal Monitoring Methods

Although still indirect and somewhat subjective, EFM gives data slightly more objective than intermittent auscultation and infers information about current and ongoing fetal oxygenation. It does this by calculating and recording an average FHR per minute, indicating the baseline rate and variability, and by providing a continuous graphic printout of rate patterns and periodic changes.

To fully appreciate EFM patterns, it is helpful to have a continuous record for interpretation. Correct application of monitor methods and an understanding of the way to properly operate the monitor help the user obtain accurate information. Fetal monitors are made by a variety of manufacturers and may have capabilities for external (indirect) monitoring only or for both external and internal (direct) monitoring of FHR and maternal contractions (Fig. 3-1). Other features, such as fetal electrocardiogram (ECG) monitoring, twin monitoring, amnioinfusion, ambulatory monitoring, electronic transmission of strips from one location to another, central displays, and computer record storage are available from most manufacturers.

External (Indirect) Monitoring

The external monitor parts are the ultrasound transducer (Fig. 3-2, *A*) for assessing FHR and the tocotransducer (Fig. 3-2, *B*) for assessing contractions. To place the transducers properly, it is important to ascertain by abdominal palpation how the baby is positioned.

External contraction monitoring

Near term, the tocotransducer should be placed over the fundus of the uterus, two to three fingerwidths below the top and slightly off center from the umbilicus on the side where the fetal back is palpated. A good rule of thumb for placement of the tocotransducer for preterm contractions is to palpate the uterus for firmness and place the tocotransducer where this is best felt. The placement may be in any quadrant,

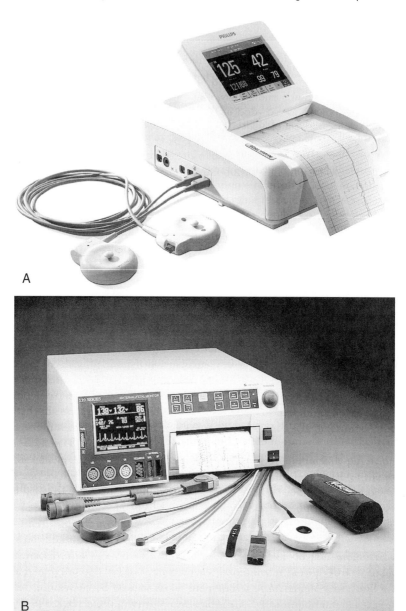

Figure 3-1 A, Avalon FM30 transducer. **B,** Corometrics Model 129 maternal/fetal monitor provides measurement of FHR, fetal oxygen saturation, UA, and maternal parameters, including SpO₂, ECG, FHR, and noninvasive BP. The audible and visual "spectra alert" option may be added to this monitor. (**A,** Courtesy Philips Medical Systems, Andover, MA. **B,** Courtesy GE Medical Systems Information Technologies, Milwaukee, WI.)

including those lower than the umbilicus. There is a pressure-sensitive area on the underside of the tocotransducer that must respond to changes in the abdominal wall when the uterus contracts against it. The tocotransducer is secured in place with a belt that is tightened only enough to keep it from slipping or it is secured with a stretchy band. The monitor has an indicated dial or button to artificially set the reference for uterine resting tone, usually between 10 and 20 mm Hg on the graph paper. Box 3-1 presents the advantages and limitations of external contraction monitoring.

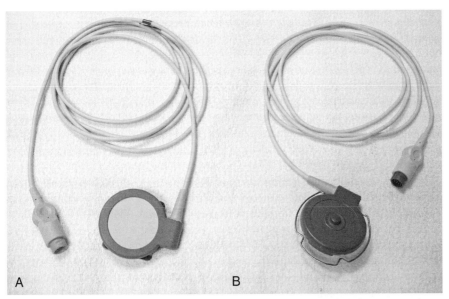

Figure 3-2 External monitoring includes the ultrasound transducer and the tocotransducer. **A,** Ultrasound transducer is placed over the fetal chest wall facing the fetal heart. **B,** Tocotransducer is placed over the best palpated area of the uterus, usually near the umbilicus near term.

Box 3-1   Advantages and Limitations of External Contraction Monitoring

Advantages
- Noninvasive
- Convenient
- Provides continuous record of frequency and duration of contractions

Limitations
- Cannot accurately measure strength (intensity)
- Restricts patient movement or must be adjusted frequently with position change

---

Modified from Tucker S, Miller L, Miller D: *Mosby's pocket guide to fetal monitoring: a multidisciplinary approach,* ed 6, St Louis, 2009, Mosby.

External fetal heart rate monitoring

The ultrasound transducer has sending and receiving crystals encased in a disk. If possible, it should be placed over the fetal back for detection of the best signal. The signal is detected from the motion of the heart valves closing between the atria and ventricles.

The ultrasound transducer selects the complex of two sound waves from the motion of the two atrioventricular valve closures, or it selects the one sound wave that is timed within the logical sequence of events; then it calculates the rate per minute. Through a system of logic, it samples a set number of valve closures, compares the previous intervals, and decides which to count. The logic system tends to give the appearance of slightly greater rate differences than are truly present. This causes the appearance of "roughness" or a "jiggle" to the line (Freeman, Garite, and Nageotte, 2003). Because there are still different generations and models of equipment in use, it is important to recognize the parameters and to know from which era the monitor in use comes. If the rate differences are not logical compared with the previous calculated rates, blanks will appear in the tracing. Blanks also occur when the signal is lost from fetal movement or shift in maternal position. Box 3-2 presents the advantages and limitations of external FHR monitoring.

Internal (Direct) Monitoring

Internal monitoring uses different components: an intrauterine pressure catheter (IUPC) (Fig. 3-3, *A*) and a fetal spiral electrode (FSE) (Fig. 3-3, *B*). An IUPC monitors the frequency, duration, and intensity of the contraction and the resting tone of the uterus. The FSE monitors the fetal electrocardiogram.

Intrauterine pressure catheter

The IUPC may be inserted by qualified registered nurses (RNs) if this is allowed according to regulations of each state's nurse licensing board. In addition, individual institutional policies and procedures are adhered to.

The IUPC catheter is inserted before the spiral electrode, in an aseptic manner, into the uterine cavity. The catheter is a flexible, narrow-gauge tube with holes along a short distance and at the proximal end. It is partially enclosed in a firmer plastic catheter introducer. Once amniotic membranes are ruptured and the cervix

---

Box 3-2   Advantages and Limitations of External Fetal Heart Rate Monitoring

Advantages
- Noninvasive
- Does not require dilation or membrane rupture
- Convenient
- Continuous recording of fetal heart rate (FHR)
- Can assess changes in baseline, variability, accelerations, decelerations

Limitations
- Tracing quality affected by maternal position, obesity, and fetal movement

Modified from Tucker S, Miller L, Miller D: *Mosby's pocket guide to fetal monitoring: a multidisciplinary approach*, ed 6, St Louis, 2009, Mosby.

is adequately dilated, the IUPC can be placed, allowing uterine pressure monitoring, amnioinfusion, and fluid sampling. The two types of IUPCs are a fluid-filled catheter (not used as commonly) or a solid catheter. The differences between these two include setting up the equipment and the procedure for zeroing the monitor. Zeroing the monitor must be accomplished according to the individual manufacturer's instructions.

The examiner's hand carefully lifts the presenting part and inserts the introducer with the catheter just through the dilated cervix. Then the catheter is carefully

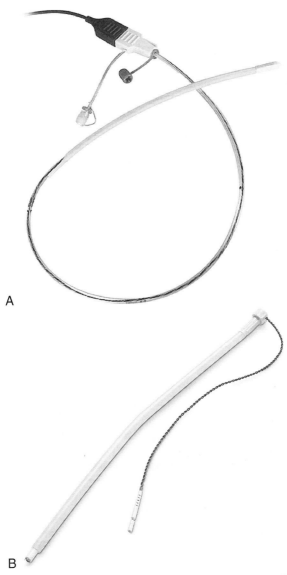

Figure 3-3 A, Intrauterine pressure catheter. **B,** Fetal spiral electrode for attachment to leg plate. (Courtesy Kendall-LTP, Chicopee, MA.)

advanced to a specific marker visualized on the outside of the perineum. The introducer is drawn back toward the distal end, and the catheter remains behind. The catheter is then secured to the patient's thigh.

As the uterus contracts and relaxes, the intercavitary pressure is reflected against the catheter. The distal end is connected to a reusable cable that connects the disposable IUPC to the fetal monitor. Pressure of contractions is measured in millimeters of mercury (mm Hg).

Fetal spiral electrode

The FSE may also be placed by qualified RNs. It is attached to the presenting part of the fetus, avoiding such potentially dangerous areas as the fontanels, facial features, or genitalia, if breech. The FSE has two color-coded wires attached to it. These are twisted together, and all are encased in an introducer. The examiner identifies the area of the presenting part and then inserts the introducer between the fingers and flush against the presenting part. The distal ends of the wires are rotated clockwise until gentle resistance is encountered; thus the FSE is attached to the fetal presenting part. The introducer is removed, the end of the FSE is connected to a leg plate on the patient's thigh, and the leg plate cord is plugged into the fetal ECG receiver on the monitor.

The monitor, in this way, directly counts from the fetal R wave (the highest amplitude electrical impulse from the fetal heart). It does not need to respond to or disregard other fetal impulses, but may count maternal R-R intervals if the fetus is dead. What is plotted on the graph paper is each rate from every R-R interval calculated, as it is, for 1 minute. Box 3-3 presents advantages and limitations of internal monitoring.

Other Features on Monitors

Electronic fetal monitors frequently have other features for monitoring the mother. It is possible to monitor the pulse, oxygenation and maternal blood pressure, and print these recordings out on the monitor strips. In addition, this patient information

---

Box 3-3   Advantages and Limitations of Internal Monitoring

Advantages

Contractions are measured accurately for:
- Strength
- Duration
- Frequency
- Resting tone

More comfortable than external monitoring

Limitations
- Requires ruptured membranes and dilation
- If prolonged, ruptured membranes may carry a small increase in infection
- Possible injury to uterine wall or fetus if improperly inserted

In the presence of a fetal demise the FSE may record the maternal heart rate

---

Modified from Tucker S, Miller L, & Miller D: *Mosby's pocket guide to fetal monitoring: a multidisciplinary approach*, ed 6, St Louis, 2009, Mosby.

can be automatically placed in a computer-based documentation system through the use of computer interfaces. Antepartum and intrapartum monitors are equipped with these capabilities. Also, there are remote devices for charting from a handheld keyboard to such things as physician visits, vaginal examinations, position changes, oxytocin (Pitocin) changes, and intravenous (IV) fluids given, and this information prints onto the monitor strip.

Electronic fetal monitors frequently have other features for monitoring twin or multiple gestations. For twins, two separate ultrasound transducers allow a continuous recording of each fetus. Easy identification of each fetus is provided electronically by the color coding on the computer screen. If a paper fetal monitor recording is used, differentiation between each fetus in a twin gestation can be identified by a thicker line tracing for one fetus and a thinner line tracing for the second fetus.

Cordless ultrasound and tocotransducers are available to allow the laboring patient to have increased freedom to ambulate while the fetus is continuously monitored. External watertight transducers are also available and can be used with wireless telemetry to allow for continued fetal surveillance during hydrotherapy or when the patient is using the shower or tub to promote relaxation.

Central fetal monitor displays allow for viewing of several fetal monitor tracings at one location. Remote viewing of these multiple displays is available on a computer screen, which may be viewed from several locations, including the nurse's station, locker room, physician's office, or the physician's home. Some of these electronic systems include audible alerts to identify a fetal heart rate outside preset fetal heart rate ranges. Alerts are also available for loss of signal if the patient moves or the fetus moves and the ultrasound transducer is unable to provide a continuous recording of the fetal heart tones (FHT).

Fetal Monitoring Terms

The 2008 NICHD updated fetal monitoring definitions defined *periodic* fetal heart patterns as those associated with uterine contractions, and *episodic* fetal heart patterns as those not associated with uterine contractions. They suggest the term hyperstimulation be replaced with the term *tachysystole*, meaning greater than 5 contractions in 10 minutes, averaged over a 30-minute window (Macones and others, 2008a,b).

Additionally the NICHD (Macones and others, 2008a,b) has developed a three-tiered system to categorize FHR tracings. This three-tiered system includes *Category I*, which is described as *normal*, suggesting normal fetal acid-base status at the time of assessment. These tracings require routine care with no specific intervention. *Category II* is described as *indeterminate* and not predictive of abnormal fetal acid-base status, but cannot be assigned as Category I or Category III (abnormal) FHR tracings. These Category II tracings require evaluation and continued surveillance and reevaluation. *Category III* FHR tracings are described as *abnormal* and are identified as predictive of abnormal fetal acid-base status at the time of evaluation. They require prompt intervention to resolve the abnormal FHR pattern such as maternal position change, application of oxygen, treatment of maternal hypotension, and discontinuation of labor stimulation as appropriate. Box 3-4 summarizes the NICHD fetal heart rate categories and the patterns included in each category.

Box 3-4   NICHD Fetal Heart Rate Categories and Patterns

Category I
Normal suggesting normal fetal acid-base status at the time of evaluation.
Includes all of the following:
- Baseline rate 110–160 bpm
- Moderate variability
- Absent—late or variable decelerations
- Present or absent—accelerations
- Present or absent—early decelerations

Category II
Indeterminate and not predictive of abnormal fetal acid-base status but they are
not able to be assigned as Category I or Category III FHR tracings.
Examples include:
- Bradycardia not accompanied by absent variability
- Tachycardia
- Minimal or marked variability
- Absent variability not accompanied by recurrent decelerations
- Absent or induced accelerations after fetal stimulation
- Recurrent variable decelerations accompanied by minimal or moderate variability
- Prolonged deceleration
- Recurrent late decelerations with moderate variability
- Variable decelerations with slow return to baseline, overshoots, or shoulders

Category III
Abnormal and are identified as predictive of abnormal fetal acid-base status at
the time of evaluation.
Include either of the following:
- Absent FHR variability and any of the following: recurrent late decelerations, recurrent variable decelerations, bradycardia
- Sinusoidal pattern

Modified from Macones GA, Hankins GD, Spong CY, Hauth J, Moore T: The 2008 National Institute of Child Health and Human Development workshop report on electronic fetal monitoring: update on definitions, interpretation, and research guidelines, *J Obstet Gynecol Neonatal Nurs,*112(3):510-515, 2008.

Can Category I, Category II, and Category III Be Applied to Intermittent Auscultation?

In an effort to support the use of a common language in the interpretation of fetal monitoring, the NICHD has also recommended the use of the three-tiered system when communicating about IA. Intermittent auscultation can be categorized as Category I *(normal)* or Category II *(indeterminate)* as stated in Box 3-5. However because Category III *(abnormal)* uses information about FHR variability it is not feasible to categorize IA in Category III (AWHONN, 2009).

The patient plan of care using the three-tiered system to categorize IA is based on a multitude of factors. A thorough and complete patient history and the events

---

Box 3-5   Intermittent Auscultation Fetal Heart Rate Categories and Patterns

Category I—*Normal*
Include ALL of the following:
- Regular rhythm with normal FHR baseline between 110 and 160 bpm
- Presence of FHR accelerations (increases) from the baseline
- Absence of FHR decelerations (decreases) from the baseline

Category II—*Indeterminate*
Include ANY of the following:
- Irregular rhythm
- Presence of FHR decelerations (decelerations) from the baseline
- Bradycardia
- Tachycardia

Category III—*Abnormal*
- Unable to specify Category III because FHR variability information is not available.

Modified from Association of Women's Health, Obstetric, and Neonatal Nurses (AWHONN): *Fetal heart monitoring: principles and practices*, ed 4, Washington, DC, 2009, AWHONN.

during the current admission must be incorporated into the communication between the members of the health care team. The plan of care can then be developed that is individualized and appropriate for the patient.

Fetal Heart Rate

The fetal CNS, specifically the ANS, controls the FHR. Because the ANS of the fetal brain is developed first, it is the most rudimentary. It requires a significant degree of hypoxia before FHR control shows the effects. Observation of Category I (*normal*) FHR patterns predicts adequate CNS oxygenation. However, Category II (*indeterminate*) features are considerably more subjective and of less predictive value for fetal oxygenation. In other words, little is known about how long it takes for what degree of hypoxia to occur (Freeman, Garite, and Nageotte, 2003).

Each examination of a fetal monitor strip should follow the same systematic steps:
- Evaluate patient history and status.
- Evaluate contraction frequency, duration, and if IUPC is used, intensity and resting tone.
- Determine the average baseline rate rounded to the nearest increment of 5.
- Describe FHR variability (fluctuations in the baseline).
- Identify accelerations, if present.
- Describe or, when possible, name patterns of periodic or episodic decelerations in the FHR.
- Describe changes in trends of the FHR pattern over 10 minutes or more.
- Diagnose fetal response to stimuli, initiate independent nursing interventions, and collaborate with the physician for medical management.

Baseline Fetal Heart Rate

Baseline fetal heart rate is identified as the approximate mean FHR rounded in increments of 5 beats per minute (bpm) lasting at least 10 consecutive minutes and excludes accelerations, decelerations, and periods of FHR variability greater than 25 bpm (marked variability). In any 10-minute window the baseline duration must be at least 2 minutes or the baseline is described as indeterminate for that period. Therefore it may be necessary to review the previous 10-minute window to determine the baseline rate. The baseline FHR is always documented as a single number (145) and not as a range (140 to 150 or 140s) (Fig. 3-4). The baseline FHR is normally 110 to 160 bpm. Rates above 160 for more than 10 minutes are termed tachycardia (Fig. 3-5), and those below 110 for more than 10 minutes are termed bradycardia (Fig. 3-6). Table 3-1 summarizes baseline fetal heart rates.

Baseline Variability

Variability is the most important FHR characteristic. It is the most important indicator of normal fetal pH or acidosis and reflects a healthy nervous system, chemoreceptors, baroreceptors, and cardiac responsiveness (Sweha, Hacker, and Nuovo, 1999). According to the National Institute of Child Health and Human Development (Macones and others, 2008a,b), variability is defined as fluctuations in the baseline FHR that are irregular in amplitude and frequency. Grades of fluctuation are based on amplitude range. Variability is classified as the peak-to-trough in bpm:

- Absent: undetectable amplitude range
- Minimal: greater than undetectable but equal to or less than 5 bpm amplitude

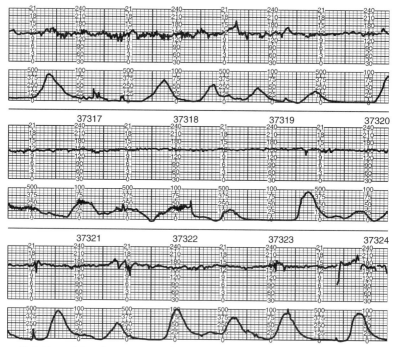

Figure 3-4 Normal baseline FHR. Baseline FHR found between contractions, in absence of periodic changes, and observed in 10-minute segments *(panels 37317 through 37319 in center)* is 150. This rate is within the normal range. *FHR,* Fetal heart rate.

- Moderate: 6 to 25 bpm amplitude range
- Marked (saltatory): more than 25 bpm amplitude

A review of abnormalities of baseline variability can be reviewed in Table 3-2.

Fetal Arrhythmia and Artifact

Fetal arrhythmias occur as a result of abnormalities in the automatic origination of impulses throughout the myocardium, a disruption of the normal impulse conduction pathway, or both. Some are benign, whereas others are pathologic.

Table 3-1 Summary of Baseline Fetal Heart Rate Abnormalities

Tachycardia (Fig. 3-5)

Description	Rate higher than 160 bpm for at least 10 consecutive minutes
Etiology	Acute, short-term hypoxia
	Drugs given to mother, such as beta sympathomimetics (terbutaline, ritodrine)
	Stress
	Arrhythmia
	Fetal infection
	Maternal fever (may be caused by epidural analgesia)
	Maternal hyperthyroid disease
Mechanism	Sympathetic response
Significance	Serious when >180 bpm
Nursing interventions	Look for cause
	Turn patient to side
	Hydrate to improve circulating volume
	O_2 at 8–10 L/min by tight face mask
	Reduce stressors: turn off oxytocin (Pitocin); treat maternal fever

Bradycardia (Fig. 3-6)

Description	Rate <110 bpm for at least 10 consecutive minutes
Etiology	Chronic long-term hypoxia
	Drugs such as beta-blockers (propranolol [Inderal])
	Arrhythmia
	Terminal event after severe stress
	Prolapsed cord
Mechanism	Parasympathetic response
Significance	Serious when <80 bpm or lasting >10 minutes
Nursing interventions	Turn side to side or to knee-chest position
	O_2 at 8–10 L/min by tight face mask
	Correct maternal hypotension
	Look for cause such as prolapsed cord
	Prepare for delivery by most expeditious means

Modified from Association of Women's Health, Obstetric, and Neonatal Nurses (AWHONN): *Fetal heart monitoring: principles and practices*, ed 4, Washington, DC, 2009, AWHONN.

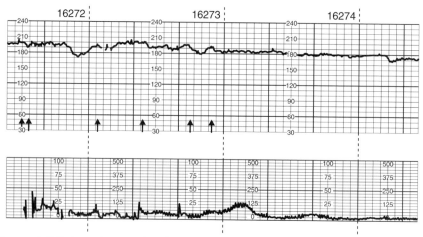

Figure 3-5 Tachycardia. Baseline fetal heart rate *between panels 16272 and 16274* is 185 bpm. Arrows are result of maternal use of remote marker to indicate fetal movement.

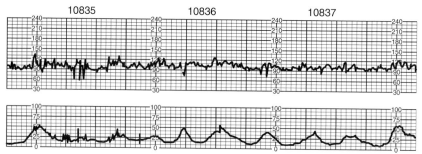

Figure 3-6 Bradycardia. Baseline fetal heart rate is 95 bpm. Moderate variability is present.

To determine benign from pathologic fetal arrhythmias, features of both must be kept in mind. Those that are benign tend to appear in labor and disappear shortly after delivery. These neonates tend to have no heart abnormalities, neither anatomic nor functional. Pathologic fetal arrhythmias tend to be associated with certain maternal conditions such as lupus, illicit drug use, infection, and hyperthyroidism or fetal cardiac abnormalities; they also tend to be present and detected prenatally and are present during labor and persist into the neonatal period (Snyder and Copel, 2005).

Fetal arrhythmias usually can be detected as vertical lines through the baseline. Although these lines are sometimes so close together that they almost appear as solid blocks, the baseline can be found through them. There are rarely other problematic features about the baseline (Fig. 3-8).

Artifact is a disruption of the normal logic system in the machine, which typically calculates the FHR by counting intervals of R wave to R wave. When it is unable to function in this way, the tracing appears as a garbled mess of vertical lines, through which one cannot identify a baseline rate or patterns. Table 3-3 describes

Table 3-2   Abnormalities of Baseline Variability*

Absent Variability (see Fig. 3-7, *panel 1*)

Description	Undetectable fluctuations in FHR
Etiology	Severe degree of hypoxia
Mechanism	Loss of interplay between branches of ANS
Significance	Category III status and indicative of fetal acidemia (pH <7.1)
Nursing interventions	Look for cause and treat by repositioning laterally
	Start and/or increase IV
	Give O$_2$ at 8–10 L/min by face mask
	Notify physician and report findings and intervention

Minimal Variability (see Fig. 3-7, *panel 2*)

Description	Baseline FHR fluctuations <5-beat amplitude
Uncomplicated causes	Sleep, narcotic, barbiturate, or other CNS depressant; usually does not persist >60 min or length of initial medication effect
Problematic causes	Early hypoxia, congenital anomalies, fetal cardiac arrhythmias, extreme prematurity
Mechanism	CNS depression during sleep or after medication
Significance	Usually benign
Nursing interventions	Continued observation
	Acoustic stimulations

Marked Variability (see Fig. 3-7, *panel 4*)

Description	Persistent cyclic fluctuations, of amplitude >25 bpm
Etiology	Recovery from previous insult
	Response to sudden stimuli
	Stimulant drugs such as cocaine or methamphetamines
	Sympathomimetic drugs such as terbutaline
	Sudden hypoxia often associated with variable decelerations with a slow return to baseline or overshoots (Table 3-5 and Fig. 3-10)
Mechanism	Increased interplay between sympathetic and parasympathetic branches of ANS or loss of ANS control
Significance	If persistent identified as a Category II fetal monitor tracing
Nursing interventions	Look for cause and treat by repositioning laterally
	Start and/or increase IV
	Give O$_2$ at 8–10 L/min by face mask

*See Figure 3-7.
ANS, Autonomic nervous system; *CNS,* central nervous system; *FHR,* fetal heart rate; *IV,* intravenous.

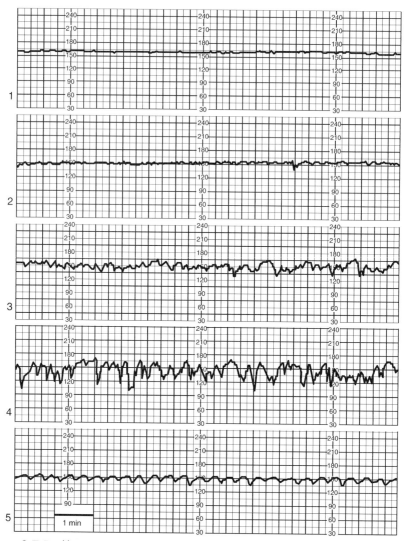

Figure 3-7 Fetal heart rate variability is depicted in each panel. All are traced from a spiral electrode. 1, Absent. 2, Minimal. 3, Moderate. 4, Marked. 5, Sinusoidal. Original scaling, 30 bpm per cm vertical axis, and paper speed 3 cm/min −1 horizontal axis.

and summarizes artifact versus arrhythmia, and Table 3-4 describes and summarizes dysrhythmias and their significance.

If a fetal arrhythmia is suspected, M-mode or spectral Doppler fetal echocardiography is most commonly used to diagnosis and monitor the arrhythmia (Snyder and Copel, 2005). Of all possible fetal arrhythmias, supraventricular tachycardia (SVT) and congenital heart block are serious. SVT may be treated in utero, whereas heart block is not treatable. Medical management of SVT consists of pharmacologic fetal cardioversion. The pharmacologic agents used are such drugs as digoxin, beta-blockers, procainamide, and quinidine.

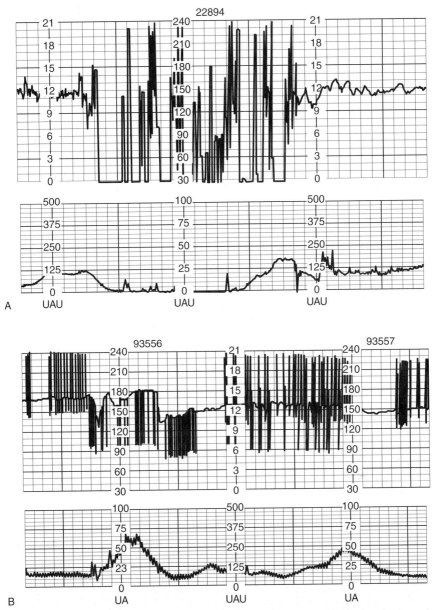

Figure 3-8 A, Artifact. Note disorganized scattering of impulses traced by fetal scalp electrode. **B,** Arrhythmia. Note organized distribution of impulses traced by fetal spiral electrode.

Fetal Heart Rate Patterns and Periodic Rate Changes

FHR patterns express the mechanism of insult to the fetus. Knowing the mechanism facilitates appropriate nursing response and intervention. It also helps predict whether a change can be made and how long it might take. Periodic changes are in response to certain stimuli. When FHR accelerations are observed, they are usually explained by

Table 3-3   Artifact versus Arrhythmia

Instrument	Artifact	Arrhythmia
Auscultation device Fetal spiral electrode	Regular rate and rhythm Perpendicular excursions irregular and baseline completely obscured	Abnormal rate or rhythm Baseline can be read despite perpendicular excursions

Table 3-4   Dysrhythmias: Appearances, Audible Features, and Significance

Dysrhythmia	Appearance	Audible Features	Significance
PACs	Excursions above and below baseline	Compensatory pauses	Benign
PVCs	Same	Same	Usually benign unless superimposed on preterminal rate or wandering baseline
PAT or continuous SVT	Rate too fast to trace	Rate >240 bpm; irregular	Serious and treatable; can be converted while in utero
			Fetal hydrops (similar to adult congestive heart failure) may be fatal
Congenital heart block	Suddenly drops by half	Fetoscope rate same as slowed rate	May result in fetal death
		Doppler rates 2 × fetoscope rate = 2:1 block	Associated with maternal connective tissue disease
			Newborn will need immediate placement of pacemaker
Sinoatrial arrest	In lowest point of variable deceleration, rectangular deflection appears	Absent audible impulse	Benign

PAC, Premature atrial contraction; *PAT,* paroxysmal atrial tachycardia; *PVC,* premature ventricular contraction; *SVT,* supraventricular tachycardia.

fetal movement or healthy response to contractions. The FHR can demonstrate patterns of acceleration or deceleration in response to most stimuli. Table 3-5 provides a summary of accelerations and decelerations. Table 3-6 describes sinusoidal pattern.

ANTEPARTUM AND INTRAPARTUM FETAL SURVEILLANCE

The latest census statistics estimate that more than two thirds of fetal deaths occur in the antepartum period (ACOG, 1999). Certainly a means of surveillance that allows detection of risk before damage occurs could greatly benefit those pregnancies.

Text continued on p. 71.

Table 3-5   Summary of Accelerations and Decelerations

Category I *(Normal)* Rate Changes
Uniform Accelerations (Fig. 3-9, A)

Description	Uniform shape
	Begin when contraction begins and end when contraction ends
	Often mirror intensity of contractions
Mechanism of insult	Sympathetic response to stimuli
Significance	Healthy CNS response
	Often associated with breech presentations
Nursing intervention	Totally benign, so none needed; document

Nonuniform Accelerations (Fig. 3-9, B)

Description	Nonuniform in shape
	Usually occur in response to fetal movement so they vary in contraction cycle
Mechanism of insult	Sympathetic response to stimuli
Significance	Healthy CNS response; reassuring
Nursing intervention	None

Early Decelerations (Fig. 3-10, A)

Description	Usually symmetric
	Frequently mirror contraction intensity
	Onset, nadir, and recovery of the deceleration occur at the same time as the onset, highest point, and recovery of the contraction.
	Begin when contraction begins and end when contraction ends
	When noted, usually occur between 4- and 7-cm dilation of cervix, but can occur at any time
Mechanism of insult	Head compression
	Parasympathetic (vagal) reflex caused by pressure on fontanels against resisting cervix
Significance	Considered normal, although they do not occur in all fetuses

Continued

Table 3-5   Summary of Accelerations and Decelerations—cont'd

Nursing interventions	Differentiate these from late decelerations
	No action necessary or helpful; document

Variable Decelerations

Description	Variable in shape, often V- or W-shaped
	Variable placement in relationship to contractions; may occur between or with contractions
	Heart rate falls abruptly (onset to the lowest point in <30 sec) and rises abruptly
	Decrease in the FHR is ≥15 bpm lasting ≥15 sec and <2 min in duration
	Defined as recurrent if they occur with ≥50% of uterine contractions in any 20-minute window
	Defined as intermittent if <50% in any 20-minute segment
Mechanism of insult	Cord compression
Significance	Category II *(indeterminate)* if recurrent or with other characteristics such as a slow return to baseline or overshoots
Nursing intervention	Change maternal position

Category II *(Indeterminate)* and Category III *(Abnormal)* Rate Changes
Variable Decelerations (Fig. 3-10, B)

Significance	Category II *(indeterminate)* if:
	Recurrent
	Followed by tachycardia
	Slow return to baseline
	"Overshoots"
	Category III *(abnormal)* if:
	Recurrent with absent baseline variability
Nursing interventions	Turn side to side or to knee-chest position
	Give O_2 at 8–10 L/min by tight face mask
	Improve circulating volume
	Expect expeditious delivery if Category III *(abnormal)*
	Document

Late Decelerations (Fig. 3-10, C)

Description	Usually symmetrical
	Gradual decrease (onset to nadir ≥30 seconds) and return to baseline associated with a uterine contraction
	Nadir of the deceleration occurs after the peak of the contraction
	Generally the onset, nadir, and recovery of the deceleration occur after the beginning, peak, and ending of the contraction

Table 3-5   Summary of Accelerations and Decelerations—cont'd

Description, cont'd	Defined as recurrent if they occur with ≥50% of uterine contractions in any 20-minute window
	Defined as intermittent if <50% in any 20-minute segment
Mechanism of insult	Uteroplacental insufficiency, leading to CNS hypoxia or myocardial depression
Significance	Always Category II *(indeterminate)* or III *(abnormal)* regardless of depth of deceleration
	Acute episodes and moderate variability are more likely to be correctable
	Chronic episodes accompanied by decreased or absent variability are less likely to be correctable; usually associated with fetal acidosis
Nursing interventions	Turn patient to side
	Give O₂ at 8–10 L/min by tight face mask
	Rapidly infuse IV fluid
	Correct hypotension
	If oxytocin (Pitocin) used, turn it off
	Expect expeditious delivery if not corrected in 30 minutes; document

Modified from American College of Obstetricians and Gynecologists (ACOG): *Antepartum fetal surveillance*, Practice Bulletin, No. 9, Washington, DC, 1999, ACOG; Association of Women's Health, Obstetric, and Neonatal Nurses (AWHONN): *Fetal heart monitoring: principles and practices*, ed 4, Washington, DC, 2009, AWHONN.
CNS, Central nervous system; *IV*, intravenous; *O₂*, oxygen.

Prolonged Deceleration (Fig. 3-10, D)

Description	Abrupt deceleration of at least 15 bpm, lasting 2–10 minutes
Mechanism of insult	Prolonged cord compression
Significance	If lasts longer than 10 minutes, fetus may become acidemic, followed by myocardial depression
Nursing interventions	Notify physician or midwife of first occurrence
	Check for cord prolapse
	Turn patient side to side or to knee-chest position until change is affected
	Give O₂ at 8–10 L/min by tight face mask
	Correct maternal hypotension; increase IV fluids
	Continually observe until delivery; document
	Be prepared for emergency delivery

Modified from Association of Women's Health, Obstetric, and Neonatal Nurses (AWHONN): *Fetal heart monitoring: principles and practices*, ed 4, Washington, DC, 2009, AWHONN.

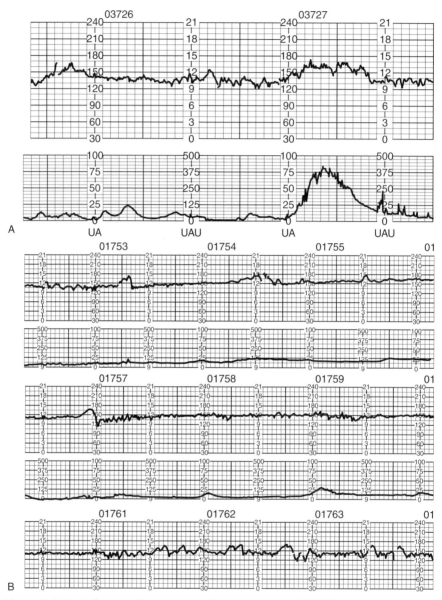

Figure 3-9 A, Uniform acceleration is noted beginning in *panel 03727* in response to contraction beneath. **B**, Nonuniform accelerations can be seen between contractions. Baseline fetal heart rate of 150 bpm with accelerations to 170 bpm.

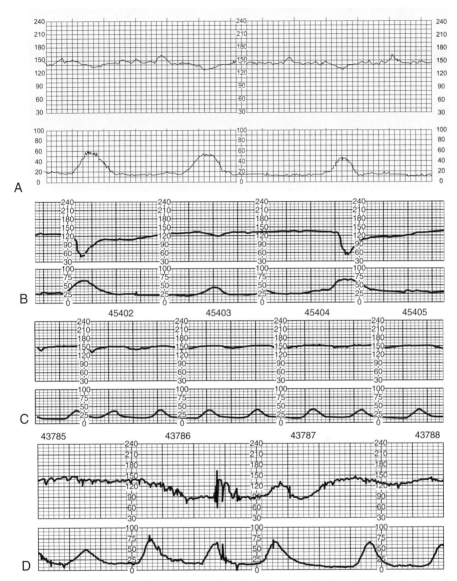

Figure 3-10 A, Early decelerations. Baseline fetal heart rate (FHR) is 145. Gradual decelerations begin when the contraction begins and end when the contraction ends. **B,** Category III *(abnormal)* variable decelerations. Note baseline of 130 bpm with a slow return to baseline and absent variability. Absent variability places this fetal monitor recording in Category III requiring prompt interventions. **C,** Late decelerations. Baseline FHR is 150 bpm. Decelerations are seen with each contraction. Nadir of the decelerations occurs after the peak of the contractions. The absence of variability places this fetal monitor recording in Category III. **D,** Prolonged deceleration in *panels 43786 and 43787.* This deceleration followed initiation of epidural anesthesia and frequently can be avoided with intravenous fluid preload.

Table 3-6   Sinusoidal Pattern (Fig. 3-11)

Description	Smooth, undulating baseline with regular (3–5) oscillations per minute that persists for ≥20 minutes
Mechanism of insult	Derangement of CNS control of FHR secondary to increased arginine vasopressin
	When severe degree of hypoxia from fetal anemia is coupled with fetal hypovolemia
Significance	Category III *(abnormal)* fetal heart rate finding
	Only way to treat successfully in utero is by fetal intrauterine transfusion
Nursing interventions	Prepare for emergent delivery
	Prepare for intrauterine transfusion
	Position patient laterally
	Infuse IV fluids rapidly
	Give O_2 at 6–10 L/min by face mask; document

Modified from Association of Women's Health, Obstetric, and Neonatal Nurses (AWHONN): *Fetal heart monitoring: principles and practices,* ed 4, Washington, DC, 2009, AWHONN.
CNS, central nervous system; *FHR,* fetal heart rate; *IV,* intravenous; *O_2,* oxygen.

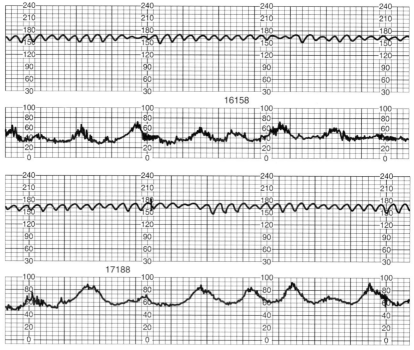

Figure 3-11 Sinusoidal heart rate. A smooth, wavelike undulating FHR pattern with a cycle frequency of 3 to 5 oscillations/minute.

Antepartum monitoring provides a means of doing just that. When fetal compromise takes place, fetal activities are lost in reverse order of their development. FHR decelerations occur first, followed by loss of, in order, accelerations, breathing movements, body movements, and muscle tone, and then death occurs (Harman, 2009). Decreased amniotic fluid can also indicate fetal compromise because decreased renal blood flow lowers fetal urinary output, resulting in decreased amniotic fluid volume. Decreased amniotic fluid, on the other hand, can cause fetal compromise because of the increased risk for cord compression (ACOG, 1999).

In gestations less than 27 weeks, causes of intrauterine death have been identified to include infection, abruption, and lethal congenital abnormalities. And in gestations at greater than 28 weeks, causes identified may include growth restriction and placental abruption. However, 27% to 60% of intrauterine fetal deaths are unexplained (Shaffer and Parer, 2007).

The most common maternal conditions associated with fetal compromise follow:
- Intrauterine growth restriction
- Hypertensive disorders of pregnancy
- Chronic hypertension
- Diabetes
- Postterm pregnancy
- Connective tissue disease
- Renal disease
- Hemolytic incompatibility
- Multiple gestation
- Placental abnormalities

The purpose of testing is to identify the fetus at risk for decreased oxygenation resulting in permanent injury or death and to identify a healthy fetus and prevent unnecessary interventions (Tucker, Miller, and Miller, 2009). The decision as to when to begin antepartum testing may be based on multiple factors, including viability, severity of the condition, and when the condition is recognized. With the availability of regionalized centers, transportation capabilities, and long-distance telemetry, early detection of fetal compromise is possible and desirable for optimal treatment and outcome. The most frequently used tests to detect early fetal compromise are presented in Boxes 3-6 through 3-13, which may serve as useful guides for nursing policies and procedures (ACOG, 1999).

Fetal Oxygen Saturation Monitoring with Fetal Pulse Oximetry Assessment During Labor

Simpson and Porter (2001) and Garite and colleagues (2000) described the benefits of taking fetal O_2 saturation measurements during labor and compared them with the benefits of EFM. In a few studies, assessing fetal status with fetal O_2 saturation measurements was found to be as accurate as with EFM. Fetal pulse oximetry added to cardiotocography showed reduced caesarean section rates for nonreassuring fetal status in a single trial, although no difference was found in the overall caesarean section rate or the mother's or newborn's health (East, Chau, and Colditz, 2004; Bloom and others, 2006).

Text continued on p. 80.

Box 3-6   Nonstress Test (NST)

Definition
An NST is a widely accepted method of evaluating fetal status by observing accelerations of the FHR following a stimulus such as fetal activity, indicating normal fetal pH and neurologic status.

Procedure
- Explain the testing procedure to the patient.
- Have the patient empty her bladder and then position herself in a semi-Fowler's, lateral tilt position. Sitting or walking may stimulate fetal reactivity (Cito and others, 2005).
- Place the ultrasound transducer and tocotransducer.
- Document the date and time the test is started, the make and model of the monitor, the external modes used, the patient's name, the reason for the test, and the maternal vital signs.
- Record maternal blood pressure at least once in 20 minutes.
- Run a 10- to 20-minute FHR contraction strip.
- If, at the end of the first 20 minutes, reactive criteria have not been met, consider vibroacoustic stimulation and then wait an additional 20 minutes for reaction that meets the criteria.
- At the end of the test, interpret and document the results and report them to the physician, midwife, or provider.

Interpretation
Reactive
- There are at least two accelerations of peak amplitude of at least 15 bpm above the baseline lasting 15 or more seconds within a 20-minute period. Other Category I (normal) features such as presence of variability and absence of Category II (indeterminate) periodic or episodic decelerations such as a prolonged deceleration or recurrent late decelerations with any spontaneous contractions or fetal movement are described and expected for a test to read as reactive (Fig. 3-12).

Nonreactive
- There are no accelerations over a 40-minute period or they fail to meet reactive criteria (Fig. 3-13).

Management
- A reactive NST should be repeated every 3 or 4 days for continued prediction of fetal well-being.
- If the NST remains nonreactive after the second 20 minutes or if any Category II periodic changes are present, another more definitive evaluation of the fetus, such as ultrasound for a biophysical profile, is indicated.

Advantages
- It is a noninvasive test requiring no initiation of contractions.
- It is quick to perform.
- There are no known side effects.
- It has a low false-negative rate (less than 1%) (ACOG, 1999).

Box 3-6   Nonstress Test (NST)—cont'd

Disadvantages

- It is not as sensitive to fetal oxygen reserves as CST.
- It has a high false-positive rate, 80% to 90% (ACOG, 1999).

CST, Contraction stress test; *FHR,* fetal heart rate; *NST,* nonstress test.

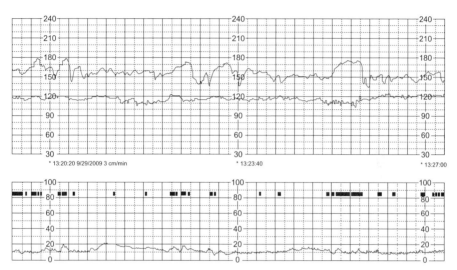

Figure 3-12 Reactive nonstress test. Baseline fetal heart rate of 150 with accelerations of greater than 15 beats lasting for more than 15 seconds.

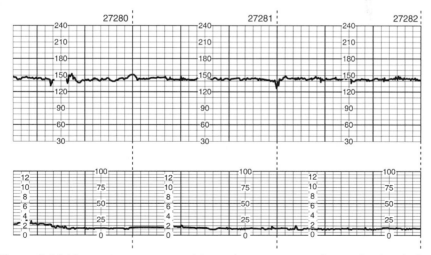

Figure 3-13 Nonreactive nonstress test. No accelerations are seen that can be described as meeting criterion of 15 beats more than baseline for 15 seconds.

Box 3-7   Vibroacoustic Stimulation

Definition
A technique used to evaluate fetal status by observing accelerations of the FHR. Often used in conjunction with a nonstress test to elicit an acceleration indicating the absence of acidosis.

Vibroacoustic stimulation is an evaluation tool only used with a baseline rate that is within normal limits. If the fetus is experiencing a deceleration or bradycardia, vibroacoustic stimulation is not an appropriate intervention.

Harman (2009) states that vibroacoustic stimulation should not be part of routine testing in high risk pregnancies.

Procedure
- If no fetal movements are observed, use an acoustic stimulation device or an electrolarynx to produce a vibratory sound stimulus.
- Explain the testing procedure to the patient and the reasons for its use; assure her it is not harmful to the fetus.
- Apply stimulus to the maternal abdomen over the fetus' head for 1 second; wait 1 minute.
- If no acceleration occurs after first stimulus, apply a second stimulus for 2 seconds; wait 1 minute.
- If no acceleration occurs after the second stimulus, apply a third stimulus for 3 seconds; wait 1 minute.
- Report results to the physician, midwife, or provider.

Interpretation
Reactive
- Indicated by the presence of an acceleration. The peak of the acceleration must be equal to or greater than 15 bpm above the baseline and the acceleration must last equal to or greater than 15 seconds from the onset to the return to the baseline.

Advantages
- It decreases NST length (Tan and Smyth, 2003).
- It decreases the incidence of nonreactive NST (Tan and Smyth, 2003).
- There are no known risks if the protocol outlined is followed.

Additional Information
- Use of vibroacoustic stimulation for assessment of fetal wellbeing during labor in the presence of a nonreassuring FHR tracing is not supported by evidence in randomized controlled trials (East, Smyth, Leader, Henshall, Colditz, Tan, 2005).

FHR, Fetal heart rate; *NST*, nonstress test.

Box 3-8   Fetal Movement Counting

Definition
Maternal perception of fetal body movement has been used as an indicator of fetal well-being. Animal studies have found a reduction in movements or the absence of movement in response to chronic hypoxia. Although there are no current human studies the principles have been applied to fetal behavior.

The goal of fetal movement counting is that when a mother identifies a decrease in her baby's normal movement pattern she can report this to her healthcare giver and additional testing can be accomplished with the hopes of preventing fetal death.

Mangesi and Hofmeyr (2007) identified the lack of data to support the practice of fetal movement counting in preventing fetal death but agree there is not enough evidence to influence practice at this time.

Procedure
- Teach patient the significance of fetal movements.
- Teach patient a fetal assessment method—count fetal movements or record time.
- Count fetal movements for a fixed period of time. Instruct the patient to lie down on her side and count all the fetal movements felt in 1 hour.
- Record time taken to count a fixed number of fetal movements. Instruct the patient to start counting at 9 A.M. and stop counting for the day and record the time when 10 fetal movements have been noted.
- Demonstrate how to record movements on a daily fetal movement record.

Interpretation
- Report decreased fetal movement compared with the previous day's counts or fewer than 10 fetal movements in any 1 hour period.

Management
- If decreased fetal movement is reported, evaluate fetal status with an NST or a biophysical profile immediately and manage according to the results.

Gestational Influences
- Gestational age: At 34 to 38 weeks fetal movements show a maturational decrease in number with the onset of typical infant behaviors of small-amplitude highly coordinated movements (Harman, 2009).
- Diurnal rhythm: Normally fetal movement is increased in the late evening.

Fetal Behavior
- State: Fetal behavioral states can be defined by the beginning of the third trimester. Other than rapid eye movements and repetitive mouthing movements there is usually no fetal movement during quiet sleep. In the middle of the 3rd trimester inactivity extends from about 220 seconds to as long as 110 minutes by 40 weeks (Harman, 2009).
- Drugs: Depressant drugs such as barbiturates, narcotics, and alcohol can reduce fetal movement. In therapeutic doses, most drugs do not reduce fetal movement.
- Fetal malformation: A fetus with a malformation is more likely to have reduced activity.

NST, Nonstress test.

Box 3-9   Contraction Stress Test

Definition
A CST is a fetal well-being test that is infrequently used to determine how the fetus responds to relative hypoxia during a contraction. A compromised fetus, with a limited ability to compensate for mild hypoxia because of limited oxygen reserves, demonstrates a consistent pattern of late decelerations during the test.

Procedure
- Explain the testing procedure to the patient.
- Have the patient empty her bladder and then position herself in a semi-Fowler's position. A wedge may be placed under her hip to prevent supine hypotension if needed.
- Place the ultrasound transducer and tocotransducer.
- Document the date and time the test is started, make and model of monitor, the external modes used, the patient's name, the reason for the test, and the maternal vital signs.
- Run a 20-minute NST for baseline information regarding FHR and uterine contractions.
- Stimulate contractions either by nipple stimulation of endogenous oxytocin or with intravenous oxytocin.
- Observe for uterine tachysystole.
- Assess maternal blood pressure every 10 to 15 minutes during the test and when the test is completed.
- Discontinue contraction stimulation when three or more contractions of more than 40 seconds duration within a 10-minute period occur.
- Interpret the test results and report findings to the provider.
- Continue monitoring until uterine and FHR activity have returned to prestimulation state.

Initiation of Contractions with Nipple Stimulation
- Have the patient begin, on one side, nipple brushing through clothing. Have her continue until a contraction begins or for 10 minutes.
- If no contraction occurs in 10 minutes of brushing, have her change sides and continue for 10 minutes. If still not effective, have her brush both nipples simultaneously.
- Have the patient continue nipple brushing on effective side or sides until a contraction occurs. Stop until the contraction is over, and then begin again until three contractions occur in 10 minutes.

Stimulation of Contractions with Oxytocin
- Start mainline intravenous normal saline or Ringer's lactate.
- Piggyback oxytocin diluted so that increments of 0.5 mU/min can be delivered.
- Start at 0.5 mU/min; double amount every 15 to 20 minutes until 4 mU and then increase by 2 mU until three contractions occur in 10 minutes or maximum dose of 16 mU is reached.

Interpretation
Negative (Fig. 3-14)
- No decelerations are noted on the entire strip. Variability is present, and there is an absence of any Category I or Category II changes.

Box 3-9   Contraction Stress Test—cont'd

Equivocal
- A test may be equivocal for one of three reasons:
  1. Suspicious: Less than 50% of the contractions on the entire strip have late decelerations: (Fig. 3-15, *A*).
  2. Tachysystole: A contraction frequency of more than five in 10 minutes, fewer than 60 seconds between contractions, or a contraction lasting longer than 90 seconds with a late deceleration occurring (Fig. 3-15, *B*).
  3. Unsatisfactory: The quality of the tracing is too poor to accurately interpret FHR with contractions; or the frequency of three contractions in 10 minutes cannot be obtained for an endpoint of the test (Fig. 3-15, *C*).

Positive (Fig. 3-16)
- Fifty percent or more of the contractions on the strip have late decelerations associated with them even if the endpoint of three contractions in 10 minutes is not obtained.

Management
- A negative CST predicts continued fetal well-being for 7 days and needs only to be repeated weekly provided maternal well-being is the same (Freeman, Garite, and Nageotte, 2003).
- An equivocal CST should be followed with another form of fetal assessment.
- A positive CST necessitates more vigorous management. If variability is present and the fetus is mature by the proper dates and in a vertex position, a very carefully monitored induction can be attempted. If the fetus is immature, treating the maternal condition that might have precipitated the problem may be the best treatment to give the baby a chance.
- With a positive CST when variability is absent, delivery by an emergency cesarean is the only chance for optimal outcome for the baby regardless of maturity.
- Regardless of test results, if variable decelerations are noted, an amniotic fluid index is recommended.

Advantages
- It is more sensitive to fetal oxygen reserves than NST.
- It has a low false-negative rate (less than 1%) (ACOG, 1999).

Disadvantages
- CST is contraindicated in such high risk conditions as preterm labor and placenta previa.
- It must be administered in a birthing setting.
- It has a false-positive rate greater than 50% (ACOG, 1999).

CST, Contraction stress test; *FHR,* fetal heart rate; *NST,* nonstress test.

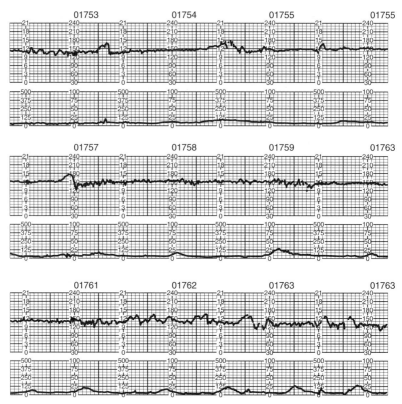

Figure 3-14 Negative and reactive contraction stress test obtained with breast stimulation. No late decelerations are noted in any panel. Moderate variability is present, and fetal heart rate accelerates periodically. Three contractions are present in 10 minutes (*panels 01761 through 01763*).

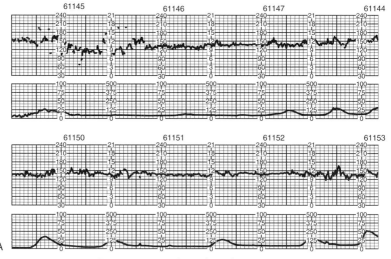

Figure 3-15 For legend see facing page.

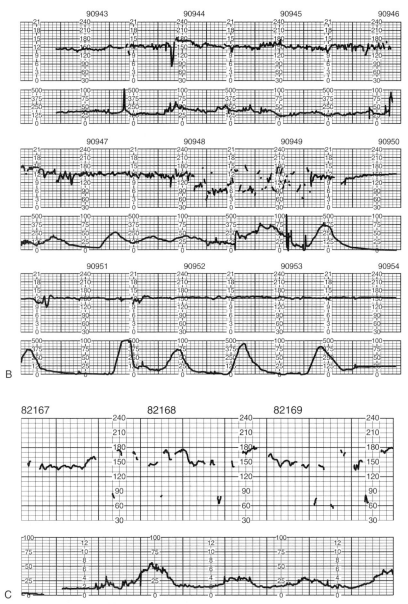

Figure 3-15 A, Equivocal contraction stress test because of one late deceleration in *Panel 61145.* Breast simulation was started to further challenge placental function and determine whether late decelerations would persist. Because remainder of test was negative for late decelerations and reactive, test was repeated the following day. **B,** Equivocal contraction stress test because of uterine activity indicting tachysystole. **C,** Equivocal contraction stress test, because tracing immediately following each contraction is unsatisfactory for accurate interpretation of fetal heart rate response.

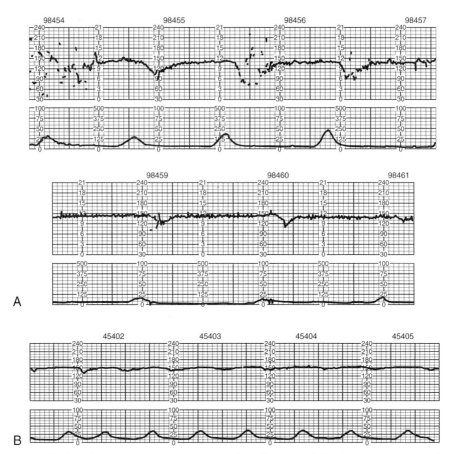

Figure 3-16 A, Positive contraction stress test with moderate variability. Tracing was continued, and reactivity was noted while decisions were made for delivery in postterm pregnancy. **B,** Positive contraction stress test with absent variability. Baby was delivered by emergent cesarean birth with Apgar scores below 6. Mother was stable with preeclampsia.

In May 2000 the Food and Drug Administration approved fetal O_2 saturation after careful consideration of the results of a multicenter randomized clinical study (Garite and others, 2000). The system used a single-use disposable sensor that was inserted into the uterus via the cervix and rests against the fetal temple, cheek, or forehead and is held in place by the uterine wall. The sensor usually rotates and descends with the fetus as labor progresses, which can affect the availability of data. Its measurements are based on the same premise as pulse oximetry in that the major light sensors in the blood are oxyhemoglobin and deoxyhemoglobin.

The American College of Obstetricians and Gynecologists did not endorse this device because of the lack of data to support improvement in clinical outcomes when compared with the potential cost with the introduction of this technology (ACOG, 2001). In January of 2009 the manufacturer discontinued the support of the N400 fetal oximeter (J.C. Reichert, personal communication, February 26, 2009).

Box 3-10   Amniotic Fluid Volume

Definition
Amniotic fluid volume (AFV) is the evaluation of the quantity of amniotic fluid. Amniotic fluid is the result of fetal urine production. Adequate placental blood flow usually promotes adequate fetal renal blood flow and therefore adequate urine output. Thus amniotic fluid volume reflects long-term uteroplacental function.

Procedure
Scan and measure the depth of the largest cord-free pocket of amniotic fluid. Research supports the technique over amniotic fluid index (AFI) (Magann and others, 2007).

Interpretation
- Less than 2 cm: Oligohydramnios
  - Indicates need for delivery or close maternal and fetal surveillance.
- 2 cm to 8 cm: Normal
- Greater than 8 cm: Polyhydramnios

AFI, amniotic fluid index; *AFV,* amniotic fluid volume.
From Harman C: Assessment of fetal health. In Creasy R, Resnik R, Iams J, Lockwood C, Moore T, editors: *Creasy and Resnik's maternal-fetal medicine: principles and practice,* ed 6, Philadelphia, 2009, Saunders.

Box 3-11   Biophysical Profile (BPP)

Definition
A biophysical profile is an evaluation of fetal well-being through the use of various reflex activities that are CNS-controlled and sensitive to hypoxia, as well as the fetal environment that can affect fetal well-being.

Procedure
Scan the abdomen and assess fetal tone, movements, breathing, fetal reactivity (cardiotocogram), and amniotic fluid.

Interpretation (Harman, 2009)
The biophysical activities that are the first to develop are the last to disappear when asphyxia occurs.
- *Fetal tone:* One or more episodes of extension of a fetal extremity with return to flexion; and/or opening and closing of hand.
- Starts to function at 7.5 to 8.5 weeks of gestation
- Is abolished at a pH less than 7.0
- *Fetal movement:* Four or more body or limb movements within 30 minutes
- Starts to function at 9 weeks of gestation
- Is abolished when the pH is between 7.1 and 7.2
- *Fetal breathing:* Intermittent, multiple episodes of hiccups or rhythmic fetal breathing movements of at least 30 seconds duration in a 30 minute observation.
- Starts to function at approximately 20 to 21 weeks of gestation
- Is abolished at a pH of 7.2

Continued

Box 3-11   Biophysical Profile (BPP)—cont'd

- *Fetal reactivity—Computerized cardiotocography (CTG)*: Two or more FHR accelerations of at least 15 bpm for at least 15 seconds within 20 minutes
- Starts to function at 26 to 28 weeks of gestation
- Is abolished at a pH of less than 7.19
- *Amniotic fluid*: Decreased amniotic fluid can be the result of chronic hypoxia or can cause hypoxia. Normal amniotic fluid is recognized as at least one cord-free vertical pocket of amniotic fluid greater than 2 cm (Harman, 2009).

Scoring
- Assign 0 or 2 points each for fetal tone, movements, breathing, reactivity (cardiotocogram), and amniotic fluid volume.
- A BPP of 8 to 10 is normal if amniotic fluid volume (AFV) is normal. The test needs be repeated in 3 to 4 days.
- A BPP of 6 is considered equivocal. The test should be repeated. A persistent score of 6 indicates delivery of a mature fetus; if fetus is immature repeat the test in 24 hours.
- A BPP score of 0 to 4 means delivery by obstetrically appropriate method.
- A BPP score of 0 to 2 means immediate delivery.
  Oligohydramnios constitutes an abnormal biophysical assessment regardless of the overall score (Harman, 2009).

Advantages
- It permits conservative therapy and prevents premature intervention.
- BPP evaluates multiple fetal variables.

AFV, amniotic fluid volume; *BPP*, biophysical profile; *CTG*, computerized cardiotocography.

Box 3-12   Modified Biophysical Profile (Modified BPP)

Definition
A modified biophysical profile is an evaluation of fetal well-being. It combines the results of a nonstress test with an amniotic fluid volume. The NST is a short-term indicator of fetal hypoxemia and the AFV is an indicator or long-term placental function.

Interpretation (Shaffer & Parer, 2007)
- Normal: Reactive NST and AFV >5 cm and absence of variable or late decelerations
- Abnormal: any **one** of the following:
  - Nonreactive NST
  - Variable or late decelerations
  - AFV <5 cm

BPP, biophysical profile; *NST*, nonstress test; *AFV*, Amniotic fluid volume

Box 3-13   Doppler Flow Studies

Definition

Doppler flow studies are noninvasive methods for studying intrauterine environment, specifically the uteroplacental blood flow in the umbilical arteries. Doppler flow studies can facilitate the decision-making process regarding delivery time in pregnancies complicated by intrauterine growth restriction.

Procedure

- The nurse should help the patient position herself in a supine position and place a wedge under her right side to facilitate adequate blood flow and reduce maternal positional side effects.
- A pulsed Doppler device is positioned over the fetus. The umbilical artery blood flow is distinguished from other blood flow by its characteristic waveform.
- The directed blood flow within the umbilical arteries is calculated using the difference between the systolic and the diastolic flow. Measurements are averaged from at least five waveforms.

Interpretation

- Elevations of the systolic/diastolic (S/D) ratio above 3.0 are considered abnormal (Shaffer & Parer, 2007).
- Elevations of the S/D ratio are seen in hypertensive disorders of pregnancy, fetal growth restriction, or other causes of uteroplacental insufficiency.

NURSING MANAGEMENT

Assessments

Antepartum

- Auscultate FHR with fetoscope or Doppler for 60 seconds and record at appropriate intervals. To identify an increase or decrease in the rate count for multiple consecutive periods of 6 seconds (multiply by 10).
- Explain to the patient the reasons for antepartum testing and the procedure.
- Discuss the significance of and the procedure for monitoring fetal movement at home on a daily basis. Teach the patient when to notify her health care provider.
- Reinforce the importance of follow-up care.
- Refer to case management and/or social services for financial concerns if the family is without health benefits.

Intrapartum

Low risk patients

- When the patient is admitted in labor, apply external EFM for 20 minutes. Then assess FHR by intermittent auscultation during and after contractions or by continuous fetal monitoring.
- Assess maternal blood pressure, pulse, and respirations every 1 to 2 hours before the onset of active labor and every hour during active labor.
- Assess maternal temperature every 1 to 4 hours, depending on the stage of labor and the status of membranes.

- During latent phase of labor, assess and record FHR every 30 to 60 minutes (AAP/ACOG, 2007; AWHONN, 2009).
- During active labor, assess and record FHR every 15 to 30 minutes (AAP/ACOG, 2007; AWHONN, 2009).
- During second-stage labor, assess and record FHR every 5 to 15 minutes (AAP/ACOG, 2007; AWHONN, 2009).

High risk patients

- When the woman is admitted in labor, apply external EFM for 20 minutes. Continuous electronic fetal monitoring is recommended for patients with high risk conditions by ACOG (AWHONN, 2009).
- During latent-phase labor, assess and record FHR pattern every 30 minutes (AAP/ACOG, 2007; AWHONN, 2009).
- During active-phase labor, assess and record FHR pattern every 15 minutes (AAP/ACOG, 2007; AWHONN, 2009).
- During second-stage labor, assess and record FHR pattern every 5 minutes (AAP/ACOG, 2007; AWHONN, 2009).
- FHR pattern assessment should include baseline heart rate, variability, and presence or absence of accelerations and decelerations (AWHONN, 2009).
- Assess maternal blood pressure, pulse, and respirations every 1 to 2 hours before the onset of active labor and every hour in active labor.
- Assess maternal temperature every 1 to 4 hours, depending on the stage of labor and status of membranes.

Interventions

On identification of a Category II *(indeterminate)* or Category III *(abnormal)* FHR pattern: (1) reposition the patient laterally, turn her from side to side, or have her get in a hands-and-knees position or modified Trendelenburg position, depending on pattern and fetal response; (2) start and/or infuse IV fluids (lactated Ringer's) rapidly; (3) discontinue labor stimulant if being administered or, if not, obtain an order for 0.25 mg subcutaneous terbutaline; (4) administer O_2 at 8 to 10 L/min by mask; (5) notify physician or midwife; and (6) vibroacoustic or fetal scalp stimulation to assess fetal response may be used as appropriate.

- Treat by position change, fluids, and medications such as terbutaline for cessation of contractions if intolerance to labor is detected and there are more than 15 to 30 minutes before delivery set up.
- Monitor maternal contractions every 30 minutes, and maintain a safe and effective labor pattern with maternal positioning (of choice and therapeutic), fluids, and comfort measures as appropriate (see Chapters 27 and 28).
- Record fetal and maternal responses to nursing interventions. Notify physician or midwife of any adverse effects on fetal response (ACOG, 1999; AWHONN, 2009).

CONCLUSION

Assessment of fetal well-being throughout pregnancy and intrapartum is paramount to achieve an optimal perinatal outcome. Nurses need skill in fetal assessment to accurately assess, develop, implement, evaluate, and document effective care to promote optimal outcomes. As we continue to add to our knowledge base we will be better equipped to provide evidence-based care to the families we encounter.

BIBLIOGRAPHY
Electronic Fetal Monitoring

Alfirevic Z, Devane D, Gyte GM: Continuous cardiotocography (CTG) as a form of electronic fetal monitoring (EFM) for fetal assessment during labour, *Cochrane Database Syst Rev* (Issue 3), Art. No.: CD006066. DOI: 10.1002/14651858, 2006.

American Academy of Pediatrics (AAP) and American College of Obstetricians and Gynecologists (ACOG): *Guidelines for perinatal care*, ed 6, Elk Grove Village, IL, 2007, AAP/ACOG.

American College of Obstetricians and Gynecologists (ACOG): *Antepartum fetal surveillance,* Practice Bulletin, No. 9, Washington, DC, 1999, ACOG.

American College of Obstetricians and Gynecologists (ACOG): *Intrapartum fetal heart rate monitoring: nomenclature, interpretation, and general management principles, Practice Bulletin,* No. 106, Washington, DC, 2009, ACOG.

Association of Women's Health, Obstetric, and Neonatal Nurses (AWHONN): *Fetal heart monitoring: principles and practices,* ed 4, Washington, DC, 2009, AWHONN.

Blackburn ST: *Maternal, fetal, & neonatal physiology: A clinical perspective,* ed 3, St Louis, 2007, Saunders.

Centers for Disease Control and Prevention (CDC): *National vital statistics system: beyond 20/20 method of delivery,* 2006. Available at: http://www.cdc.gov.

Cunningham F, Leveno K, Bloom S, Hauth J, Rouse D, Spong C: *Williams obstetrics,* ed 23, New York, 2010, McGraw-Hill Medical.

Feinstein N, Sprague A, Trepanier M: *Fetal heart rate auscultation,* ed 2, Association of Women's Health Obstetric and Neonatal Nurses, 2008.

Freeman K: Problems with intrapartum fetal heart rate monitoring interpretation and patient management, *Obstet Gynecol* 100(4):813–826, 2002.

Freeman R, Garite R, Nageotte M: *Fetal heart rate monitoring,* ed 3, Baltimore, 2003, Lippincott Williams & Wilkins.

Haggerty L, Nuttall R: Experienced obstetric nurses' decision-making in fetal risk situations, *J Obstet Gynecol Neonatal Nurs* 29(5):480–490, 2000.

Hamilton B, Martin J, Ventura S: Births: preliminary data for 2007, *Nat Vital Stat Report* 57(12):1–23, 2009. Retrieved from http://www.cdc.gov/nchs/data/nvsr/nvsr57/nvsr57_12.pdf.

Knox GE, Simpson KR, Garite TJ: High reliability perinatal units: an approach to the prevention of patient injury and medical malpractice claims, *J Health Risk Manage* 19(2):24–32, 1999.

Kochanek K, Martin J: *Supplemental analyses of recent trends in infant mortality,* Hyattsville, MD, 2005, National Center for Health Statistics (NCHS).

MacDorman M, Mathews TJ: Recent trends in infant mortality in the United States, *National Center for Health Statistics (NCHS) Data Brief ,* October 2008.

Macones GA, Hankins GD, Spong CY, Hauth J, Moore T: The 2008 National Institute of Child Health and Human Development workshop report on electronic fetal monitoring: update on definitions, interpretation, and research guidelines, *J Obstet Gynecol Neonatal Nurs* 112(3):510–515, 2008a.

Macones GA, Hankins GD, Spong CY, Hauth J, Moore T: The 2008 National Institute of Child Health and Human Development workshop report on electronic fetal monitoring: update on definitions, interpretation, and research guidelines, *Obstet Gynecol* 112(3):661–666, 2008b.

Magann EF, Chauhan SP, Doherty DA, and others: The evidences for abandoning the amniotic fluid index in favor of the single deepest pocket, *Am J Perinatol* 24:549–555, 2007.

Mahlmeister L: Legal implications of fetal heart assessment, *J Obstet Gynecol Neonatal Nurs* 29(5): 517–526, 2000.

McKeon LM, Cunningham PD, Detty Oswaks JS: Improving patient safety: patient focused, high-reliability team training, *J Nurs Care Qual* 20(5):1–7, 2008.

Meschia G: Placental respiratory gas exchange and fetal oxygenation. In Creasy R, Resnik R, Iams J, Lockwood C, Moore T, editors: *Creasy and Resnik's maternal-fetal medicine: principles and practice,* ed 6, Philadelphia, 2009, Saunders.

Phelan J, Kim J: Fetal heart rate observations in the brain-damaged infant, *Semin Perinatol* 24(3): 221–229, 2000.

Radin T, Harmon J, Hanson D: Nurses' care during labor: its effect on the cesarean birth rate of healthy, nulliparous women, *Birth* 20(1):14–21, 1993.

Schmidt J: The development of AWHONN's fetal heart monitoring principles and practices workshop, *J Obstet Gynecol Neonatal Nurs* 29(5):509, 2000.

Simpson K: Standardized language for electronic fetal heart monitoring, *MCN Am J Matern Child Nurs* 29(5):336, 2004.

Simpson K, Creehan P: *Perinatal nursing*, ed 3, Philadelphia, 2008, Lippincott.

Snyder C, Copel J: Fetal cardiac arrhythmias: diagnosis and therapy. In James D and others, editor: *High risk pregnancy: management options*, ed 3, Philadelphia, 2005, Saunders.

Society of Obstetricians and Gynecologists of Canada (SOGC): *Clinical practice guidelines: fetal health surveillance in labour*, No. 112, 2002.

Sweha A, Hacker TW, Nuovo J: Interpretation of the electronic fetal heart rate during labor, *Am Fam Physician* 59(9):2487–2500, 1999.

Thacker SB, Stroup D, Chang M: Continuous electronic heart rate monitoring for fetal assessment during labor, *Cochrane Database Syst Rev* (Issue 2), Art. No.: CD000063. DOI: 10.1002/14651858. CD000063, 2001.

Tucker S, Miller LA, Miller DA: *Mosby's pocket guide to fetal monitoring: a multidisciplinary approach*, ed 6, St Louis, 2009, Mosby.

Antepartum Fetal Surveillance

American College of Obstetricians and Gynecologists (ACOG): *Antepartum fetal surveillance*, Practice Bulletin, No. 9, Washington, DC, 1999, ACOG.

Cito G, and others: Maternal position during non-stress test and fetal heart rate patterns, *Acta Obstet Gynecol Scand* 84(4):335–338, 2005.

Devoe LD: Antenatal fetal assessment: contraction stress test, nonstress test, vibroacoustic stimulation, amniotic fluid volume, biophysical profile, and modified biophysical profile—an overview, *Sem Perinatol* 32(4):247–252, 2008.

East CE, Smyth RMD, Leader LR, Henshall NE, Colditz PB, Tan KH: Vibroacoustic stimulation for fetal assessment in labour in the presence of a nonreassuring fetal heart rate trace, *Cochrane Database Syst Rev*, (Issue 2), Art. No.: CD004664.

Freeman R, Garite R, Nageotte M: *Fetal heart rate monitoring*, ed 3, Baltimore, 2003, Lippincott Williams & Wilkins.

Harman C: Assessment of fetal health. In Creasy R, Resnik R, Iams J, Lockwood C, Moore T, editors: *Creasy and Resnik's maternal-fetal medicine: principles and practice*, ed 6, Philadelphia, 2009, Saunders.

MacDorman MF, Matthews TJ: *Recent trends in infant mortality in the United States. NCHS data brief*, No 9, Hyattsville, MD, 2008, National Center for Health Statistics.

Mangesi L, Hofmeyr GJ: Fetal movement counting for assessment of fetal well-being. *Cochrane Database Syst Rev* 2007, (Issue 1), Art. No.: CD004909. DOI: 10.1002/14651858.

Manning F: Fetal biophysical profile: a critical appraisal, *Clin Obstet Gynecol* 45(9):975–985, 2002.

Shaffer B, Parer J: Antepartum fetal monitoring. In Queenan J, Spong C, Lockwood C, editors: *Management of high-risk pregnancy*, ed 5, Malden, MA, 2007, Blackwell.

Tan KH, Smyth RMD: Fetal vibroacoustic stimulation for facilitation of tests of fetal well being, *Cochrane Database Syst Rev 2003*, (Issue 4), Art. No.: CD002963.

United Health Foundation: *American Public Health Association (APHA), and Partnership for Prevention: America's health ranking, 2005*, Minnetonka, MN, 2005, United Health Foundation.

Wyatt S, Rhoads S: A primer on antenatal testing for neonatal nurses: Part 2. Tests of fetal well-being, *Adv Neonatal Care* 6(5):228–241, 2006.

Fetal Oxygenation Saturation

American College of Obstetricians and Gynecologists (ACOG): Fetal pulse oximetry, Committee Opinion, No. 258, *Obstet Gynecol* 98(3):523–524, 2001.

Bloom SL, and others: Fetal pulse oximetry and cesarean delivery, *N Engl J Med* 355(21):2195–2202, 2006.

East CE, Chan FY, Colditz PB: Fetal pulse oximetry for fetal assessment in labour, *Cochrane Database Syst Rev* (Issue 2), Art. No.: CD004075. DOI: 10.1002/14651858.CD004075. pub3, 2004.

Garite T, and others: A multicenter controlled trial of fetal pulse oximetry in the intrapartum management of non-reassuring fetal heart rate patterns, *Am J Obstet Gynecol* 183(5):1049–1058, 2000.

Simpson K, Porter M: Fetal oxygen saturation monitoring: using this new technology for fetal assessment during labor, *AWHONN Lifelines* 5(2):26–33, 2001.

4

Perinatal Screening, Diagnoses, and Fetal Therapies

Advances have been made in antepartum fetal surveillance, diagnosis, and medical therapies. These advances include the following:

- Prenatal genetic screening
- Prenatal diagnostic tests
- Prenatal therapies such as transfusion, surgery, and multifetal pregnancy reduction

PRENATAL GENETIC SCREENING

Prenatal genetic screening is performed for events that occur in less than 1% of pregnancies (Wapner, Jenkins, and Khalek, 2009). Down syndrome is the most common clinically significant chromosomal abnormality and occurs at a rate of 1 in 650 live births in the general United States population (Armour, 2008). Historically, screening for this genetic abnormality has focused on women over age 35; however, growing evidence emphasizes the need for prenatal screening of all women regardless of maternal age (Alldred and others, 2008). Prenatal care includes various prenatal screening and diagnostic tests to evaluate for congenital abnormalities and genetic disorders.

Purpose

Prenatal genetic screening is used to detect or define risk for fetal congenital malformations and inherited disorders.

Indications

Prenatal genetic screening starts with a risk assessment that includes maternal age, a family history, and ethnicity. Table 4-1 identifies the at-risk population groups that should be offered screening for certain high-risk genetic conditions. Other indications for prenatal genetic screening:

- Abnormal genetic history of mother or father
- Previous child with genetic defect
- Maternal phenylketonuria (PKU) or congestive heart disease
- Maternal history of two or more miscarriages
- Extreme parental anxiety/concern about potential for genetic abnormalities

Table 4-1   Population Groups at High Risk for a Genetic Condition

Population Group	Genetic Condition	Available Screening Test
All women seeking genetic screening	Down syndrome	Quad Screen, nuchal translucency, urine test, triple screen
Positive family history	Positive disease found in the history	Disease-specific test
Ashkenazi Jewish descent	Tay-Sachs disease Canavan disease	Hexosaminidase A level, DNA mutation
French Canadian or Cajun descent	Tay-Sachs disease	Hexosaminidase A level
Southeast Asian descent	α-Thalassemia	Mean corpuscular volume (MCV)
Middle Eastern/ Mediterranean descent	β-Thalassemia	MCV
African-American descent	Sickle cell disease α-Thalassemia β-Thalassemia	Hb electrophoresis MCV, DNA mutation
Hispanic descent	Sickle cell disease	Hb electrophoresis MCV, DNA mutation
All women seeking pre-conception counseling (especially whites of European origin)	Cystic fibrosis	DNA mutation

Modified from March of Dimes Defects Foundation: Integrating genetics into your practice. *Contemp Ob Gyn* Nov. 1, 2003; Wapner R, Jenkins T, Khalek N: Prenatal diagnosis of congenital disorders. In Creasy R, Resnik R, Iams J, Lockwood C, Moore T, editors: *Creasy & Resnik's maternal-fetal medicine: principles and practice*, ed 6, Philadelphia, 2009, Saunders; Alldred K, and others: Antenatal screening for Down's syndrome (protocols), *Cochrane Database Syst Rev*, Issue 4, 2008.

Resources

Informative online resources:
- ACOG— *http://www.acog.net*
- Gene Tests— *http://www.genetests.org*
- March of Dimes— *http://www.marchofdimes.com/gyponline*
- National Society of Genetic Counselors— *http://www.nsgc.org*

SCREENING METHODS

Since most genetically abnormal children are born at varying ages to parents without a history of abnormality, routine screening is recommended and is cost effective. Traditionally routine prenatal genetic screening has been performed during the second trimester of pregnancy. However, to facilitate the detection of fetal abnormalities earlier, first trimester screening has increased in use since the completion of two large studies in 2005 that validated its reliability. To date, there is no agreed gold standard screening test; as a result, women are still offered a variety of screening tests based on geographic location and practitioner preference.

Second Trimester Screening

Definition

One marker is maternal serum alpha-fetoprotein (MSAFP), a protein produced by the fetal liver. MSAFP screening is useful in identifying certain developmental defects in the fetus. High levels may indicate neural tube defects with 70% to 80% accuracy, ventral abdominal wall defects with 40% accuracy, esophageal and duodenal atresia, and some renal or urinary tract anomalies and STI syndrome (AWHONN, 2008). Abnormally low levels have been noted in some cases of Down syndrome.

Other serum markers are also measured. *Triple marker screening* is another method of screening that can be performed in the second trimester. The triple screen detects the MSAFP, human chorionic gonadotropin (hCG), and unconjugated estriol (uEST). Combining all three chemical markers with the mother's age allows a detection rate of some trisomies at two to three times the detection rate with MSAFP alone. Low MSAFP, low uEST, and high hCG are associated with Down syndrome, with approximately 65% accuracy in women under 35 years of age and with 70% accuracy in women 35 years of age and older (Armour, 2008). A low value in all three markers is associated with trisomy 18 with 60% to 75% accuracy. In addition to the trisomies, triple marker screening detects 85% to 90% of open neural tube defects (Wilson, 2000; Jorde, Carey, Bamshad, and White, 2006).

The *quad-screen* adds a fourth marker, inhibin A (a placental hormone), to enhance the accuracy of screening for Down syndrome in women younger than 35 years of age. It has a lower false-positive rate of 5% or less (Wald, Huttly, and Hackshaw, 2003; AWHONN, 2008). Low inhibin A levels indicate the possibility of Down syndrome.

Timing

The optimal time for MSAFP, triple marker screening, or quad-screen is 16 to 18 weeks of gestation (AWHONN, 2008).

Method

Maternal serum is routinely drawn as a screen between 16 and 18 weeks of gestation. It is necessary to have accurate information about gestational dating, maternal weight, race, number of fetuses, and insulin dependency.

The following can cause falsely elevated levels of MSAFP:
- Low birth weight
- Oligohydramnios
- Multifetal gestation
- Decreased maternal weight
- Underestimated fetal gestational age

The following can cause false low levels of MSAFP:
- Fetal death
- Increased maternal weight
- Overestimated fetal gestational age

Interpretation of Results

Second trimester maternal serum marker levels are not diagnostic; instead, they serve as a screen for fetal risk factors. Elevated or low levels indicate a need to follow up with other diagnostic studies, such as ultrasound, chorionic villus sampling, or amniocentesis, to help make specific diagnoses. Normal maternal serum markers indicate that there is a low risk for specific abnormalities, but they do not ensure a perfect, normal baby.

First Trimester Screening

Definition

First trimester screening uses ultrasound for measuring the nuchal translucency (NT), a fluid collection at the nape of the fetus' neck, and two serum protein markers: plasma protein-A (PAPP-A) and free beta subunit of human chorionic gonadotropin (β-hCG). Increased nuchal translucency, greater than 3 mm between 10 and 14 weeks of gestation, with decreased serum PAPP-A and β-hCG levels indicates a possible increased risk for certain trisomies such as 21 (Down syndrome), 18 (Edwards syndrome), and 13 (Patau syndrome). Increased nuchal translucency alone indicates a 10% to 15% risk for fetal cardiac disease (ACOG, 2004).

Timing

The optimal time for first trimester screening is 10 to 14 weeks of gestation (ACOG, 2004).

Interpretation of Results

First trimester maternal serum marker levels and nuchal translucency are not diagnostic, but rather serve as a screen for fetal risk factors. Elevated or low levels indicate a need to follow up with other diagnostic studies, such as ultrasound, chorionic villus sampling, or amniocentesis. Normal maternal serum markers and nuchal translucency measurements indicate that there is a low risk for specific abnormalities, but they do not ensure a perfect, normal baby.

Combining First and Second Trimester Screening

Combining first and second trimester screening lowers false-positive rates from 8.5% to 5.6% as indicated by results of the FASTER trial (Malone and others, 2003).

ULTRASOUND EVALUATION FOR FETAL ABNORMALITIES

Many practices use ultrasound routinely in the first two trimesters. First, it is used to validate or establish the estimated date of delivery. It is particularly useful for this purpose when done before 20 weeks. Second, it is used between 16 and 20 weeks of gestation (as a level II ultrasound) to evaluate the fetal anatomy and check for certain markers of chromosomal abnormalities (ACOG, 2008). Some aneuploidy ultrasound markers are listed in Box 4-1.

Box 4-1   Fetal Aneuploidy Tissue Markers Identified by Ultrasound
• Brachycephaly
• Increased nuchal thickness
• Congenital heart defects
• Hyperechoic bowel
• Shortened femur or humerus
• Renal anomalies
• Duodenal atresia
• Holoprosencephaly
• Choroid plexus cyst
• Diaphragmatic hernia
• Ventriculomegaly
• Posterior fossa cyst
• Omphalocele
• Intrauterine growth restriction
• Talipes
• Shortened or absent nasal bone
• Widened ischial spine angle

From Wapner R, Jenkins T, Khalek N: Prenatal diagnosis of congenital disorders. In Creasy R, Resnik R, Iams J, Lockwood C, Moore T, editors: *Creasy & Resnik's maternal-fetal medicine: principles and practice,* ed 6, Philadelphia, 2009, Saunders.

In a level II ultrasound, the anatomy is evaluated from head to extremities. Evaluations include the following (ACOG, 2008):
- Ventricles of the head for size—the middle cerebral artery may be evaluated for blood flow after 24 weeks of gestation
- Face, profile, and full-on views
- Nuchal translucency
- Heart and its four chambers—blood flow through valves may be evaluated with a fetal echocardiogram after 20 to 22 weeks of gestation
- Abdominal contents, including the intestines, liver, spleen, and kidneys
- All four extremities, including hands and feet

Ultrasound is useful in other stages of pregnancy to evaluate growth parameters, cerebral artery blood flow, and already known abnormalities for progressive or worsening trends. It also may be useful for the opposite; that is, to evaluate for therapeutic procedures or treatment effects that help confirm reasons to continue the pregnancy (ACOG, 2008).

PRENATAL DIAGNOSTIC TESTS

When a screening test is positive or a prior history of a fetus with a chromosomal abnormality exist, the diagnosis is confirmed or ruled out by diagnostic testing. According to the American College of Obstetrics and Gynecology (2007), diagnostic testing should be offered to all women regardless of maternal age. The rapid rate of technological advancements in this field has led to an explosion of diagnostic procedures and laboratory testing options. The procedures can be split into two groups,

Table 4-2   Diagnostic Procedures and Laboratory Testing Options

Invasive Diagnostic Procedures	Laboratory Tests
Chorionic villus sampling	Traditional cytogenetic testing
Amniocentesis	Multiplex ligation-dependent probe amplification (MLPA)
Percutaneous umbilical blood sampling	Quantitative fluorescent polymerase chain reaction (QF-PCR)
Fetal skin biopsy	Polymerase chain reaction (PCR)
Fetal muscle biopsy	Chromosome microarray (CMA)
Fetal kidney biopsy	Fluorescence in situ hybridization (FISH)
Fetal urine aspiration	Array comparative genomic hybridization (CGH)
Preimplantation genetic screening	Array based genomic hybridization (AGH)
Noninvasive Procedures	
Free Fetal DNA	

From Wapner R, Jenkins T, Khalek N: Prenatal diagnosis of congenital disorders. In Creasy R, Resnik R, Iams J, Lockwood C, Moore T, editors: *Creasy & Resnik's maternal-fetal medicine: principles and practice,* ed 6, Philadelphia, 2009, Saunders; Ogilvie C, and others: Current controversies in prenatal diagnosis 3: for prenatal diagnosis, should we offer less or more than metaphase karyotyping? *Prenat Diagn* 29:11-14, 2009.

invasive diagnostic testing and noninvasive diagnostic testing. Table 4-2 shows the different diagnostics procedures and testing options currently being used.

Chorionic Villus Sampling

Definition

In chorionic villus sampling (CVS), a portion of the chorion is aspirated and ana-lyzed for evidence of genetic, chromosomal, or biochemical abnormalities.

Routes

CVS is done by transabdominal aspiration (needle) or transcervical aspiration (catheter).

Risks

The benefit of diagnosing fetal disorders earlier must be weighed against the risks. Risk of fetal loss, maternal RH immunization, infection, and possible limb abnor-malities resulting from the CVS procedure is 0.5% to 2% (AWHONN, 2008). Postprocedural bleeding is the most common complication occurring in 7% to 10% of patients undergoing the transcervical route; whereas postprocedural bleeding is rare in patients who undergo the transabdominal approach (Wapner, Jenkins, and Khalek, 2009). The transcervical CVS approach is contraindicated in the presence of a cervical infection such as chlamydia or herpes.

Timing

Transabdominal CVS needle aspiration is done in the first or second trimester. Trans-abdominal CVS needle aspiration or transcervical CVM aspiration is done ideally at 10 to 13 weeks of gestation (Cunningham and others, 2010).

Procedure for Abdominal Route

Before the start of the procedure ultrasound examination is performed to confirm fetal heart rate activity and placental location. Then with continuous ultrasonographic guidance, a 19- to 20-gauge spinal needle with stylet is inserted through the maternal abdominal wall and myometrium into the chorion. The stylet is withdrawn, and a 20-ml syringe is attached to an aspiration device. Chorionic villi are obtained by repeated (15 to 20) rapid aspirations of the syringe plunger to 20-ml negative pressure. Simultaneously the needle tip is redirected three to four times within the placenta. The needle is withdrawn under continuous 20-ml negative pressure. The villi are sent to a laboratory with the ability to perform cytogenetic testing.

Procedure for Transcervical Route

Before the start of the procedure, an ultrasound examination is performed to confirm fetal heart rate, gestational age, and placental location. The location of the cervix and the uterus are identified and the catheter path is mapped. In the transcervical approach, the patient is placed in a lithotomy position and the vulva and vaginal are prepped with a povidone-iodine solution. A speculum is placed in the vagina and the cervix is prepped in a similar fashion. A 20-mm catheter with a pliable stainless steel obturator is then passed through the cervix and into the chorion. The obturator is removed, and a 10-ml syringe is attached to the catheter. Chorionic villi are obtained by applying 2 to 5 ml of negative pressure at several sites on the chorion. The specimen is then transferred to a Petri dish for inspection under a microscope to judge quantity of tissue. The villi are sent to a laboratory with the ability to perform cytogenetic testing.

Interpretation of Results for Transabdominal and Transcervical Routes

CVS is now considered a reliable method of prenatal diagnosis with a 99.7% rate of successful cytogenetic diagnosis (Wapner, Jenkins, and Khalek, 2009). However, in its initial development errors occurred in the results secondary to maternal cell contamination and misinterpretation of mosaicism isolated to the placenta (Ledbetter and others, 1990). Results can be obtained in as little as 24 hours when direct testing methods are used and in 5 to 8 days when cells are growing and harvested; in the indirect testing method cells are harvested at 5 to 8 days (Hunter and Soothill, 2006; Wapner, Jenkins, and Khalek, 2009). Currently the direct method of villi testing has the advantage of providing rapid results with decreased risk of maternal cell contamination. This contamination appears to occur more frequently in specimens obtained with the transcervical approach. As a result is it highly recommended that both the direct and indirect testing method be performed on villi specimens (Simoni and others, 1983; Wapner, Jenkins, and Khalek, 2009).

Postprocedure Care

The fetal heart rate (FHR) is auscultated twice in 30 minutes. Unsensitized Rh D-negative patients are given 300 mg of Rho (D) immune globulin. A repeat ultrasound is scheduled to be performed at 16 weeks of gestation.

Amniocentesis

Definition

Amniocentesis is the transabdominal needle aspiration of 10 to 20 ml of amniotic fluid for laboratory analysis.

Timing

There are two types of amniocentesis, early and second trimester (sometimes called conventional). The second trimester/conventional amniocentesis is preferred for genetic screening and is performed between 15 and 20 weeks of gestation (ACOG, 2008; Alfirevic, Mujezinovic, and Sundberg, 2008). Early amniocentesis, performed between 11 and 14 weeks, results in significantly higher rate of pregnancy loss (2.5% compared with 1%), other complications such as talipes equinovarus (1.6% compared with 3.1%), and postprocedural amniotic fluid leakage of 3.5% compared with 1.7% (Whitworth, Bricker, and Neilson, 2008).

Risks

Risks with amniocentesis include the following:
- Spontaneous abortion
- Trauma to the fetus or placenta
- Bleeding
- Preterm labor
- Maternal infection
- Rh sensitization from fetal bleed into maternal side of circulation

Preparation

In preparation for amniocentesis, the nurse explains the procedure to the patient. The patient is encouraged to urinate just before the procedure to avoid the risk for bladder puncture. Usually a 20-minute electronic fetal monitoring (EFM) strip is run or an ultrasound evaluation is made before the procedure to explore the potential site for probability of obtaining the fluid.

Procedure

First a detailed ultrasound is performed to take fetal measurements, obtain an anatomic survey of the fetus, locate the placenta, and choose an amniocentesis site. Then the abdomen is prepped with an antiseptic such as povidone-iodine (Betadine). Most practitioners do not use lidocaine (Xylocaine). A spinal-gauge needle is then inserted into the site selected under ultrasound guidance. Approximately 20 to 30 ml of fluid is withdrawn for a genetic analysis and alpha-fetoprotein (AFP) screen. If the procedure is being used as a method of draining excess amniotic fluid, the needle is anchored, tubing is attached, and the necessary amount of fluid is removed by gravity (Wilson, 2000; Hunter and Soothill, 2006; Jorde, Carey, Bamshad, and White, 2006).

Interpretation of Results

Amniocentesis has an accuracy rate of 99%. After 3 to 7 days of cell growth there exist enough fetal cells for staining or karyotype analysis. Chromosomal mosaicism occurs in approximately 0.1% to 0.3% of amniocentesis specimens. Although true fetal mosaicism is rare, ultrasound assessment should be performed to evaluate fetal growth and possible structural anomalies.

Postprocedural Care

After amniocentesis, if performed after 24 weeks, an EFM strip is run, primarily to detect contractile patterns suggestive of preterm labor or abruption. The FHR is monitored and evaluated as appropriate for the gestational age (Wilson, 2000; Hunter and Soothill, 2006; Jorde, Carey, Bamshad, and White, 2006). The Rh D-negative woman should receive Rho (D) immune globulin (300 mg) because there is potential for a procedure-associated fetal-maternal hemorrhage.

The woman should be advised not to lift anything heavy for 2 days and to report any amniotic fluid leakage, fever, severe cramps, or vaginal bleeding. Slight cramping for the first day or two is normal.

Percutaneous Umbilical Blood Sampling

Purpose

Historically percutaneous umbilical blood sampling (PUBS) was done to obtain rapid karyotype results. However, with recent advancements in the field of cytogenetic the indications for PUBS have changed. Now the rationale for the use of PUBS is to evaluate mosaic results discovered in CVS and amniocentesis testing. The procedure is also done to measure fetal hemoglobin in case of erythroblastosis fetalis, for a fetal platelet count in alloimmune thrombocytopenia or thrombocytopenia purpura, or to assess for a fetal infection (Wapner, Jenkins, and Khalek, 2009).

Risks

There is a 2% higher than background risk for fetal loss with percutaneous umbilical blood sampling; however, this number is difficult to qualify because of the severe congenital malformations of these fetuses (Wapner, Jenkins, and Khalek, 2009). Associated complications of this procedure are bleeding, cord hematomas, transient fetal bradycardia, infection, and fetal-maternal hemorrhage (James and others, 2004).

Timing

The blood sample may be drawn as early as an early amniocentesis, but is generally done late in the second trimester when such diagnoses may change options and recommendations for medical management (James and others, 2004).

Method

With concurrent ultrasonographic visualization, a 23- or 25-gauge spinal needle is directed into the umbilical vein about 1 cm from the site of cord insertion into the placenta (Jorde, Carey, Bamshad, and White, 2006). In regard to intrafetal insertion sites, the hepatic vein is the safest and most accessible location. In cases where oligohydramnios exist, color Doppler imaging enhances vessel visualization and accurate needle insertion (Wapner, Jenkins, and Khalek, 2009).

Interpretation of Results

Recommendations for biochemical testing on the blood should include a complete blood count with a differential analysis, anti-1 and anti-i cold agglutinin, ß-hCG, factors IX and VIIIC, and AFP levels. It is important to note that because a gold standard currently does not exist for the biochemical evaluation of fetal blood, it is not common practice for all of these tests to be performed (Jorde, Carey, Bamshad, and White, 2006; Wapner, Jenkins, and Khalek, 2009).

Postprocedure Care

External fetal monitoring is done for 1 to 2 hours after the procedure. Also, the nurse should instruct the mother how to count fetal movements so that she can count them when she is discharged home.

OTHER INVASIVE DIAGNOSTIC FETAL PROCEDURES

There are rare occasions in which other invasive diagnostic procedures are performed. Because of the low number of cases performed and the congenital malformations of the fetuses undergoing the procedures, there is little statistical information related to fetal mortality and morbidity secondary to these invasive diagnostic procedures.

Skin Biopsy

Purpose

Fetal skin biopsy is performed to diagnosis genetic skin disorders when molecular testing is not available (Wapner, Jenkins, and Khalek, 2009). Other purposes for skin biopsy are to diagnosis mosaicism.

Method

Using continuous real-time sonographic guidance, a 21-gauge biopsy forceps is inserted through a 19-gauge angiocath. Fetal skin is manually removed from various sites, usually the fetus' back. The skin cells are then sent to a laboratory for cytogenetic testing (Vincenzo and others, 1998).

Postprocedure Care

If the procedure is performed after 24 weeks, external fetal monitoring is done for 1 to 2 hours after the procedure. Also, the nurse should instruct the mother how to count fetal movements so that she can count them when she is discharged home.

Muscle Biopsy

Purpose

Fetal muscle biopsy is performed for dystrophin analysis to diagnosis muscular dystrophy when molecular testing is not available or results are ambiguous (Wapner, Jenkins, and Khalek, 2009).

Method

Fetal muscle biopsies are done under continuous sonographic guidance. The biopsy process is similar to other fetal biopsy procedures (Yoram and others, 1999).

Timing

The accuracy of the test is based on gestational age of the fetus. After 20 weeks' gestation the skeletal muscle is relatively mature and dystrophin production is high, which should result in accurate testing results (Yoram and others, 1999).

Postprocedure Care

If the procedure is performed after 24 weeks, external fetal monitoring is done for 1 to 2 hours after the procedure. Also, the nurse should instruct the mother how to count fetal movements so that she can count them when she is discharged home.

Kidney Biopsy

Purpose

A fetus at risk of congenital nephrosis can be identified by three markers:
- Markedly elevated amniotic alpha-fetoprotein
- Negative acetylcholinesterase
- Unremarkable ultrasound evaluation.

However, diagnosis of congenital nephrosis is only possible with a kidney biopsy. The renal cells are then examined under an electron microscope for tissue anomalies (Wapner and others, 2001).

Method

Before the procedure it is necessary to map the entire renal vascular supply with color Doppler and the needle pathway is plotted, thereby decreasing the chance of damaging the kidney's vasculature. Once ready, a 22-gauge needle is used to deliver an intramuscular injection of pancuronium to the fetus. Then with continuous sonographic guidance an 18- to 20-gauge biopsy needle is guided into the renal cortex and negative pressure is applied with a syringe. The fetal tissue obtained is assessed to ensure glomeruli tissue is obtained (Wapner and others, 2001).

Timing

The accuracy of the test is affected by the size of the renal fossa. After 20 weeks gestation the success rates improve in regard to obtaining glomeruli tissue (Wapner and others, 2001).

Postprocedure Care

If the procedure is performed after 24 weeks, external fetal monitoring is done for 1 to 2 hours after the procedure. Also, the nurse should instruct the mother how to count fetal movements so that she can count them when she is discharged home.

Urine Aspiration

Purpose

Fetal urine aspiration is performed on fetuses that have a congenital lower urinary tract obstruction (LUTO) and are under evaluation for prenatal shunt placement. If left untreated LUTO has a mortality rate of 45% and a chronic renal failure rate of 25% to 30% of those infants who survive the neonatal period (Morris, 2007).

Method

Using ultrasound guidance, fetal urine is obtained directly from the renal pelvis with the use of a 20-gauge needle. The sample is obtained from the side where the kidney appears to be least compromised (Miguelez, 2005). Urinalysis is then performed. There is growing controversy over the reliability of the analytes being tested and their ability to reflect postnatal renal function (Morris, 2007).

Timing

There is no defined window of testing in the literature. It is important to note that analyte levels change throughout the gestational development of the fetus; therefore, accurate information related to the gestational age of the fetus is essential (Morris, 2007).

Postprocedure Care

If the procedure is performed after 24 weeks, external fetal monitoring is done for 1 to 2 hours after the procedure. Also, the nurse should instruct the mother how to count fetal movements so that she can count them when she is discharged home.

Preimplantation Genetic Diagnosis

Purpose

The desired outcome of preimplantation genetic diagnosis (PGD) is to produce a healthy pregnancy free from inherited genetic disease, thereby avoiding pregnancy termination. The procedure is noninvasive to the women but it is invasive to the embryo.

Since the 1990s the use of PGD has grown significantly and offers benefits to the following populations (Fragouli, 2007):

- Carriers of a single gene disorder, which is dominant or recessive, autosomal or X-linked
- Carriers of structural chromosome abnormalities
- Women of advanced maternal age
- Couples with repeated implantation failure following assisted reproduction treatments
- Couples with repeated and unexplained miscarriages

Method

There are two different methods used to complete PGD. These methods vary based on the time passed since in vitro fertilization (IVF); however, the literature indicates that regardless of the biopsy, timing the procedure is well tolerated and normal embryonic development is possible. Following are the two different scenarios (Fragouli, 2007; Wapner, Jenkins, and Khalek, 2009):

- Biopsy of one to two blastomeres from cleavage stage of three day-old embryo
- Biopsy of 5 to 12 trophectoderm from the oocyte during meiosis progression

The cells retrieved from the biopsy are analyzed for genetic disorders by either polymerase chain reaction (PRC) or fluorescence in situ hybridization (FISH). Results from the procedures can be obtained 90% of the time; however, errors have occurred in the interpretation of the result because of the mosaic nature of the early embryo (Wapner, Jenkins, and Khalek, 2009).

Noninvasive Prenatal Diagnosis

Procedure

Numerous studies have identified both intact fetal cells and free fetal DNA (ffDNA) circulating in the maternal serum. The amount of ffDNA in the maternal plasma exists in greater quantity and is easier to obtain than intact fetal cells from maternal serum (Wapner, Jenkins, and Khalek, 2009). However, improvements in retrieving and concentrating both intact fetal cells and ffDNA are required to enhance the efficiency and reliability of cytogenetic testing.

Method

Both intact fetal cells and ffDNA can be obtained from maternal serum obtained by routine venipuncture. Using diffusion gradients, fluorescent cell sorting, and magnetic cell separation, the concentration of intact fetal cells (fetal nucleated red blood cells) can be increased to allow for analysis for specific aneuploids by FISH (Wapner, Jenkins, and Khalek, 2009).

The method for retrieving ffDNA requires the maternal serum to be separated into intact cellular components and maternal plasma. The laboratory uses automated DNA extraction methods to isolate and concentrate the ffDNA, which can then undergo cytogenetic testing (Clausen and others, 2007). Research is currently being done to decrease the rate of maternal DNA contamination of the ffDNA and improve the testing reliability.

Timing

Historically because of the limited sample size of intact fetal cells and ffDNA, these diagnostic procedures were done and studied in the second trimester of pregnancy. However, the goal of the noninvasive diagnostic procedure is to be the first line diagnostic testing option. Because ffDNA is the most abundant fetal sample in the maternal circulation, 3% to 6% of the maternal plasma, it has become the source of most research studies in this field. Great energy is being put forward to improve the retrieval process, and some recent studies have shown successful identification of fetal aneuploidy as early as 7 weeks' gestation (Hyett and others, 2005; Clausen and others, 2007).

PRENATAL THERAPY

Fetal Intrauterine Transfusion

Definition

Fetal intrauterine transfusion is an accepted procedure that is associated with increased success, new clinical applications, and more common uses; however, it is not a new concept. In the 1970s, fetal intrauterine transfusions were being done experimentally only as a last resort in the most technologically sophisticated level III facilities. The procedure was fraught with risks of maternal infection, fetal injury, and poor success. At the time, ultrasound technology made placement difficult, and a safe procedure for fetal direct intravenous transfusion was improbable. Now, the direct intravascular routes have become the primary route of transfusion. The intrahepatic route for fetal blood transfusion has been associated with higher fetal survival rates than transfusion into the umbilical vein (Dodd, Windrim, and van Kamp, 2008).

Purpose

The purpose of direct intrauterine fetal transfusion is to ensure appropriate fetal blood volume, thereby decreasing fetal morbidity and mortality. Direct intrauterine fetal transfusion is indicated for the severely hydropic fetuses before 33 weeks of gestation in an Rh D-negative sensitized pregnant woman, fetuses with decreasing fetal hemoglobin or hematocrit, or in fetuses with rising bilirubin levels and delta optical density in the amniotic fluid.

Risks

The overall risk of complications associated with intrauterine fetal transfusion is 1.3% to 2.5%. Overall survival for fetuses that require intrauterine blood transfusion for anemia is 85% to 90%; however, this rate decreases significantly for infants suffering from hydrops.

Risks associated with intrauterine fetal transfusion include the following:
- Maternal infection (1.2% to 3%)
- Overtransfusion
- Fetal vascular trauma
- Onset of preterm labor (.1% to 2%)
- Premature rupture of membranes (.1% to 2%)
- Fetal distress (Dodd, Windrim, and van Kamp, 2008)

Method

Careful aseptic preparation of the maternal abdomen is necessary. The nurse should premedicate the mother with enough narcotics and tranquilizers to render the fetus quiet. Another option is to administer a paralytic to the fetus. The fetal vein of choice is located using ultrasound. A 22-gauge long spinal needle is guided toward the vessel. Once the tip is placed correctly, blood—20 to 50 ml/kg (depending on gestation), cross-matched to the mother, and spun down to a hematocrit greater than 70%—is then instilled slowly. Other studies have transfused enough group O Rh-negative and seronegative for cytomegalovirus to achieve a post-transfusion Hct of 40% (Tanawattanacharoen, 2001; Dodd, Windrim, and van Kamp, 2008).

Postprocedure Care

EFM is used for 1 to 2 hours after the procedure. The mother is instructed to continue fetal movement counts, weekly obstetrical ultrasounds, and non-stress tests (Dodd and others, 2008).

Fetal Intrauterine Surgery

Definition

Therapeutic advances in technology that led to fetal intrauterine surgical corrections evolved from interventions for Rh D sensitization and for effects on the fetus (Weiner, 2005; Wapner, Jenkins, and Khalek, 2009). Initially therapy was directed at diseases acquired in utero. In the early 1980s, therapies for congenital disorders began to be attempted (Wapner, Jenkins, and Khalek, 2009).

All forms of fetal surgery remain experimental, although some trends are becoming evident:

- Surgical correction of obstructive uropathies: The rationale for such therapy is to bypass the site of the obstruction and thereby prevent progressive renal damage.
- Surgical placement of shunts for pleural effusions
- Surgical correction of obstructive hydrocephalus: The rationale is to reduce ventricular size and expansion to minimize compression damage to the cerebral cortex.
- Surgical correction of anastomotic vessels in a monochorionic twin pregnancy: The rationale is to stop the twin-twin transfusion and prevent the 80% fetal mortality related to the condition.
- Repair of a myelomeningocele before neuronal damage
- Repair of fetal diaphragmatic hernia: Presumably, repair of the hernia provides release of compressive forces and restores normal lung development. The following fetal surgery has not proved very successful:
    - In utero plastic repair of such abnormalities as cleft palate and lip: Theoretically, plastic repairs before birth would heal with less scarring.

All but the last three surgical procedures are performed with a fiberoptic scope and ultrasonic guidance for placement.

Methods

Surgical corrections may be accomplished by ultrasound-guided percutaneous placement of catheter shunts or by hysterotomy with direct visualization and surgical repair. The type of congenital malformation, as well as the skill and training of the perinatologist, determine the exact method (Bindman and others, 2001; Weiner, 2005; Jorde, Carey, Bamshad, and White, 2006; Roberts, Neilson, Kilby, and Gates, 2008; Wapner, Jenkins, and Khalek, 2009).

Risks

Problems arise when assessing the success and benefit of fetal intrauterine surgical corrections, not the least of which are ethical dilemmas. Because of increased fetal and neonatal survival and the nature of accompanying disabilities, with surgical corrections of some disorders, more fetuses survive as infants with disabilities. Therefore it appears that increased survival will increase the societal problems of caring for infants with disabilities.

Some repairs corrected with intrauterine fetal surgery have higher success than others. Infants with diaphragmatic hernia repair have the lowest survival rate. Those with repair of uropathologic conditions have the highest survival, although the best is with posterior urethral valve syndrome and the worst is with urethral atresia.

The recent advancements in the treatment of twin-twin transfusion syndrome have involved the use of endoscopic lasers to cause the coagulation of anastomotic vessels. This new approach has resulted in less fetal and neonatal death than traditional amnioreduction and septostomy (Roberts, Neilson, Kilby, and Gates, 2008).

Hydrocephalic disorders are generally well screened for the amount of adequate cerebral cortical tissue before attempting the repair. If other associated neural tube defects accompany hydrocephalus, the degree of handicap in surviving infants also varies (Wapner, Jenkins, and Khalek, 2009).

When hysterotomy is the chosen route for accomplishing the repair, there are other attendant problems. First the incision into the uterus generally is as risky as, and requires similar treatment to, the uterine incision of a classic cesarean. Second, as the procedure is being carried out, loss of amniotic fluid and interruption of the integrity of the amnion occur. Stapling the amnion to the uterine wall as the incision is being made compensates for interruption of the integrity of the amnion. Loss of amniotic fluid is restored by warmed normal saline as the cavity is closed. Third, keeping the head and upper respiratory system of the fetus out of the fluid during the procedure is essential to prevent stimulating the switch from fetal cardiopulmonary circulation to neonatal circulation.

The number and type of fetal therapies for congenital disorders probably are limited by the difference in the relative size of the fetus and the available technology and surgical instruments. Those problems can be expected to be overcome as innovative and creative solutions are found to manage them.

Multifetal Pregnancy Reduction

Definition

Multifetal pregnancy reduction is a procedure to reduce the number of multiple embryos conceived, usually by one of the fertility modalities. It is done by injecting high doses of potassium chloride into the fetuses that are easiest to reach after carefully evaluating a complete fetal survey to determine that healthy fetuses, those most likely to survive, have remained. The procedure carries a risk for causing preterm labor, previable delivery, and infection.

Fertility procedures are fraught with multiple concerns. Through manipulation outside the uterus, they more often result in monoamniotic twins and thus carry a higher risk for twin-to-twin transfusion. Other concerns are generally related to the ethical dilemmas presented to the family and care providers. Because of their decision to selectively terminate or carry multiple embryos and risk losing all, parents are at high risk for complicated grief, potentially requiring referral for therapeutic psychologic support.

NURSING MANAGEMENT

Prevention

The main functions of nursing care are to prevent uninformed decisions by parents, fetal compromise after intrauterine therapies, and unnecessary distress of the human spirit because of decisions for fetal testing or therapy.

Counselors and teachers are of prime importance. The ultimate goal is to empower families to make difficult decisions considering their ability to parent and the quality of life for their unborn child.

Assessment

Assessment of stressors, coping styles, general knowledge, and locus of control related to physical and emotional health helps in formulating nursing diagnoses. The nurse must articulate diagnoses and collaborative problems related to alterations in, risks to, complicating factors in, and strengths and deficiencies of the individuals and the family as a unit as follows:

- Assess for coping styles.
- Assess parents' need for comforting spiritual rituals (see Chapter 7).

Intervention

The nurse should help the parents come to an understanding of the potential risks and benefits of the various methods of prenatal genetic screening and of essential fetal therapy. The nurse should help them cope in the event of an unanticipated fetal outcome as follows:

- Prepare for potential unexpected result.
- Establish a trusting relationship.
- Encourage and foster open communication with health providers.
- Coordinate a multidisciplinary conference with parents in attendance.
- Assist with preparations for extended family visitation while the patient is hospitalized.
- Encourage questions.
- Give anticipatory guidance.
- Be prepared to repeat information more than once.
- Provide more than one viewpoint or opinion.
- Provide accurate information about fetal tests and therapy.
- Encourage and facilitate close family contact; eliminate separation.
- Refer to parents' spiritual or psychologic support person(s).
- Communicate acceptance of expressed spiritual pain.
- Encourage expression and exploration of feelings.
- Support parents' decisions without expressing personal conflict and attitudes that may be in opposition to parents' attitudes.

CONCLUSION

The continued rapid growth in technologic and innovative advances in fetal evaluation and therapies has exceeded considerations of physical, psychologic, and social consequences. It has become increasingly difficult for parents with a high risk pregnancy to obtain adequate information about expected benefits and negative consequences of fetal evaluation and therapies. The rapid growth also contributes to difficulty in keeping current with information needed to counsel and guide parents in making thoroughly informed decisions about fetal evaluation or therapy. Nurses have a professional responsibility to seek, be receptive to, and be intelligently critical of information that is on the cutting edge of the future.

BIBLIOGRAPHY

Alfirevic Z, Mujezinovic F, Sundberg K: Amniocentesis and chorionic villus sampling for prenatal diagnosis, *Cochrane Database Syst Rev* (Issue 2), Art. No.: CD003252, 2008.

Alldred SK, Alfirevic Z, Deeks JJ, Neilson JP: Antenatal screening for Down's syndrome (Protocol), *Cochrane Database Syst Rev* (Issue 4), Art. No.: CD007384, 2008.

American College of Obstetricians and Gynecologists (ACOG): *First-trimester screening for fetal aneuploidy, Committee Opinion,* No. 296, Washington, DC, 2004, ACOG.

American College of Obstetricians and Gynecologists (ACOG): *Invasive prenatal testing for aneuploidy,* Practice Bulletin, No. 88, Washington, DC, 2007, ACOG.

American College of Obstetricians and Gynecologists (ACOG): *Ultrasonography in pregnancy,* Practice Bulletin, No. 98, Washington, DC, 2008, ACOG.

Armour K: Recent developments in prenatal screening: removing advanced maternal age as a qualifier. Symposium conducted at the meeting of Association of Women's Health, Obstetrics and Neonatal Nurses 2008, Los Angeles.

Association of Women's Health Obstetrics and Neonatal Nursing (AWHONN): Antenatal Care. In Rice K, Creehan P, editors: *Perinatal nursing,* 3 ed, Philadelphia, 2008, Lippincott Williams & Wilkins.

Bindman R, and others: Second-trimester ultrasound to detect fetuses with Down syndrome: a meta-analysis, *JAMA* 285(8):1044–1055, 2001.

Clausen FB, and others: Improvement in fetal DNA from maternal plasma. Evaluation of NucliSens magnetic extraction system and the QIAamp DSP virus kit in comparison with the QIAamp DNA blood mini kit, *Prenat Diagn* 27(1):6–10, 2007.

Cunningham F, Leveno K, Bloom S, Hauth J, Rouse D, Spong C: *Williams obstetrics,* ed 23, New York, 2010, McGraw-Hill.

Dodd JM, Windrim RC, van Kamp IL: Techniques of intrauterine fetal transfusion for women with red-cell isoimmunisation for improving health outcomes (Protocol), *Cochrane Database Syst Rev* (Issue 2), Art. No.: CD007096, 2008.

Fragouli E: Preimplantation genetic diagnosis: present and future, *J Assist Reprod Genet* 24(6):201–207, 2007.

Hunter A, Soothill P: Invasive procedure for antenatal diagnosis. In James D, and others, editors: *High risk pregnancy: management options,* ed 3, Philadelphia, 2006, Saunders.

Hyett J, and others: Reduction in diagnostic and therapeutic interventions by non-invasive determination of fetal sex in early pregnancy, *Prenat Diagn* 25(12):1111–1116, 2005.

James D, Mahomed K, Stone P, Van Wijngaarden W, Hill L, editors: *Evidence-based obstetrics: a companion volume to high risk pregnancy,* ed 2, Philadelphia, 2004, Saunders.

Jorde L, Carey J, Bamshad M, White R: *Medical genetics,* ed 3, St Louis, 2006, Mosby.

Ledbetter DH, and others: Cytogenetic results of chorionic villus sampling: high success rate and diagnostic accuracy in the United States collaborative study, *Am J Obstet Gynecol* 162:495, 1990.

Malone F, and others: First- and second-trimester evaluation of risk (FASTER) trial: principal results of the NICHD Multicenter Down Syndrome Screening Study, *Am J Obstet Gynecol* 189:S56, 2003.

Miguelez J: Fetal obstructive uropathy: is urine sampling useful for prenatal counseling? *Prenat Diagn* 26(1):81–84, 2005.

Morris RK: Systemic review of accuracy of fetal urine analysis to predict poor postnatal renal function in cases of congenital urinary tract obstruction, *Prenat Diagn* 27(10):900–911, 2007.

Ogilvie C, and others: Current controversies in prenatal diagnosis 3: for prenatal diagnosis, should we offer less or more than metaphase karyotyping? *Prenat Diagn* 29(1):11–14, 2009.

Roberts D, Neilson JP, Kilby M, Gates S: Interventions for the treatment of twin-twin transfusion syndrome, *Cochrane Database Syst Rev* (Issue 1), Art. No.: CD002073, 2008.

Simoni G, and others: Efficient direct chromosome analyses and enzyme determinations from chorionic villi samples in the first trimester of pregnancy, *Hum Genet* 349(63):376–381, 1983.

Tanawattanacharoen S: Intrauterine rescue transfusion in monochorionic multiple pregnancies with recent single intrauterine death, *Prenat Diagn* 21(4):274–278, 2001.

Vincenzo B, and others: Prenatal confirmation of true fetal trisomy 22 mosaicism by fetal skin biopsy following fetal blood sampling, *Prenat Diagn* 18(4):384–389, 1998.

Wald N, Huttly W, Hackshaw A: Antenatal screening for Down syndrome with the quadruple test, *Lancet* 361(9360):835–836, 2003.

Wapner R, Jenkins T, Khalek N: Fetal disorders: diagnosis and therapy. In Creasy R, Resnik R, Iams J, Lockwood C, Moore T, editors: *Creasy & Resnik's maternal-fetal medicine: principles and practice*, ed 6, Philadelphia, 2009, Saunders.

Wapner R, and others: Prenatal diagnosis of congenital nephrosis by in utero biopsy, *Prenat Diagn* 21(4):256–261, 2001.

Weiner C: Fetal hemolytic disease. In James D, and others, editors: *High risk pregnancy: management options*, ed 3, Philadelphia, 2005, Saunders.

Whitworth M, Bricker L, Neilson J: Ultrasound for fetal assessment in early pregnancy, *Cochrane Database Syst Rev* (Issue 2), 2008.

Wilson R: Amniocentesis and chorionic villus sampling, *Curr Opin Obstet Gynecol* 12(2):81–86, 2000.

Yoram N, and others: Fetal muscle biopsy as a diagnostic tool in Duchenne muscular dystrophy, *Prenat Diagn* 19(10):921–926, 1999.

5

Integrative Therapies in Pregnancy and Childbirth

S ince the 1990s, complementary and alternative medicine has been rapidly gaining in popularity for both consumers and health care practitioners. This chapter is intended to acquaint nurses with some of the alternative and complementary therapies that are frequently requested by families experiencing high risk pregnancies. Surveys indicate that patients find complementary and alternative therapies congruent with their own values, beliefs, and philosophical orientation toward health and life. Each year more people are using these services (Petrie and Peck, 2000).

This chapter is simply an introduction to these therapies; readers are strongly encouraged to refer patients to a complementary and alternative medical specialist for treatment. The listed therapies are safe and effective during pregnancy when administered by a person who is properly trained. Although complementary and alternative therapies are generally not supported by solid scientific research, most are based on empirical use and have been practiced for hundreds or even thousands of years. In the case of traditional Chinese medicine (TCM), Chinese herbs and acupuncture have been used for more than a thousand years, and the applications, cautions, and contraindications are well known but only now being scientifically proved.

Therefore these therapies should not be discarded based on the lack of solid scientific evidence. To set such a standard would be disadvantageous; for instance, although much of conventional allopathic medicine is also unsupported by solid, evidence-based literature, it still produces desired results.

When conventional medical treatment is combined with alternative or complementary therapies, the term *integrative medicine* is commonly used. In 1992, the Office of Alternative Medicine was established by the National Institutes of Health to begin to investigate the safety and efficacy of integrative medicine. In 1999, this office was renamed the National Center for Complementary and Alternative Medicine (NCCAM). According to the NCCAM (2006), there are five complementary and alternative fields of practice:

- *Alternative medical systems.* Alternative medical systems are complete systems of medical theory and practice. They include TCM, ayurvedic medicine (India's traditional medicine), homeopathy, naturopathy, and Native American healing.
- *Mind-body interventions.* Mind-body interventions are various techniques designed to enhance the capacity of the mind. Examples are biofeedback, yoga, meditation, hypnotherapy, dance, music and art therapy, relaxation therapy, integrated guided imagery, aromatherapy, spirituality and prayer, humor, journaling, and dream work.
- *Biologic-based therapies.* These therapies include herbal, dietary, and nutritional therapies, including vitamin, mineral, and other supplements, as well as exercise and other lifestyle changes.
- *Manipulative and body-based methods.* These include various hands-on healing techniques such as acupressure, massage, osteopathy, chiropractic, reflexology, and kinesiology.
- *Energy therapies.* Energy therapies include acupuncture, healing touch, therapeutic touch, polarity, Reiki, jin shin jyutsu, external qi gong, touch for health, and reflexology.

BRIEF OVERVIEW OF SELECTED INTEGRATIVE THERAPIES IN PREGNANCY

Alternative Medical Systems

Traditional Chinese Medicine (TCM) and Acupuncture

TCM is a complete medical system that originated in China more than 4000 years ago to diagnose and treat illness, prevent disease, and improve well-being. TCM developed independently from the Western view of anatomy, physiology, and pathology. Qualified practitioners observe, diagnose, and treat illness using a different set of principles and vocabulary than those commonly used in conventional Western medicine.

TCM, on the most fundamental level, is the harmony and balance of qi (pronounced *chee*) in the body. *Qi* can be defined as the essence and the basis of all life, or the vital energy. It warms the body, keeps the mind active, creates breath, expels a baby during birth, and gives us each a distinct personality. Qi is not only part of the human body but also part of the surrounding environment. The general category of qi can be broken down into *yin* and *yang*, which represent the dualistic poles of nature. The sign of the *tai ji* is used to illustrate the nature of yin and yang. Yin and yang maintain the homeostasis of the body. *Yin* represents the dark, inclusive, night, material, cold, inactive, and interior pole. *Yang*, in contrast, is the bright, exclusive, day, immaterial, warm, active, and exterior pole.

TCM is based on the theory of the normal functioning of the human body and its relationship to the environment. The environment includes weather (cold, hot, arid, humid), lifestyle (type of work and hours, exercise, diet), pathogens (viruses, bacteria, fungi, pollens), and relationships (married, single, death of close family), all which affect health and balance. Any aberration is considered a disharmony, which is ultimately a precursor to disease. Once an imbalance or disease has arisen, the TCM methods of diagnosis such as pulse and tongue assessments are used to identify the pattern of disharmony. The treatment principle is formed, and the appropriate modalities are applied.

The most recognized TCM treatment modality in the United States is *acupuncture*. Acupuncture is the insertion of fine (32- to 38-gauge) solid needles into the skin at acupuncture points, which are located along and independent of the meridian system. There are more than 2000 different acupuncture points on the body, situated along the limbs, chest, abdomen, back, spine, ears, face, and scalp. There are 12 major *meridians* (channels of energy flow), each connecting to an organ and running distally throughout the body. The energy that flows through the meridians is qi. The depth of puncture varies, depending on the location and treatment effect desired. Once placed, the needles are retained for a varied length of time, most commonly between 15 and 45 minutes. The number of acupuncture treatments in a course of therapy varies based on the disease being treated and the overall health of the individual. Certain points are contraindicated for use in pregnancy because they can stimulate uterine contractions and result in premature labor.

Chinese herbal medicine is an integral part of TCM. In China, herbal prescriptions are used more frequently and for a wider range of conditions than acupuncture. The theories of Chinese herbal medicine are identical to those of acupuncture. The practitioner obtains a TCM diagnosis using the techniques of observation, auscultation and olfaction, interrogation, and palpation. A treatment plan is then devised, and an herbal prescription is constructed that is very specific to the state of the individual.

Herbal prescriptions usually contain between 2 and 14 individual herbs selected from a pharmacopoeia of thousands. Over hundreds of years of prescribing herbs, the Chinese have empirically and, more recently, scientifically studied the effects of herbs on the human body. Information has been obtained regarding the toxicity levels, preparation procedures, contraindications, and cautions of using Chinese herbs. Chinese herbal medicine is advanced and traditionally used with many disorders. It is complementary to acupuncture therapy, as well as to most prescription drugs.

Other TCM therapies include (Fontaine, 2005):

- *Tui na.* This manipulative or therapeutic bodywork uses massage techniques to treat physical problems.
- *Cupping.* This is a treatment technique whereby suction is applied to the skin surface using small jars in which a vacuum is created. The cups are commonly retained for 1 to 15 minutes. Cupping is frequently used to treat disorders of the musculoskeletal system.
- *Moxibustion.* This is a common adjunctive technique used in TCM. The name refers to the technique with which heat is applied to the acupuncture points by igniting products made from the dried leaves of the mugwort plant (*Artemisia vulgaris*). There are many ways to warm the "moxa" on the acupuncture point. Sometimes the moxa pole can be used to warm acupuncture needles that have already been inserted. This method is commonly used to turn a baby from the breech position.
- *Chinese nutritional therapy.* In this system, foods are categorized by their energetic properties and their effect on organ systems. A diet of beneficial foods is prescribed to treat disease, and recommendations are given about foods that should be avoided or eaten in moderation.

- *Gua sha.* This is a manual technique that uses a coin or spoon to scrape the surface of the skin. It promotes the circulation of qi and blood and is also used to treat musculoskeletal pain syndromes.
- *Plum blossom needling.* This is a form of cutaneous needle therapy. The acupuncture points are stimulated by lightly tapping an instrument that has a head composed of a bundle of five or seven small, short needles attached to a handle. This tapping causes a reddening of the skin and promotes circulation. It is most applicable for disorders of the skin and nervous system.
- *Electrical stimulation.* The most common form of electrical stimulation uses a machine similar to a TENS (transcutaneous electrical nerve stimulation) unit with clips attached to the end of retained needles. Therapy is used in conjunction with acupuncture and lasts from 10 to 30 minutes; the presence of the current may or may not be felt by the patient. Electroacupuncture is most often used as analgesia and is applicable during labor and delivery.

Homeopathy

Homeopathy is an energy-based, pharmacologic system of medicine that uses a set of principles and laws for prescribing specifically prepared medicines to correct disease. Developed by Dr. Samuel Hahnemann (1755-1843) of Germany, the basic theory of homeopathy is "like cures like" or the "Law of Similars." For example, for constipation, a homeopathic remedy that in crude form is known to *produce* constipation can actually treat the same condition when used in minute doses.

Homeopathic remedies are prepared from almost anything that can be used to help relieve disease. The process of preparing homeopathic remedies is complex and includes the process of dilution in a solution of water and alcohol. Frequently, the remedy dilution is so great that no trace of the original substance remains. The process of dilution imprints the energetic pattern of the material into the solution.

The homeopathic approach toward disease is different from the allopathic approach. Homeopaths take into consideration all aspects of health, including the physical, mental, emotional, and spiritual life. Every occurrence that is connected with the onset of the ailment is considered. The information gathered during case taking is extensive. Once a treatment plan is made, a single remedy or a combination remedy is administered, most often in the form of a liquid or small pills that are placed sublingually.

Mind-Body Interventions

Aromatherapy

Aromatherapy is described as the therapeutic application of essential oils through the skin using the mediums of lotions, creams, or baths or the methods of inhalation or massage. Essential oils are highly concentrated complex essences obtained from flowers, leaves, stems, barks, fruits, seeds, and resins. Each of the hundreds of oils has specific effects and different properties. As the oils are absorbed into the body, there are pharmacologic, physiologic, and psychologic reactions. The ancient practice of aromatherapy has been found in Chinese and Greek literature, and it has experienced a revival in Europe, the United States, and Canada.

Only a trained aromatherapist should administer aromatherapy; many essential oils should be avoided during pregnancy because they have uterine-stimulating and emmenagogic effects (Box 5-1).

Hypnotherapy

Hypnotherapy is a form of deep relaxation with an alert mind producing alpha waves. In this state, critical faculties are suspended and the subconscious mind can be more easily accessed (Tiran and Mack, 2000). Hypnotherapy can be likened to deep relaxation, daydreaming, or meditation in which a similar state is experienced. This state of mind is a naturally occurring phenomenon that we have all experienced; therefore it can be assumed that there is no intrinsic danger when administered by a highly trained professional.

Spiritual Healing and Prayer

Spiritual healing and *prayer* are terms that define a wide range of different belief systems and the power that these beliefs have to heal the body and spirit. Spirituality is a basic human need. Although spirituality is believed to be associated with religion, the concept of spirituality goes beyond religion. Conventional medicine has traditionally ignored the mind-body connection and its impact on health and healing; prayer and spiritual healing are avenues to incorporate this type of healing system into the mainstream. It is important for health care professionals to be sensitive to all the belief systems that exist.

Benefits of spiritual healing and prayer include availability of an increased support system and community, increased self-esteem and self-love, and increased connectedness to the divine. Increased spirituality has been associated with decreased maternal complications in labor and delivery and fewer neonatal intensive care unit admissions (Petrie and Peck, 2000).

Box 5-1	Aromatherapy Oils That Are Completely Contraindicated During Pregnancy		
Arnica	Deer tongue	Rue	
Bitter almond	Dwarf pine	Sassafras	
Boldo leaf	Elecampane	Savin	
Broom	Exotic basil	Summer savory	
Buchu	Fennel (bitter)	Tansy	
Calamus	Horseradish	Thuja	
Camphor	Jaborandi leaf	Tonki	
Cassia	Mugwort (armoise)	Vanilla	
Chervil	Mustard	Wintergreen	
Cinnamon bark	Origanum	Wormseed	
Clove	Pennyroyal	Wormwood	
Costus			

From Tiran D, Mack S: *Complementary therapies for pregnancy and childbirth*, ed 2, London, 2000, Bailliere Tindall.

Yoga

Yoga is a mind-body exercise based on East Indian philosophy, and it has been practiced for nearly 6000 years. It has been said that the highest level of yoga is the recognition of the true self. There are many types of yoga, each including a vast repertoire of asanas (postures, positions, or connections) that establish a relationship to the earth. These are performed while standing, sitting, or lying on the floor. Prenatal yoga is a subspecialty.

Benefits of yoga include increased flexibility, increased muscle strength and cardiorespiratory endurance, improved mental attitude, increased self-esteem, better sleep, healthier eating habits, and better communication pathways between body, mind, and spirit. As with any new exercise program, there are basic guidelines to keep in mind: go slowly, listen to the body, pay attention to warning signals, and, most important, keep at it.

Biologic-Based Therapies

Herbal Medicine

Herbal medicine is defined as the use of crude plant-based products to treat, prevent, or cure a disease. It is undoubtedly the earliest form of medicine. In the United States there are two main systems used for prescribing botanical medicine: TCM and Western herbalism. This section focuses on the application of herbs according to the system developed in the West. Chinese herbs are covered in the Traditional Chinese Medicine section.

In the United States, herbs are not classified as drugs by the Food and Drug Administration, but they can be considered drugs from the medical perspective because many provoke a pharmacologic response within the body. This dispels the myth that because herbs are natural, they are always safe. When used by a trained practitioner, herbal therapy can provide effective treatment with low risk for side effects. Herbal medicine is health-oriented rather than disease-oriented and can be administered by infusions, decoctions, tinctures, and oils.

Box 5-2 lists herbs that should be avoided or used only with caution by a trained herbalist. Many of the herbs listed are abortifacients and are used to induce labor. For more specific and exhaustive lists of components and properties of herbs produced in Western medicine and their effects on pregnancy, refer to the book *Natural Medicines: Comprehensive Database, 2000* (Pharmacist's Letter, 2000). Herbal remedies can be used during pregnancy to treat many ailments, such as hypertension, dysglycemia, nausea and vomiting, threatened miscarriage, varicose veins, hemorrhoids, constipation, anemia, heartburn, cystitis, herpes, fatigue, mood changes, and bacterial, fungal and yeast infections.

Nutritional Therapy

Nutritional therapy includes the use of vitamins, minerals, amino acids, enzymes, and natural food supplements to maintain health or treat disease. Vitamins are essential to all life and contribute to good health by regulating the metabolism and assisting the biochemical processes that release energy from digested food.

Box 5-2   Herbal Remedies That Are Contraindicated or to Be Used with Caution During Pregnancy

Common Name	Latin Name
Arborvitae	*Thuja occidentalis*
Barberry	*Berberis vulgaris*
Beth root	*Trillium erectum*
Black cohosh	*Cimicifuga racemosa*
Blue cohosh	*Caulophyllum thalictroides*
Cinchona bark	*Cinchona* spp.
Cotton root bark	*Gossypium herbaceum*
Goldenseal	*Hydrastis canadensis*
Juniper	*Juniperus communis*
Motherwort	*Leonurus cardiaca*
Mugwort	*Artemisia vulgaris*
Pennyroyal	*Mentha pulegium*
Poke root	*Phytolacca americana*
Rue	*Ruta graveolens*
Sage	*Salvia officinalis*
Squaw vine	*Mitchella repens*
Tansy	*Tanacetum vulgare*
Wormwood	*Artemisia absinthium*

From Tiran D, Mack S: *Complementary therapies for pregnancy and childbirth*, ed 2, London, 2000, Bailliere Tindall.

Minerals are needed by every living cell to ensure proper function and structure. They are needed for proper composition of body fluids, formation of blood and bone, maintenance of healthy nerve function, and regulation of muscle tone, including that of the muscles of the cardiovascular system. Amino acids are the chemical units or building blocks that make up protein. Protein is a necessary part of every living cell in the body, including the muscles, ligaments, tendons, organs, glands, nails, hair, bones, and many vital body fluids. Enzymes are energized protein molecules that act as catalysts to hundreds of thousands of biochemical reactions that control life's processes. They are essential for digesting food, stimulating the brain, providing cellular energy, and repairing all tissues, organs, and cells. Natural food supplements include a wide variety of products. In general, they can be high in certain nutrients, contain active ingredients that aid in the digestive or metabolic processes, or provide a combination of nutrients and active ingredients.

Manipulative and Body-Based Methods

Chiropractic

The science of *chiropractic* focuses on the relationship of the nervous system to the mechanical framework of the body. Chiropractors generally manipulate only the protruding parts of the spinal vertebrae, but the focus is on attaining a holistic balance of the body.

The aims of chiropractic treatment during pregnancy (Tiran and Mack, 2000) are to:

- Improve spinal alignment and stability of the pelvis
- Minimize musculoskeletal and related discomforts
- Optimize neurologic function
- Improve posture
- Provide a better space and environment for the baby
- Reduce stress
- Enhance self-image and feelings of well-being
- Enable the body to work at its optimum during and after labor
- Accelerate postpartum recovery

Massage Therapy

Therapeutic massage is defined as: The scientific art and system of the assessment of and manual application to the superficial soft tissue of skin, muscles, tendons, ligaments, fascia, and the structures that lie within the superficial tissue by using the hand, foot, knee, arm, elbow, or forearm through the systematic external application of touch, stroking (effleurage), friction, vibration, percussion, kneading [pétrissage], stretching, compression, or passive and active joint movements within the normal physiologic range of motion. Also included are adjunctive external applications of water, heat, and cold for the purposes of establishing and maintaining good physical condition and health through normalizing and improving muscle tone, promoting relaxation, stimulating circulation, and producing therapeutic effects on the respiratory and nervous systems, and the subtle interactions between all body systems. These intended effects are accomplished through the energetic and mind-body connections in a safe, nonsexual environment that respects the client's self-determined outcome for the session (Fritz, 2004).

The benefits of therapeutic massage therapy are vast and include physical, emotional, and mental effects. Gentle massage can be especially beneficial for the woman with a high risk pregnancy complicated by multiple gestation, preterm labor, or both (see Chapter 23). Massage and manual therapies are safe during pregnancy when administered gently, avoiding pressure on the abdomen and uterus and prolonged supine positioning during therapy sessions.

Physically, massage can reduce cortisol levels and blood pressure, increase the flow of lymph through the body, and increase immunity. It can also stretch and loosen muscles, improve blood flow, facilitate the removal of metabolic waste, and increase the flow of oxygen and nutrients to cells and tissue. Most important, massage stimulates the release of endorphins and decreases pain. On a mental level, massage therapy increases relaxation, reduces mental stress, and enhances clarity and creative thinking. Emotionally, massage satisfies the need for human touch and caring, which increases the sense of well-being and reduces anxiety levels.

Osteopathy

Osteopathy focuses on restoring and maintaining balance in the neuromusculoskeletal systems of the body. In comparison with chiropractors, osteopaths use arms and legs as fulcrums to bend and twist the body; this is called *long-lever manipulation.* The osteopath aims to preserve the balance between joints, muscles, ligamentous structures, and nerves, which allows the body to function at its most optimal capability. Osteopathic treatment is safe, gentle, and noninvasive and therefore appropriate for pregnant women. There are a few side effects and a few contraindications to treatment, including (Tiran and Mack, 2000) any history of or threatened miscarriage, active pathology, inflammatory conditions, and some cases of joint hypermobility. Conditions that can benefit from osteopathy include sciatica, carpal tunnel syndrome, neuralgia paraesthetica, diabetes, symphysis pubis pain, coccydynia, edematous ankles, indigestion and heartburn, and round ligament pain.

Energy Therapies

Cranial Sacral Therapy

The osteopathic physician John Upledger pioneered cranial sacral therapy in the United States. *Cranial sacral therapy* is a gentle, hands-on method of evaluating and enhancing the functioning of a physiologic body system called the *craniosacral system*, which is comprised of the membranes and cerebrospinal fluid that surround and protect the brain and spinal cord.

By complementing the body's natural healing process, cranial sacral therapy is increasingly used as a preventative health measure for its ability to bolster resistance to disease, and it is effective for a wide range of medical problems associated with pain and dysfunction.

Polarity

Polarity is a holistic, natural health care system, founded by Dr. Randolph Stone, combining the discoveries of quantum physics with the wisdom of the ancients. It is based on the premise that we are fields of pulsating life-force energy made up of specific frequencies known as the five elements: ether, air, fire, water, and earth. Each element relates and flows in a balance of positive and negative attractions arising from a neutral center. Imbalances and blockages can arise when our thoughts, emotions, and physical body are out of alignment. Polarity teaches that pain and discomfort are signals for us to learn, change, and realign our lives.

A polarity practitioner works together with the client using the tools of bodywork, exercise, nutrition, and verbal guidance to evaluate and balance life-force energy. Polarity bodywork involves gentle rocking, stretching, and pressure-sensitive touching based on energy flow. Polarity exercises are easy yoga-type stretching postures that combine sound, breath, and self-massage. Polarity nutrition views food as energy and develops an ongoing, ever-changing, and creative nutritional awareness rather than a rigid set of rules. Polarity verbal guidance is based on the assumption that "right thinking" is the cornerstone of good health. Verbal processes involve understanding and feeling our emotions, taking responsibility for our lives, and creating life-enhancing thoughts.

Benefits of polarity therapy include release of pain and stiffness, increased relaxation, clearer thinking, greater flexibility, amplified energy levels, enhanced ability to cope with stress, improved communication and relationships, healthier lifestyle, and elevated levels of self-acceptance.

MANAGEMENT OF ALTERNATIVE AND COMPLEMENTARY THERAPIES IN PREGNANCY

Only those people who are trained in specific certified programs of study should apply the therapies and treatment modalities described in this section. No traditional providers should experiment with the use of therapies that are unfamiliar; they could cause harm if they do. It is essential that all providers of traditional therapies are aware of when to refer and to whom they should refer for certain conditions in high risk pregnancies.

Hyperemesis

Traditional Chinese Medicine

In TCM, hyperemesis occurs when there is a relative imbalance in the organ systems and meridians associated with digestion. The aim of treatment is to restore proper balance and stop nausea and vomiting. As with any TCM treatment, a collection of points is selected according to the individual pattern of disharmony.

Stimulation of the acupuncture point P6 (Nei guan) has been shown in multiple trials to be effective in reducing nausea and vomiting. This point is therefore added to almost all acupuncture protocols. The number of acupuncture treatments varies greatly according to the individual patient and severity of illness. In most cases, there is improvement after the first treatment. Three to five points are usually chosen. The intensity and duration of the sickness has a direct relationship to the state of the woman's digestive system (spleen and stomach meridians) before conception. The effects of the acupuncture calm the digestive system, decrease fatigue, expel phlegm, and decrease nausea and vomiting. To prevent hyperemesis in future pregnancies, it is recommended to start acupuncture treatments a couple of months before conception to balance and build the digestion and the spleen-stomach organ system.

In a study conducted in China of a formula consisting of 11 herbs, about 90% of patients with nausea and vomiting showed improvement within 2 days. Most symptoms disappeared within 10 days (Jin, 2003).

Homeopathic Approaches

Homeopathy can be an excellent choice for treatment of hyperemesis because small tasteless pills are dissolved under the tongue with little chance of inducing nausea and vomiting. *Sepia* is the remedy most helpful for ordinary nausea and vomiting of pregnancy. It is indicated when nausea is intensified by the smell or thought of foods, and/or when the woman is regarded as irritable, emotional, and selfish because of her need to be alone and quiet. *Pulsatilla* is another excellent remedy that should be used when symptoms include intolerance of warm rooms, improvement in the open air, and sensitivity to fatty or rich foods, bread, milk, or fruit. *Nux Vomica* is the remedy of choice when the patient exhibits nervous hyperstimulation with a history of drug abuse or intolerance, constipation, insomnia or ailments from lack of sleep or emotional excitement. *Ignatia* is given when there is evidence of acute grief, sorrow or disappointment. *Phosphorus* is very effective for ailments of pregnancy and is recommended when there are complaints related to an overactive imagination with exaggerated fears, burning pains, and thirst for cold drinks. Homeopathic *Ipecac* is most likely to be helpful when the condition is characterized by severe and constant nausea unrelieved by vomiting; undiluted ipecac is a very strong purgative and should never be used in pregnancy (Moskowitz, 1992). These remedies can be used alone or in combination, but caution needs to be used to ensure the homeopathic preparations of these substances are not confused with herbal products.

Hypnotherapy

When emotional factors are implicated in the cause of hyperemesis, the use of hypnosis with positive suggestions can be helpful. One approach involves the removal of any fears of hypnosis, along with an explanation of the role of the vomiting center in the brain and how it works, coupled with a general discussion about the value of good nutrition in pregnancy. Guided imagery can also be used with the mother imagining herself eating, enjoying, and retaining familiar foods in a relaxed environment where she feels safe and secure.

Herbal Therapy

The cutaneous application of wild yam cream has been anecdotally reported to reduce nausea and vomiting (Petrie and Peck, 2000). Dandelion root tea calms and strengthens the stomach, improves the appetite, and supports the liver. An infusion of ginger (in small amounts), chamomile, peppermint, catnip, fennel, red raspberry, or lemon balm can also help.

Nutritional Therapy

Food therapy includes recommendation of eating small portions of bland cooked foods frequently. Eating protein can help sustain blood sugar levels. Avoiding greasy, fatty, and sugary foods can be beneficial. Carbonated or noncarbonated water with a squeeze of lemon, grape, grapefruit, or orange juice can be a palatable way to replenish fluids. It is best to avoid coffee, soda, and other caffeine- or sugar-laden drinks. Herbal formulas also can be administered.

Common nutritional deficiencies include too little iron, vitamin B (specifically B_6, pyridoxine) (Petrie and Peck, 2000), magnesium, calcium, and protein. It can be difficult for a woman with hyperemesis to take vitamins. It is best for her to take vitamins with food because they are easier to digest and less likely to induce nausea and vomiting (see Chapter 1 for more specific traditional nutritional approaches).

Cranial Sacral and Polarity Therapy

Cranial sacral and polarity therapies can be used together energetically to normalize the adaptational processes of the body. If anxiety or any other emotional subjects are at the root of the sickness, these therapies allow the body, mind, and spirit to integrate and relax in a nurturing environment.

Breech Presentation

Traditional Chinese Medicine

The use of acupuncture and TCM to correct breech presentation has attracted much attention. The technique involves stimulation of acupuncture point UB 67, located on the lateral edge of the small toe, with laser, acupuncture, electroacupuncture, or moxibustion. The technique using moxibustion involves gently heating UB 67 for 15 minutes once a day for 10 days total. It is recommended to pause after the fifth day for a couple of days and to check for change in fetal positioning. If the fetal position has not corrected, the treatment can be resumed for another 5 days (Maciocia, 2005).

It is believed that this technique increases corticoadrenal secretion through the increase of placental estrogens and changes in prostaglandin levels. This, in turn, raises the basal tone and enhances uterine contractility, thus stimulating fetal activity (Maciocia, 2005). Studies conducted in China report varying success ranging from 80.9% to 90.3% (Tiran and Mack, 2000). Studies conducted in Italy reported success rates of 66.6% (Cardini and Marcolongo, 1993) and 75.4% (Cardini and Weixin, 1998). Most research papers on moxibustion show the highest rate of success to occur at 34 weeks of gestation, making this the optimal time to administer the technique (Yelland, 2004).

Auricular stimulation therapy using a seed of *Vaccaria segetalis* on seven acupuncture points located on the ear was shown to increase the rotation to a cephalic position (Petrie and Peck, 2000).

Homeopathy

The homeopathic remedy *Pulsatilla* may potentially be successful in encouraging babies to turn.

Hypnotherapy

Hypnotherapy techniques using imagery can be helpful. It has been demonstrated that patients may experience successful turning of the baby when they attend weekly office hypnosis sessions providing suggestions for general relaxation and release of anxiety and fear in addition to listening to relaxation tapes at home. Hypnosis has been used to facilitate both spontaneous and external versions (Petrie and Peck, 2000).

Constipation

Traditional Chinese Medicine

There is a physiologic disposition for constipation during pregnancy. From the TCM point of view, it can be caused by an insufficient amount of qi and nutrients or an excess of stagnated qi. It is difficult to treat constipation during pregnancy, whether by acupuncture or herbs, because the basic treatment principle of moving qi downward is absolutely forbidden during pregnancy. Treatment is further complicated because no acupuncture points on the abdomen can be used. A skilled TCM practitioner will make dietary recommendations, prescribe safe herbal formulas, and manipulate approved points with gentle acupuncture.

Aromatherapy

The use of essential oils during pregnancy is controversial. Some aromatherapy schools condone the use of essential oils throughout pregnancy, even during the critical first three months, whereas others question the safety of their use during pregnancy at all. Citrus oils, including mandarin orange and grapefruit, used in conjunction with the massage technique described in the following text can help relieve constipation.

Yoga and Exercise

Lifestyle changes, such as adding a brisk walk each morning, can be a great boost to the digestion as well as promoting regular bowel movements. Many yoga exercises may also be beneficial. It is helpful to set aside time each day to sit on the toilet to encourage regularity. During this time, relaxation methods focusing on releasing the abdominal and pelvic floor muscles may help.

Herbal Therapy

Herbal medicine offers a variety of herbs to aid in the relief of constipation. It is important to avoid botanicals that act as strong laxatives, purgatives, and cathartics. Herbs such as dandelion root, yellow dock, flax or psyllium seeds, catnip, or cramp-bark can all be used.

Nutritional Therapy

Nutritional therapies can play an important part in relieving constipation. Eating an abundance of fresh vegetables and two pieces of fresh fruit a day can add bulk to the stool. It may also help to add a fiber supplement for this purpose. Congesting foods such as cheese, meat, and greasy foods should be avoided or eliminated. Water is also very important; a half to a whole gallon of water should be consumed daily.

Massage Therapy

Massage, especially gentle abdominal massage following the route of the large intestine in a clockwise direction, can help stimulate peristaltic movement.

Mental and Emotional Problems

Traditional Chinese Medicine

In Chinese medical theory, mental and emotional problems have a connection to the organ systems. Energetic disharmonies on the physical level can give rise to mental and emotional disharmonies, just as long-standing mental and emotional problems can give rise to physical problems.

Depression during pregnancy and the postpartum period are common, but it is imperative to refer a patient with severe symptoms to a qualified health care professional for immediate evaluation and care. Both acupuncture and Chinese herbs are generally effective for the treatment of minor mental and emotional problems. Acupuncture is preferred during the first 3 months of pregnancy. Prognosis depends on the TCM diagnosis. Depression related to pregnancy responds better to treatment than long-standing clinical depression and inherited chemical imbalances. The University of Arizona is conducting a study on acupuncture and the treatment of depression. So far, the results have been favorable. Stanford University is also beginning to research the efficacy of acupuncture treatment for depression during pregnancy.

Homeopathy

There are many different remedies that can treat mental and emotional problems; this is one of the biggest strengths of homeopathy. The diagnosis and treatment is intricate and individualized. Many factors are taken into account when a remedy is prescribed. Because of this, specific remedies will not be listed.

Aromatherapy

Neroli essential oil works as an antidepressant and is effective in alleviating nervousness, tension, and anxiety. *Chamomile* has a soothing and calming nature and helps promote sleep and rest. *Geranium* and *lavender essential oils* can also be used for their antidepressant qualities during the third trimester.

Hypnotherapy

Hypnotherapy promotes deep relaxation and offers a way to get in touch with deeper emotions in a safe atmosphere. Many techniques may promote the reduction of stress and anxiety.

Spiritual Healing and Prayer

Getting in touch with the divine and acknowledging a higher purpose in life can promote a general sense of stability and well-being. Counseling within the patient's religion or spirituality of choice can also be beneficial.

Yoga

Practicing yoga fosters an improvement in self-awareness and self-image. It also promotes physical health that is interconnected with mental-emotional health.

Herbal Therapy

Western herbs that can help promote relaxation include chamomile, oatstraw, lemon balm, lavender flowers, skullcap, dandelion, and valerian. All of these herbs are commonly prescribed by trained practitioners.

Cranial Sacral and Polarity Therapy

Both cranial sacral and polarity therapies work on integrating the mind, body, and spirit while promoting relaxation and stimulating the body to heal itself.

Nutritional Therapy

Nutritional deficiencies, dehydration, and lack of exercise can also contribute to mental and emotional problems. Maintaining a nutritious diet with adequate fruits, vegetables, whole grains, and lean meats can prevent mood swings caused by low blood sugar levels. Daily intake of six to eight glasses of water along with daily walking or other exercise can promote mental and physical health. Holistic theory believes that mental health is congruent with physical health and vice versa.

Low Back Pain

Traditional Chinese Medicine

Low back pain is a common problem in the last trimester of pregnancy. Acupuncture is recognized for its success in treating musculoskeletal pain, including low back problems. Low back pain is often improved within a few treatments and usually has lasting effects. The etiology of the pain is diagnosed primarily through assessments of pulse and tongue characteristics, and sensitivity of acupuncture points, which are chosen to alleviate discomfort. Both distal and local points are selected.

Yoga and Exercise

Yoga is also beneficial in balancing and strengthening the musculoskeletal system. For the best results, yoga should be started before conception or at the beginning of the pregnancy to strengthen the body in preparation for the increased weight of the baby in the third trimester. Yoga can promote good posture, which can help prevent sciatic nerve discomfort as well as back pain.

Swimming can also help relieve back pain and is quite refreshing toward the end of pregnancy. It is a great way to become weightless and provides an effective low-impact exercise. Exercise in general is a good way to relieve muscular and emotional tension and can significantly improve back problems.

Herbal Medicine

Topically, arnica can be used to relieve low back pain. A warm bath with Epsom salt and aromatherapy oils such as lavender, rosemary, chamomile, and lemon balm can help relax the muscles. Some Western herbs that can help relieve low back pain during labor are skullcap, St. John's wort, black haw, and crampbark (Petrie and Peck, 2000).

Nutritional Therapy

Nutritional deficiencies such as insufficient calcium and magnesium can lead to muscle aches and lowered threshold of discomfort. Food sources of calcium include milk, hard cheeses, yogurt, leafy green vegetables, almonds, sea vegetables, salmon, and blackstrap molasses. It is best to avoid coffee, chocolate, cola, cocoa, and red meats.

Chiropractic

Chiropractic care has been proven to be effective in the treatment of acute low back pain and can be safely administered during pregnancy (Petrie and Peck, 2000).

Massage and Bodywork

Massage and bodywork can also treat low back pain. Most pregnancy body-workers have special pillows that can accommodate comfortable positions for the end of the pregnancy. Benefits of massage and bodywork are twofold: massage can not only reduce pain and increase circulation, but also relax and promote well-being.

Osteopathy

Osteopathy is excellent at correcting sacroiliac problems and sciatica. Manipulations are used based on an accurate diagnosis and mostly involve long-leverage techniques.

Hypertensive Disorders

Traditional Chinese Medicine

There is no TCM category that encompasses pregnancy-induced hypertension, pre-eclampsia, and eclampsia. In the book *Obstetrics and Gynecology in Chinese Medicine,* Maciocia (2005) categorized these diseases according to their symptoms in pregnancy, which include edema, dizziness, headache, and convulsions. Hospital admission and careful evaluation may be necessary. Acupuncture should be used only as an adjunctive therapy to enhance the effects of conventional medical treatment.

Nutritional Therapy

Diet and food therapy have a role in the treatment of hypertension, and a thorough dietary evaluation should be included in the initial assessment of all patients. General recommendations are increased consumption of whole grains, high-quality protein (100 g/day), calcium, and potassium-rich foods such as beets, greens, and bananas with the avoidance of refined foods. Specific foods for reducing high blood pressure include cheese, yogurt, nuts, seeds, fish, watermelon, cucumbers, parsley, buckwheat, raw onions, and garlic. It is also important to drink at least eight cups of liquid daily.

Yoga and Exercise

Daily exercise helps to improve circulation. Yoga, walking, swimming, or any exercise that stimulates circulation is excellent for prevention of high blood pressure. Yoga gives the added benefit of incorporating relaxation therapy, which in turn also reduces the risk for increased blood pressure. For more benefit, add 20 minutes of relaxation therapy to daily exercise.

Herbal Therapy

If a rise in blood pressure is caused by stress and anxiety, herbs can help. Western herbs for the treatment of hypertension include dandelion leaf and root, nettles, red raspberry, hawthorn berry, lemon balm, chamomile, lavender, hops, oat straw, lime blossom, skullcap, valerian, passion flower, lady's slipper, and wood betony.

Massage Therapy

Massage therapy can promote deep relaxation and stimulate the removal of fluids from the body. Massage therapy is applicable for mild hypertensive disorders.

Preterm Labor

Traditional Chinese Medicine

Premature labor is generally considered a deficiency condition; the body does not have enough qi to "hold" the baby in position. Acupuncture and Chinese herbal therapy are aimed at tonifying the qi of the body, thus stopping premature contractions.

The stimulation of the acupuncture point Spleen 4 has been shown to help the body carry the baby to term (Petrie and Peck, 2000).

Hypnotherapy

Audio-guided relaxation sessions combined with pharmacologic treatments have been demonstrated to postpone labor better than pharmacologic therapies alone (Petrie and Peck, 2000).

Induction of Labor

Traditional Chinese Medicine

Acupuncture, acupressure, and Chinese herbs have been found to be effective in the induction of labor. Women choose to be induced for various reasons, ranging from elective to mandatory. In approximately 12 separate clinical studies of the induction of labor with acupuncture, no negative side effects have been reported or identified (Tiran and Mack, 2000). One to three acupuncture treatments in conjunction with Chinese herbs can induce labor within 2 to 72 hours. Elective induction is not recommended before 38 weeks of gestation because success rates are higher closer to term.

Induction of labor by acupuncture involves using electroacupuncture equipment to intensely stimulate the "forbidden" points of pregnancy. Contractions are usually felt immediately and most often have lasting effects. There are specific acupuncture points for cervical dilation and for production of uterine contractions. If uterine contractions do not persist after the first treatment, another treatment is recommended within the next 48 hours, followed by ingestion of a Chinese herbal prescription. Acupuncture can be used to complement conventional medical induction techniques.

Homeopathy

Remedies such as *Pulsatilla, Secale cornutum, Caulophyllum thalictroides, Cimicifuga,* and *Arnica montana* can be used daily for 1 to 2 weeks before the due date. These can limit false labor, protracted first stages, and postpartum blood loss. Homeopathy remedies such as blue cohosh and *Pulsatilla* can be given during labor to stimulate progress.

Herbal Therapy

Blue cohosh and black cohosh are Western herbs often used to stimulate the uterus, ripen the cervix, and induce or augment labor. These herbs should **never** be used in conjunction with Pitocin. Evening primrose oil, taken orally or applied locally to the cervix, can also augment labor.

Analgesia in Labor

Traditional Chinese Medicine

The use of acupuncture as analgesia began in the 1950s in China with the integration of TCM and conventional medical care. *Acupuncture analgesia* refers to the pain-relieving effects and the physiologic regulatory effects obtained after stimulation of specific acupuncture points on the patient (Tureanu and Tureanu, 1999).

Both distal and local points are used, including points on the ear, limbs, and lower back. The amount of pain relief is subjective and therefore hard to ascertain precisely and objectively. Study results vary tremendously. In most cases, pain relief is significant.

Hydrotherapy

Water and baths offer a soothing and relaxing form of pain relief, which also help soften the perineal tissues. Women have been using water therapy for as long as they have had access to baths and hot water. Most women find water to be comforting and, once immersed, they have an easier time letting go and allowing labor to take its course. Access to a water bath may be easier to attain at a birth center than in the hospital. If a water birth is an option, it is important to plan ahead. Some considerations follow (Wesson, 2000):

- Hospital or birth center policy
- Birth attendant's clinical experience with water births
- Cost
- Type of pool
- Floor strength, space requirements, heating and electrical safety subjects

Herbal Therapy

Some Western herbs help decrease pain and tone the uterus for labor and delivery. Raspberry leaf tea has been consumed to help women have an easier labor. It tones the uterus and is a source of iron and vitamin C. Most women drink three cups a day during the last trimester. Skullcap is an antispasmodic that relaxes muscles and acts as a tonic to the nervous system. Motherwort is an herb that can be used for pain relief in the early part of a regular labor. St. John's wort can be useful for controlling anxiety and spasms. The practitioner must always obtain a thorough medication history and be aware of potential drug and herb interactions during labor and childbirth.

Aromatherapy

There are essential oils that can tone the uterus, encourage contractions, reduce pain, relieve tension and spasms, diminish fear and anxiety, and enhance the feeling of well-being. Clove bud oil can help reduce pain and is a stimulant and antispasmodic. Rose oil acts as an antidepressant, sedative, and uterine tonic. Clary sage is a specific pain reliever for labor and also acts as an antidepressant and sedative. It should not be used during pregnancy, but it is valuable during labor. Neroli oil helps to reduce fear, anxiety, and inhibitions. Jasmine oil strengthens contractions and reduces feelings of pain and panic.

Homeopathy

Homeopathy can be used to help relieve pain in labor. *Caulophyllum* may help when contractions are ineffective or when the cervix is too rigid. It can also be used during the last trimester of pregnancy to prepare for childbirth. *Pulsatilla* promotes irregular contractions and has also been used to turn a malpositioned baby. *Kali carbonicum* decreases pain in the back, buttocks, and thighs. *Cimicifuga* is effective in reducing feelings of fear and despair, as well as alleviating the pain of contractions that improve when the mother lies on her left side.

Massage Therapy

Massage and counterpressure techniques can be applied during contractions to reduce lumbar and sacroiliac pain. A variety of massage techniques have been shown to be safe and effective during labor (Petrie and Peck, 2000).

Addictions

Traditional Chinese Medicine

In 1985, substance abuse counselors and acupuncturists formed the National Acupuncture Detoxification Association to support treatment of addictions. A treatment protocol was developed at the Lincoln Hospital Substance Abuse Clinic and is being used in hundreds of settings across the country. Acupuncture detoxification can assist recovery in many ways. Biochemical effects include increased endorphin production, which results in an improved ability to cope with stress, withdrawal symptoms, and cravings. The body's natural detoxification process is strengthened. Psychologically, acupuncture enhances the sense of vitality and well-being and reinforces the ability to stay clean. Benefits include reduced cravings and stress, increased ability to solve the problems of daily living, and increased feelings of relaxation and self-confidence.

The treatment protocol consists of bilateral insertion of needles into five ear points. The duration of the treatment can be 25 to 45 minutes, depending on the need of the patient. In the acute withdrawal phase, which can last from 1 to 30 days, acupuncture is recommended five times a week or more. During the postacute withdrawal phase, which may last 6 months or longer, treatment is recommended for a minimum of three times a week. Follow-up treatments are assessed on an individual basis to prevent relapse. As with any other addiction therapy, support groups and counseling are recommended.

Hypnotherapy

Hypnotherapy and other relaxation techniques can be used in conjunction with conventional therapies to increase the success of addiction recovery.

Postpartum Bleeding

Traditional Chinese Medicine

There are acupuncture points that specifically stop bleeding, in particular Spleen 1, which can be used in conjunction with conventional methods to increase effectiveness.

Herbal Therapy

The Western herb Shepherd's purse can be administered in tea or tincture form to help control postpartum bleeding. Yarrow is also regarded as an excellent homeostatic agent and is often used with Shepherd's purse. Cinnamon and cayenne have also been used effectively.

Table 5-1 Evidence-Based Databases

Database	Description	Web Address
Combined Health Information Database (CHID)	Easy retrieval of journal citations for professionals, patients, and the general population about different health topics	http://cehn.org/cehn/resourceguide/chid.html
CRISP	Searchable database of federally funded biomedical research projects	http://crisp.cit.nih.gov
IBIDS Database	Database of published, international, scientific literature on dietary supplements, including vitamins, minerals, and botanicals	http://grande.nal.usda.gov/ibids/index.php
Consumer Lab	Reports of product reviews	http://consumerlab.com/
Clinical Trial	Reports of clinical trials	http://clinicaltrials.gov

CHID, Combined health information database; *CRISP*, computer retrieval of information on scientific projects; *IBIDS*, international bibliographic information on dietary supplements.

CONCLUSION

Nurses and other health care practitioners should be aware of this growing body of knowledge and recognize when to refer patients for complementary or alternative treatment. When making a referral, the health care practitioner needs information about the education, training, credentialing, and licensing of the practitioner to whom they are referring the patient. In order to keep abreast of this ever-changing body of medicine, refer to Table 5-1 for evidence-based databases.

BIBLIOGRAPHY
General

Fontaine K: *Complementary and alternative therapies for nursing practice*, ed 2, Upper Saddle River, NJ, 2005, Prentice Hall.

National Center for Complementary and Alternative Medicine (NCCAM): *What is complementary and alternative medicine?* Gaithersburg, Md, 2006, National Institutes of Health. Retrieved from http://nccam.nih.gov.

Petrie P, Peck M: Alternative medicine in maternity care, *Prim Care* 27(1):117–136, 2000.

Tiran D, Mack S: *Complementary therapies for pregnancy and childbirth*, ed 2, London, 2000, Bailliere Tindall.

Wesson N: *Labor pain: a natural approach to easing delivery*, Rochester, VT, 2000, Healing Arts Press.

Traditional Chinese Medicine

Abouleish E, Depp R: Acupuncture in obstetrics, *Anesth Analg* 54(1):82–88, 1975.

al-Sadi M, Newman B, Julious S: Acupuncture in the prevention of postoperative nausea and vomiting, *Anaesthesia* 52(7):658–661, 1997.

Cardini F, Marcolongo A: Moxibustion for correction of breech presentation: a clinical study with retrospective control, *Am J Chin Med* 21(2):133–138, 1993.

Cardini F, Weixin H: Moxibustion for correction of breech presentation: a randomized controlled trial, *JAMA* 280(18):1580–1584, 1998.

de Aloysio D, Penacchioni P: Morning sickness control in early pregnancy by Neiguan point acupressure, *Obstet Gynecol* 80(5):852–854, 1992.

Holland A: *Voices of qi: an introductory guide to traditional Chinese medicine*, Seattle, 1997, Northwest Institute of Acupuncture and Oriental Medicine.

Jin Y: *Handbook of obstetrics and gynecology in Chinese medicine: an integrated approach*, Seattle, 2003, Eastland Press.

Li Q, Wang L: Clinical observation on correcting malposition of fetus by electro acupuncture, *J Tradit Chin Med* 16(4):260–262, 1996.

Maciocia G: *Obstetrics and gynecology in Chinese medicine*, ed 2, New York, 2005, Churchill Livingstone.

Martoudis S, Christofides K: Electroacupuncture for pain relief during labor, *Acupunct Med* 8(2):51, 1990.

Moskowitz, R: *Homeopathic medicines for pregnancy and childbirth*, 1992, North Atlantic Books.

Tureanu V, Tureanu L: *Acupuncture in obstetrics and gynecology*, St Louis, 1999, Warren H. Green.

West Z: *Acupuncture in pregnancy and childbirth*, London, 2001, Churchill Livingstone.

Yelland S: *Acupuncture in midwifery*, ed 2, Cheshire, England, 2004, Books for Midwives Press.

Zhao CX: Acupuncture treatment of morning sickness, *J Tradit Chin Med* 8(3):228–229, 1988.

Relaxation Therapy

Benson H, Stuart E: *The wellness book: the comprehensive guide to maintaining health and treating stress-related illness*, Boston, 1992, Mind Body Institute, New England Deaconess Hospital at Harvard Medical School.

Kolkmeier L: Relaxation: opening the door to change. In Dossey B, and others, editors: *Holistic nursing: a handbook for practice*, ed 2, Gaithersburg, Md, 1995, Aspen.

Massage and Bodywork

Fritz S: *Fundamentals of therapeutic massage*, St Louis, 2004, Mosby.

Yoga

Baker JP: *Prenatal yoga and natural birth*, ed 3, Monroe, UT, 2002, Freeston Publishing.

Balaskas J: *Preparing for birth with yoga*, London, 2003, Thorsons Publishers.

Homeopathy

Jacobs J, Moskowitz R: Homeopathy. In Micozzi M, editor: *Fundamentals of complementary and alternative medicine*, New York, 1996, Churchill Livingstone.

Lockie A, Geddes N: *Homeopathy: the principles and practice of treatment*, London, 2000, Dorling Kindersley.

Aromatherapy

Tiran D: *Clinical aromatherapy for pregnancy and childbirth*, London, 2000, Bailliere Tindall.

Tiran D, Mack S: *Complementary therapies for pregnancy and childbirth*, ed 2, London, 2000, Bailliere Tindall.

United States Essential Science Publishing: *People's desk reference for essential oils*, 2005, Essential Science Publishing.

Western Herbs

McIntyre A: *The herbal for mother and child*, Rockport, Mass, 2003, Elements Books.

Mills S, Bone K: *The essential guide to herbal safety*, New York, 2005, Churchill Livingstone.

Pharmacist's Letter and Prescriber's Letter: *Natural medicines: comprehensive database*, Stockton, Calif, 2000, Therapeutic Research Faculty.

6

Psychologic Adaptations

To understand the emotional work and psychologic adjustments a high risk mother and her family must accomplish, certain concepts should be examined. Understanding concepts of attachment, the tasks of pregnancy, and the concept of adaptation in relation to crisis, anxiety, and frustration can be helpful when developing a plan of care for a high risk pregnant family.

ATTACHMENT

Attachment is a process influenced by many complex factors and is a permanent, interactional, emotional bond that exists for life. Parent-infant attachment usually begins at the time the pregnancy is planned or during the pregnancy, even in many high risk pregnancies (Klaus and Kennell, 1982; Kemp and Page, 1987a).

Maternal

For the mother, attachment to the fetus is enhanced when the baby begins to move, the mother's body begins to change shape, and the uterus grows. Her focus is usually turned to the baby and its well-being, at which time she establishes a relationship with the fetus (Rubin, 1970; Gay, Edgil, and Douglas, 1988). If the mother is afraid the fetus may die, this attachment may not take place because she is too fearful to establish a relationship. If family relationships are strained, it is more difficult for an expectant mother to form a positive attachment with her baby (Gupton, Heaman, and Cheung, 2001).

Paternal

The father's attachment to the fetus differs from that of the mother's. Most of his attachment centers on acceptance and support of the mother's changing physical and emotional state. When a threat to maternal or fetal health develops, the father may feel guilty for his inability to protect the mother and the fetus and ensure a safe passage for them (Wohlreich, 1987). This may affect his attachment.

Influencing Factors

Parental attachment to the fetus and newborn depends on the following factors:

- Emotional maturity
- Experience in being nurtured
- Interpersonal relationships with significant others
- Ability to cope with physiologic and psychologic stressors
- Desire for pregnancy and self-concept of parenthood
- Fears and fantasies during the pregnancy

There is a sensitive period immediately after birth when attachment is enhanced through the interactions of parents with their infant. These interactions are categorized into observable sensory levels (Rubin, 1984; Sherwen, 1987).

Tactile

When given the opportunity, most parents will make immediate tactile contact with their infant. The initial contact is exploratory and is made with the fingertips. Progression of tactile contact follows an orderly pattern but can vary in its length of time. After the fingertips, the palms of the hands are used to stroke and massage the baby. Then the baby is drawn into close contact with the mother and encompassed (Tulman, 1985).

Verbal

Some parents make early verbal contact by carrying on a continual stream of soft, high-pitched verbalization (Tomlinson, 1990). The context usually involves relating how the infant resembles other family members.

Visual

Early eye-to-eye contact is sought even when the infant is not being held. The parents usually try to position themselves so that they and the infant are en face. If the infant does not open his or her eyes, they implore him or her to do so.

Entrainment

The speech pattern of either parent has a powerful influence on the infant's activity. The infant very soon forms activity patterns in a reciprocal relationship that resembles a dance. The infant's response in this manner seems to lock the parent into repeating speech over and over.

Synchrony

The first act of synchrony occurs in the feeding process. The mother responds to the infant's sucking bursts and pauses for breath. Mothers learn to respond in the cycles of sucking and pausing at the appropriate points to stimulate or discourage sucking.

If the neonate is sick and the parents' interactions and caregiving opportunities are limited, attachment may lag behind. However, according to Klaus and Kennell (1984), these parents become attached to their babies, but the attachment might be delayed.

MATERNAL TASKS

A series of developmental tasks must be accomplished in pregnancy for the mothering attachment behaviors to occur (Rubin, 1975; Gay, Edgil, and Douglas, 1988; Patterson, Freese, and Goldenberg, 1990).

Pregnancy Acceptance

Pregnancy validation or acceptance usually takes place during the first trimester when the woman determines that she is pregnant and begins securing acceptance of the pregnancy from significant others. During this time, she is concerned about herself and seeking "safe passage" for herself.

Establishing a Relationship with the Fetus

The pregnant woman begins to establish a relationship with the fetus when she can look beyond her concern about herself and focus on the fetus being part of her (fetal embodiment). This is when she becomes more dependent and wants to socialize with other pregnant women. As her relationship with her fetus grows, she begins to view the fetus as a separate individual from her (fetal distinction). The focus of safe passage at this time is for the fetus as well as for herself through prenatal care and making lifestyle changes.

Role Transition

Role transition involves preparing for the birth and early motherhood. Now the mother is seeking safe passage for herself and her baby during the delivery process.

PATERNAL TASKS

The expectant father's unconscious feelings and early memories of childhood play an important part in his emotional adjustment to the pregnancy. His involvement in the birth promotes and enhances nurturing behavior (Colman and Colman, 1971; Sherwen, 1987). The father's involvement and accomplishment of paternal tasks can be divided into three phases: the announcement phase, moratorium phase, and focusing phase (May, 1982; Diamond, 1986).

Announcement Phase

The announcement phase is the period when the pregnancy is first recognized and the father informs others of the pregnancy. This period varies in length from a few hours to a few weeks. It may be characterized by strong feelings of elation or shock, depending on the desire for the pregnancy. However, the father's response is usually mixed with pride, joy, concern, and conflict.

Moratorium Phase

The moratorium phase also varies in length, but typically spans from the 12th to the 25th week of gestation. The pregnancy does not seem real to the father during this time and is characterized by emotional distancing. Distancing allows the man to work through any ambivalence about what he will give up because of the pregnancy, such as an exclusive relationship with the mother-to-be, privacy, quiet home, and social freedom. He often spends more time at work because of his financial concerns. Marital tension and disrupted communication are common during this phase.

Focusing Phase

The focusing phase begins around the 25th to 30th week of gestation and extends to the onset of labor. The expectant father focuses on his experience, begins to feel more in tune with the mother, and redefines his world in terms of his future fatherhood role.

HIGH RISK STRESSORS

Stress is defined as any real or perceived difficulty that results in the release of stress hormones. Recent studies (Wadhwa and others, 1998; Teixeira, Fisk, and Glover, 1999) reconfirm a correlation between maternal stress during pregnancy and increased risk for a small-for-gestational-age baby and preterm delivery. It appears that it is the woman's perception of stress that affects her and her fetus' overall health (Adler and others, 2000).

Situational and Maturational Stressors

Pregnancy itself is a situational stressor. The cognitive process of pregnancy is one of questioning and uncertainty (Rubin, 1970; Affonso and Sheptak, 1989). When a pregnancy becomes high risk and the expectant mother or her fetus is at risk for illness or death, the family is faced with a far greater situational stressor. At the same time, the family is also faced with maturational stressors.

The development of a high risk condition may disrupt the accomplishment of maternal or paternal tasks, and added stressors may result. Fears for the mother's well-being can cause heightened ambivalence about the pregnancy. Previous pregnancy losses may be recalled. This may complicate acceptance of the reality of a current pregnancy and increase the risk for prenatal and postpartum depression (PPD) (Hughes, Turton, and Evans, 1999). If signs of bleeding or other ominous physical signs occur, it might be difficult to validate the pregnancy. Preparations for the baby may be halted. Prenatal education for self and partner also might not be an option offered to an ill or hospitalized mother. Unmet expectations for the pregnancy may be a source of frustration at a time when activities would otherwise be directed at preparation for parenthood.

Preparation for the birth process might be totally out of the parents' control if the mother's well-being is in question. Fears about procedures and care may take precedence over the usual plans. The growth rate of the mother's body may be a great concern. Choices for infant feeding, the birth process, or the coach's support might differ from what were desired.

When all or any of the developmental tasks are thwarted or interfered with, bonding can be slow in the neonatal period. If either the neonate or mother is ill immediately after delivery, early contact may not occur. When the neonate is premature or is connected to machinery, the parents might fear touching the infant. The appearance and behavior of the neonate can be so new to the parents that their visual inspection finds nothing with which to identify. Finally if the pregnancy was thought to be in jeopardy, efforts might have been devoted to "letting go" rather than "attaching to." If this is so, the parents must resolve these feelings before they can begin to attach. The depth of emotion surrounding the possible death of the baby can be so strong as to permanently interfere with attachment if feelings are not explored.

Hospitalization Stressors

Antepartal hospitalization can cause added stressors for the family of a high risk pregnancy. These stressors include separation from home, family, and other support persons, which can cause increased loneliness. Other stressors are feelings of added loss of control or powerlessness, boredom, changes in family circumstances causing stress on family functioning, and concern for the family members at home (Mercer and others, 1988; Loos and Julius, 1989; Gupton, Heaman, and Cheung, 2001). Dependency needs may not be fulfilled. Socialization with other pregnant women can be limited.

PSYCHOLOGIC RESPONSES TO A HIGH RISK PREGNANCY

A high risk pregnancy affects the whole family (Coffman and Ray, 2002). The family may react in a variety of ways to the diagnosis of a high risk pregnancy. It depends on what significance they place on the condition, their experience with coping skills, their ability to effectively problem solve, and available situational supports (Aguilera, 1998).

Anxiety

Anxiety can arise when expectations are not met. In a high risk pregnancy, the expectation of a normal pregnancy culminating in delivery of a healthy baby is threatened. The strength of the unmet needs and degree of awareness about them determine the extent of anxiety.

Threat to Self-Esteem

If the expectant mother feels the diagnosis is a blow to her self-confidence, she may experience a sense of low self-esteem (Kemp and Page, 1987b). This may cause her to feel she has failed as a woman (loss of a perfect pregnancy) and as a mother (fear of loss of a perfect baby), lowering her confidence in her ability to be a mother.

Self-Blaming

The parents may react by blaming themselves for real or imagined wrongdoing, or one parent may blame the other.

Frustration

Frustration occurs when obstacles prevent the achievement of a goal. The behavioral effects of frustration include anger, aggression, withdrawal, fixation, or finally, even learning. Frustration occurs in a high risk pregnancy when goals such as a healthy pregnancy, having a perfect baby, or having the perfect birth experience are impeded by the obstacles of illness, separation, and rigid rules.

Conflict

Conflict results when there are simultaneous, opposing goals of equal strength. If the desired pregnancy causes physical restrictions requiring financial strains or imposes difficulty in mothering tasks with other children, conflict can result. The choices offered to the mother might all be unappealing. If her goal is to have a vaginal delivery and a cesarean delivery is the only safe option for her, conflict occurs.

Crisis

A crisis occurs when an important life goal is threatened and no immediate solution is apparent (Aguilera, 1998). Inability to function results, and a state of disequilibrium ensues.

HORMONAL RESPONSE TO A HIGH RISK PREGNANCY

Placental corticotrophin-releasing hormones blunt the hypothalamic-pituitary-adrenal (HPA) axis. Suppression of the HPA axis can affect mood and increase the risk for postpartum depression. Skin-to-skin mother-infant contact stimulates hormonal production that promotes the return of normal HPA axis functioning, minimizing risk for PPD (Dombrowski, 2001). If mother-infant skin-to-skin contact is not possible because there are maternal or infant health problems, the risk for PPD is increased.

HIGH RISK ADAPTATION

The ability to restore equilibrium depends on three balancing factors. First, an individual must have a realistic perception of an event resulting in psychologic crisis. Second, there must be adequate support from significant others. Third, an individual must have developed adequate coping mechanisms in the past or the ability to problem solve (Aguilera, 1998).

To deal with the multiple crises a high risk pregnancy imposes, the mother and her family must call on past coping mechanisms and also must learn new ones. The nurse should discuss with parents ways they have responded in the past and encourage the use of tactics that have previously worked. Prior pregnancy loss should be discussed early in a current pregnancy to assess for coping strategies.

Information must be provided repeatedly about the disease or condition the woman is facing and should be explained thoroughly to provide autonomy and choices where possible. Information facilitates a realistic appraisal of the events and prepares the couple for potential future events. Significant people, especially the partner, should accompany the mother when information is given. Hospitalization should include flexible rules to allow for the father's presence whenever he can be there, and separations should be minimized whenever possible.

When both the woman and her partner can be given choices in care, personal strategies for coping are less limited and thus more effective. Skill in encouraging these coping mechanisms is necessary in a high risk obstetric setting because of the psychologic impact on the entire family. To maintain the unity of the family when the pregnancy is over, it is important to facilitate the sharing of events. Interventions in a crisis should be aimed at restructuring the present by suppressing negative uses of energy and supporting positive efforts.

Sittner, DeFrain, and Hudson (2005) found that similar themes emerge from their descriptive narratives related to the psychosocial impact of a high risk pregnancy on the family. These themes are mixed emotions, adjustments and support, and information care. From their research, Sittner, Defrain, and Hudson (2005) identified five characteristics that facilitate family coping: positive communication, enjoyable time together, appreciation and affection for each other, spiritual well-being, and commitment to the family.

NURSING MANAGEMENT DURING A HIGH RISK PREGNANCY

Prevention

A high risk pregnancy carries with it a threat not only to the physical well-being of the mother and fetus, but also to the emotional well-being of the entire family unit. Therefore serious consideration must be given to assisting all family members. The nurse must assess and assist the high risk family in the use of previously learned, effective coping styles and the development of new coping skills. To do this, the focus of nursing care must be on identifying and exploring feelings of fear, anxiety, and frustration and the resolution of conflicts in needs. Maintaining the family as a unit as much as possible, especially the mother and her partner, is paramount. Except for situations in which the mother's life may be in jeopardy, the father should be encouraged to spend normal family time with the hospitalized woman. Other children should be brought in for frequent supervised visits. Socialization needs and nesting preparations should be encouraged in creative and innovative ways.

Assessment

An initial and ongoing assessment to determine the individual's and family's functioning response to the actual threat to optimal physical and emotional pregnancy outcome is paramount. This is the basis for formulating appropriate nursing diagnoses and an individualized plan of care. This eliminates making assumptions regarding how the expectant parents are feeling and how they are coping. A prenatal psychologic assessment guide, using the functional health patterns, has been developed (Box 6-1).

Nursing Interventions to Allay Fear and Facilitate Coping During a High Risk Pregnancy

- Provide time for the patient and her family to express their concerns regarding the possible outcome for the baby and discuss the inconvenience to the mother and family of the treatment. Encourage them to vent any apprehension, uncertainty, fear, anger, and worry they may be experiencing. Talking can help them identify, analyze, and understand the events causing the fear. Beginning such discussion with a mother can be facilitated with statements such as "Many women in your situation feel. ..."

Box 6-1   Psychologic Assessment for High Risk Pregnancy

Health-Perception and Health-Management Pattern
- What choices in your birth plan have been limited, such as attendance at childbirth education classes, type of delivery, need for anesthesia, or other medical interventions, because of the development of a high risk condition?
- Do you feel your control has been affected?

Nutritional and Metabolic Pattern
- What dietary changes need to be made because of your high risk condition?
- Why do you need to make these dietary changes?

Elimination Pattern
- What kinds of elimination changes, if any, have developed because of your high risk condition or treatment?

Activity and Exercise Pattern
- What activity changes have been necessary because of your high risk condition?
- Why do you need to make these activity changes?
- What does bedrest or limited activity, if ordered, mean to you and your family?

Sleep and Rest Pattern
- Have you had any disturbing dreams?
- How do you feel after sleeping or resting at night?
- Does this high risk condition affect your normal sleeping pattern? If so, how?

Cognitive and Perceptual Pattern
- What is your understanding of the high risk condition, proposed plan of treatment, and possible effects on self, fetus, and neonate?

Self-Perception and Self-Concept Pattern
- What does this high risk condition mean to you and your family?
- Are you or your family experiencing any guilt feelings, or asking questions such as "What did we do to cause this?"
- Is anyone upset at you or blaming you for this high risk condition?
- How do you feel it has affected your self-confidence, maternal role, and acceptance of the pregnancy?

Role and Relationship Pattern
- What are the family stressors?
- Who lives in the home?
- How has this high risk condition affected your home, work, and other responsibilities?
- How can the nurse help you and your family plan any needed restructuring of roles and activities?
- What are your financial concerns because of this high risk condition such as medical bills, child care expenses, traveling and lodging expenses for out-of-town family?

Continued

Box 6-1   Psychologic Assessment for High Risk Pregnancy—cont'd

Sexuality and Reproductive Pattern
- Assess the patient and her significant other of the need to modify or restrict sexual activity.
- How does the modified or restricted sexual activity affect you and your significant other?

Coping and Stress-Tolerance Pattern
- What are you most worried or fearful about?
- Identify stressors that are affecting you and your family because of this high risk condition.
- How is this hospitalization affecting your life?
- How supportive is the baby's father and your family and friends?
- What coping techniques have been effective for you in the past?
- What resources are available to you?
- What referral services would be helpful?

Value and Belief Pattern
- Which values, if any, are being affected or threatened by this high risk condition?

- Encourage the father to release his fear and anxiety in a positive way instead of keeping it to himself. Couples who do not receive help together might otherwise increase each other's fear and anxiety.
- Help parents discuss their feelings with the other children in the family so that the siblings can understand why their parents are upset. Allow the children to express any guilt they may be experiencing. If they wished that the fetus would "go away," provide reassurance that they did not cause the situation and that the parents still love them.
- Encourage the expectant family to express feelings and concerns about the anticipated labor and delivery experience.
- Explain the high risk condition, all treatment modalities, and reasons for each.
- Define terms that health professionals use in talking to the family.
- Clarify misconceptions. Explain causes of the condition and, if causes are unknown, any associations or lack of association with patient activities.
- Keep the patient informed of her health status, results of tests, and fetal well-being.
- Encourage bedrest exercises.
- Help the family obtain needed social support (Logsdon and Davis, 1998).
- Refer the family to a community support group such as Sidelines (*http://www.sidelines.org*).
- Refer the family to a perinatal clinical nurse specialist, counselor, social worker, or pastoral care, whichever they desire.

Nursing Interventions to Enhance Self-Esteem During a High Risk Pregnancy

- Encourage verbalization of feelings by "active listening."
- Provide emotional support as needed.
- Help the patient identify strategies for accomplishing pregnancy acceptance, fetal embodiment, fetal distinction, and role transition.
- Encourage the patient to participate in her own care and decision making as much as possible. For example, allow her to self-administer medications and encourage her and her partner's involvement in the treatment plan.
- Support, encourage, and enhance information gathering for childbirth preparation and acquisition of parenting skills. Special childbirth education classes designed to meet the unique needs of the high risk pregnant couple are clearly beneficial (Soeffner and Hart, 1998).
- Alter the environment to enable the mother and father to meet their needs for acquiring parenting skills and for parent-child interaction.
- Allow the mother to choose her own foods within the restrictions, and encourage foods to be brought from home.
- Develop flexible visiting policies for the high risk unit. Provide extra beds for fathers-to-be to feel welcome to spend the night. Encourage siblings-to-be to visit.
- Make needed referrals, such as to social service and mental health specialists, if problems are identified.

Nursing Interventions to Promote Family Processes During a High Risk Pregnancy

- Assess the patient's responsibilities to determine difficulties she will face in implementing prescribed bedrest or limited activity.
- Teach the patient and her significant others about the importance of bedrest or limited activity for her high risk condition.
- Help the family problem solve difficulties in implementing maternal bedrest or limited activity.
- Make needed referrals, such as to the social worker, if problems are identified that the family cannot work out.
- Provide and encourage extended and private visiting time.
- Encourage couple closeness.
- Promote spiritual well-being as the family defines spirituality.
- Involve appropriate family members in decisions.

Diversional Activity Interventions During a High Risk Pregnancy

- Assess the patient's interest in various diversional activities within the activity limit.
- Provide crafts, reading, games, and puzzles that can be done in bed, or encourage the patient to have these things brought in.
- Provide classes in preparation for childbirth by way of video, a hospital television, or group classes that can be attended while reclining.

- Encourage writing in a journal.
- Refer to a divisional therapist or volunteer to provide reading materials, handicrafts, or other interesting things.

PRENATAL DEPRESSION

Definition

High risk pregnant women are at increased risk of prenatal and postpartum depression. Prenatal depression can further compound the high risk condition, increasing the risk of substance use, poor eating habits, and preterm labor (Dayan and others, 2006).

Screening

Effective screening is divided into two components. The first component is risk factor screening for which a history of depression is the strongest predictor (Dietz and others, 2007) along with a high level of life stressors. The second component is early detection using a screening tool. The American College of Obstetricians and Gynecologists (ACOG, 2006) recommends a psychosocial screen to be done each trimester. One effective method (ICSI, 2008) is a quick two-question screen simply asking the women these two questions:

- Over the past 2 weeks, have you felt down, depressed, or hopeless?
- Over the past 2 weeks, have you felt little interest or pleasure in doing things?

Kroenke and Spitzer (2002) found this approach to have a sensitivity of 96% and specificity of 57%. A positive result indicates further assessment needed to determine a diagnosis.

POSTPARTUM DEPRESSION

Definition

High risk pregnant women are at risk for PPD, one of the postpartum mood disorders. PPD can occur in the antenatal or postpartum period. Understanding this, the provider and nurses should assess for predictors in the antenatal or postpartum period by the 6-week check-up and intervene early with appropriate referrals. It is also important to be able to recognize the difference between the normal "blues" and one of the four postpartum mood disorders: PPD, postpartum panic disorder, obsessive-compulsive disorder, and postpartum psychosis (Beck, 1999; Currid, 2004; Doucet, Dennis, Letourneau, and Blackmore, 2009).

Types

The blues affect approximately 80% of postpartum women (Dossett, 2008). The onset is within the first week and lasts up to 6 weeks. Self-limiting symptoms include dysphoria, mood lability, irritability, tearfulness, anxiety, and insomnia.

PPD affects 10% to 15% of postpartum women (Dietz and others, 2007), and the risk is higher for women with a history of previous mood disorder. According to two meta-analyses (Beck, 1996; O'Hara and Swain, 1996) and summarized by Beck (1999), the most common predictors follow:

- Prenatal depression
- Child care stress related to health problems, difficult temperament, difficulty sleeping, or difficulty feeding the infant
- Life stress factors such as divorce, job change, death of a loved one, and hospitalization
- Lack of social support
- Prenatal anxiety
- Ambivalence about the pregnancy
- Maternity blues
- Marital dissatisfaction
- History of previous depression

The onset of PPD is usually insidious, and it may take 2 to 3 months to fully manifest itself. Symptoms include depressed mood, excessive anxiety, irritability, fatigue, changes in appetite, somatic complaints, insomnia, feelings of worthlessness or guilt, and difficulty making decisions or concentrating lasting well beyond the first 1 to 2 weeks (Rice and others, 2001; Bozoky and Corwin, 2002). Ambivalent or negative feelings toward the infant are often reported, as is suicidal ideation. The sooner the identification, the earlier the referral and treatment can begin. Earlier treatment has a better prognosis than later treatment (Mills, 2001).

Metz and colleagues first described postpartum onset panic disorder in 1988. Symptoms include extreme anxiety, fear, and sense of doom accompanied by the physical manifestations of difficulty breathing, heart palpitations, dizziness, or shaking.

Sichel and associates identified postpartum obsessive compulsive disorder in 1993. Symptoms include repetitive thoughts of harming the baby leading to compulsive overprotection of the child.

Postpartum psychosis may result from unrecognized and untreated depression or independent of it. It affects 0.1% to 2% of postpartum women. The onset is usually within the first 2 to 4 weeks, but in acute onset, it may occur as early as 48 to 72 hours postpartum. Symptoms include agitation, irritability, depressed mood or excessive euphoria, delusions, depersonalization, inability to sleep, and disorganized behavior. Infanticide can be as high as 4%, and suicide is also very high in this group (Scottish Intercollegiate Guidelines Network, 2002; Cantwell and Cox, 2003).

Differential Diagnoses of Postpartum Depression

Differential diagnoses include the following:

- Hypothyroidism
- Anemia
- Preexisting psychiatric illness
- Sheehan syndrome
- Autoimmune disorders
- Human immunodeficiency virus (HIV)
- Intoxication or withdrawal states
- Intracranial mass

Neonatal Effects

Untreated PPD may influence mother-infant attachment, mothering role, and family functioning. According to Beck (2002), Currid (2004), and Ryan, Millis, and Misri (2005), adverse effects on the infant include problems such as:

- Cognitive and emotional development
- Infant attachment
- Infant behavior
- Cognitive development

USUAL MEDICAL MANAGEMENT AND PROTOCOLS FOR NURSE PRACTITIONERS

Management of Baby Blues

Provide reassurance and validation of what the mother describes as her feelings. Problem-solve for support in caring for herself, the home, and the baby. This is usually sufficient to facilitate resolution in 80% of the patients (Suri and Altshuler, 2004).

Screening for Postpartum Depression

The first step is to identify who is at risk for developing PPD. Assess for precursors or risk factors in the antenatal period (Beck, 1999; ICSI, 2008).

- History of previous depression, including PPD
- Stressful life events occurring presently, such as divorce, job change, or death of a loved one
- Lack of spousal or partner support
- Lack of adequate social support system
- Previous pregnancy loss through miscarriage, stillbirth, or neonatal death
- Previous pregnancy complicated by an unexpected or unintended outcome
- Current pregnancy, which is complicated with or without potential unintended outcomes

The next step in the management of postpartum depression is early detection. Several screening tools are available to health care providers to screen for PPD, such as the Postpartum Depression Predictors Inventory (PDPI), Postpartum Depression Screening Scale (PDSS), Beck Depression Inventory-II (BDI-II), and Edinburgh Postnatal Depression Scale (EPDS) (Beck, 1999, 2002; Beck and Gable, 2001a,b; Clemmens, Driscoll, and Beck, 2004; Hanna and others, 2004) (Box 6-2). Screening is imperative and should be carried out by all health care providers managing the woman's health during the first year following childbirth. It can start as early as 2 to 3 days postpartum (Dennis, Janssen, and Singer, 2004). Assessment can also be carried out during well-child visits (Chaudron and others, 2004).

Diagnosis of Postpartum Depression

It is also important to identify timing of onset of symptoms in relation to the delivery, and providers must recognize their own limitations. Providers of women's health care and nurses caring for women in these areas are gatekeepers. We are there to know how to identify the problem and make the appropriate referrals in a timely manner. Depression After Delivery Inc. (*http://www.depressionafterdelivery.com*) provides a

Box 6-2   Edinburgh Postnatal Depression Scale

Instructions to the Provider or Nurse Administering the Screen
- The mother is asked to underline the response that comes closest to how she has been feeling the last 7 days.
- All 10 items must be completed.
- Care should be taken to avoid the possibility of the mother discussing her answers with others.
- The mother should complete the scale herself, unless she has limited English skills or has difficulty with reading.
- The EPDS may be used at 6 to 8 weeks to screen postnatal women.

Scoring
Response categories are scored 0, 1, 2, and 3, according to increased severity of the symptom. Items marked with a bullet are reverse-scored (e.g., 3, 2, 1, and 0). The total score is calculated by adding together the scores for each of the 10 items. Users may reproduce the scale without further permission providing they respect copyright (which remains with the *British Journal of Psychiatry*) by quoting the names of the authors, the title, and the source in all reproduced copies.

Edinburgh Postnatal Depression Scale Tool
J.L. Cox, J.M. Holden, R. Sagovsky
Department of Psychiatry, University of Edinburgh
From *Br J Psychiatry* 150(6):782, 1987
Name _____
Date of birth _____
Address _____
Phone _____
Insurance _____
Baby's(ies') age(s) _____

Instructions to the Patient
You have recently had a baby, and we are interested in how you are feeling. Please underline the answer that comes closest to how you have felt in the past 7 days, not just how you are feeling today. Here is an example, already completed:
- I have felt happy:
  - Yes, all of the time
  - Yes, most of the time
  - No, not very often
  - No, not at all

This means: "I have felt happy most of the time" during the past week.
Please complete the other questions in the same way. In the past 7 days:
- I have been able to laugh and see the funny side of things:
  - As much as I always could
  - Not quite so much now
  - Definitely not so much now
  - Not at all

Continued

Box 6-2   Edinburgh Postnatal Depression Scale—cont'd

- I have looked forward with enjoyment to things:
  - As much as I ever did
  - Rather less than I used to
  - Definitely less than I used to
  - Hardly at all
- I have blamed myself unnecessarily when things go wrong:
  - Yes, most of the time
  - Yes, some of the time
  - Not very often
  - No, never
- I have been anxious and worried for no good reason:
  - No, not at all
  - Hardly ever
  - Yes, sometimes
  - Yes, very often
- I have felt scared or panicky for no very good reason:
  - Yes, quite a lot
  - Yes, sometimes
  - No, not much
  - No, not at all
- Things have been getting on top of me:
  - Yes, most of the time I haven't been able to cope at all
  - Yes, some of the time I haven't been coping as well as usual
  - No, most of the time I have coped quite well
  - No, I have been coping as well as ever
- I have been so unhappy that I have had difficulty sleeping:
  - Yes, most of the time
  - Yes, sometimes
  - Not very often
  - No, not at all
- I have felt sad or miserable:
  - Yes, most of the time
  - Yes, quite often
  - Not very often
  - No, not at all
- I have been so unhappy that I have been crying:
  - Yes, most of the time
  - Yes, quite often
  - Only occasionally
- The thought of harming myself has occurred to me:
  - Yes, quite often
  - Sometimes
  - Hardly ever
  - Never

From Cox JL, Holden JM, Sagovsky R: Detection of postnatal depression: development of the 10 item Edinburgh Postnatal Depression Scale, *Br J Psychiatry* 150:782-786, 1987.

Box 6-3   Criteria for Major Depressive Syndrome

The patient must have at least five of the symptoms listed below during one 2-week period:

Dysphoria
Useful Question for Screening
- "Have you been feeling sad ... down in the dumps?"

Anhedonia
Useful Questions for Screening
- "What do you do to enjoy yourself?"
- "Have your interests in these things changed recently?"

Insomnia or Hypersomnia
Fatigue or Loss of Energy
Psychomotor Agitation or Retardation
Change in Appetite or Weight
Low Self-Esteem or Guilt
Useful Question for Screening
- "Have you been really down on yourself recently?"

Poor Concentration or Indecisiveness
Thoughts of Death/Suicidal Ideation
Useful Questions for Screening
- "How does the future look to you?"
- "Do you sometimes feel life is not worth living?"
- "Do you ever wish you were dead?"
- "Do you have thoughts of hurting yourself?"
- "Do you have a plan?"

Modified from American Psychiatric Association: *Diagnostic and statistical manual of mental disorders DSM-IV-TR*, ed 4, Washington, DC, 2000, APA.

---

current list of health care providers, such as psychiatrists, psychologists, psychologist and psychiatric nurse practitioners, licensed professional counselors, and clinical social workers, who specialize in postpartum depression. Use the ICD-9 code definition for a major episode of depression with the postpartum onset specifier (Box 6-3) when the diagnosis is determined.

TREATMENT OF PRENATAL AND POSTPARTUM DEPRESSION

Treatment for prenatal depression centers on referral to a prenatal depression provider. Psychotherapy may be appropriate for mild to moderate depression. If the woman was on a psychiatric medication before pregnancy, careful evaluation is needed before stopping any psychiatric medication because of the up to 68% risk of relapse (Cohen and others, 2006). Support groups can be beneficial.

Treatment for PPD should be evidence-based, using national clinical guidelines. The Scottish Intercollegiate Guideline Network (SIGN) (2002) guideline on Postnatal Depression and Puerperal Psychosis is one such guideline and can be accessed by way of the Internet (*http://www.sign.ac.uk/guidelines/fulltext/60/index/html*). Treatment includes:
- Medical workup to rule out a physiologic cause such as thyroid or anemia
- Psychiatric evaluation
- Counseling and psychotherapy
- Involvement in a PPD support group for social support and coaching (Maley, 2002)
- Family-focused interventions
- Possibly, pharmacologic supplementation

A recent systematic Cochrane review indicated that such interventions as cognitive behavior therapy, nondirective counseling, interpersonal psychotherapy, and telephone-based support may be effective treatment options (Dennis and Hodnett, 2007).

Pharmacologic Considerations During Pregnancy and Lactation

General prescribing principles during pregnancy or breastfeeding include the need to establish a clear indication for the drug treatment, use the lowest effective dose for the shortest period necessary, and use drugs with a better evidence base of least harm. Assess the benefit/risk ratio of depression and pharmacologic risk for both mother and fetus/breastfed infant (SIGN, 2002). Both maternal depression and pharmacotherapy have risks. When pharmacologic therapy is deemed necessary, consider the following pharmacologic principles according to ACOG (2008) and SIGN's (2002) evidence-based review of prescribing in pregnancy and during the breastfeeding period:
- Avoid lithium, antiepileptic drugs such as valproate sodium and carbamazepine, and benzodiazepines during pregnancy and lactation, if possible.
- Selective serotonin reuptake inhibitors (SSRIs) except paroxetine (Paxil) and tricyclic antidepressants (TCAs), except doxepin, are usually considered first-line agents if antidepressants are necessary. Preferred choices of a SSRI are fluoxetine (Prozac), or sertraline (Zoloft). Preferred choices of a TCA are nortriptyline (Pamelor) or desipramine (Norpramin). The dose may need to be increased to maintain efficacy during pregnancy (Weiner and Buhimschi, 2009). A systematic review of randomized controlled trials by Lewis-Hall and others (1997) conclude that SSRIs appear to have fewer side effects than do TCAs.
- Provide patient education to expectant parents as to the possible effect of psychiatric medications on their neonate. Studies have indicated limited evidence of increased teratogenic risk (Alwin, Reefhuis, and Rasmussen, 2007; Louik and others, 2007; Ramos, St-Ande, Rey, Oraichi, and Berard, 2008). Use of SSRIs near term has been associated with Neonatal Withdrawal Syndrome (30% risk), manifesting such symptoms as jitteriness, mild respiratory distress, transient tachypnea of the newborn, weak cry, poor muscle tone, increased motor activity, and hypoglycemia (Kallen, 2004; Zeskind and Stephens, 2004; Moses-Kolko and others, 2005; Courtney, 2009). Rare but serious association of prolongation of the QT interval, a marker for sudden cardiac death, and persistent pulmonary

hypertension have been related to fetal exposure to an SSRI (Chambers and others, 2006; U.S. Food and Drug Administration, 2006; Dubnov-Raz and others, 2008). TCA exposure can lead to transient neonatal withdrawal symptoms as well (ACOG, 2008).

- When prescribing antidepressants during breastfeeding, it is best to prescribe a single dose to be taken before the baby's longest sleep period. Sertraline is considered the safest (Dossett, 2008).
- All women of childbearing age on an antiepileptic drug should take a daily dose of 5 mg folic acid. These drugs are folic acid antagonists.
- Postpartum hormonal treatment with transdermal estrogen patch has been used to treat PPD with some success (Albert, 2002).

Nursing Management

Prevention

To reduce mental illness and complications as outlined in *Health People 2010*, prevention and early recognition of prenatal and postpartum depression are imperative.

Assessment and Interventions for Postpartum Depression

- Institute formal screening using the EPDS (Cox, Holden, and Sagovsky, 1987) (see Box 6-2) or another appropriate screening tool such as Postpartum Depression Predictors Inventory (PDPI), Postpartum Depression Screening Scale (PDSS), Beck Depression Inventory-II (BDI-II), or Postpartum Adjustment Questionnaire (Davis, Cross, and Lind, 2008).
- Provide educational materials about signs and symptoms of PPD to let patients know that you are concerned about their emotional as well as physical health.
- Refer to support groups such as Depression After Delivery; (*http://www.depressionafterdelivery.com*), Postpartum Support International (800-944-4PPD; *http://www.postpartum.net*), Postpartum Education for Parents (*http://www.sbpep.org*).
- If there are signs of clinical depression or PPD, make referrals for individual or family counseling.
- Promoting physical activity and mindfulness based yoga during the pregnancy has been shown to promote mental health and decrease the risk of postpartum depression (Beddoe and others, 2009; Ersek and Huber, 2009).
- Assess for suicidal ideation or plans to harm self or another to determine whether referral is emergent or can wait for an opening in a schedule. It is most helpful to have interviewed prospective referral sources to determine their comfort and competencies in these two highly specialized areas of depression.
- Provide family support because PPD affects the entire family.

CONCLUSION

A high risk pregnancy imposes a myriad of psychologic stressors on individuals and the family unit. Supportive care that considers the needs of the family is a must. Without adequate support, families experiencing a high risk pregnancy are also at high risk for permanent separation, divorce, substance abuse, and physically and emotionally abusive situations. With adequate support, family members can achieve a sense of accomplishment in the face of adversity and become emotionally closer to one another.

BIBLIOGRAPHY

Adler N, and others: Perspective on life can affect women's health, according to new studies, *Health Psychol* 19:544, 2000.

Affonso D, Sheptak S: Maternal cognitive themes during pregnancy, *MCN Am J Matern Child Nurs* 18:147, 1989.

Aguilera D: *Crisis intervention: theory and methodology*, ed 8, St Louis, 1998, Mosby.

Albert C: The dark days of postpartum depression, *Adv Nurse Pract* 6:67, 2002. Retrieved from http://www.advanceforNP.com.

Alwin S, Reefhuis J, Rasmussen S: Use of selective serotonin-reuptake inhibitors in pregnancy and the risk of birth defects, *N Engl J Med* 356:2684–2692, 2007.

American College of Obstetricians and Gynecologists (ACOG): *Psychosocial risk factors: perinatal screening and intervention*, Committee Opinion, No. 343, Washington, DC, 2006, ACOG.

American College of Obstetricians and Gynecologists (ACOG): *Use of psychiatric medications during pregnancy and lactation*, Practice Bulletin, No. 92, Washington, DC, 2008, ACOG.

American Psychiatric Association: *Diagnostic and statistical manual of mental disorders: DSM-IV-TR*, ed 4, Washington, DC, 2000, APA.

Beck C: A meta-analysis of predictors of postpartum depression, *Nurs Res* 45:297, 1996.

Beck C: *Postpartum depression: case studies, research, nursing care*, Washington, DC, 1999, Association of Women's Health, Obstetric, and Neonatal Nurses.

Beck C: Revision of the postpartum depression predictors inventory, *J Obstet Gynecol Neonatal Nurs* 31(4):394–402, 2002.

Beck C, Gable R: Postpartum Depression Screening Scale: development and psychometric testing, *Nurs Res* 49(5):272–282, 2000.

Beck C, Gable R: Comparative analysis of the performance of the postpartum depression screening scale with two other depression instruments, *Nurs Res* 50(4):242–250, 2001a.

Beck C, Gable R: Further validation of the Postpartum Depression Screening Scale, *Nurs Res* 50(3):155–164, 2001b.

Beddoe A, Yang C, Kennedy H, Weiss S, Lee K: The effects of mindfulness-based yoga during pregnancy on mental psychological and physical distress, *J Obstet Gynecol Neonatal Nurs* 38(3): 310–319, 2009.

Bozoky I, Corwin E: Fatigue as a predictor of postpartum depression, *J Obstet Gynecol Neonatal Nurs* 31(4):436–443, 2002.

Cantwell R, Cox J: Psychiatric disorders in pregnancy and the puerperium, *Curr Obstet Gynaecol* 13:7, 2003.

Chambers C, Hernandez-Diaz S, Van Marter L, Werler M, and others: Selective serotonin-reuptake inhibitors and risk of persistent pulmonary hypertension of the newborn, *N Engl J Med* 354:579–587, 2006.

Chaudron L, and others: Detection of postpartum depression symptoms by screening at well-child visits, *Pediatrics* 113(3):551–558, 2004.

Clemmens D, Driscoll J, Beck C: Postpartum depression as profiled through the depression screening scale, *MCN Am J Matern Child Nurs* 29(3):180–185, 2004.

Coffman S, Ray M: African American women describe support processes during high-risk pregnancy and postpartum, *J Obstet Gynecol Neonatal Nurs* 31(5):536–544, 2002.

Cohen L, Altshuler L, Harlow B, Nonacs R, and others: Relapse of major depression during pregnancy in women who maintain or discontinue antidepressant treatment, *JAMA* 295:499–507, 2006.

Colman A, Colman L: *Pregnancy: the psychological experience*, New York, 1971, Herder & Herder.

Courtney K: Use of SSRIs in pregnancy, *Nurs Womens Health* 13(3):234–238, 2009.

Cox JL, Holden JM, Sagovsky R: Detection of postnatal depression: development of the 10-item Edinburgh Postnatal Depression Scale, *Br J Psychiatry* 150:782–786, 1987.

Currid T: Improving perinatal mental health care, *Nurs Stand* 19(3):40–43, 2004.

Davis S, Cross J, Lind B: Exploring the postpartum adjustment questionnaire as a predictor of postpartum depression, *J Obstet Gynecol Neonatal Nurs* 37:622–630, 2008.

Dayan J, Creveuil C, Marks N, and others: Prenatal depression, prenatal anxiety, and spontaneous preterm birth: a prospective cohort among women with early and regular antenatal care, *Psychosom Med* 68:938–946, 2006.

Dennis C, Hodnett E: Psychosocial and psychological interventions for treating postpartum depression, *Cochrane Database Syst Rev* (Issue 4), Art. No.: CD006116, 2007.

Dennis C, Janssen P, Singer J: Identifying women at-risk for postpartum depression in the immediate postpartum period, *Acta Psychiatr Scand* 110(5):338–346, 2004.

Diamond M: Becoming a father: a psychoanalytic perspective on the forgotten parent, *Psychoanal Rev* 73(4):445–468, 1986.

Dietz P, Willams S, Callaghan W, and others: Clinically identified maternal depression before, during, and after pregnancies ending in live births, *Am J Psychiatry* 164:1515–1520, 2007.

Dombrowski M: Kangaroo (skin-to-skin) care with a postpartum woman who felt depressed, *MCN Am J Matern Child Nurs* 26(4):214–216, 2001.

Dossett E: Perinatal depression, *Obstet Gynecol Clin North Am* 35:419–434, 2008.

Doucet S, Dennis C, Letourneau N, Blackmore E: Differentiation and clinical implications of postpartum depression and postpartum psychosis, *J Obstet Gynecol Neonatal Nurs* 38(3):269–279, 2009.

Dubnov-Raz G, Juurlink D, Fogelman R, Merlob P, Ito S, and others: Antenatal use of selective serotonin-reuptake inhibitors and QT interval prolongation in newborns, *Pediatrics* 122(3):e710–e715, 2008.

Epling J: FPIN's clinical inquiries: antidepressant medications in pregnancy, *Am Fam Physician* 70(11):2195, 2004. Retrieved from http://www.aafp.org/afp/20041201/fpin.html.

Ersek J, Huber B: Physical activity prior to and during pregnancy and risk of postpartum depressive syndrome, *J Obstet Gynecol Neonatal Nurs* 38(5):556–566, 2009.

Gay J, Edgil A, Douglas A: Reva Rubin revisited, *J Obstet Gynecol Neonatal Nurs* 17(6):394–399, 1988.

Gentile S: The safety of newer antidepressants in pregnancy and breast feeding, *Drug Saf* 28(2):137–152, 2005.

Gupton A, Heaman M, Cheung L: Complicated and uncomplicated pregnancies: women's perception of risk, *J Obstet Gynecol Neonatal Nurs* 30(2):192–201, 2001.

Hanna B, and others: The early detection of postpartum depression: midwives and nurses trial: a checklist, *J Obstet Gynecol Neonatal Nurs* 33(2):191–197, 2004.

Hughes P, Turton P, Evans C: Stillbirth as risk factor for depression and anxiety in the subsequent pregnancy: cohort study, *BMJ* 318(7200):1721–1724, 1999.

Institute for Clinical Systems Improvement (ICSI): *Health care guidelines: Routine prenatal care*, ed 12, Bloomington, MN, 2008, ICSI. Retrieved from http://www.icsi.org.

Kallen B: Neonate characteristics after maternal use of antidepressants in late pregnancy, *Arch Pediatr Adolesc Med* 158:312–316, 2004.

Kemp V, Page C: Maternal prenatal attachment in normal high-risk pregnancies, *J Obstet Gynecol Neonatal Nurs* 16(3):179–184, 1987a.

Kemp V, Page C: Maternal self-esteem prenatal attachment in high-risk pregnancy, *Matern Child Nurs J* 16:195, 1987b.

Klaus M, Kennell J: *Parent-infant bonding*, ed 2, St Louis, 1982, Mosby.

Klaus M, Kennell J: Bonding: another view, *Perinatol Neonatol* 8(2):72, 1984.

Kroenke K, Spitzer R: The PHQ-9: a new depression diagnostic severity measure, *Psychiatric Annals* 32:509–521, 2002.

Lewis-Hall F, and others: Fluoxetine versus tricyclic antidepressants in women with major depressive disorder, *J Womens Health* 6(3):337–343, 1997.

Logsdon M, Davis D: Guiding mothers of high-risk infants in obtaining social support, *MCN Am J Matern Child Nurs* 23(4):195–199, 1998.

Loos C, Julius L: The client's view of hospitalization during pregnancy, *J Obstet Gynecol Neonatal Nurs* 18(1):52–56, 1989.

Louik C, Lin A, Werler M, and others: First-trimester use of selective serotonin-reuptake inhibitors and the risk of birth defects, *N Engl J Med* 356:2675–2683, 2007.

Maley B: Out of the blue: creating a postpartum depression support group, *AWHONN Lifelines* 6(1):62–65, 2002.

May K: Three phases of father involvement in pregnancy, *Nurs Res* 31(6):337–342, 1982.

Mercer R, and others: Effect of stress on family functioning during pregnancy, *Nurs Res* 37(5):268–275, 1988.

Metz A, Sichel D, Goff D: Postpartum panic disorder, *J Clin Psychiatry* 49(7):278–279, 1988.

Mills M: In *The moody blues: mood disorders in pregnancy*. Presentation at Obstetrical Challenges of the New Millenium, Phoenix, AZ, April 2001.

Moses-Kolko E, Bogen D, Perel J, Bregar A, and others: Neonatal signs after late in utero exposure to serotonin reuptake inhibitors: literature review and implications for clinical applications, *JAMA* 293:2372–2383, 2005.

O'Hara M, Swain A: Rates and risk of postpartum depression: a meta-analysis, *Int Rev Psychiatry* 8:37, 1996.

Patterson E, Freese M, Goldenberg R: Seeking safe passage: utilizing health care during pregnancy, *Image J Nurs Sch* 22(1):27–31, 1990.

Ramos E, St-Andre M, Rey E, Oraichi D, Berard A: Duration of antidepressant use during pregnancy and risk of major congenital malformations, *Br J Psychiatry* 192(5):344–350, 2008.

Rice M, and others: Postpartum depression: identification, treatment, and prevention in primary care, *Clin Lett Nurse Pract* 5(4):1, 2001.

Rubin R: Cognitive style in pregnancy, *Am J Nurs* 70(3):502–508, 1970.

Rubin R: Maternal tasks in pregnancy, *MCN Am J Matern Child Nurs* 4:143, 1975.

Rubin R: *Maternal identity and the maternal experience*, New York, 1984, Springer.

Ryan D, Millis L, Misri N: Depression during pregnancy, *Can Fam Physician* 51:1087–1093, 2005.

Scottish Intercollegiate Guidelines Network (SIGN): *Postnatal depression and puerperal psychosis: a national clinical guideline, Edinburgh (Scotland): Scottish Intercollegiate Guideline Network (SIGN)*, 2002, June 28, SIGN publication; No. 60, Retrieved from http://www.sign.ac.uk/guidelines/fulltext/60/index/html.

Sherwen L: Maternal role attainment. In Sherwen L, editor: *Psychosocial dimensions of the pregnant family*, New York, 1987, Springer.

Sichel D, and others: Postpartum obsessive compulsive disorder: a case series, *J Clin Psychiatry* 54(4):156–159, 1993.

Sittner B, DeFrain J, Hudson D: Effects of high-risk pregnancies on families, *MCN Am J Matern Child Nurs* 30(2):121–126, 2005.

Soeffner M, Hart MA: Back to class: helping high-risk moms cope with hospitalization, *AWHONN Lifelines* 2(3):47–51, 1998.

Suri R, Altshuler L: Postpartum depression: risk factors and treatment options, *Psychiatric Times* XXI(11), 2004. Retrieved from http://www.psychiatrictimes.com/p041064.html.

Teixeira J, Fisk N, Glover V: Association between maternal anxiety in pregnancy and increased uterine artery resistance index: cohort based study, *BMJ* 318(7177):153–157, 1999.

Tomlinson P: Verbal behavior associated with indicators of maternal attachment with the neonate, *J Obstet Gynecol Neonatal Nurs* 19(1):76–77, 1990.

Tulman L: Mothers and unrelated persons' initial handling of newborn infants, *Nurs Res* 34(4):205–210, 1985.

U.S. Food and Drug Administration (FDA): Treatment Challenges of Depression in Pregnancy and the Possibility of Persistent Pulmonary Hypertension in Newborns, *FDA Public Health Advisory*, 2006. Retrieved from http://www.fda.gov/cder/drug/advisory/SSRI_PPHN200607.htm.

Wadhwa P, and others: Maternal corticotrophin-releasing hormone levels in the early trimester predict length of gestation in human pregnancy, *Am J Obstet Gynecol* 179(4):1079–1085, 1998.

Weiner C, Buhimschi C: *Drugs for pregnant and lactating women*, ed 2, Philadelphia, 2009, Saunders.

Wohlreich M: Psychiatric aspects of high-risk pregnancy, *Psychiatr Clin North Am* 10(1):53–68, 1987.

Zeskind P: Depression during pregnancy: are antidepressants safe for the fetus?, *Womens Health Prim Care* 7(3):142, 2004.

Zeskind P, Stephens L: Maternal selective serotonin reuptake inhibitor use during pregnancy and newborn neurobehavior, *Pediatrics* 113:368–375, 2004.

7

Perinatal Death and Bereavement Care

I n the past few decades, increased awareness and sensitivity to the special needs of bereaved parents has changed hospital-based intervention—from *shielding* parents from the death of their baby to *supporting* parents through the experience. As a result, the modern standard of care is to engage parents in ongoing conversations about their baby, their experience of pregnancy and parenting, and their grief. Obstetric and neonatal nurses have a unique opportunity to support parents in their desire to affirm their baby's importance and spend time with their baby.

This chapter offers a brief history of bereavement care, the parent's experience of grief and adjustment, and quality standards of care, including Practice Guidelines produced by the Pregnancy Loss and Infant Death Alliance (*PLIDA*). *PLIDA* is a nonprofit organization that offers education, support, and networking opportunities for professionals and advocates whose work supports bereaved families.

BRIEF HISTORY OF PERINATAL BEREAVEMENT CARE

During the past 150 years, there have been dramatic changes in our culture's management of birth and death. Up until the late 1800s, these important relationship-altering experiences occurred in the context of social networks and in the home environment. The birthing mother was typically attended by women in the community who trusted (and had experienced) the natural progression of labor and delivery; the newborn was put to the breast and kept in the mother's care with ongoing assistance from family and friends (Kitzenger, 1987). If the baby died before or after birth, the mother was tended to by this community of women, the baby's body was cared for in the home, and sometimes a photograph was made (Hochberg, 2003).

During the period of 1890 to 1940, as medical interventions were developed to accompany birth and death, a transition from home to hospital started to occur. But instead of treating birth and death as naturally unfolding experiences that happened in the context of important relationships, medical practices focused on sterile control by technically skilled medical practitioners who followed one-size-fits-all protocols. These practices also ignored the holistic and unique needs of the individual woman,

By Deborah L. Davis, PhD, Suzanne Helzer, RNC, LCCE.

downplayed the significant emotional, social, spiritual, and relational aspects of these experiences, and considered family members to be unsterile and meddling (Walzer Leavitt, 1986; Wertz and Dorothy, 1989). So by the mid-1900s, mothers who gave birth in a hospital were routinely separated from their babies after birth, hospitalized for extended periods, and isolated by rigid visiting restrictions. With the advent of neonatal intensive care in the 1960s, these policies were strictly enforced in the NICU, as they were considered essential to the care of vulnerable newborns.

Whereas intrusive medical management of uncomplicated birth became firmly entrenched in the culture and in hospital policies, the death of a baby became hushed and hidden from view. In a westernized medical culture that looked upon death as failure, health care practitioners typically did not receive training or support on how to deal with the death of a patient nor a family's grief, much less how to cope with these experiences themselves. This lack led to medical practices for perinatal bereavement that was designed to "protect the parents"—as well as the practitioners in the name of efficiency and professionalism—by hiding the evidence, avoiding grief, and offering platitudes. Common discharge instructions were "get on with life, don't dwell on it, and have another baby."

Then in the 1960s, as parents became more informed and assertive, they began to question standards of obstetric and neonatal care that ignored their emotional needs. Medical professionals too, some affected by their own personal experiences as "patient," started to reflect on the practices that took control away from families and inadvertently interfered with holistic health, development, and healing. Since the 1970s, research on postpartum and NICU care has consistently shown that isolation could interfere with the parents' bonding and attunement to their newborn, and compromise the newborn's health and development, from successful breastfeeding to intact recovery from the rigors of intensive care (Bowlby, 1982; Klaus and Kennel, 1982; Gorski, 1991; Als, 1992; Luddington-Hoe and Golant, 1993; Als and Gilkerson, 1997; Maroney, 2003; Lawrence, 2005). Research and thoughtful analysis has also examined how and why parents were affected by death of a baby, for any reason and at any time during pregnancy or infancy, and demonstrated that is was a profound experience that required a full expression of grief (Lewis, 1976; Peppers and Knapp, 1980; Klaus and Kennell, 1982; Bowlby, 1982; Leon, 1992a, 1992b, 1992c; Kluger-Bell, 1998; Brier, 2008). Most significantly, for parent and practitioner alike, avoiding death and grief created misery, not relief. More harm than good has come from practices purported to "protect" babies from parents, grieving parents from pain, and practitioners from feeling much of anything.

What followed has been a revolution in obstetric, postpartum, neonatal, and bereavement care. Innovation has led to current standards of care for all new parents that focus on the importance of building an empathic relationship that supports both parents, honors and affirms their relationship with their baby, and fosters each parent's unique process of adjustment, whatever the circumstances or outcome. Cultivating a caring relationship with parents is what makes individualized care possible, and care can actually be *more* efficient and professional when the emotional landscape is acknowledged (Barnsteiner and Gillis-Donovan, 1990). This focus on relationships is known as *relationship-based care*, and is a way to ensure parent satisfaction with care, particularly during a crisis (Leon, 1992a, b, c; Swanson, 1993; Als and Glikerson, 1997; Davis and Stein, 2004; Koloroutis, 2004).

CONTINUING DEVELOPMENT OF BEREAVEMENT CARE

In the area of bereavement care, a concerted collaboration between parent-advocates and health care practitioners has led to new standards of comprehensive, compassionate care for grieving families. Now, instead of the well-intentioned but misguided shielding of parents from the death of their baby, quality care means supporting parents through this experience. Instead of avoiding grief and removing the baby from the parents' arms, practitioners are inviting parents to talk about their baby's life and death, share their emotions, and have open-ended conversations about spending time with their baby. Practitioners are offering parents unbiased information and decision-making support to ensure truly informed decisions, from end-of-life medical care to whether and how to spend time with their baby's body. Parents are no longer routinely dismissed with advice to have another baby, and more practitioners are providing follow-up care and support through the subsequent pregnancy and beyond.

After researchers in England found that mothers who felt coerced into seeing their deceased babies were traumatized by this experience (Hughes and others, 2002), the discussions that followed served to renew efforts to refine bereavement care (Walling, 2002; Davis, 2004; Gold, Dalton, and Schwenk, 2007). This refinement has been accompanied by an overdue acknowledgement that health care practitioners require—and desire—training, experience, and support for their work with bereaved families (Jansen, 2003; Chan and others, 2007, 2008; Fenwick and others, 2007; Gold, 2007; Cameron, Taylor, and Greene, 2008; Gold, Kuznia, and Hayward, 2008; Roehrs and others, 2008). By facing their own feelings about death and learning how to engage effectively with grieving families, practitioners can feel confident and competent as they face the challenges—and reap the rewards—of this important work. All the while, willing parents have continued to report that being able to spend time with their baby validates their role as mother and/or father, and enables them to ultimately embrace their baby's life and death as a meaningful, cherished, albeit bittersweet experience (Geerinck-Vercammen and Kanhai, 2003; Kuebelbeck, 2005; Cacciatore and Bushfield, 2007; Kobler, Limbo, and Kavanaugh, 2007; Brier, 2008; Kuebelbeck and Davis, 2010).

To the benefit of parents and practitioners alike, state-of-the-art bereavement care is returning to the emotionally attuned, relationship-based care that was naturally provided in the home more than a century ago. As in the past, grieving families can experience extended and nurturing contact with their dying or dead infants, unlimited visitation by family and friends, participation in social and religious rituals of mourning, and the opportunity to take cherished photographs. The most modern care also offers palliative treatment, perinatal hospice, and information about providing after-death care in the home, all of which expand the health care practitioner's ability to provide comprehensive and compassionate care to bereaved families.

Overview of the Grieving Process

Grieving is a natural and necessary process of coming to terms with loss (Bowlby, 1982). It involves gradually letting go of *what might have been*, and adjusting to *what is* (Rando, 1991; Davis, 1996).

When a baby dies, parents grieve intensely because their bond with this baby has already deepened. This process of bonding or emotionally investing in a baby can start even before conception as parents dream of having a baby someday (Klaus and Kennell, 1982). After pregnancy is confirmed, even if unplanned, parents can start envisioning this particular child. Throughout the pregnancy, this vision and their bond grows stronger as parents talk to their baby, feel the kicks and hiccups, admire ultrasound pictures, collect infant clothing and supplies, and pick out names. When parents invest in their baby, they invest in the opportunity to raise this child.

When a baby dies, parents experience profound grief for this child and their shattered dreams. The parents' grieving process includes:
- Facing the reality of their baby's death
- Learning to cope with an unpredictable ebb and flow of many intense emotions
- Holding onto memories and keepsakes in order to experience a gradual letting go of their baby
- Integrating this baby into their family as "one who is not with us anymore"
- Adjusting to the vision of a different future

The emotions of parental grief include a wide range of pronounced and bewildering feelings, such as numbness, yearning, betrayal, failure, anger, guilt, sadness, and despair. Parents may also experience physical symptoms such as aching arms, tightness in the chest, poor appetite, restlessness, and fatigue. It is normal for parents to have hallucinations of hearing a baby cry or feeling the baby move inside the womb, and to feel preoccupied with their baby. Particularly during the first year, many parents feel distractible, irritable, isolated, and depressed, and wonder if they will ever recover. These are all natural parts of grief.

Grieving parents, regardless of their baby's gestational age or length of life, share much common ground, but each parent's timetable and path through grief will be unique. Grief can be affected by circumstances surrounding the baby's death, personal history, temperament, health, culture, spiritual beliefs, social support, and previous loss (Peppers and Knapp, 1980; Bowlby, 1982; Kirkley-Best and Kellner, 1982; Miller, 2002). Some parents move through their grief primarily by expressing, writing, sharing, or talking about their feelings; others move through their grief by jumping into action. Many couples see these emotional versus action-oriented differences in each other, and benefit from understanding and accepting both styles as valid (Martin and Doka, 1999).

As parents grieve, they are simultaneously, even if erratically, moving along a continuum of healing. For many parents, healing involves a bittersweet feeling of manageable sadness that death happened, mixed with happiness that they were blessed by this child's brief life (Davis, 1996).

Parents benefit from being informed about grief and assured that their reactions are shared by other grieving parents. This information and reassurance can help them to make sense of their emotional experience and navigate the difficult terrain. Most parents also benefit from having written support materials, which can be perused when they are ready to absorb and process the information, insights, and encouragement contained therein.

CONTACT WITH THE BABY'S BODY

Consistent with their bond and devotion to their baby, bereaved parents report that close contact with their baby after death is an invaluable experience (Peppers and Knapp, 1980; Kirkley-Best and Kellner, 1982; Harmon and Cicchinelli, 1985; Davis, Stewart, and Harmon, 1988; Saflund, Sjogren, and Wredling, 2004; Gold, Dalton, and Schwenk, 2007). Contact affirms both the baby's life and the reality of death (Davidson, 1977). Contact also allows the parents to transform their bond from the unseen but loved baby in the womb to the visible and held child in their arms, and to establish the particular identity of this child in the family, including who he or she looked like (Leon, 1992a, b, c). Spending time with their baby can help parents feel connected to their child, and loving contact with their baby can meet an intense spiritual need (Capitulo, 2005).

Many parents find it meaningful to demonstrate their love in physical ways, including touching, examining, holding, cuddling, and kissing, before (if possible) and after their baby has died. Parents can also find comfort in rituals such as baptism or blessing, bathing and dressing the baby *themselves*, as well as collecting keepsakes, such as locks of hair, foot and hand prints, and photographs. Parents also report that these experiences can help them acquire positive memories and comforting mementos, which affirm their baby's existence and validate their grief (Peppers and Knapp, 1980; Davis, Stewart, and Harmon, 1988; Harmon, Plummer, and Frankel, 2000; Workman, 2001; Capitulo, 2005; Kobler, Limbo, and Kavanaugh, 2007).

If a baby is in poor condition because of anomalies, early gestational age, or having been dead for longer than a few days, parents can still benefit from seeing their baby, particularly when the health care practitioner can openly and honestly describe the normal and beautiful parts of their baby's body, and then explain any anomalies or deterioration. Even when their baby is undeveloped, deformed, or deteriorated, parents tend to focus on the special beauty in their baby, looking through the eyes of love and seeing past what others may find difficult to view (Harmon and Cicchinelli, 1985).

Because parents vary on whether, when, and how they want to spend time with their baby, and because there is no empiric evidence that refusing to see the baby interferes with grief, parents must be supported in making their own decisions and doing what they believe is best (Hughes and others, 2002; Davis, 2004; Gold, Dalton, and Schwenk, 2007). Determining how to spend time with their baby affirms their parental bond and being in charge of whether or when to spend time with their baby can also restore some sense of control over what happens to them even as they face the trauma of their baby's death. Health care practitioners must remain unbiased, supporting parents in whatever they choose to do.

PLIDA Practice Guidelines (Boxes 7-1 and 7-2) expand on how to implement this aspect of bereavement care and address related issues, such as the benefits of delaying postmortem evaluation and the insignificance of infection risks.

SUPPORT DURING SUBSEQUENT PREGNANCY

The bygone advice, "Forget about this baby and go have another one" only serves to belittle the parent's grief and the baby who died. When published case studies illustrated how bereaved mothers with chronic or repressed grief could have disturbed

Text continued on p. 162.

Box 7-1   When Bereaved Parents Want to Hold Their Baby

PLIDA Practice Guidelines: When Bereaved Parents Want to Hold Their Baby
Related PLIDA Position Statements:

- **Infection Risks Are Insignificant:** Infection risks are insignificant for bereaved parents who have close contact with their deceased baby's body.
- **Delaying Postmortem Pathology Studies:** When bereaved parents hold their baby's body for any length of time after death, there is little or no impact on postmortem pathology studies.

Guidelines for the Bereavement Care Provider
Remember that after death, the body does not produce new pathogens.
If a baby has contracted an infection before death, those pathogens may proliferate slightly after death, but in most circumstances that proliferation will pose an insignificant risk to the parents. The parents can kiss and cuddle their baby, and the parents can keep their baby with them for extended periods of many hours.

Protective clothing can be used by health care providers to prevent extended contact with bodily fluids when hazardous infection is suspected. Careful cleaning of the baby's body will protect the parents from any residual risk, and swaddling with a cloth can protect others who hold the baby. For any person who has an impaired immune system, standard precautions (gown and gloves) are advisable.

If others elect to be gowned and gloved, and parents want to know why, they can be gently informed and reassured that these precautions are to protect "outsiders" from the remote chance of infection, but that they, the parents, belong in the inner circle with their baby, and bear no risk.

Whatever the condition of the baby, touch and carry the baby with gentle caring. Your tenderness and reverence is affirming, validating, and comforting to the parents.

Delay autopsy whenever possible. When parents are able to have extended and repeated opportunities to spend time with their baby's body, the psychosocial and emotional benefits to them can significantly outweigh the benefits of prompt postmortem evaluation.

Encourage meetings between parents and the pathologist. Personal contact enables the pathologist to give the parents realistic and reassuring information about the autopsy. If samples need to be collected within 24 hours, the pathologist can assure them the baby will be well cared for and returned promptly.

Let parents know they can keep their baby with them. After delivery and until the mother is discharged, the baby's body can stay in the room with the parents as much as they desire.

Refrigeration is advised when the baby is not with the parents, to maintain the integrity of the skin and reduce the normal, although minor, proliferation of any pathogens. The baby can be placed in a warming unit or wrapped in a warm blanket before being held by the parents.

For more information on these guidelines, please refer to the *PLIDA* Position Statements listed above.

Box 7-2   PLIDA Practice Guidelines: Offering the Baby to Bereaved Parents

PLIDA Practice Guidelines: Offering the Baby to Bereaved Parents
Related PLIDA Position Statements:

- **Bereaved Parents Holding Their Baby:** After their baby dies, it is the parents' right to decide how much time, if any, to spend with their baby, and to determine when and how to use this precious time.
- **Offering the Baby to Bereaved Parents:** When a baby dies, parents should be offered their baby within the context of an empathic relationship, where the health care provider engages parents in periodic conversations, eliciting their thoughts and feelings about spending time with their baby, and then supports the parents in doing what they believe is best, whether or not they elect to spend time with their baby.

Guidelines for the Bereavement Care Provider
First and foremost, cultivate an empathic relationship with parents. Ask them about the pregnancy, and particularly for early pregnancy loss or pregnancy termination, listen to the parents' conceptualization of this event, so that you are able to honor their perceptions and wishes. Whenever parents see their loss as "the death of our baby," ask them about their baby and provide care accordingly. Also inquire about their physical well-being and comfort. Cultivating an empathic relationship with parents gives them a caring context within which to process their experiences and emotions, and thoughtfully explore their options.

Understand the benefits parents can experience in spending time with their baby. For grieving parents, contact with their baby can:
- Validate their role as parents to this child
- Offer opportunities to express their love and devotion *(such as holding, kissing, bathing, dressing)* and engage in rituals *(such as blessing, baptism, naming ceremonies)*
- Cultivate cherished memories *(such as how their baby looked and felt)* and keepsakes *(such as hair, footprints, photographs)*
- Rally the support of family and friends who can meet their baby too
- Help them process the traumatic events surrounding their baby's death as they share this parenting experience with others, including other grieving families in post-discharge support settings
- Allow for a more gradual goodbye

All of these benefits can foster productive grieving for those parents who want and need contact, memories, and keepsakes. If denied this experience, some parents will harbor lasting and significant regrets. However, for parents who do not want or don't feel the need for contact, they may not reap these benefits, and some may harbor lasting regrets if pressed to have contact with their baby. Understanding the complexities of perinatal bereavement and the long-term effects of contact with the baby requires further systematic research. In any case, the complexities underline the importance of individualizing care for each parent.

Work to individualize care. Every parent is unique, every family is different, and you will encounter much variety in parents' responses and desires. So rather than trying to fit parents into a rigid protocol, or deciding whether they should see their baby, or directing their involvement with their

Continued

Box 7-2   PLIDA Practice Guidelines: Offering the Baby to Bereaved Parents—cont'd

baby, ask parents about their needs and preferences and accommodate each family's process and timeframe.

- Some parents will know right away whether or not they want to see their baby; others need time to weigh their options.
- Some parents will decide not to see their baby; others will welcome the opportunity.
- Some parents will embrace their baby without hesitation, others will be more cautious about seeing, touching, or holding their baby.
- Some parents will need more time with their baby; others will need less.
- Some parents will want to keep the baby with them for extended periods; others will want short or multiple viewings on different days.
- Some parents will find your presence reassuring; others will want privacy.
- Some will want family and friends to see their baby; others will prefer to be alone with their baby.

Parents benefit from making their own decisions in their own time. If parents decide to see their baby, they benefit from pacing themselves instead of having arbitrary constraints placed on them.

Follow the parents' lead. Be an unbiased sounding board for their thoughts and feelings, offer them options and individualized guidance, address their concerns, and leave the decision-making to them. By listening, responding, and respecting parents' choices, you are:

- Honoring their self-knowledge
- Recognizing their competence to navigate this difficult terrain; even as they may feel temporarily incompetent, your confidence in them can be a reassuring boost
- Giving them room to make satisfying choices
- Averting the regrets that can accompany being directed or pushed
- Reminding them that they can still exert some control over what happens after their baby dies
- Alleviating trauma and the accompanying feelings of helplessness

Practice cultural and religious sensitivity. In some cultures, close contact with a dead body is prohibited, while in other cultures, it is considered the highest form of respect to remain with a body until burial. Likewise, some religions specify that a body needs to be buried or cremated in a short time window, which may affect the parents' ability or need to be with their baby.

- Assess each family's practices, keeping in mind that they may or may not wish to observe their traditions.
- Never assume—always ask.
- Remember that even if parents look, talk, and act like you, they may hold very different beliefs and preferences.
- To find out their wishes, you might ask, "Can you tell me about your family's traditions when someone dies?" or "Are there any religious or cultural traditions that you would like to observe?" or "It would be helpful for me to know what is most important to you as you consider spending time with your baby."

Box 7-2   PLIDA Practice Guidelines: Offering the Baby to Bereaved Parents—cont'd

- If parents want guidance from elders or religious practitioners, help them receive this counsel, while letting them know that you will honor whatever the parents themselves decide to do.
- As you build a rapport with each parent, you can gauge what types of information and support are welcome.

Honor the parent-baby bond. Central to your mission is to honor the parent-baby relationship, and make room for each parent to nurture their baby and/or their baby's memory.

- Observe and acknowledge the unique bond each parent feels with her or his baby, no matter the gestational age or whether the baby lived after delivery.
- Whether they want contact or not, you can affirm their baby's existence and importance by acknowledging their baby's life and their loving bond. Ask them to tell you about their baby, the pregnancy, their dreams for this child, and how they plan to honor their baby's memory. "Tell me about your baby (pregnancy, delivery, dreams.)" "Have you thought about doing (making, buying, keeping) anything special to remember this baby by?"
- Many parents find it comforting to hear that they have been, and always will be, this child's mother or father. Refer to them as such.
- If parents elect to spend time with their baby, step back so that the *parents* can bathe, groom, dress, and generally take care of their baby whenever possible. Even if the mother is bed-bound, you can ensure her proximity and participation—all of these activities can take place on her lap or next to her. For many parents, taking care of their baby is a meaningful and memorable way for them to nurture and feel close to their little one.
- Parents who see their baby can also find it therapeutic to play a primary or participatory role in clipping locks of hair, making molds or prints of tiny hands, feet, and other body parts, or taking photographs of their baby. Collecting these mementos provides additional opportunities to feel close to their baby and lets parents have a creative role in determining what their keepsakes look like.

Engage parents in open-ended conversations about their baby and their options. When you listen to parents, you are able to accompany them as they evaluate their options, communicate their needs, and figure out what is best for themselves. For some hesitant parents, simply having an opportunity to express their feelings and tell their story can help them recognize the benefits of seeing their baby. For others, the chance to share their thoughts and feelings can affirm their decision to not view their baby.

- In general, rather than dispensing advice or directing, ask them what they are feeling and thinking about with regard to their baby, the circumstances, and their options. It is far more therapeutic for them to gather their own insights than to have you set the pace or plan.
- Ask, "Have you thought about seeing your baby?" or "How do you feel about seeing your baby?" This will help them consider what they want and need.
- Resist directly asking, "Do you want to see your baby?" as this will only elicit a simple "yes" or "no" answer.

Continued

Box 7-2   PLIDA Practice Guidelines: Offering the Baby to Bereaved Parents—cont'd

- During these conversations, listen to their thoughts, desires, and feelings about their baby and their ideas about having contact.
- Let them know that they can hold, undress, dress, bathe, rock, and photograph their baby, and that you can provide a rocking chair, disposable cameras, blankets, clothing, a small tub, and bathing accessories.
- As they consider contact with their baby, ask them how they would want to use this precious time.
- Let parents know that friends and other family members can be involved in rituals, photographs, and keepsakes. Parents can find it comforting to be surrounded by loved ones, including the baby's siblings, grandparents, aunts, uncles, and family friends. By inviting others into the circle, parents are essentially holding their baby inside a loving community, which can help them hold onto their baby's memory.
- Whether or not they want contact with their baby, tell them, "I'm here to listen if you'd like to talk about your baby, your pregnancy and delivery, and how you're doing."
- About their baby's name, ask the open-ended question, "Had you picked out names for this baby?" Find out the meaning or source of this name, and then ask, "Do you feel comfortable using this name for this baby?" If they are considering saving the intended name for a future baby, reassure them that many other parents have done the same, and the measure of their devotion is not the particular name they choose, but the care they are taking to pick the best name for this child. If they choose a name, use it when referring to their baby.

When you engage with and listen to parents, you are better able to understand and respond to their needs and wishes.

Engage parents in conversations proactively, when possible. If the baby has died before birth, or if the baby is likely to die during or shortly after delivery, ask the parents, "Have you thought about seeing your baby?" so that they can think proactively about how to make the most of this time. For instance, you'll know whether to hand the baby to the parents immediately after delivery. You'll also be giving mother and father time to:

- Confront the unknown and become informed
- Make a decision and come up with creative ideas
- Decide whether to have family and friends present
- Consider their other children, as including their baby's siblings can be particularly touching, meaningful, and beneficial

Remind parents that making plans can help them prepare and can offer guidance to their health care providers. Assure them that these plans are not set in stone, and they are free to adjust to unforeseen circumstances or change their minds and improvise.

Continually assess what the parents are thinking and feeling with regard to seeing their baby. In your ongoing conversations with parents about their baby, listen to their thoughts, feelings, and ideas, and continually assess where they are in their decision-making process.

- What are their feelings about holding their baby?
- Have they ever seen a dead body before?

Box 7-2   PLIDA Practice Guidelines: Offering the Baby to Bereaved Parents—cont'd

- What are their fears?
- What are their regrets?
- What do they want from this opportunity?

Then you can tailor your guidance and support to fit their needs.

Utilize a checklist that makes room for qualitative answers. Rather than simply checking "yes" or "no," document the parents' thoughts, feelings, and fears, as well as your responses. These notes can help you and your team assess and respond to their needs for time, information, support, and reassurance. These notes can also assist you in providing a comprehensive and compassionate continuity of care.

Offer unbiased, balanced information that helps parents figure out what is best for themselves. During your conversations with the parents, tell them, "Some parents find it comforting and helpful to spend time with their baby, while others decline, but the choice is yours to make." If the parents are worried that seeing their baby is strange or morbid, you can inform them that some parents would rather remember their baby as what they imagined during pregnancy or as the live baby they once held, but many parents find it reassuring to see their baby and express their love and nurturing in physical ways. Let parents know that it is normal and natural for them:

- To feel a connection to their baby
- To be curious about what their baby looks like
- To notice family resemblances
- To be nurturing—cuddling, dressing, or bathing their baby
- To want keepsakes such as a lock of hair, hand and footprints
- To want photographs that record their baby's appearance and their love for this child
- To name their baby

Reassure parents by addressing their fears or concerns. Parents can benefit from knowing that many parents feel uncertain or scared about seeing a dead body or a baby who might have an unusual appearance.

- Inquire, "Do you have any concerns about what your baby looks like?" Then you can address their fears by describing their baby's appearance, letting them know they may find family resemblances, and telling them that their baby will be brought to them, warmed and wrapped in a warm blanket.
- Inform parents of their baby's condition. Even the most fragile babies can be touched and held by parents if the body is carefully and respectfully prepared, and the parents are honestly and reassuringly informed about their baby's tiny size, discoloration, the delicate nature of their baby's skin, or bodily fluids.
- Comfort parents by telling them that their baby is treated with respect and dignity at all times.
- Whatever the baby's gestational age or condition, when you are open and accepting toward the baby's appearance and condition, this can be tremendously comforting and validating for parents.

Remain accommodating and impartial to the wide range of parental responses. Some parents will know right away that they want to see and hold their baby. Other parents will remain adamant that they do not wish to do so,

Continued

Box 7-2   PLIDA Practice Guidelines: Offering the Baby to Bereaved Parents—cont'd

preferring to remember their baby alive (whether before or after birth). And some parents will be undecided and may simply need time to recover from delivery and the initial shock in order to come to a decision. Rather than trying to convince all parents to see their baby, focus on exploring the options with each parent.

- Be aware of your own biases, so that you can resist convincing or pushing them to do what *you* believe is best.
- Be mindfully accepting of all requests and actions by parents, particularly when their choices are different from what you believe to be most meaningful, or from what you've observed or experienced with other families.
- Encourage parents to communicate their needs and focus on helping parents figure out what's best for themselves.
- When parents are unsure about whether they want to see their baby, you can simply inform them of their options, address their concerns, and assure them that they can take their time to decide.
- Let parents know that their baby will continue to be available to them, if and when they are ready.
- Some parents will warm up to the idea over time and with your reassuring conversations about seeing a dead body or how normal their feelings are.
- Sometimes a baby's parents have different ideas and make different choices. Offer them the freedom to pursue their own experiences.
- Whatever a parent's choices and pace, continue to engage, listen, and support.

Encourage parents to do what is meaningful to them. Some parents will have lots of ideas and engage freely in rituals and nurturing behaviors. Others will be grateful for your culturally sensitive suggestions or reassurance. If parents want to see their baby or are considering it:

- Ask parents about their ideas of how they might want to spend this time and then offer the support they need to carry out their desires.
- Describe what other parents have found meaningful to do during this time; doing so gives parents a framework and permission to think broadly about what they want to do.
- Offer ideas that expand on their own and fit with their expressed preferences; this individualized guidance can help them consider their options and explore the possibilities.
- Let parents know that they can stay with their baby for as long as they wish, and that they can have multiple viewings over time as well.
- Ask them if they want you to stay with them or if they'd rather have their privacy. Let them know that you are available and how to reach you.

Find creative ways to honor the bond between multiple babies. Many parents are keenly aware of the bond between babies who spent time together in the womb. Whether all of their babies are deceased or some are living, parents may want affirmation of this bond by having the opportunity to hold all of their babies together in their arms. Photographs of this time with the babies together can be treasured keepsakes.

Box 7-2   PLIDA Practice Guidelines: Offering the Baby to Bereaved Parents—cont'd

Let parents know that their baby is always available to them. A significant way to individualize care is by making the baby freely available to parents for as long as they and their circumstances require.

- Keeping the baby available allows parents more time to move through the normal shock that can hinder decision-making or blur their memory of seeing the baby right away or only once.
- When you make the baby available to parents, they can determine when and how to spend time with their baby.
- Parents can decide whether to keep their baby in the mother's room continuously, or they can have the baby brought to them periodically.
- No matter how many days have passed since the death occurred, it can still be important and appropriate for parents to want to view or spend time with their baby, even as the body changes.
- Lengthy availability is especially important for mothers who experience a traumatic or surgical delivery, or who are in intensive care or at a different hospital due to their baby's transport.
- It is important to have an institutional policy in place whereby a baby is accessible to the parents for as long as the mother is hospitalized and until the parents consent to transfer to a funeral home or final disposition.
- There should be a process in place whereby a nurse, chaplain, or social worker can retrieve and warm the baby when the parents request.
- Follow-up with families who leave the hospital soon after their baby dies is critical, as they may be overcome with shock and trauma, and need at least a day to process the reality of their baby's death.
- Funeral arrangements for the baby may be completed prior to the mother's discharge or it could take several days up to a week, depending on the family's circumstances. The bereavement care provider should provide follow-up to the family *and* work individually with families who want their baby to stay at the hospital after the mother is discharged and final disposition for the baby is pending. The bereavement care provider can be instrumental in helping families transition to working with their funeral director to arrange additional time with the baby.
- Some hospitals will have the morgue space, staff time, and other resources available that support your efforts to individualize care even further by making the baby available to parents even after the mother is discharged and final disposition arrangements are made for the baby.
- Your effort to individualize care will occur in the context of many factors, including the gestational age and condition of the baby, state policies, institutional procedures and facilities, and the parent's cultural or religious practices. For more related information that can guide policy, please refer to other PLIDA Position Statements and PLIDA Practice Guidelines.

Respect the process of letting go. Letting go of their baby is a process, and for many parents, an important piece of this process is coming to the realization that the body is empty of life. As one mother said, "She feels different now. This is not *her* anymore. It is just her body now." Individualize care, in order to give each parent the time they need to come to terms with this reality. Some parents need more time, some need less. For some parents, this process of letting go

Continued

Box 7-2   PLIDA Practice Guidelines: Offering the Baby to Bereaved Parents—cont'd

can involve multiple interactions with their baby over several days. Continued access to their baby can help parents face the reality of their baby's death within the context of their bond with their baby.

Know that your empathic relationship with parents can aid their adjustment. Whether parents want to see their baby or not, your kindness and understanding are key to supporting parents as they do the emotional, spiritual, and cognitive work they need to do. Providing follow-up care to parents after discharge is a natural extension of this relationship. Follow-up allows you to check in as their shock wears off and they're confronting the reality of their baby's death, and you can make the appropriate referrals to local and online support groups, professional counseling, and other resources. While families may be overwhelmed immediately after the baby's death, it is important to provide written information and access to these various discharge-support options, as well as the contact information for a hospital representative who might be available post-discharge to help with community support referrals.

These Practice Guidelines were approved June 26, 2008 by the Board of Directors of PLIDA, the Pregnancy Loss and Infant Death Alliance. PLIDA is solely responsible for the content.

---

relationships with children born subsequently, the standard advice changed to, "Wait 6 to 12 months so you can emotionally recover first." The observed psychopathology included overprotectiveness or "vulnerable child syndrome," coined by Green and Solnit (1964); disappointment in the new baby as an inadequate replacement for the dead baby or "replacement child syndrome," coined by Cain and Cain (1964); and being emotionally unavailable to the new baby because of chronic grief (Davidson, 1977; Peppers and Knapp, 1980). But the new advice to "emotionally recover first" promoted unrealistic expectations that grief should end, that a year was sufficient time to "finish grieving," and that the mother should resist her ongoing desire to bear a healthy baby until she was done grieving. In reality, mothers report that emotional recovery is not synonymous with a complete end to grief; a number of years passed before they could feel "at peace" with their baby's death; and waiting that long to embark on another pregnancy was out of the question (Davis and others, 1989).

Further research over the years has pointed out that mothers' emotion-laden experience of subsequent pregnancy and parenting is not necessarily psychopathology caused by unresolved grief, but a normal reaction to the trauma of perinatal death. Anxiety and resistance to bonding during subsequent pregnancy, feeling protective of the new baby after delivery, and wondering about the resemblance between babies are all common, natural reactions that do not always lead to disturbed relationships; after all, with firsthand experience that tragedy can happen to her, the bereaved mother cannot be expected to remain blissful or naïve about her prospects for a healthy baby or one who will continue to thrive (Chez, 1995; Davis, 1996). Instead, she will likely feel fearful, depressed, hypervigilant, vulnerable, have lowered expectations for a healthy baby, and continually struggle to find a balance between hope and fear (Côté-Arsenault, and others, 2001; DeBackere, Hill, and Kavanaugh, 2008; O'Leary and Thorwick, 2008). The bereaved mother can be affected throughout her pregnancy, whether her previous baby died earlier or later in pregnancy or after birth, whatever the cause of her baby's death, or whether she has living children (Côté-Arsenault and Morrison-Beedy, 2001; Wollenschein and others, 2007; Bergner and others, 2008). Anxiety may increase as the due date approaches, particularly for mothers with multiple or late-term losses, and many mothers report a temporary resurgence of grief with the delivery of the new baby, as they are flooded with memories of the baby who died (Davis, 1996; Côté-Arsenault and Donato, 2007). In spite of the negatives, being pregnant again and giving birth to a healthy baby can be healing (Davis, 1996; Barr, 2006).

The prescription for physical recovery depends on the mother's unique medical history and condition, and there are no consistent findings on a "best time" emotionally for getting pregnant after a baby dies (Rowland and Goodnight, 2009). This indicates the importance of individualized care, including emotional support around the issue of a subsequent pregnancy. In fact, mothers report wanting and benefiting from accurate information about their own physical and emotional recovery rather than generalized prescriptions, so that they can decide for themselves after assessing and balancing their own unique needs and circumstances (Davis and others, 1989). Mothers can also benefit from comprehensive and compassionate support during the pregnancy, delivery, and postpartum follow-up, including acknowledgment of their emotional experience, validation of both positive and negative feelings, information and reassurance, more frequent monitoring and phone calls, longer office visits, and referrals to support groups (Côté-Arsenault and Freije, 2004; Côté-Arsenault, and others, 2006; DeBackere, Hill, and Kavanaugh, 2008; O'Leary, 2009). Instead of avoiding the topic of the last pregnancy, the practitioner's affirmation of their deceased baby and their devoted parenting of this child may help parents move forward in bonding to the new baby during the next pregnancy (O'Leary, 2004.) Mothers can also benefit from reviewing the events surrounding their baby's death with their practitioner so as to understand their maternity care and gain a sense of control going forward. Counseling that reinforces positive approaches to coping, remembering, and grieving for the baby who died, restoring confidence, reducing anxiety, individualizing the babies, and investing in the new baby may help the mother find a better balance between her hopes and fears and facilitate a healthy relationship with the babies born subsequently (DeBecker, 1999; Douglas and Sussman, 2000; Lamb, 2002; Jeffers, 2003; Follette and Pistorello, 2007; Forsyth and Eifert, 2008; Gamble and Creedy, 2009; O'Leary 2009).

CUTTING-EDGE TOPICS IN PERINATAL BEREAVEMENT CARE

Perinatal Hospice Care after Prenatal Diagnosis of a Life-Limiting Condition

When a baby is diagnosed prenatally with a fatal condition, the standard of care has been to recommend termination of the pregnancy. This recommendation has roots in the outdated approach of "protecting" parents, but in fact, pregnancy termination does not spare parents from grief (Kersting and others, 2009; Korenromp and others, 2009). A new alternative, perinatal hospice, also sometimes called perinatal palliative care, is a safe, innovative, and compassionate model of support that can be offered to parents (Calhoun and Hoeldtke, 2000; Calhoun and others, 2003). Perinatal hospice is not a place, nor does it need to be a formal program. It is the provision of care that supports parents through the rest of their pregnancy, through planning for the gentle birth and death of their baby whenever that might happen, through medical decision making before and after birth, and through their grief. Perinatal hospice does not insist that parents go to term. Depending on the baby's condition, the mother's health, or family circumstances, parents may choose to induce labor before term, but their focus remains on giving their baby a gentle birth, affirming their baby's life, and continuing to take care of their baby before and after death.

If a baby lives longer than a few minutes or hours after birth, perinatal hospice also incorporates conventional hospice care, such as managing pain or discomfort. It is a continuum of comprehensive, coordinated care that honors the baby as well as the parents in their role as devoted nurturers.

The time is ripe for perinatal hospice, as modern bereavement care can support parents through this emotional experience, neonatal palliative care can offer treatment to reduce or eliminate suffering, and with the advent of more nuanced medical decisions in the neonatal intensive care unit (NICU), parents do not have to fear that they will be forced to hand over their dying newborn to painful and protracted intensive care (Kuebelbeck and Davis, 2010).

Palliative Care for the Dying Baby

Palliative care is a comprehensive, multidisciplinary approach that aims to relieve suffering by managing pain and other symptoms of a condition or disease, and attends to the holistic needs of the infant as well as the family (Carter, Hubble, and Weise, 2006). It affirms life and regards dying as a natural process, intending neither to hasten nor postpone death, the goal being to enable the dying baby to have the best possible quality of life. When willing and able, parents are supported and integrated into the baby's care as the primary caregivers and decision makers (Brosig and others, 2007; De Lisle-Porter and Podruchny, 2009).

Palliative care can include end-of-life care for the dying baby in or out of the NICU, as well as medical treatments such as supplemental oxygen or a feeding tube for a baby whose death is not imminent or whose comfort will be improved by these measures. Ideally, DNR language is replaced by the new "Allow Natural Death" (AND) language (Knox and Vereb, 2005). DNR focuses on withholding or withdrawing medical treatment and is often confusing to implement or explain to bereft families. In contrast, AND is more descriptive and definitive, making it clear to parents and caregivers alike that medical treatment is to focus on comfort for the dying baby and on allowing a natural death to occur without the interference of aggressive or painful intervention.

After-Death Care in the Home

As part of the "green burial" and "home funeral" movements, more families are reclaiming traditions of caring for the dead in the intimacy of home. Instead of relinquishing their baby to strangers in the hospital morgue or funeral home, parents can take their baby home and continue their role as caregivers. This not only circumvents the often heart wrenching relinquishment of the baby's body in the hospital, but also gives parents the opportunity to spend additional time with their infant, gather memories, and experience a more gradual goodbye, which can decrease parental grief (Wijngaards-de Meij and others, 2008). Parents may find it more comfortable and meaningful to have a vigil at home, and invite family and friends to meet their baby and say goodbye (Kuebelbeck and Davis, 2010). Home care is also far less costly, which is often a consideration for young families (Gonzalez and Hereira, 2008).

Legal requirements vary, but it is legal across the United States and many other countries to provide at least some after-death care, including transporting the body from hospital to home, or to the cremation or burial site (Carlson, 1998). For example, embalming is rarely required by law and is prohibited by some religions. Caring for the body is mostly as simple as bathing, dressing, and keeping the body cool with dry ice hidden underneath blankets (Crossings, 2009). Health care practitioners can assist parents by providing the necessary paperwork and information on practical matters such as keeping the body cool, as well as the local legal requirements. More information is available from home funeral advocacy groups, such as the Funeral Consumers Alliance, and Crossings at *www.crossings.net*.

Pregnancy Loss and Infant Death Alliance Practice Guidelines

Practice guidelines (see Boxes 7-1 and 7-2) for state-of-the-art perinatal bereavement care were created by PLIDA in 2008. These guidelines are evidence based, rooted in the academic research training programs and professional experience of nationally renowned experts in the field of perinatal bereavement, many of whom reviewed these guidelines and shared their expertise. These guidelines explain the what, why, and how of relationship-based bereavement care. Free copies of these and other PLIDA Practice Guidelines and their accompanying PLIDA Position Statements can be downloaded from the organization's web site, *www.plida.org*.

CONCLUSION

The primary goals of the nurse in providing nursing care at the time of pregnancy loss or infant death are to maintain the integrity of the family unit and promote healthy, uncomplicated grief. This is best accomplished through compassionate, sensitive caring at the time of the death and by referring for appropriate follow-up during the first year after the loss.

BIBLIOGRAPHY

Als H: Individualized, family-focused developmental care for the very low birthweight preterm infant in the NICU. In Friedman SI, Sigman MD, editors: *Advances in applied developmental psychology, The psychological development of low-birth-weight children*, vol 6, Norwood, NJ, 1992, Ablex Publishing, pp. 341–388.

Als H, Gilkerson I: The role of relationship-based developmentally supportive newborn intensive care in strengthening outcome of premature infants, *Semin Perinatol* 21:178–189, 1997.

Armstrong DS: Perinatal loss and parental distress after the birth of a healthy infant, *Adv Neonatal Care* 7(4):200–206, 2007.

Barnsteiner JH, Gillis-Donovan J: Being related and separate: a standard for therapeutic relationships, *Matern Child Nurs J* 15(4):223–224, 226–228, 1990.

Barr P: Relation between grief and subsequent pregnancy status 13 months after perinatal bereavement, *J Perinat Med* 34:207–211, 2006.

Bergner A, Beyer R, Klapp BF, Rauchfuss M: Pregnancy after early pregnancy loss: a prospective study of anxiety, depressive symptomatology and coping, *J Psychosom Obstet Gynaecol* 29(2):105–113, 2008.

Bowlby J: *Loss: sadness and depression*, New York, 1982, Basic Books.

Brier N: Grief following miscarriage: a comprehensive review of the literature, *J Womens Health (Larchmt)* 17(3):451–464, 2008.

Brosig CL, Pierucci RL, Kupst MJ, Leuthner SR: Infant end-of-life care: the parents' perspective, *J Perinatol* 27(8):510–516, 2007.

Cacciatore J, Bushfield S: Stillbirth: the mother's experience and implications for improving care, *J Soc Work End Life Palliat Care* 3(3):59–79, 2007.

Cain AC, Cain BS: On replacing a child, *J Am Acad Child Psychiatry* 3:443–456, 1964.

Calhoun BC, Hoeldtke NJ: The perinatal hospice: ploughing the field of natal sorrow, *Frontiers in Fetal Health* 1(2):16–33, 2000.

Calhoun BC, and others: Perinatal hospice: comprehensive care for the family of the fetus with a lethal condition, *J Reprod Med* 48(5):343–348, 2003.

Cameron J, Taylor J, Greene A: Representations of rituals and care in perinatal death in British midwifery textbooks 1937-2004, *Midwifery* 24(3):335–343, 2008.

Capitulo KL: Evidence for healing interventions with perinatal bereavement, *MCN Am J Matern Child Nurs* 30(6):389–396, 2005.

Carlson L: *Caring for the dead: your final act of love*, Hinesburg, VT, 1998, Upper Access Books.

Carlson R, Weber-Dennigmann K, Lammert C: *Sharing and caring: establishing and maintaining an effective share program*, St Charles, MO, 2007, Share Pregnancy and Infant Loss Support, Inc.

Carter BS, Hubble C, Weise KL: Palliative medicine in neonatal and pediatric intensive care, *Child Adolesc Psychiatr Clin North Am* 15(3):759–777, 2006.

Chan MF, and others: Attitudes of midwives towards perinatal bereavement in Hong Kong, *Midwifery* 23(3):309–321, 2007.

Chan MF, and others: Investigating factors associated to nurses' attitudes towards perinatal bereavement care, *J Clin Nurs* 17(4):509–518, 2008.

Chez R: After hours, *Obstet Gynecol* 85(6):1059–1061, 1995.

Côté-Arsenault D: Weaving babies lost in pregnancy into the fabric of the family, *J Fam Nurs* 9:23–37, 2003.

Côté-Arsenault D: Threat appraisal, coping, and emotions across pregnancy subsequent to perinatal loss, *Nurs Res* 56(2):108–116, 2007.

Côté-Arsenault D, Bidlack D, Humm A: Women's emotions and concerns during pregnancy following perinatal loss, *MCN Am J Matern Child Nurs* 26(3):128–134, 2001.

Côté-Arsenault D, Donato KL: Restrained expectations in late pregnancy following loss, *J Obstet Gynecol Neonatal Nurs* 36(6):550–557, 2007.

Côté-Arsenault D, Donato K, Earl SS: Watching and worrying: early pregnancy after loss experiences, *MCN Am J Matern Child Nurs* 31:356–363, 2006.

Côté-Arsenault D, Freije MM: Support groups helping women through pregnancies after loss, *West J Nurs Res* 26:650–670, 2004.

Côté-Arsenault D, Marshall R: One foot in-one foot out: weathering the storm of pregnancy after perinatal loss, *Res Nurs Health* 23:473–485, 2000.

Côté-Arsenault D, Morrison-Beedy D: Women's voices reflecting changed expectations for pregnancy after perinatal loss, *J Nurs Sch* 33:239–244, 2001.

Crossings: *Resource guide: a manual for home funeral care*. Retrieved at www.crossings.net/resourceguide030109.pdf.

Davidson GW: Death of the wished-for child: a case study, *Death Educ* 1:265–275, 1977.

Davis DL: *Empty cradle, broken heart: surviving the death of your baby*, rev. ed. Golden, CO, 1996, Fulcrum.

Davis DL: Reflections on the Lancet Stillbirth Study, *The Forum, Association for Death Education and Counseling* 30:2,4–5, 2004.

Davis DL, Stein MT: *Parenting your premature baby and child: the emotional journey*, Golden, CO, 2004, Fulcrum.

Davis DL, Stewart M, Harmon RJ: Perinatal loss: providing emotional support for bereaved parents, *Birth* 15(4):242–246, 1988.

Davis DL, Stewart M, Harmon RJ: Postponing pregnancy after perinatal death: perspectives on doctor advice, *J Am Acad Child Adolesc Psychiatry* 28:481–487, 1989.

DeBackere KJ, Hill PD, Kavanaugh KL: The parental experience of pregnancy after perinatal loss, *J Obstet Gynecol Neonatal Nurs* 37(5):525–537, 2008.

DeBecker G: *Protecting the gift: keeping children and teenagers safe (and parents sane)*, New York, 1999, Random House.

De Lisle-Porter M, Podruchny AM: The dying neonate: family-centered end-of-life care, *Neonatal Netw* 28(2):75–83, 2009.

Douglas A, Sussman JR: *Trying again: a guide to pregnancy after miscarriage, stillbirth, and infant loss*, Dallas, TX, 2000, Taylor Trade Publishing.

Fenwick J, and others: Providing perinatal loss care: satisfying and dissatisfying aspects for midwives, *Women Birth* 20(4):153–160, 2007.

Follette VM, Pistorello J: *Finding life beyond trauma*, Oakland, CA, 2007, New Harbinger.

Forsyth JP, Eifert GH: *The mindfulness and acceptance workbook for anxiety*, Oakland, CA, 2008, New Harbinger.

Gamble J, Creedy DK: A counseling model for postpartum women after distressing birth experiences, *Midwifery* 25(2):e21–e30, 2009. Epub 2007 Jul 27.

Geerinck-Vercammen CR, Kanhai HH: Coping with termination of pregnancy for fetal abnormality in a supportive environment, *Prenat Diagn* 23(7):543–548, 2003.

Gold KJ: Navigating care after a baby dies: a systematic review of parent experiences with health providers, *J Perinatol* 27(4):230–237, 2007.

Gold K, Dalton V, Schwenk T: Hospital care for parents after perinatal death, *Obstet Gynecol* 109(5):1156–1166, 2007.

Gold KJ, Kuznia AL, Hayward RA: How physicians cope with stillbirth or neonatal death: a national survey of obstetricians, *Obstet Gynecol* 112(1):29–34, 2008.

Gonzalez F, Hereira M: Home-based viewing (el velorio) after death: a cost-effective alternative for some families, *Am J Hosp Palliat Care* 25(5):419–420, 2008.

Gorski PA: Developmental intervention during neonatal hospitalization: critiquing the state of the science, *Pediatr Clin North Am* 38(6):1469–1479, 1991.

Green M, Solnit AJ: Reactions to the threatened loss of a child: a vulnerable child syndrome, *Pediatrics* 34:58–66, 1964.

Harmon RJ, Cicchinelli DG: Fetal and neonatal loss. In Simons RC, editor: *Understanding human behavior in health and illness*, Baltimore, 1985, Williams & Wilkins.

Harmon RJ, Plummer NS, Frankel KA: Perinatal loss: parental grieving, family impact, and intervention services. In Osofsky JD, Fitzgerald HE, editors: *WAIMH handbook of infant mental health: Infant mental health in groups at high risk*, vol 4, New York, 2000, Wiley and Sons.

Hochberg T: Touching souls: Healing with bereavement photography, The Forum, *Association for Death Education and Counseling* 29(2):6, 2003.

Hughes P, Turton P, Hopper E, Evans CD: Assessment of guidelines for good practice in psychosocial care of mothers after stillbirth: a cohort study, *Lancet* 13:360(9327):114–118, 2002.

Hughes P, Riches S: Psychological aspects of perinatal loss, *Curr Opin Obstet Gynecol* 15:107–111, 2003.

Jansen JL: A bereavement model for the intensive care nursery, *Neonatal Netw* 22(3):17–23, 2003.

Jeffers S: *Embracing uncertainty: breakthrough methods for achieving peace of mind when facing the unknown*, New York, 2003, St. Martin's Press.

Kavanaugh K, Hershberger P: Perinatal loss in low-income African American parents, *J Obstet Gynecol Neonatal Nurs* 34(5):595–605, 2005.

Kavanaugh K, Moro T: Supporting parents after stillbirth or newborn death: there is much that nurses can do, *Am J Nurs* 106(9):74–79, 2006.

Kavanaugh K, Moro TT, Savage TA, Reyes M, Wydra M: Supporting parents' decision making surrounding the anticipated birth of an extremely premature infant, *J Perinat Neonatal Nurs* 23(2):159–170, 2009.

Keeling J, editor: *Fetal and neonatal pathology*, London, 2001, Springer.

Kersting A, and others: Grief after termination of pregnancy due to fetal malformation, *J Psychosom Obstet Gynaecol* 25(2):163–169, 2004.

Kersting A, and others: Psychological impact on women after second and third trimester termination of pregnancy due to fetal anomalies versus women after preterm birth—a 14-month follow up study, *Arch Womens Ment Health* 12(4):193–201, 2009.

Kirkley-Best E, Kellner KR: The forgotten grief: a review of the psychology of stillbirth, *Am J Orthopsychiatry* 52(3):420–429, 1982.

Kitzenger S: *Your baby, your way: making pregnancy decisions and birth plans*, New York, 1987, Pantheon.

Klaus M, Kennel J: *Parent-infant bonding*, St Louis, 1982, Mosby.

Kluger-Bell K: *Unspeakable losses: understanding the experience of pregnancy loss, miscarriage, and abortion*, New York, 1998, W.W. Norton.

Knox C, Vereb J: Allow natural death: a more humane approach to discussing end-of-life directives, *J Emerg Nurs* 31(6):560-561, 2005.

Kobler K, Limbo R, Kavanaugh K: Meaningful moments: the use of ritual in pediatric and perinatal death, *MCN Am J Matern Child Nurs* 32(5):288–296, 2007.

Koloroutis M, editor: *Relationship-based care: a model for transforming practice*, Minneapolis, 2004, Creative Health Care Management.

Korenromp MJ, and others: Adjustment to termination of pregnancy for fetal anomaly: a longitudinal study in women at 4, 8, and 16 months, *Am J Obstet Gynecol* 201(2):160, 2009.

Kuebelbeck A: Perinatal hospice: a holistic approach when death comes at the beginning of life, The Forum, *Association for Death Education and Counseling* 31(1), 2005.

Kuebelbeck A, Davis DL: *A gift of time: continuing your pregnancy after prenatal diagnosis of a life-limiting condition*, Baltimore, 2010, Johns Hopkins University Press.

Lamb EH: The impact of previous perinatal loss on subsequent pregnancy and parenting, *J Perinat Educ* 11(2):33–40, 2002.

Lawrence RA: *Breastfeeding: a guide for the medical profession*, ed 6, New York, 2005, Mosby.

Leon IG: Providing versus packaging support for bereaved parents after perinatal loss, *Birth* 19(2):89–91, 1992a.

Leon IG: Perinatal loss: a critique of current hospital practices, *Clin Pediatr (Phila)* 31(6):366–374, 1992b.

Leon IG: *When a baby dies: psychotherapy for pregnancy and newborn loss*, New Haven, CT, 1992c, Yale University Press.

Lewis E: The management of stillbirth: coping with an unreality, *Lancet* 11(7986):619–620, 1976.

Limbo RK, Wheeler SR: *When a baby dies: a handbook for healing and helping*, rev ed, La Crosse, WI, 1998, Gundersen Lutheran Medical Foundation, Inc.

Luddington-Hoe SM, Golant SK: *Kangaroo care: the best you can do to help your preterm infant*, New York, 1993, Bantam Doubleday Dell.

Mander R: *Loss and bereavement in childbearing*, Oxford, 1994, Blackwell Scientific.

Martin TL, Doka KJ: *Men don't cry, women do: transcending gender stereotypes of grief*, New York, 1999, Brunner-Routledge.

Maroney DI: Recognizing the potential effect of stress and trauma on premature infants in the NICU: how outcomes are affected? *J Perinatol* 23:679–683, 2003.

Meert KL, Thurston CS, Briller SH: The spiritual needs of parents at the time of their child's death in the pediatric intensive care unit and during bereavement: a qualitative study, *Pediatr Crit Care Med* 6(4):420–427, 2005.

Miller S: *Finding hope when a child dies: what other cultures can teach us*, New York, 2002, Fireside Books.

O'Leary J: Grief and its impact on prenatal attachment in the subsequent pregnancy, *Arch Womens Ment Health* 7(1):7–18, 2004.

O'Leary J: Never a simple journey: pregnancy following perinatal loss, *Bereavement Care* 28(2):12–17, 2009.

O'Leary J, Thorwick C: Parental attachment to the unborn child and parental mental representations during pregnancy following perinatal loss, *Attachment: New Directions in Psychotherapy and Relational Psychoanalysis Journal* 2:292–320, 2008.

Peppers LG, Knapp RJ: *Motherhood and mourning: perinatal death*, Westport, CT, 1980, Praeger.

Rando TA: *Grieving: how to go on living when someone you love dies*, New York, 1991, Bantam.

Roehrs C, and others: Caring for families coping with perinatal loss, *J Obstet Gynecol Neonatal Nurs* 37(6):631–639, 2008.

Rowland A, Goodnight WH: Fetal loss: addressing the evaluation and supporting the emotional needs of parents, *J Midwifery Womens Health* 54(3):241–248, 2009.

Royal College of Obstetricians and Gynaecologists and Royal College of Pathologists: *Fetal and perinatal pathology: Report of a joint working party*, London, 2001, RCOG Press. Retrieved from www.rcp.gov. bc.ca/guidelines/Master%5B1%5D.PM5.InvestAssesStillbirths.May2000.pdf.

Saflund K, Sjogren B, Wredling R: The role of caregivers after a stillbirth: views and experiences of parents, *Birth* 31(2):132–137, 2004.

Swanson KM: Nursing as informed caring for the well-being of others, *Image J Nurs Sch* 25(4):352–357, 1993.

Walling AD: Tips from other journals: should mothers see their infants after stillbirth? *Am Fam Physician* Nov 15, 2002. Retrieved from www.aafp.org/afp/2002/1115/p1956.html.

Walzer Leavitt J: *Brought to bed: childbearing in America, 1750-1950*, New York, 1986, Oxford University Press.

Wertz R, Dorothy C: *Lying-in: a history of childbirth in America*, New Haven, CT, 1989, University Press.

Wigglesworth JS, Singer DB, editors: *Textbook of fetal and perinatal pathology*, Boston, 1998, Blackwell Science.

Wijngaards-de Meij L, and others: The impact of circumstances surrounding the death of a child on parents' grief, *Death Stud* 32(3):237–252, 2008.

Wollenschein M, Gustke M, Woopen C, Rohde A: A subsequent pregnancy after a termination of pregnancy because of fetal anomaly—all forgotten and a new beginning? *Prax Kinderpsychol Kinderpsychiatr* 56(9):741–757, 2007.

Wisconsin Stillbirth Service Project (WiSSP): *Most often asked questions about stillbirth evaluation* Retrieved from www2.marshfieldclinic.org/wissp/commonly.htm.

Workman E: Guiding parents through the death of their infant, *J Obstet Gynecol Neonatal Nurs* 30(6):569–573, 2001.

Wright C, Lee REJ: Investigating perinatal death: a review of the options when autopsy consent is refused, *Arch Dis Child Fetal Neonatal Ed* 89:F285, 2004. Retrieved from http://fn.bmjjournals.com/cgi/content/full/89/4/F285.

Young SEJ, Healing TD: Infection in the deceased: a survey of management, *CDR Review Communicable Disease Report* 5(5):R69–R73, 1995.

Zeanah CH, Dailey JV, Rosenblatt MJ, Saller DN Jr: Do women grieve after terminating pregnancies because of fetal abnormalities? A controlled investigation, *Obstet Gynecol* 82(2):270–275, 1993.

8

Ethical Decision Making

Perinatal nurses are confronted daily with ethical dilemmas. This chapter examines the nature of values clarification, introduces a framework for ethics, provides a model for ethical decision making, outlines the individual nurse's responsibility for participation and involvement, and lists the relevant clinical perinatal examples that commonly confront the perinatal nurse.

VALUES CLARIFICATION

Educators, psychologists, anthropologists, sociologists, and theologians have influenced the definition of values. They consider values to be attitudes, beliefs, and moral judgments that are chosen freely and thoughtfully and are prized and acted on (Albert and others, 2006; Beauchamp and Childress, 2008).

Process of Valuing

The process of valuing has three aspects: choosing, prizing, and acting.

Choosing

Choosing involves the cognitive component of valuing. Logical, critical, creative thinking and moral judgment development are included. Important elements of choosing include the following:
- Choosing freely
- Choosing from available alternatives
- Choosing after considering the consequences of each alternative
- Complements other values previously internalized

Prizing

Prizing involves the affective component. This feeling component of valuing includes the following aspects (Beauchamp and Childress, 2008):
- Being aware of one's position on the matter
- Expressing one's value

- Experiencing positive self-esteem as a result of the expression of the value
- Communicating and sending clear messages about the value
- Empathetic listening
- Feeling pride and happiness with the choice

Acting

Acting involves the behavioral component and results in the following (Beauchamp and Childress, 2008):

- Personal, professional, and academic competence
- Conflict resolution
- Willingness to affirm the choice publicly
- Assimilation of the choice as part of personal behavior
- Consistent repetition of the choice

MORAL JUDGMENT DEVELOPMENT

The moral judgment development theory complements valuing. Kohlberg (1981) contributed to the study of moral development by expanding on the work of Piaget and describing six stages of moral development.

Stages

Preconventional Level

The child at the preconventional level is responsive to cultural rules and labels of good and bad, right and wrong. These labels are considered by the child in the context of punishment, reward, or exchange of favors. This level is divided into two stages.

Stage 1

Stage 1 is the stage of punishment and obedience. Avoidance of punishment and deference to power are ends in themselves. The physical consequences of an action determine whether it is good or bad. For example, the reason for doing right is to avoid punishment from those with more power.

Stage 2

Stage 2 is the stage of instrumental purpose and exchange. Right action is that which pragmatically satisfies one's own needs and occasionally the needs of others. Right is following the rules because it is in the immediate interest. Right is also what is fair, equal, a deal, or an agreement. Reciprocity is given for the actual reward rather than out of loyalty or gratitude.

Conventional Level

At the conventional level of moral judgment development, the person considers the expectations of others and conformity as valuable in their own right, regardless of the immediate consequences. There is an attitude of not only conformity but also active maintenance, support, and justification of the order. Stages 3 and 4 are at this level.

Stage 3

Stage 3 is the stage of mutual interpersonal expectations, relationships, and conformity. Good behavior is that which pleases and helps others and is approved by them.

Conformity to stereotypes is common. Behavior is frequently judged by intention, as in meaning well. Right behavior is being nice and living up to what is expected.

Stage 4

Stage 4 is the stage of social system and conscience maintenance. Right action is doing one's duty in a group, showing respect for authority, and upholding the prescribed social order for its own sake. Orientation is toward authority, fixed rules, and maintenance of the social order.

Postconventional Level

The postconventional level is also called the autonomous or principled level. The individual attempts to define moral values and principles that have validity and application apart from the authority of society and the individual's identity with societal groups. There are two stages at this level.

Stage 5

Stage 5 is the stage of 'a priori' rights and social contract or utility. This stage has utilitarian overtones. Right action is defined in terms of standards that have been agreed on by society in terms of individual rights. Right action is described as upholding basic rights, values, and legal contracts of society even when they conflict with concrete rules and laws of the group.

Awareness of relativism of personal values and opinions exists, with an emphasis on reaching consensus. Right action is also a matter of personal values aside from what is constitutionally agreed on. There is an emphasis on the legal point of view, with the possibility of changing law in terms of rational consideration of societal utility (Douglas, 2001).

Stage 6

Stage 6 is the stage of universal ethical principles. Right action is defined by a decision of conscience in accord with self-chosen ethical principles. Specific laws usually rest on these principles. When, however, laws violate these principles, acts must be in accord with principles rather than law. Principles are abstract, ethical, and universal, such as the principles of justice, reciprocity, equality, and respect for human dignity.

Qualities

In addition to the six stages of moral development, Kohlberg (1981) described six qualities of the stages of moral development:

- The development of morality proceeds in an invariant sequence as the individual matures and as the environment offers the necessary stimulation and opportunities to learn.
- Subjects cannot comprehend moral reasoning at a level more than one stage beyond their development.
- Subjects are cognitively attracted to reasoning one level above their own predominant level.
- Movement through stages is effected when cognitive disequilibrium is created by conflicting values.
- Although the time it takes to move through the stages varies, the sequence is always the same.
- Movement to higher stages of moral development is advantageous for the individual and society.

FRAMEWORK FOR ETHICS

Definitions

Ethics

Ethics is the study of values in human conduct or the study of right conduct. It is a branch of philosophy that attempts to state and evaluate principles by which ethical dilemmas may be resolved. It is not a science with right or wrong answers but rather a systematic, critical, rational, defensible, intellectual approach to determining what is best in a situation with conflicting values. The result will ultimately be unfavorable and pit one or more ethical principles against another (Albert and others, 2006).

Metaethics

Metaethics is the part of ethics that focuses on the extent to which ethical judgments are reasonable or justifiable.

Normative Ethics

Normative ethics is the part of ethics that raises questions about what is right or ought to be done in a situation that calls for an ethical decision.

Ethical Principles

Several basic principles help to identify values, morals, beliefs, and attitudes and to clarify ethical dilemmas (Table 8-1). Ethical principles comprise the sixth stage of Kohlberg's (1981) moral development. The characteristics of ethical principles follow:
- They suggest direction or propose certain behaviors.
- They serve as guides to organizing and understanding ethically relevant information in an ethical dilemma.
- They propose how to resolve competing claims.
- They are the reasons justifying moral actions.
- They are universal in nature. They are not absolute; they do have exceptions.
- They are neither rules (means) nor values (ends).
- They are unchangeable and discovered by human beings rather than invented.

MODEL FOR ETHICAL DECISION MAKING

Characteristics of Ethical Dilemmas

We live in an era in which technologies develop faster than we can consider consequences. Changes affect clinical practice before guidelines for use are developed and before the social and ethical impact can be considered. Recent technologic advances in endocrinology, genetics, reproductive therapy, neonatal and maternal-fetal medical care, and fetal therapy have created numerous ethical dilemmas for the recipient of care and the caregiver. These dilemmas and the resultant decisions have a considerable impact on society.

The characteristics of an ethical dilemma follow (Albert and others, 2006):
- The choice is between equally undesirable alternatives.
- Real choices exist between possible courses of action.

Table 8-1   Definitions of Ethical Principles

Ethical Principle	Definition
Autonomy	Being one's own person without constraints by another's action or psychologic and physical limitations
Beneficence	Duty to do good
Confidentiality	Holding information entrusted in context of special relationships as private
Fidelity	Duty to keep one's promise or word
Finality	May override demands of law and custom
Generality	Must not refer to specific people or situations
Informed consent	Contains four elements: Disclosure of sufficient information Comprehension Voluntary agreement Competency to make decision
Justice	Equitable distribution of risks and benefits
Nonmaleficence	Duty to do no harm
Ordering	Ethical principles must be prioritized even though they may be conflicting
Publicity	Principles must be known and recognized by all
Reparation	Duty to make up for a wrong
Universality	Same principle must hold for everyone, regardless of time, place, or people involved
Utility	Greatest good or least harm for the greatest number
Veracity	Duty to tell the truth

- The people involved place a significantly different value judgment on possible actions or the consequences.
- Data alone do not help to resolve the dilemma.
- "Answers" to the dilemma come from a number of different disciplines, such as psychology, sociology, and theology.
- Actions taken in an ethical dilemma result in unfavorable outcomes or constitute a breach of one's duty to another individual.
- The choices made in an ethical dilemma have far-reaching effects on our perception of human beings and our definition of personhood, our relationships, and people and society as a whole.
- Any ethical decision involves the allocation and expenditure of resources that are finite.
- Ethical dilemmas are not solvable but rather resolvable.
- There is no right or wrong when dealing with two equally unfavorable actions.

Theories in Ethics

Two classic schools of thought—teleology and deontology—dominate ethical theory (Follin, 2004).

Teleology

According to the theory of teleology, the rightness or wrongness of an action is determined by the consequences, not by whether it is inherently right or wrong. This approach to decision making is risk-to-benefit-based. It is also called utilitarianism or consequentialism.

Deontology

The theory of deontology holds that the inherent characteristics of the decision can be judged independent of its outcome or consequences. Duty-based or rights-based approaches are examples of deontologic thoughts.

Moral Relativism

A pure application of either teleology or deontology may not be useful. Aspects of both theories are usually combined when making ethical decisions blended with moral relativism. Moral relativism adds the notion of personal interpretation. The application of paradigm cases, anecdotal experiences, and ethical principles to clinical problems exemplifies relativism.

The root principles of ethical theory are beneficence, justice, and autonomy (see Table 8-1). Decision making is always colored by the individual's values, attitudes, knowledge, desires, cultural mores, experiences, and background (Beauchamp and Childress, 2008).

Steps in Decision Making

The steps in ethical decision making are described in Box 8-1.

Nursing Responsibility

The concepts central to nurses' responsibility in participation in ethical decision making are caring, coordination, and advocacy. These concepts are based on the unique relationship between the nurse and the patient. Clinical ethics, existing aside from medical ethics, incorporates the ethical problems the nurse encounters in the independent and collaborative domains of practice. Nursing is owned by society and as such is an essential part of society with a responsibility to the whole.

Caring

Caring, described by Swanson (1993), provides the first mandate for nurses' participation in and assumption of ethical practice. The second mandate is derived from the social contract and the American Nurses Association (ANA) code for nurses (Box 8-2). The third mandate for participation in ethical decision making is the pivotal position of nursing within the health care organization. Professional nursing practice is ethical nursing practice.

Conscience Clauses

Nurses are occasionally placed in situations where physician orders or patient requests may conflict with their own professional ethic and moral codes. Conscience

Box 8-1   Steps in Ethical Decision Making

Identify the Problem
- Who are the people involved?
- How are they interrelated?
- What is involved?

Identify the Values, Issues, or Ethical Dilemmas, and Make a Concise Statement of the Problem and Conflicts in Values
- State your values and ethical position related to the case.
- Generate alternatives for resolving the dilemma or dilemmas.

Examine and Categorize the Alternatives
- List alternatives.
- Identify those consistent and those inconsistent with your own values and ethics.

Predict the Possible Consequences for Those Acceptable Alternatives
- Identify physical, psychologic, social, spiritual, and short- and long-range consequences.
- Identify those consequences consistent with your values and ethics.

Prioritize Acceptable Alternatives
- Develop a plan of action.
- Implement the plan.
- Evaluate the action taken.

clauses are statutory provisions that allow healthcare personnel or institutions the right to refuse provision of medical care because of religious or moral beliefs. Unfortunately, many of these clauses do not take into consideration the responsibilities of healthcare providers to the general public or their own colleagues. Because of this, professional organizations such as the ANA and the Association of Women's Health, Obstetric, and Neonatal Nurses (AWHONN) have published position statements which support patients' rights to information and treatment that they may require or ask for, while taking into consideration a nurse's personal code of ethics. Obstetrical units may wish to research policies within their own institutions, provide open discussions regarding conscience clauses, and develop written guidelines which will protect nurses, support staff, and patients (Tillett, 2008).

PATIENT SELF-DETERMINATION ACT

A federal law, the Patient Self-Determination Act, went into effect in December 1991 for all health care facilities receiving federal monies. This act requires that all patients be informed of their rights to make decisions concerning their health care.

Box 8-2 American Nurses Association Code of Ethics

- The nurse, in all professional relationships, practices with compassion and respect for the inherent dignity, worth, and uniqueness of every individual unrestricted by consideration of social or economic status, personal attributes, or nature of the health problems.
- The nurse's primary commitment is to the patient, whether an individual, family, group, or community.
- The nurse promotes, advocates for, and strives to protect the health, safety, and rights of the patient.
- The nurse is responsible and accountable for individual nursing practice and determines the appropriate delegation of tasks consistent with the nurse's obligation to provide optimum care.
- The nurse owes the same duties to self as to others, including the responsibility to preserve integrity and safety, to maintain competence, and to continue personal and professional growth.
- The nurse participates in establishing, maintaining health care environments and conditions of employment conducive to the provision of quality health care and consistent with the values of the profession through individual and collective action.
- The nurse participates in the advancement of the profession through contributions to practice, education, administration, and knowledge development.
- The nurse collaborates with other health professionals and the public in promoting community, national, and international efforts to meet health needs.
- The profession of nursing, as represented by associations and their members, is responsible for articulating nursing values, for maintaining the integrity of the profession and its practice, and for shaping social policy.

From American Nurses Association: *Code of ethics for nurses with interpretive statements*, Silver Springs, MD, 2001, American Nurses Publishing. Retrieved from *www.nursingworld.org/ethics/chcode.htm.*

ADVANCE DIRECTIVE

An advance directive, also known as a living will or a durable power of attorney, recognizes the patient's right to control decisions relating to acceptance or refusal of aspects of his or her own medical care. When the patient has decision-making capacity, that control can be exercised by formulating an advance directive.

If the patient loses decision-making capacity, a durable power of attorney can appoint another person to make those decisions. A living will can direct the physician to provide, withhold, or withdraw life-sustaining care.

In the case of a pregnant woman, however, the advance directive does not allow her to make decisions in advance that may affect fetal survival or quality of life. For example, if a pregnant woman is involved in a motor vehicle accident and sustains a head injury that permanently affects her cardiorespiratory center, she may be kept on life-sustaining care despite instructions in her living will to the contrary. If sustaining her on life support can successfully maintain the pregnancy, which shows no evidence of fetal compromise, her living will requesting no life support will be disregarded. In such situations it has been determined that postponement of maternal death does less harm to her when balanced against the fetal right to survive.

ETHICS COMMITTEE

Most tertiary institutions have a review board or ethics committee in place for situations in which individuals/families need assistance in dealing with difficult decisions regarding what is right or fair care or when ethical decisions collide with legal and moral obligations of the institution. These committees are usually multidisciplinary and composed of physicians and nurses from the various settings where many of the dilemmas arise, along with allied health care professionals such as an administrator, a member of the clergy, a social services representative, an attorney or risk management representative, and an ethicist (who actually may be one of the professionals previously listed) (Beauchamp and Childress, 2008). A layperson may be asked to serve on the committee as well.

In the beginning of the formation of a board, there are usually some requirements for the prospective members to receive formalized education in the process of ethical decision making. There typically is also some time set aside to educate the members and for them to become accustomed as a group to the processes they will follow. The main functions of the committee are:

- To develop and revise ethical policies and procedures such as informed consent, confidentiality, and advance directives
- To assist with difficult ethical decisions related to health care

It is recommended that there be a process in place for handling emergency situations and specified people who must serve on the board to make decisions. The family should always be invited to provide input and to attend some part of the session when possible and when desired.

CLINICAL EXAMPLES OF ETHICAL DILEMMAS

Some clinical examples of ethical dilemmas that perinatal nurses face are listed in Box 8-3.

CONCLUSION

The list of perinatal ethical decisions is much longer than that given in Box 8-3. Some dilemmas are everyday issues. Others are likely to be encountered infrequently and then only in select tertiary perinatal centers. However, it is impossible to work in perinatal nursing and not become involved in ethical dilemmas or participate in ethical decision making. The nurse must not only examine issues in light of the level of participation she or he is willing to have but also facilitate an environment in which colleagues and patients can participate in ethical decisions. The nurse functions as educator, support person, counselor, administrator, researcher, and care provider. Nurses spend more time with patients than any other health care team members do. As a result, nurses must take an active and assertive role in the development of ethical guidelines for areas of perinatal practice (Follin, 2004; Beauchamp and Childress, 2008).

Box 8-3	Clinical Examples of Perinatal Ethical Dilemmas

- Voluntary pregnancy termination
- Second trimester abortions
- Selective reduction in multiple gestation
- Emergency contraception
- Previable termination of pregnancy for maternal reasons
- Termination of pregnancy by telemedicine (Lupton, 2008)
- Harvesting of fetal organs or tissue
- In vitro fertilization and decisions for disposal of remaining fertilized ova
- In vitro fertilization with multiple eggs
- In vitro fertilization in mothers with advanced maternal age
- Allocation of resources in pregnancies complicated by substance abuse and other antisocial behaviors
- Allocation of resources in pregnancy care during previable period
- Fetal surgery
- Treatment of genetic disorders or fetal abnormalities found on prenatal screening
- Routine use of electronic fetal monitoring (EFM) for cesarean delivery indication in cases of previous cesarean delivery
- Routine use of electronic fetal monitoring (EFM) on low-risk intrapartum patients
- Equal access to prenatal care
- Health care rights
- Maternal rights versus fetal rights
- Extraordinary medical treatment for pregnancy complications
- Court-ordered cesarean section
- Using organs from an anencephalic infant
- Genetic engineering/gender selection
- Cloning
- Surrogate motherhood
- Mandatory drug testing
- Sanctity of life versus quality of life for extremely premature or severely disabled infant

BIBLIOGRAPHY

Albert R and others: *Clinical ethics: a practical approach to ethical decisions in clinical medicine*, ed 6, New York, 2006, McGraw-Hill.

American College of Obstetricians and Gynecologists: *Position statement: ethical decision making in obstetrics and gynecology*, Washington, DC, 2007, ACOG.

American College of Obstetricians and Gynecologists: *Position statement: the limits of conscientious refusal in reproductive medicine*, Washington, DC, 2007, ACOG.

American College of Obstetricians and Gynecologists: *Position statement: surgery and patient choice*, Washington, DC, 2008, ACOG.

American Nurses Association: *Code of ethics for nurses with interpretive statements*, Silver Springs, MD, 2001, American Nurses Publishing. Retrieved from http://www.nursingworld.org/Main MenuCategories/EthicsStandards/CodeofEthicsforNurses.aspx.

Association of Women's Health, Obstetric, and Neonatal Nurses: *Position statement: access to health care issues*, Washington, DC, 2005, AWHONN.

Association of Women's Health, Obstetric, and Neonatal Nurses: *Position statement: role of the registered nurse in support of patients as related to genetic testing*, Washington, DC, 1998, AWHONN.

Association of Women's Health, Obstetric, and Neonatal Nurses: *Position statement: nurses' rights and responsibilities related to abortion and sterilization*, Washington, DC, 1999, AWHONN.

Association of Women's Health, Obstetric, and Neonatal Nurses: *Position statement: fetal assessment*, Washington, DC, 2000a, AWHONN.

Association of Women's Health, Obstetric, and Neonatal Nurses: *Position statement: pregnancy discrimination act*, Washington, DC, 2000b, AWHONN.

Beauchamp T, Childress T: *Principles of biomedical ethics*, ed 6, New York, 2008, Oxford University Press.

Bendikson K, Racowsky C: *Gender selection,* UpToDate, 2008. Retrieved from http://www.uptodate.com.

Bergeron V: The ethics of cesarean section on maternal request: a feminist critique of the American College of Obstetricians and Gynecologists' position on patient-choice surgery, *Bioethics* 21(9):478–487, 2007.

Douglas M: Ethics in nursing practice. In Brent N, editor: *Nurses and the law: a guide to principles and applications*, ed 2, Philadelphia, 2001, Saunders.

Follin S, editor: *Nurse's legal handbook*, ed 5, Philadelphia, 2004, Lippincott Williams & Wilkins.

Kalish RB, McCullough LB, Chervenak FA: Patient choice cesarean delivery: ethical issues, *Curr Opin Obstet Gynecol* 20(2):116–119, 2008.

Kohlberg L: Essays on moral development. Vol I, *The philosophy of moral development;* Vol II, *The psychology of moral development: moral stages the life cycle;* Vol III, *Education and moral development: moral stages and practice,* San Francisco, 1981, Harper & Row.

Lupton M: Termination of pregnancy by telemedicine: an ethicist's viewpoint, *Br J Obstet Gynecol* 115:1071–1073, 2008.

Swanson K: Nursing as informed caring for the well-being of others, *Image J Nurs Sch* 25(4):352–357, 1993.

Tillett J: "Conscience" clauses: the rights and responsibilities of a nurse, *J Perinatal Neonatal Nurs* 22(3):179–180, 2008.

9

Legal Issues and Risk Management

*P*rofessional liability* is a concept that explains a system of accountability. This system is expected to compensate for losses and deter negligent or substandard practices by the professional. Unfortunately, the professional liability system does a poor job of both compensation and deterrence.

The system does not focus so much on poor performance and incompetence as it does on unexpected outcomes. Litigation in health care fields has increased sharply in the past 15 years, both in the number of lawsuits and in the amount of awards.

From the establishment of the National Practitioner Data Bank (NPDB) in 1990 through 2006, there have been 6208 malpractice claims imposed against professional nurses. Cases related to obstetrics and surgery comprised a significant number of these claims (NPDB, 2006). In 2005, the United States Department of Health and Human Services (USDHHS) found that a mean payment of more than $675,000 was paid out per perinatal nursing-related malpractice lawsuit (McCaffrey and others, 2008).

Obstetric-related cases for physicians generated 8.7% of all medical Malpractice Payment Reports (NPDB, 2006). According to the American College of Obstetrics and Gynecology's (ACOG) 2006 Professional Liability Survey, 7.2% of obstetricians quit practicing obstetrics, 28.5% increased their cesarean deliveries, 26.4% refused to perform vaginal birth after cesarean delivery, and 25.6% stopped taking high-risk patients because of an increase in liability and malpractice costs (ACOG, 2006).

Experiencing a deposition and potential lawsuit can be traumatic and frightening. If nurses can gain an understanding of potential obstetrical risks, their role in prevention, and knowledge of the litigation process, it will assist them in dealing with the liability system that is currently in place.

MALPRACTICE INSURANCE

Nurses are more frequently being included among separately named parties in lawsuits (Brent, 2001). As a result, more nurses carry their own malpractice insurance. Insurance premiums are higher for specialty nursing practice, such as perinatal care, than for other less litigious nursing specialties. Nurses in the specialty of perinatal care find themselves in a difficult position because they are part of a team; therefore, they do not often act independently to reduce personal risk (AWHONN, 1999).

Some issues that a nurse needs to examine before deciding to carry a personal insurance policy (Brent, 2001) are:

- Is there a high frequency of exposure to lawsuits in the setting in which I practice? High exposure may occur where there are high risk patients more than 25% of the time.
- Do the policies and procedures represent a safe standard of care?
- Do I sometimes practice outside a hospital setting in independent practice or always as an employee where liability insurance includes nurse practice? A physician's malpractice insurance does not cover the practice of office nurses. Examples of practice outside the hospital setting include teaching childbirth preparation classes, giving frequent telephone advice, doing outreach education, or providing contract care.
- Am I working in a setting where physician response is not timely or where physicians are overworked?
- Is the staff-to-patient ratio commonly lower than standard?
- Are continuing education programs encouraged, and are they supported?

According to Brous (2008), a nurse and attorney, not all claims requiring representation involve malpractice. Employers may bring charges against nurses for unprofessional conduct, as well as alleged departures from stated policies and procedures. For these reasons, the American Association of Nurse Attorneys recommends that all nurses carry their own insurance protection.

REASONS PARENTS SUE

One reason for increased frequency and severity of perinatal litigation is that patients have unrealistic and inflated expectations of the health care system to correct all ills. Another cause is the health care professional's overconfidence.

Reasons parents sue vary. Some common reasons (Brent, 2001) include:

- Injured or dead infant
- Advice of family and friends, who believe that if fault can be found, parents will feel better or at least feel that justice has been done
- Monetary concerns related to the expense of continued care for an injured infant
- Anger, a need to blame, and belief that the provider is at fault
- Complicated grief
- Surprise that anything could go wrong, unrealistic expectations, or inadequate information before giving consent for care
- Belief that litigation will be profitable
- Poor communication with health care providers

When parents sue because their child is injured, the award sought is generally for the expenses involved in the continued and future care of that child. A small amount of the award may be for the emotional damages the parents have suffered; this must be proved separately from the child's damages. When parents sue because their child is dead, the award is almost solely for the emotional damages suffered from loss of the relationship and for any impairment in other relationships. The nurse must assess the family to discover whether any of the members are unable to deal with death constructively, to meet their basic needs, to accept and receive needed help, or to express and accept various family members' individualized expressions of feelings.

LITIGATION RISK

There are three common sources of litigation risk:
- Failure to keep current
- Inadequate supervision, management, or administration of services
- Communication inadequacies, errors, or inaccuracies

Failure to Keep Current
Ways to keep current include the following:
- Exercising professional responsibility by attending continuing education programs consistently
- Participating in a detailed orientation program when employed in a new setting
- Maintaining familiarity with relevant policies and procedures (AWHONN, 2000a)
- Being aware of sources of and relevant guidelines for standards of care
- Keeping abreast of current relevant legal issues and decisions (Simpson and Knox, 2003)

Inadequate Supervision
The following aspects help to make sure that supervision is adequate:
- The immediate supervising nurse who is present (head nurse, charge nurse, team leader, designee, or nurse of other similar title) is required to respond to all questions the nurse at the bedside has regarding supervision. This includes responding to issues related to who was informed of any difficulties or immediate identification of problems.
- Nurses must know the chain of command to follow when a problem is identified; this is especially important when there is conflict regarding who should respond to patient care issues.
- Nurses should consult with other staff members who are more experienced or who are experts; in cases of litigation, this may help their defense.
- Nurses should report problematic staffing patterns or ratios to the supervisor. Areas that are potentially problematic include nurse-to-patient ratios that are too low, staff shifts on rotation or on call that are too long, inadequate staff orientation, too many inexperienced staff members, and staff members who are not qualified for their assignments. These problematic patterns must be considered and responded to by the supervisor.

Lynn, Redman, and Zomorodi (2006) cited six reasons for dissatisfaction in the health care system which contributes to the current nursing shortage:
- Lack of advancement opportunities
- Verbal abuse on the job
- Stress and overload
- Physically demanding work

- Understaffing coupled with an overwhelming number of patients with increased care requirements
- Increased paperwork which takes nurses away from patient care

This nursing shortage and the reasons definitely affect the legal climate. The nursing shortage contributes to increased personal liability and to the liability of the institution in which the nurse is practicing. It affects the physician's practice and liability secondary to dependence on adequate patient supervision and collegiality in practice.

Inadequate Communication

Patient/Family and Nurse

Some areas of patient and nurse communication risks are described in the following sections.

Patient education and childbirth preparation

There may be risks associated with misinformation, incomplete information, or no information provided in patient education and childbirth preparation situations.

Telephone advice

Generally, it is best to view a patient's telephone call requesting advice as an opportunity to help the patient focus on the main elements of the complaint and to empower the patient in self-advocacy with the concerns. When much of the nurse's time is used to take calls and give telephone advice, clear guidelines should be established for what the nurse is allowed to discuss and what the patient is supposed to do with the advice. The advice and recommendations, any consultation with the physician, and the patient's statement of understanding should be documented on a specific form intended for this purpose. This form should then be filed in the permanent record.

Amount of information

Exercise caution when giving information; providing too little or too much information, giving vague responses, giving misinformation or conflicting information, and withholding information are all practices to avoid.

Nurse to Physician

When there is disagreement between a nurse and physician, the nurse should do the following:

- Settle it privately.
- Get agreement before documenting.
- Use "I" messages rather than "you" messages. For example, "I am concerned that this problem is not being evaluated" or "I need a physician to see this strip and evaluate the patient."
- Utilize SBAR (Situation Background Assessment Recommendation) communication for efficient interactions between staff members and physicians (Mann and Pratt, 2008).
- Follow the chain of command if "the provider is absent, impaired, or clearly wrong in their plan of care or treatment, and fetal or maternal jeopardy appears to be likely" (Murray and Huelsmann, 2007) or if differences cannot be immediately resolved.
- Document the situation (just the facts), but not in the patient record.

Verbal Orders

There are increased risks involved with giving verbal orders because of issues related to translation and transmission. Also, some risk exists with telephone orders because the physician relies entirely on relayed information to diagnose the problem. This increases potential errors in treatment decisions. The Joint Commission (TJC) has instituted a national patient safety goal which states "that the recipient of a verbal or telephone order should write down the complete order or enter it into a computer while the physician is still on the phone and then read it back and receive confirmation from the individual who gave the information" (Grissinger and Munn, 2007). Ultimately, the nurse receiving the order has a responsibility to acknowledge that the physician's response seems to be in error.

Refusal or Inability to Comply

If a nurse clearly believes that to follow physician orders, to fail to obtain orders, or to fail to convince a physician of the necessity to see the patient will result in harm, he/she has an obligation to follow through with a series of actions in a timely manner, commensurate with the potential for harm. The nurse should first attempt to resolve the conflict by firmly stating the expectation of a response from the physician involved. If that response is not quickly forthcoming, the nurse must follow the administrative chain of command with alternative notification of medical team members.

MID-LEVEL PROVIDERS

Midlevel providers (nurse practitioners, midwives, nurse anesthetists, clinical nurse specialists) have only one clear thing in common from state to state and from specialty to specialty: all midlevel providers are registered nurses who have completed an advanced level of education and therefore have an increased level of responsibility and accountability as advanced practice nurses (APNs). Different states regulate the level of educational degree required to practice as an APN. More than 30 states now require APNs to have a graduate (i.e., master's) degree in their specialty. Many of those states also require these individuals to take and pass a certification examination from a specified certifying agency and to hold a current registered nurse licensure.

   If the APN is prepared in adult health areas, he or she may not practice in pediatrics and vice versa. An adult health nurse practitioner may practice in all areas of adult health but not in obstetrics. A family nurse practitioner may remain generalized or choose to primarily specialize in one or two areas. However, a family nurse practitioner may not certify by examination in any of the specialty areas if one of the usual certifying agencies is used and can only certify as a generalist. Scope of practice issues vary little from state to state for APNs.

   Certified nurse midwives must be RNs, must obtain a master's degree, and must pass certification consisting of oral and written board examinations. There is a great deal of consistency in practice privileges for nurse anesthetists from state to state, but the educational degree granted varies. Physician assistants may or may not start out as nurses. They usually have a master's degree, which is required by most states, and do not hold an independent license from their copractice physician. Again, state laws vary as to privileges granted and withheld.

States vary in how and what they regulate for APNs who have prescribing privileges. They usually describe the degree of autonomy the APN may have, from requiring the APN to list a supervising physician, to not requiring them to do so at all. In the latter case, the APN has even greater legal responsibility and accountability for understanding the law in the state in which he or she practices. An APN must seriously consider the ethical and legal obligation to practice and provide optimal care within those laws, understand the scope of practice, and not overstep the boundaries of that practice as defined by the state and certifying agencies involved in the licensure (Brent, 2001).

EFFECT OF INCREASED LITIGATION ON HEALTH CARE

The following risks and the failure to reduce them affect cost and practice in health care:
- Increased cost of health care premiums
- Increased cost of health care
- Increased cost of malpractice/liability insurance
- Decreased access to prenatal care as physicians limit their practice
- Decreased quality of care as access is limited, especially for the medically indigent for whom risk is often the greatest

Rather than deterring incompetent or substandard care, increased litigation has led to defensive medical practices that include costly and often questionably indicated testing. In addition, the personal, trusting relationship patients once shared with providers has become less trusting, with referrals to specialists who do not have a long-term care relationship with the patient. Fragmented care with increased referrals may actually result in less continuity and increased risk for negligence (Sinclair, 2000; Brent, 2001).

SYSTEMS OF LAW

The four systems of law in the United States are martial, military, criminal, and civil law.

Martial Law

Martial law is invoked only in times of social emergency. An example of a social emergency is a national disaster. Under martial law, civil rights can be selectively suspended.

Military Law

Military law operates in the military services and supersedes laws of states or other countries.

Criminal Law

Criminal law is the system by which the state prosecutes criminal behavior. It is subject to the court of appeals and is based on precedent. Intent is an important element of proof, as is proof of the criminal act itself. The defendant is considered innocent until proved guilty by the state as plaintiff (Brent, 2001).

Civil Law

Civil law serves for noncriminal behavior and seeks to recover compensation for proven damages. Negligence is a civil wrong and falls under the law of torts. In order for negligence to occur, a person must fail to act as a reasonably prudent person in similar circumstances would act. In order for there to be sufficient proof of medical malpractice, the plaintiff's claim must prove that four elements of negligence have occurred. These elements to be proved and defended are: duty, breach of duty, proximate cause, and damages (Iyer, 2003).

Duty

Duty is that special relationship, recognized by law that establishes the duty of the health care professional to render a degree of care that can be reasonably expected by a professional with the same or similar experience in the same or similar situation.

Breach of Duty

Breach of duty is a failure to meet the minimum standard of care as defined by the bodies that set the standards.

Proximate Cause

Proximate cause is an act or omission that, unbroken by any intervening cause, produces an injury. In a medical malpractice case, failure to adhere to the minimum standard of care must be the proximate cause of the injury.

Damages

Damages are the sum of money a court or jury awards as compensation. The law recognizes certain, often imprecise and inconsistent, categories of damages (Brent, 2001):

- *General damages.* Typically intangible damages such as pain and suffering, disfigurement, and interference with ordinary enjoyment of life.
- *Special damages.* Out-of-pocket expenses for medical expenses, lost wages, and rehabilitation.
- *Punitive exemplary damages.* Damages awarded to the plaintiff for intentional acts or gross negligence and used to punish the defendant or act as a deterrent to others.

Table 9-1 defines common terms used during the litigation process, terms with which nurses may be unfamiliar.

LITIGATION SEQUENCE

Once parents decide to sue, the following sequence of events occurs:

- Parents seek the services of a lawyer. They explain their view of the situation and events. During that conference, the parents name the physicians, one or more hospitals, and the nurses involved. They may bring medical records from current providers with documentation of existing problems.
- The attorney reviews the information, files the complaint, and requests records. The defense attorneys are notified.

Table 9-1   Definitions of Commonly Used Legal Terms

Terms	Definitions
Accreditation	The official authorization providing credentials for maintaining standards and ensuring quality of care
Case law	Legal principles derived from judicial decisions; differs from statutory law
Complaint	Legal document that is initial pleading on part of plaintiffs in a civil lawsuit; purpose is to give defendant notice of alleged facts constituting cause of action
Court trial	Trial without jury
Credentialing	System based on accepted standard criteria for determining competence and capabilities of a professional to provide consistent quality care and to minimize risks
Defendant	Individual who is named in a suit by plaintiff; medical malpractice or professional negligence cases usually include multiple defendants, such as hospital, physician or physicians, and potentially nurse or nurses if they are insured separately from the hospital
Deposition	A discovery procedure whereby each party may question the other party or any person who may be a possible witness
Evidence	Facts presented at trial through witnesses, records, documents, and concrete objects for purpose of proving or defending a case, such as standard of care testimony in medical malpractice case or opinion, which is testimony of an expert witness based on special training or background, rather than on personal knowledge of facts at issue
Expert opinion	Testimony of person who has specialized knowledge, training, skill, and experience in area relevant to resolution of the legal dispute
Foreseeability	Requirement that case be judged on facts as they were known at the time of the occurrence, not in retrospect, with hindsight, or with knowledge gained since that time
Incident report	Term for report of situation that is not consistent with entire operation of hospital or routine care of patient; more appropriately termed *occurrence* or *situation report*; usually privileged, protected from discovery unless described in patient record
Malpractice and negligence	Legal cause of action involving failure to exercise degree of diligence and care that a reasonable and ordinarily prudent person in same specialty would exercise acting under similar circumstances
Plaintiff	Individual initiating lawsuit; in case of injured minor, parents or state brings suit

Table 9-1   Definitions of Commonly Used Legal Terms—cont'd

Terms	Definitions
Professional negligence	In medical terms, malpractice is failure to exercise that degree of care, as it is used by reasonably careful health care professionals in same or similar situation or with like qualifications; failure to meet this acceptable standard of care must be direct cause of injury
Respondent superior	Legal principle that makes employer liable for civil wrongs committed by employees within course and scope of their employment
Risk management	Systems approach to prevention of malpractice claims; involves identification of system problems, analysis, and treatment of risks before a suit is brought, as well as identification of patients who may sue
Standards of care	Norms of behavior and action defined by a particular profession and described and applied by professional and accrediting organizations
Statutory law	Law enacted by legislature
Statute of limitations	Time period in which plaintiff may file lawsuit; varies from state to state and is extended in most states for birth injury for discovery to take place after school age has been reached; then time is specified for complaint to be filed after discovery

- The attorney notifies the court of intent to bring suit and states the elements of the complaint.
- During this period, called *discovery* (Brent, 2001), a list of all possible parties to be deposed is reviewed.
- The defense attorneys for the listed parties also begin discovery.
- Potential experts for the physicians, the hospital, and the nurses are contacted to begin reviewing records.
- Some depositions are taken. The plaintiff's attorney takes the depositions of the physician(s) and the most closely involved nurses. The defense attorneys are present.
- The defense attorney or attorneys take depositions of the parents. The plaintiff's attorney is present.
- Experts are named with the court after their agreement is obtained. Some attorneys give the experts an affidavit, which is a legal document stating in general terms what the expert is prepared to stipulate as expert opinion. This statement usually involves his or her opinion of whether the standards of care were met.
- Depositions are taken from experts and from other persons listed in the medical records.
- Some states have a system for screening cases before deciding to settle or go to court.

- The attorneys for both sides begin to make offers and counteroffers for settlement out of court.
- If no settlement is reached, the plaintiff's attorney files a court date.
- All filings of complaints, experts named, and court dates have deadlines that need to be met in order to be within the statute of limitations.
- The attorneys orchestrate the timetable for presentation of witnesses and experts. The plaintiff has the first and last word in presentation of the case.
- Subpoenas are issued to the witnesses. The attorneys who issue the subpoenas pay experts. The defense attorney recovers those costs from the insurance companies for the physicians, the hospital, or the nurse or nurses (Brent, 2001).

NURSE'S DEPOSITION

Players

People involved in the nurse's deposition are the hospital's attorney, plaintiff's attorney, physician's attorney, various paralegals and nursing consultants, a court recorder, and the witness.

Process

Swearing In

The court recorder swears in the witness by having the witness state name and current address and then swear or promise to tell the truth.

Introductory Questioning

The plaintiff's attorney begins by asking general questions such as name, marital status, current and past employment, and schooling. These questions are designed to put the nurse at ease, gain his or her trust, and evaluate body language when telling the truth for comparison against later answers about sensitive issues.

Questioning Regarding the Case

The rest of the questions are related to the care given by that nurse to the mother. These questions usually are designed to nail down the facts from the witness or the opinions of the expert. They vary in style and associated pitfalls.

Helpful Guidelines

- *Answering "yes or no" questions*: If the plaintiff's attorney asks for a "yes or no" response, and the question does not lend itself to either, the best answer is "I don't understand the question" or "I don't know." It is not wise to rephrase the question or answer "yes or no" and then try to explain the conditions. Sometimes the questions are fired in rapid succession, with the goal of eliciting a string of "yes or no" answers. The tendency in this situation is to answer "yes or no"; however, if the witness stops to think, the answer might vary. The best strategy is to stop, rephrase the question silently, and then answer thoughtfully.

- *Answering long, difficult, complex questions*: Do not answer the question in its long form. State that the question is confusing. If asked to explain the confusion, ask for the question to be separated into smaller parts; do not rephrase it.
- *Response when hospital's attorney objects to question*: If the hospital's attorney objects to a question, remember that there is no judge to arbitrate. You must have a response. Consider the objection to be a clue to think carefully about your response. Two common problems that may cause the attorney to object are (1) the question is phrased to force you to contradict yourself, or (2) the question asks for an opinion that is not in your purview. In either of these cases, the two best answers are "I don't know (understand)" and "the question is confusing."
- *Always answer truthfully*: Even when the answer is perceived by you as less than helpful to the defense, a truthful answer is always best.
- Always look directly at the plaintiff's attorney.
- *Dress professionally and comfortably*: Position your body to occupy all of your allotted space with glasses, tissues, small purse, or a glass of water to mark boundaries. Do not curl into a small space in the chair; *occupy* it. Avoid caffeinated beverages before or during the deposition.
- *Never argue*: Do not argue with the attorney if he or she mistakenly rephrases your responses; state that you did not understand your response to have been given as repeated.
- *Simply answer the question being asked*: Never explain unless specifically requested to do so.
- *Preparation before deposition*: Study the scientific principles underlying the situation. Study the applicable standards and policies and procedures in force at the time of the incident (Ramos, 2003).

TRIAL

Players
The same players exist for the trial as for the deposition; in addition, a judge and jury are present. There may be some onlookers, including the parents and hospital staff, if approved by both attorneys.

Process
- All attorneys read opening statements.
- The plaintiff presents his or her case first; then the defense presents. The plaintiff has some rebuttal time.
- The judge may sustain or overrule attorneys' objections. If the objection is overruled, you answer; if it is sustained, you do not.
- Look at the attorney when he or she questions you, and look at the jury when you answer.

The trial can be very threatening to self-esteem. A lawsuit may require giving information to the state board of nursing, and you may be required to take continuing education or assertiveness training and your practice scope may be limited. View the experience as an opportunity for professional growth. Support groups or individual therapy is available through many employee assistance programs. Be aware of vulnerability in the practice concurrent with the events of the lawsuit. Avoid discussing the case with any other involved staff members for your protection and theirs.

Prevention

Nurses have the following professional and personal responsibilities for preventing litigation and for assisting in the reduction of awards:
- Use practice that is evidence-based (Kardong-Edgren, 2001; Simpson and Knox, 2003)
- Know the sources of standards of care and what the specific standards are. Table 9-2 describes relevant sources.
- Participate in formulating and writing nursing policies and procedures. Box 9-1 describes elements of policies and procedures to be considered.
- Know and apply components of risk management and quality assurance in clinical practice. Box 9-2 describes components of risk management and quality assurance.

Table 9-2   Sources of Standards

Organization	Description
The Joint Commission (TJC) (formerly Joint Commission on the Accreditation of Healthcare Organizations)	TJC accreditation is a voluntary and paid-for service. Among other things, it scrutinizes specialty services and requests proof of quality assurance, staff education, policies and procedures, staff ratios, and nursing procedures.
American Nurses Association (ANA)	The ANA provides statements of standards of maternal child nursing care and the Code for Nurses, 1976. It provides guidelines for minimum care standards in the specialty area of maternal child nursing.
Association of Women's Health, Obstetric, and Neonatal Nurses* (AWHONN)	AWHONN promotes excellence in nursing practice to improve the health of women and newborns. It publishes standards of practice and education.
Community standards	Community standards are superseded by a national standard. However, a like-level designation is compared with similar-level designations. Where designation has not been requested by state accreditation such as through health department or perinatal association, the facility remains undesignated. It is compared to the level I (primary care) facilities in that state.

*For more information, contact AWHONN, 2000 L Street NW, Suite 740, Washington, DC, 20036; (800) 673-8499.

- Establish a mutually agreed upon language for fetal heart rate pattern interpretation and medical record documentation (Feinstein, Torgersen, and Atterbury, 2003). Ideally, terminology as set forth by the National Institute of Child Health and Human Development (NICHD) should be instituted to facilitate consistent communication and documentation among care givers (Simpson and Creehan, 2008).
- Document clinical practice in a complete, concise, and accurate manner, including communication among health team members and with patients and family. There is some controversy regarding whether charting on monitor strips should be done at all beyond identifying the patient and medical record. This

---

Box 9-1   Policy and Procedure Writing

Practice Statements
- Write policies so that a wide range of acceptable practice is possible and flexibility is allowed.
- When restrictions or limitations for acceptable practice are necessary, they should be specified (AAP & ACOG, 2007).

Policy Statements
- Specific care to be rendered

Staff
- Patterns of staffing
- Educational preparation
- Special credentialing/certification/validation
- New orientation and continuing education

Equipment
- Care, repair, and testing
- Cleaning and storage
- Environment where care can or cannot be provided

Suggested Organization of Policy and Procedure
- Institution name
- Department
- Title
- Dates of origination, review, and revision
- Approval signature/committee
- Date of approval
- Purpose and patient's desired outcomes
- Practice and policy statements
- Equipment
- Procedure
- Additional information
- Cross index
- References

Box 9-2   Components of Risk Management: Continuous Quality Assurance

Policy Revision
- Write new or review/revise existing policies and procedures based on national evidence-based guidelines, when available.
- Reflect achievable goals that can lead to reliable patient outcomes.
- Update the policy to reflect current practice and to meet current standards of care.
- Have a policy regarding staffing ratios and chain of command for conflict resolution.
- Educate and provide in-service education for staff about new or revised policies and procedures.
- Keep old policies until the statute of limitations expire.

Monitoring Quality Assurance
- Document a quality assurance program with provision for monitoring patient outcomes, process outcomes if patient outcomes do not meet established levels, and operational and administrative outcomes.
- Conduct patient satisfaction surveys.
- Utilize Perinatal Safety Nurse to assist in decreasing preventable adverse outcomes.

Risk Management Plan for Problematic Perinatal Clinical Risks
- Fetal heart rate (FHR) monitoring as to method, frequency, and documentation data
- Oxytocin administration and safe use of labor stimulants
- Fundal versus suprapubic pressure
- Nursing response to obstetric emergencies such as:
  - Fetal intolerance to labor or antepartum events
  - Maternal hemorrhage
  - Eclamptic seizures
  - Hypertensive emergencies
  - Precipitous delivery
  - Uterine rupture
  - Umbilical cord prolapse
  - Hypoglycemia
  - Maternal and fetal resuscitation
- Cardiac and respiratory emergencies
- HIV issues of reasonable accommodations and privacy
- Newborn safety (e.g., kidnapping)
- Perinatal grief support
- Advice during telephone triage
- Staffing

Sources of Liability (Simpson and Knox, 2003)
- Failure to give proper telephone advice to patients
- Failure to comply with the Emergency Medical Treatment and Active Labor Act (EMTALA)

Box 9-2   Components of Risk Management: Continuous Quality Assurance—cont'd

- Failure to accurately interpret, communicate, and document fetal heart pattern (see section below)
- Failure to inform patient of risks and benefits associated with elective induction of labor
- Failure to institute cesarean section in a timely manner—30-minute rule
- Failure to utilize Centers for Disease Control and Prevention (CDC) guidelines for prevention of Group B Streptococcal (GBS) infection
- Failure to administer cervical ripening or labor induction medications in a safe manner
- Application of fundal pressure with shoulder dystocia
- Failure to provide appropriate equipment and personnel for neonatal resuscitation

Documentation
- Patient status
- Care provided according to the nursing process and professional standards of care
- Quality assurance indicators
- Monitoring results
- Correction plan and implementation

Adapted from Rostant and Cady, 1999; Sprague and Trepanier, 1999; Simpson and Knox, 2003; Will and others, 2006.

is particularly true when it pertains to recording time for certain events. Most experts agree that, in general, charting needs to be simplified so that events do not have to be charted in multiple places. Multiple charting increases the likelihood of inconsistencies in the time something was recorded on various charts. Times are recorded from a variety of sources such as a clock on a graph, a nurse's watch, and clocks on the walls of any room the patient occupies or to which she may be moved in an emergency. On the other hand, there are those who argue that the increased use of computerized charting with use of checklists and little space for narrative leave only a small amount of room to document emergent events in sequential order and detail. Therefore the thinking processes that went into nursing decisions are easily overlooked and misinterpreted, and the timing of actions is often impossible to determine. If, during an emergent situation, nurses feel they must document on the fetal monitor strip, it is important to make sure the information and times documented in the electronic record coincide with the fetal monitor strip annotations. Documentation of routine care in multiple places is not recommended because of liability issues (Feinstein and others, 2003). Box 9-3 describes guidelines for documentation.
- Be aware of potential risks in clinical practice. Box 9-4 lists some clinical examples of common issues.

Box 9-3   Guidelines for Documentation

Documentation in Maternal Record
- Time electronic fetal monitor (EFM) was applied and mode of monitoring
- Patient status and activity
- Fetal heart rate (FHR): baseline rate, variability, presence/absence of accelerations and/or decelerations (document per NICHD recommendation)
- Uterine activity: presence, frequency, and duration (document per NICHD recommendation)
- Intensity and resting tone if intrauterine pressure catheter (IUPC) is used
- Assessment
- Vital signs
- Cervical assessments
- Interventions, including patient response and time of physician notification
- Communication between nurse and physician
- Antepartum and postpartum patient education, verbalization and demonstration of understanding
- Referrals

Storage
- Safe and confidential storage of patient records must be provided by the hospital to last for at least the statute of limitations; fetal monitor strips not electronically stored are the fetal record and should be stored with the maternal record.

Purpose of Documentation
- Provides record of patient assessment and assists with planning care
- Evaluates patient condition and ongoing response to treatment
- Allows assessment of developing patterns in patient condition
- Provides a history for future admissions
- Provides communication among health care professionals contributing to patient care and documents that communication
- Explains diagnosis and course of illness management and treatment
- Assists in utilization review for appropriate use of hospital and resources
- Provides data in continuing education and research
- Provides information for The Joint Commission
- Provides information for billing and reimbursement
- Possibly constitutes a legal document
- Identifies and provides necessary information for incident management

From Rostant and Cady, 1999; Sprague and Trepanier, 1999; Brent, 2001; Simpson and Creehan, 2008.

PERINATAL SAFETY NURSE

Some obstetrical departments have created a Perinatal Safety Nurse (PSN) position to oversee safety issues in their daily operations. The role of this nurse is to keep patient safety as a focus within the unit, thereby decreasing preventable adverse outcomes. Duties may include patient care record reviews, collaborative work with

Box 9-4   Clinical Examples of Common Issues

- Amniotomy and placement of internal fetal electrode through intact membrane
- Electronic fetal heart rate monitoring: continuous or intermittent
- Nurse's responsibilities and management of induction/augmentation
- Nurse's response to obstetric, cardiac, or respiratory emergencies
- Patient education for self-care antepartum and postpartum
- Birth plans
- Childbirth education and patient expectations
- Vacuum-assisted deliveries
- Preterm labor response to need for treatment
- Precipitous delivery
- Role of the nurse in the care of the pregnant woman receiving analgesia and anesthesia
- Nursing care impact on cesarean birth rate
- Maternal stabilization and transport; regionalized care
- Standards for three levels of perinatal care
- Informed consent
- Adverse drug events

From Sprague and Trepanier, 1999; Haggerty and Nuttall, 2000; Mahlmeister, 2000; Maloni, 2000; Brent, 2001; Kardong-Edgren, 2001; AWHONN, 2002; Mahlmeister, 2005a,b; Stevenson, 2006; Mahlmeister, 2007.

management, staff, and interdisciplinary departments, cultivation of an environment of safety, and assistance in initiation of departmental safety goals, policies, and procedures. Although not all institutions may be able to provide a full-time PSN position, the role can be developed to be flexible in order to meet the needs of each individual department (Will and others, 2006).

EXPERT WITNESS

Nurses have an evolving role as expert witnesses. In the past, physicians most often gave expert testimony about the nurse's duty and standard of care. As nurses have become better educated about the process and their responsibilities as professionals and as citizens, it is appropriate for them to give expert testimony in malpractice cases involving specific nurses or the hospital's quality of nursing care.

CONCLUSION

With high expectations for the outcome of any pregnancy being the norm for human nature, and with forces promoting increased numbers of and amounts of awards in birth injury cases, it is little wonder that health care costs have soared. Defensibility is improved when nurses provide care based on current evidence, national standards, and guidelines, thus increasing patient safety (Simpson and Creehan, 2008).

As nurses are increasingly exposed to the risk for being named as a party to a birth injury case, it is important to realize that being found liable does not necessarily mean one is considered incompetent or likely to be punished by loss of employment or licensure. Becoming educated in terminology and the litigation process can help the nurse to maintain his or her self-esteem in this difficult and threatening experience.

BIBLIOGRAPHY

American Academy of Pediatrics (AAP) and Association of Obstetricians and Gynecologists (ACOG): *Guidelines for perinatal care*, ed 6, Elk Grove Village, III, 2007, AAP and Washington DC, 2007, ACOG.

American College of Obstetrics and Gynecology (ACOG). *2006 Professional liability survey.* Available at 222.acog.org. Retrieved March 6, 2009.

Association of Obstetricians and Gynecologists: *Position statement: quality improvement in women's health care*, Washington, DC, 2000a, ACOG.

Association of Women's Health, Obstetric, and Neonatal Nurses (AWHONN): *Access to health care issues*, Washington, DC, 2000b, AWHONN.

Association of Women's Health, Obstetric, and Neonatal Nurses (AWHONN): *Clinical position statement: amniotomy and placement of internal fetal spiral electrode through intact membranes*, Washington, DC, 2002, AWHONN.

Association of Women's Health, Obstetric, and Neonatal Nurses (AWHONN): *Fetal assessment, fetal monitoring, principles and practices*, Washington, DC, 1997, AWHONN.

Association of Women's Health, Obstetric, and Neonatal Nurses (AWHONN): *Position statement: insurance coverage*, Washington, DC, 1999, AWHONN.

Association of Women's Health, Obstetric, and Neonatal Nurses (AWHONN): *Position statement: translating standards and guidelines into practice*, Washington, DC, 2000, AWHONN.

Association of Women's Health, Obstetric, and Neonatal Nurses (AWHONN): *Standards for professional nursing practice in the care of women and newborns*, ed 6, Washington, DC, 2003, AWHONN.

Brent N: *Nurses and the law: a guide to principles and applications*, ed 2, Philadelphia, 2001, Saunders.

Brous E: Malpractice insurance and licensure protection, *Am J Nurs* 108(5):34–36, 2008.

Feinstein N, Torgersen K, Atterbury J: *Fetal heart monitoring: principles and practices*, ed. 3, Dubuque, IA, 2003, Kendall/Hunt.

Grissinger M, Munn J: Verbal orders can communicate trouble. *Nursing Spectrum/Nurse Week,* 2007. Available at http://news.nurse.com/apps/pbcs.dll/article?AID=200770621002. Retrieved March 3, 2009.

Haggerty L, Nuttall R: Experienced obstetric nurses' decision-making in fetal risk situations, *J Obstet Gynecol Neonatal Nurs* 29(5):480–490, 2000.

Iyer P: *Legal nurse consulting principles and practice*, ed 2, Boca Raton, 2003, CRC Press.

Kardong-Edgren S: Using evidenced-based practice to improve intrapartum care, *J Obstet Gynecol Neonatal Nurs* 30(4):371–375, 2001.

Lynn M, Redman R, Zomorodi M: The canaries in the coal mine speak: why someone should (and should not) become a nurse, *Nurs Adm Q* 30(4):340–350, 2006.

Mahlmeister L: Cervical ripeners and the induction of labor, *J Perinatal Neonatal Nurs* 19(2):97–99, 2005.

Mahlmeister L: Legal implications of fetal heart assessment, *J Obstet Gynecol Neonatal Nurs* 29(5):517–526, 2000.

Mahlmeister L: Preventing adverse drug events in perinatal settings, *J Perinatal Neonat Nurs* 21(1):6–8, 2007.

Mahlmeister L: Vacuum-assisted vaginal delivery, *J Perinat Neonatal Nurs* 19(1):9–11, 2005.

Maloni J: Preventing preterm birth: evidenced-based interventions shift toward prevention, *AWHONN Lifelines* 4(4):26–33, 2000.

Mann S, Pratt S: Team approach to care in labor and delivery, *Clin Obstet Gynecol* 51(4):666–679, 2008.

McCaffrey M, Neumann D, Furniss K, and others: The loneliness of the perinatal nurse in litigation, *Mat Child Nurs* 33(5):281–286, 2008.

Murray M, Huelsmann G: Perinatal morbidity and mortality: Root causes and common themes in labor and delivery litigation, *J Legal Nurs Consult* 18(4):13–18, 2007.

National Practitioner Data Bank 2006 Annual Report. Available at www.npdb-hipdb.hrsa.gov/pubs/ stats/2006_NPDB_Annual_Report.pdf. Retrieved March 1, 2009.

Ramos F: Preparing for a deposition, *Adv Nurs Pract* 11(11):23, 2003.

Rostant D, Cady R: *AWHONN: liability issues in perinatal nursing*, Philadelphia, 1999, Lippincott Williams & Wilkins.

Simpson K, Creehan P: *AWHONN perinatal nursing*, ed 3, Philadelphia, 2008, Lippincott Williams & Wilkins.

Simpson K, Knox G: Adverse perinatal outcomes: Recognizing, understanding, and preventing common accidents, *AWHONN Lifelines* 7(3):224–235, 2003.

Sinclair B: Where are the nurses? Perspectives, *AWHONN Lifelines* 4(4):7, 2000.

Sprague A, Trepanier M: Charting in record time, *AWHONN Lifelines* 3(5):25–30, 1999.

Steevenson G: Informed consent, *J Perioper Pract* 16(8):384–388, 2006.

Will S, Hennicke K, Jacobs L, and others: The perinatal patient safety nurse: a new role to promote safe care for mothers and babies, *J Obstet Gynecol Neonatal Nurs* 35(3):417–423, 2006.

10

Diabetes

D
iabetes is a disease characterized by the inability to produce or use sufficient endogenous insulin to metabolize glucose properly. This inability to metabolize glucose leads to altered metabolism. Pregnancy is a diabetogenic state. Metabolism of glucose, fats, and proteins is altered, and anti-insulin forces are present. This may affect the already altered metabolism.

According to the National Diabetes Data Group Classification, there are three types of diabetes: type 1, type 2, and type 3, gestational diabetes mellitus (GDM) (ADA, 2008). Types 1 and 2 diabetes are pregestational; that is, the woman has diabetes before becoming pregnant. In type 1 diabetes mellitus, there is absolute insulin deficiency related to a cellular-mediated autoimmune destruction of the islet cells. In type 2 diabetes mellitus, there is insulin resistance because receptor sites at the tissue level are not responsive to insulin. Therefore it takes more insulin to shut off the release of glucose from the liver. Furthermore, it takes higher levels of insulin to open the receptors and facilitate muscle glucose uptake. The pancreas is overworked to meet the increased demand of extra insulin, and hyperglycemia develops.

GDM is defined as carbohydrate intolerance that is first recognized during pregnancy (ADA, 2004b) or undiagnosed type 2 diabetes (Langer, 2007). *Impaired glucose tolerance (IGT) and impaired fasting glucose (IFG)* are levels of impaired glucose metabolism that are not severe enough to be diagnosed as type 1 or 2 or GDM but indicate prediabetes (ADA, 2009). *IGT* is defined as a 2-hour postprandial blood sugar level higher than 140 mg/dl but lower than 200 mg/dl. *IFG* is defined as a fasting blood sugar level that is 100 mg/dl or higher but lower than 126 mg/dl.

During pregnancy, IFG and IGT are considered to be clinical entities of their own. Otherwise they are considered risk factors for future diabetes and cardiovascular disease because they are associated with the insulin resistance syndrome, also referred to as *syndrome X* or *metabolic syndrome.* This syndrome consists of insulin resistance and compensatory hyperinsulinemia. Inherent characteristics are obesity (especially abdominal), dyslipidemia that includes high triglycerides, low high-density lipoprotein (HDL) and high low-density lipoprotein (LDL), hypertension, prothrombotic state, and impaired glucose tolerance (ADA, 2009; Kahn and others, 2005).

Table 10-1   Guide to Classification of Perinatal Diabetes: Revised White's
Classification

Class	Description	Vascular Disease	Treatment
A1	GDM characterized by abnormal GTT without other symptoms; fasting glucose normal	None	Diet control
A2	GDM characterized by abnormal GTT; fasting glucose elevated; insulin required to control	None	Diet and insulin
B	Diabetes onset at age 20 years or older or diabetes of less than 10-year duration	None	Diet and insulin
C	Diabetes onset between ages 10 and 19 years or duration of 10–19 years	None	Diet and insulin
D	Diabetes onset before 10 years of age or duration of more than 20 years	Benign retinopathy	Diet and insulin
E	Diabetes onset at any age	Pelvic vascular disease	Diet and insulin
F	Diabetes onset at any age	Nephropathy	Diet and insulin
R	Diabetes onset at any age	Proliferative retinopathy	Diet and insulin
RF	Diabetes onset at any age	Nephropathy and retinopathy	Diet and insulin
H	Diabetes onset at any age	Atherosclerotic heart disease	Diet and insulin
T	Diabetes onset at any age	After renal transplant	Diet and insulin

Data from American College of Obstetricians and Gynecologists (ACOG): Management of DM in pregnancy, *ACOG Technical Bulletin*, No. 92, Washington, DC, 1986, ACOG Resource Center.
GDM, Gestational diabetes mellitus; *GTT*, glucose tolerance test.

In pregnancy, diabetes is also classified according to the age at which it was diagnosed, the length of time the disease has been present, and the degree of vascular changes that have occurred. This classification was helpful in the past to provide prognostic indicators for neonatal outcome (Table 10-1). Research indicates that the degree of metabolic control and the presence or absence of long-term complications better delineate maternal and fetal risk (Kitzmiller and others, 2008).

INCIDENCE

Diabetes in pregnancy has long been recognized as a serious problem for both the mother and fetus. Before the availability of insulin in the 1920s, women with diabetes rarely became pregnant. Those who did rarely carried a fetus to viability. According to the National Health and Nutrition Examination Survey (CDC, 2008), diabetes now occurs in approximately 4% to 14% of pregnant women. GDM represents almost 90% of this group (ACOG, 2005; Mulholland and others, 2007).

CAUSES

The causes of diabetes are inherent in pancreatic inability to produce sufficient insulin to transport glucose into the cells. Insulin deficiency may result from pancreatic beta-cell damage, inactivation of insulin by inflammatory mediators or antibodies, or increased insulin requirements. Type 1 diabetes is a chronic autoimmune disorder of the pancreatic islet cells that develops in individuals who carry a genetic marker that has been identified on chromosomes 6 and 11 and possibly 10 other genes (EPGO, 2004; ADA, 2008). Viral-induced, immune-stimulated antibodies against the beta cells form. This autoimmune response causes gradual destruction of the pancreatic beta cells.

People with type 2 diabetes do not carry a genetic marker, but rather have a genetic susceptibility. Insulin resistance and pancreatic islet cell dysfunction characterize type 2 diabetes. When insulin resistance occurs, there is increased insulin secretion but ineffective insulin postreceptor binding (ADA, 2008). Thus glucose uptake by cells is decreased and hyperglycemia results. In 80% to 85% of patients with type 2 diabetes, obesity, especially in the abdominal region, causes increased inflammatory cytokines (TNF-a) to release free fatty acid causing insulin resistance (Richardson and Carpenter, 2007).

NORMAL PHYSIOLOGY

Pregnancy is a diabetogenic state characterized by mild fasting hypoglycemia, postprandial hyperglycemia, and hyperinsulinemia. These changes occur to ensure a continuous supply of glucose to the fetus. There is marked individual variation in the renal threshold for glucose.

Hyperinsulinemia: Increased Insulin Production

Estrogen and progesterone stimulate pancreatic beta-cell hyperplasia. As insulin secretion is increased, peripheral glucose utilization is enhanced, leading to a decreased fasting blood glucose level in the first trimester. During the second and third trimesters, rising placental hormones and cellular immune inflammatory cytokines (TNF-a) increase insulin resistance (Richardson and Carpenter, 2007); decreased hepatic glycogen stores and an increased hepatic production of glucose cause elevated postprandial blood sugar levels. This increased glucose presence further stimulates pancreatic islet cell hypertrophy, increasing insulin levels.

Increased Tissue Resistance to Insulin

During the second and third trimesters, pregnancy hormones (estrogen, progesterone, human placental lactogen hormone, and cortisol) antagonize insulin's effectiveness because of postreceptor cellular changes and stimulate hepatic glucose production. In addition, the placental enzyme *insulinase* accelerates degradation of insulin. The net effect is decreased insulin effectiveness, causing reduced peripheral uptake of glucose, which facilitates glucose availability to the fetus for accelerated fetal growth (Moore and Catalano, 2009).

Table 10-2   Long-Standing Vascular Effects of Hyperglycemia

Consequences	Manifestations
Microvascular	
Autonomic neuropathy	Gastrointestinal, genitourinary, cardiovascular, sexual dysfunction
Peripheral neuropathy	Decreased perception of pain; foot ulcers
Nephropathy	Proteinuria, oliguria, renal failure
Retinopathy	Visual changes that can lead to blindness
Macrovascular	
Atherosclerotic heart changes	Cardiovascular disease, coronary artery disease
Atherosclerotic peripheral vascular changes	Hypertension, hyperlipidemia; poor healing and gangrene

PATHOPHYSIOLOGY

Pregestational Diabetes

In theory, the cause of faulty metabolism in the person with diabetes is one or more of the following:

- Production of defective insulin
- Overproduction of insulin antagonist
- Increased tissue resistance to insulin
- Underproduction of insulin
- Inappropriate timing of insulin release

When insulin is not available or effective in transporting glucose into the cell, glucose remains in the bloodstream in abnormal quantities. Because of cellular starvation, the body begins breakdown of fats (*ketogenesis*) and proteins (*gluconeogenesis*) for energy.

If hyperglycemia is allowed to become severe, ketoacidosis can develop. The resultant diuresis causes loss of water and electrolytes, hyperosmolarity, and volume depletion. This in turn causes a release of stress hormones such as glucagon, catecholamines, cortisol, and growth hormones; impairs insulin action; and contributes to insulin deficiency.

When hyperglycemia becomes a long-term or recurrent event, long-standing vascular effects (Table 10-2) can occur.

When glucose is low in relation to the amount of insulin, a person with diabetes experiences different physiologic responses, manifested by hypoglycemia. During pregnancy, hypoglycemia is characterized by rapid onset. Hypoglycemia can also be exaggerated in early control of hyperglycemia. A high blood sugar level rapidly brought down to normal ranges can cause an excessive blood sugar response, and wide variations from low to high blood sugar levels can result. It is extremely important that hypoglycemia be treated with a measured amount of complex carbohydrate and protein. Thus the body does not rapidly use the glucose and then drop blood sugars even lower than the previous levels because no other source of glucose is being gradually formed and released from fats and proteins.

Women with Gestational Diabetes

GDM is defined as carbohydrate intolerance of variable severity with onset or first recognition during pregnancy, particularly in the third trimester (ADA, 2009). The pancreatic beta-cell functions are impaired in response to the increased stimulation and induced insulin resistance. This is frequently related to chronic insulin resistance that occurs more commonly in obese patients.

SIGNS AND SYMPTOMS

Gestational Diabetes

Signs of GDM in a previous pregnancy are as follows:
- Prior delivery of an infant weighing more than 9 pounds
- Previous stillbirth or an infant with congenital defects
- History of polyhydramnios
- History of recurrent monilial vaginitis

Signs of GDM in the current pregnancy are as follows:
- Recurrent monilial vaginitis
- Macrosomia of the fetus on ultrasound
- Polyhydramnios

Pregestational Diabetes

In the woman with pregestational diabetes, diabetic symptoms vary by trimester. Acanthosis nigricans (AN), a hyperpigmentation and thickening of the skin of the neck or axilla area, is a common sign of insulin resistance (Daitchman, Vermeulen, and Ray, 2008). Table 10-3 outlines the trimester manifestations and consequences.

Ketoacidosis

Signs and symptoms of ketoacidosis in the pregnant woman include the following:
- Hyperventilation or Kussmaul respirations
- Mental lethargy
- Dehydration
- Hypotension unless complicated by pregnancy-induced hypertension
- Abdominal pain; nausea and vomiting
- Fruity odor to the breath
- Ketonuria

MATERNAL EFFECTS

In general, the diabetic state in the mother does not deteriorate because of the pregnancy itself. In fact, most women, regardless of their classification during pregnancy, are in better control of their diabetes than when they are not pregnant. Despite the antagonistic forces of hormones, control is often better because of the close observation of blood sugar levels by the patient and health care team.

However, a diabetic pregnancy is more vulnerable to certain complications. The woman with diabetes who develops hyperemesis gravidarum is at risk for severe metabolic disturbances. In addition to the obvious risks of dehydration and electrolyte

Table 10-3   Trimester Manifestations and Consequences of Diabetes

	Insulin Requirements	Blood Glucose Alterations	Complicating Factors
First trimester	Reduced, related to inhibition of anterior pituitary hormones; developing embryo is glucose drain; decreased maternal caloric intake; increased insulin production	Frequent low blood glucose levels, leading to increased numbers of hypoglycemia episodes, increased incidence of starvation, ketosis, and ketonemia	Loss of appetite, nausea, or vomiting common in any early pregnancy. Recovery from an acidemic state is more difficult because of insulin antagonists.
Second trimester	Increase related to placental hormones (cortisol, insulinase) and their antiinsulin properties	Hyperglycemia leading to ketonemia, aminoacidemia	Exaggerated ketone response to caloric restriction. Decreased renal threshold from increased blood flow makes urine sugar levels meaningless. Body produces lactose or milk sugar, which further increases urinary sugar
Third trimester	Marked increase related to increased placental hormones but level off after 36 weeks of gestation	Hyperglycemia leading to ketonemia, acidemia	Same as second trimester
Labor	Decrease related to workload of labor and increased metabolism	Hypoglycemia, acidemia from starvation ketosis	Usually nothing by mouth pending cesarean delivery
Postpartum	Decrease markedly related to loss of placental hormones	Hypoglycemia	Lactation lowers insulin; can initially complicate because supply is established and scheduled

imbalance that are always encountered with hyperemesis, starvation ketosis becomes a very real threat to the mother and the developing fetus. Hospitalization with appropriate intravenous (IV) therapy for fluids and calories is essential to prevent complications.

A pregnancy complicated by diabetes is at significant risk for the complications outlined in the following. However, the risk is directly related to glucose control initiated before conception and continued throughout the pregnancy (Kitzmiller and others, 2008).

Spontaneous Abortion

Diabetes mellitus increases the risk for miscarriage related to inadequate glycemic control during the embryonic phase (first 7 weeks of gestation) indicated by an elevated Hb A1c (Kitzmiller and others, 2008). A pregnant woman with poorly controlled diabetes has a 30% to 60% risk for spontaneous abortion (Dudley, 2007).

Preeclampsia

The pregnant woman with diabetes has a significantly increased risk of preeclampsia (Hawkins and Casey, 2007). This is particularly true when there is already evidence of chronic hypertension.

Preterm Labor

A woman with diabetes has a 25% risk for developing preterm labor if she has increased uterine volume, has a hypertensive disorder, develops a kidney or urinary tract infection (UTI), or has vascular compromise (Walkinshaw, 2004).

Polyhydramnios

Polyhydramnios is also more frequently encountered in the pregnant woman with diabetes than in the general population. Approximately 18% of all women with diabetes develop polyhydramnios during pregnancy. Although the mechanism for this is not fully understood, fetal hyperglycemia is thought to result in increased fetal diuresis. The significance of polyhydramnios varies depending on its source. Polyhydramnios may threaten premature rupture of the membranes because of uterine overdistention, and polyhydramnios is known to be associated with an increased incidence of fetal anomalies. In women with severe polyhydramnios, repeated therapeutic amniocenteses can be performed to relieve the pressure. Amniocentesis, when repeated, places the mother at increased risk for rupture of the membranes and infection.

Infection

The pregnant woman with diabetes is at significant risk for development of an infection involving almost any organ system. These infections can occur during the antepartum or postpartum period. Vaginitis, especially monilial, occurs frequently. This is related primarily to the altered pH of the vaginal canal common in all pregnancies. Because of the increased incidence of vaginitis, which makes a prime medium for bacterial growth, the pregnant woman with diabetes has an increased risk for pyelonephritis and UTIs. These infections can be dangerous to health and increase the likelihood of preterm labor. Women with insulin-dependent diabetes are 2.5 times more likely to develop postpartum endometritis or a wound infection (Takoudes and others, 2004).

Related to the increased susceptibility and the increased risk for morbidity related to influenza, the American Diabetes Association (ADA, 2009) recommends that persons with diabetes be immunized yearly against influenza. Pregnant women can be vaccinated with the inactivated influenza vaccine (CDC, 2007).

Diabetic Ketoacidosis

Because of the increased risk for infection, added stress, and antiinsulin placental hormones of pregnancy, diabetic ketoacidosis (DKA) is a real risk, especially in patients with type 1 diabetes. Maternal mortality is about 2% (Carroll and Yeomans, 2005). In DKA, glucose cannot enter the cell because of insufficient active insulin; therefore the cell starves. The result is increased lipolysis (breakdown of fat in adipose tissue). Free fatty acids are then produced in the liver and ultimately more ketone bodies are produced and build up in the bloodstream. A vicious cycle is created: The increase in ketone bodies leads to dehydration, acidosis, further breakdown of fats, and increased ketones; thus the cycle begins again. This cycle ultimately ends with decreased cardiac preload, hypertension, and shock followed by death (Foley, 2004).

Cesarean or Instrumental Birth and Induction

The pregnant woman with diabetes is more likely to deliver by the cesarean route because of concurrent complications, fetal distress, fetal macrosomia, and induction failures before term.

Retinopathy

Diabetic retinopathy may accelerate during pregnancy, especially if hypoglycemia develops with rapid institution of strict glucose control (ACOG, 2005; Kitzmiller and others, 2008). This risk can be controlled by gradual attainment of normal glycemic levels and preconceptual laser photocoagulation therapy if indicated.

Hypoglycemia

The Diabetes Control and Complications Trial Research Group (1996) demonstrated that there is a greater risk for hypoglycemia when tight control is attempted (Kitzmiller and others, 2008).

FETAL AND NEONATAL EFFECTS

The effects of maternal diabetes on the fetus depend somewhat on the presence of maternal vascular complications. If the mother has class D or more advanced disease, vascular deficits can affect the sufficiency of the placenta. Placental insufficiency can also cause varying degrees of nutritional or hypoxic damage to the fetus. It is manifested by intrauterine growth restriction (IUGR) and oligohydramnios.

Hypoglycemia

Hypoglycemia normally has a minimal effect on the fetus if the mother is treated appropriately. The embryo draws its glucose from stores in the lining of the uterus, and the fetus draws from stores in the placenta. In selective transfer, glucose is transferred across the placental membrane. The immediate effects of maternal hypoglycemia on the fetus are therefore minimized over time. However, severe episodes of maternal hypoglycemia that result in ketosis have been shown to cause abnormal postnatal neurologic development (Kitzmiller and others, 2008).

Hyperglycemia

Hyperglycemia can have numerous deleterious and sometimes fatal effects.

Congenital Defects

The risk for congenital defects occurring in the infant of a mother with diabetes is three to five times more often than in the general population (Leguizamon and others, 2007). Hyperglycemia can be teratogenic by directly effecting the yolk sac development and interfering with free radical functioning (Walkinshaw, 2004; Kendrick and others, 2005). Faulty carbohydrate, protein, and fat metabolism also occur in the embryo and adversely affect organ development. Common fetal anomalies found in infants of mothers with diabetes include skeletal and central nervous system defects such as neural tube defects, congenital cardiac anomalies, gastrointestinal malformations, and congenital renal anomalies. Congenital anomalies are directly related to diabetic control in the 3 months before conception and during the first 2 months of pregnancy, as indicated by glycosylated hemoglobin levels (ACOG, 2005; Leguizamon and others, 2007; Kitzmiller and others, 2008).

Macrosomia

Elevated maternal glucose results in elevated fetal glucose. This stimulates fetal pancreatic production of insulin, which causes fetal hyperinsulinemia. Hyperinsulinemia increases growth and fat deposition, which are referred to as *macrosomia.* This is seen especially in classes A to C diabetes. These large-for-gestational-age (LGA) infants are at greater risk for birth trauma, particularly shoulder dystocia, brachial plexus injuries, facial nerve injuries, and asphyxia.

Intrauterine Growth Restriction

Intrauterine growth restriction (IUGR) is less frequent than macrosomia, occurring in conjunction with placental insufficiency resulting from maternal diabetic vascular disease. This is seen especially in women with class D or higher diabetes and in those with existing vascular disease before their pregnancy.

Intrauterine Fetal Death

There is an increased risk for unexplained and explainable stillbirths in women with diabetes. When placental insufficiency occurs as the result of vascular complications or an abruption, there is a clear reason for stillbirth. However, stillbirth occurs at times without obvious placental insufficiency as would be indicated by decreased fetal growth and oligohydramnios. These infants are usually LGA with polyhydramnios. It appears that severe prolonged hyperinsulinemia interferes with the transport of oxygen and carbon dioxide, leading to decreased fetal pH and increased Pco_2, lactate, and erythropoietin incompatible with life (Dudley, 2007).

Ketoacidosis

DKA can be life threatening to the mother and fetus. Fetal mortality is approximately 10% if ketoacidosis develops (Carroll and Yeomans, 2005). The acidotic state of DKA leads to decreased uterine blood flow, which thereby reduces fetal oxygenation.

Delayed Lung Maturity

Various studies have suggested that hyperglycemia and hyperinsulinemia cause a delay in fetal lung maturity (Walkinshaw, 2004). Elevated blood glucose appears to interfere with the production of phosphatidyl glycerol. This indicates that a mature fetal surfactant may not be present until 38 weeks of gestation (Hawkins and Casey, 2007).

Neonatal Hypoglycemia

The fetus is programmed to produce high quantities of insulin, and the neonate does not turn this off immediately. At birth, the supply of increased glucose is suddenly cut off, but increased production of insulin continues, resulting in neonatal hypoglycemic episodes.

Neonatal Hyperbilirubinemia

Because of possible long-term stress, the compensatory mechanism of increased production of red blood cells is stimulated. After delivery the increased red blood cell breakdown frequently overworks the young hepatic system, resulting in hyperbilirubinemia.

Neonatal Polycythemia

Polycythemia is the result of decreased oxygenation, stimulating the fetal kidneys to release glycoprotein hormone. This hormone stimulates the production of erythrocytes as a compensatory mechanism to increase the oxygen-carrying capacity of the blood. Therefore in the presence of uteroplacental insufficiency, the newborn may have polycythemia.

Learning Disabilities

Fetal brain cell damage and decreased brain growth result from prolonged exposure to hyperglycemia and resulting ketonemia. This will increase the incidence of learning disabilities, lower intelligence quotient (IQ), and motor impairment (Kitzmiller and others, 2008).

Childhood Obesity and Type 2 Diabetes Later in Life

The risk for a child of a mother with type 2 diabetes to develop type 2 diabetes later in life is 70% (Dabelea, Knowler, and Pettitt, 2000; Dabelea, 2007). Children who were exposed to hyperglycemia in utero have a greater risk for developing childhood obesity and childhood type 2 diabetes because they may have suffered islet cell injury (Nathanielsz, Poston, and Taylor, 2007). Breastfeeding, diet, exercise, and prevention of obesity decrease the child's risk significantly (Barclay and Murata, 2006, 2007).

DIAGNOSTIC TESTING

Diabetes Mellitus, Type 1 and Type 2

Criteria for the diagnosis of diabetes mellitus (Expert Committee, 2001) follow:
- Fasting plasma glucose (FPG) 126 mg/dl or greater after at least an 8-hour fast
- Two-hour postprandial glucose (PG) greater than 200 mg/dl after a 75-g glucose load
- Symptoms of diabetes such as polyuria, polydipsia, and unexplained weight loss plus casual plasma glucose concentration greater than 200 mg/dl

The diagnosis is made after these criteria are confirmed by a repeat positive test on a different day.

Gestational Diabetes

It is current practice to screen all patients for GDM between 24 and 28 weeks and is supported by the American Association of Clinical Endocrinologists (AACE, 2007). The USPSTF (2008) and American Diabetes Association (ADA, 2004b) recommend a more individualized screening approach and suggest not screening women at low risk. The low risk group (ADA, 2004b) includes women who meet the following criteria:
- Younger than 25 years
- Normal body weight before pregnancy
- Negative family history of diabetes (no first-degree relative with the disease)
- No history of IGT or IFG
- No history of poor obstetric outcome
- Not a member of a high risk ethnic or racial group, such as African American, Asian, Hispanic, or Native American

According to the AHRQ (2008a) literature review, there is limited evidence to support early screening for GDM before 24 weeks. Screening for GDM between 24 and 28 weeks' gestation takes one of two forms.

Two-Step Approach: Glucose Challenge Test

The two-step approach is the most common screening method for GDM. A glucose challenge test is performed by initially giving 50 g of oral glucose and 1 hour later testing the blood sugar. A blood sugar level of 139 mg/dl or less rules out GDM. A blood sugar level of 130 to 199 mg/dl should be followed up with an oral glucose tolerance test (OGTT) to confirm GDM. If the patient has a blood sugar level of 200 mg/dl or greater, treat as a gestational diabetic without further testing.

One-Step Approach: Oral Glucose Tolerance Test

An OGTT is performed without prior glucose challenge test to screen for GDM.

Two- or Three-Hour Glucose Tolerance Test

In either approach, GDM is diagnosed with an OGTT of either a 3-hour, 100-g glucose load or a 2-hour, 75-g glucose load. The 100-g OGTT is preferred because the 75-g glucose load is not as well validated. Before either OGTT, 150 g of complex carbohydrate should be eaten for 3 days. Instruct the woman to abstain

Table 10-4 Normal Serum Blood Glucose Values (mg/dl) Following 100 g Oral Glucose Tolerance Test in Pregnancy

Time of Measurement	*Carpenter and Coustan Criteria	National Diabetes Data Group
Fasting	<95	<105
1 hr	<180	<190
2 hr	<155	<165
3 hr	<140	<145

Data from American Diabetes Association: Position statement: gestational diabetes mellitus, *Diabetes Care* 27 (Suppl 1):S88-S90, 2004; Mulholland E, Njoroge T, Mersereau P, Williams J: Comparison of guidelines available in the United States for diagnosis and management of diabetes before, during, and after pregnancy, *J Womens Health* 16(6):90-801, 2007.
*Preferred.

from eating, drinking, and smoking for 8 hours before the test. Have her rest for approximately 30 minutes before the test. Begin the test by drawing a fasting blood sugar sample. Start the timer and have the patient drink 100 g of glucose solution within 5 minutes. Subsequent blood samples are drawn at 1, 2, and 3 hours. During the test, the patient should rest and abstain from smoking. GDM is diagnosed if two or more plasma glucose blood values exceed the values using the Carpenter and Coustan criteria or the National Diabetes Data Group criteria guidelines listed in Table 10-4 (ADA, 2004b; Mulholland and others, 2007). A single abnormal value indicates IGT and the patient should be retested in 2 weeks.

Detection of Maternal Complications

Women who have already been diagnosed with diabetes, either during a previous pregnancy or in the absence of pregnancy, are usually classified as previously described (see Table 10-1). If the woman is insulin-dependent, she should be screened for hypertension; dyslipidemia; peripheral and autonomic neuropathy; and renal, retinal, peripheral, vascular, and cardiac involvement. Some commonly ordered tests are blood urea nitrogen (BUN) and serum creatinine, fasting lipid profile, microalbuminuria with a 24-hour albumin excretion with creatinine clearance or collection for albumin-to-creatinine ratio, electrocardiogram (ECG), ophthalmic examination for retinopathy, and treadmill test. Women with type 1 diabetes should have thyroid function studies.

Glycosylated Hemoglobin

Hemoglobin A is normal minor hemoglobin that has a glucose link. Glucose attaches to this hemoglobin during its normal 120-day life span. The amount depends on the glucose in the bloodstream. Glycosylated hemoglobin (Hb A1c) is a blood test to determine the level of hemoglobin A that has become "sugar coated." Therefore the test reflects adequacy of glucose control for the previous 4 to 6 weeks. Hb A1c levels above 6% indicate elevated glucose during the past 4 to 6 weeks and are associated with an increased incidence of congenital anomalies. Therefore this test is used to screen women with diabetes before conception or at the initial prenatal visit and every 2 to 3 months throughout the pregnancy.

USUAL MEDICAL MANAGEMENT AND PROTOCOLS FOR NURSE PRACTITIONERS

Preconception Management

Preconception planning is the key to a successful pregnancy. Tight glycemic control before and during pregnancy decreases risks and complications for the woman and her fetus and fetal congenital abnormalities with pregestational diabetes. This involves evaluating the treatment of any existing complications of DM, as outlined in the following.

Hypertension

Ideally blood pressure should be stabilized before pregnancy. In the nonpregnant person with diabetes, angiotensin-converting enzyme inhibitors (ACE inhibitors), diuretics, or angiotensin II receptor blockers (ARBs) are the drugs of choice. However, none of these drugs should be used during pregnancy. ACE inhibitors and ARBs increase the risk for congenital malformations. Diuretics may decrease maternal plasma volume, decreasing uteroplacental perfusion. Beta-blockers are not recommended because they can interfere with glucose control. Approximately 5% to 10% of pregnant patients with diabetes have chronic hypertension (Hinton and Sibai, 2004). The antihypertensive medications of choice during pregnancy are methyldopa, calcium channel blockers such as nifedipine, or alpha-adrenergic blockers. Ideally the blood pressure should be kept between 110 and 129 mm Hg systolic and 65 and 79 mm Hg diastolic (ADA, 2009). Pregnant patients with diabetes and hypertension are at increased risk for preeclampsia, uteroplacental insufficiency (UPI), and stillbirth if the blood pressure is elevated. In contrast, a blood pressure that is too low may interfere with uteroplacental perfusion, thus interfering with fetal growth as well.

Preeclampsia is a common complication in the pregnant patient who has diabetes, with or without chronic hypertension, especially if glucose control is poor. Therefore close monitoring of the blood pressure throughout pregnancy is important.

Dyslipidemia

Many patients with diabetes are on a lipid-lowering agent such as a HMG-CoA reductase inhibitor (statin) to decrease coronary and cerebrovascular events. However, statins are a pregnancy category X drug, and their use should be stopped before pregnancy. Dyslipidemia is a chronic disorder. Cessation of therapy during pregnancy does not significantly affect the long-term sequela (Weiner and Buhimschi, 2009).

Platelet Aggregation

Many patients with diabetes have increased production of thromboxane, a potent vasoconstrictor and platelet aggregate. Low-dose aspirin (81 mg) is being used as a primary and secondary prevention strategy for patients with diabetes who have cardiovascular risk without contraindications such as aspirin allergy, bleeding disorder, hepatic disease, or are on anticoagulant therapy (ADA, 2009). Low-dose aspirin use in the second and third trimester may decrease the risk for preeclampsia and intrauterine growth restriction (IUGR) (see Chapter 22). High-dose aspirin therapy should be avoided during the third trimester related to the risk for bleeding and prolonged pregnancy (Weiner and Buhimschi, 2009).

Autonomic Neuropathy

Autonomic neuropathy can cause cardiovascular, gastrointestinal tract, or bladder dysfunction and increase the risk for pregnancy complications. Orthostatic blood pressure changes, a flat pulse rate during position change, dizziness, light-headedness, and weakness on standing are signs of possible cardiovascular neuropathy, indicating a referral. Bloating, epigastric pain, nausea, vomiting, diarrhea, and postprandial hypoglycemia are signs of gastroparesis indicating a referral to the gastroenterologist.

Peripheral Sensory Neuropathy

Because diabetes can cause peripheral sensory neuropathy leading to nerve damage to the feet, conduct a comprehensive foot screen using the LEAP assessment. The assessment includes sensory testing of the feet for position sense, vibratory sensation, and monofilament tactile perception (ADA, 2009). Details about the LEAP assessment can be found online (*http://www.hrsa.gov/leap/fivestep.htm*). Assess also the dorsalis pedis pulse, posterior tibialis pulse, capillary refill, and ankle reflexes. Any negative finding indicates a referral.

Nephropathy

Renal insufficiency can increase the risk to mother and fetus during pregnancy. Therefore all patients with diabetes should be screened before conception or at the first prenatal visit. Serum creatinine, creatinine clearance, or microalbuminuria are tests that evaluate renal function.

Retinopathy

A preconception dilated retinal examination by an ophthalmologist is recommended to assess for microaneurysms, small retinal hemorrhages, cotton wool spots, and exudates. Pregnancy can cause retinopathy to worsen.

Antepartum Glycemic Management

According to the American Diabetes Association (ADA, 2009), the goals of management of the pregnant woman with diabetes using whole blood values are as follows (add 15% if plasma values are used):

- Maintain fasting, premeal, and bedtime glucose levels between 60 and 99 mg/dl
- Keep postprandial glucose levels between 100 and 129 mg/dl
- Keep the 2 AM to 4 AM blood glucose between 60 and 99 mg/dl
- Achieve a treatment Hb A1c concentration (6% or below)
- Prevent episodes of hypoglycemia
- Prevent DKA

Home monitoring and control consist of the following six facets in the patient with diabetes: blood glucose monitoring, urine testing, insulin management, diet management, exercise recommendations, and antepartum fetal surveillance. Hospitalization may become necessary if euglycemia cannot be maintained with home monitoring and outpatient surveillance. Care is provided in collaboration with an endocrinologist and obstetrician or perinatologist.

Blood Glucose Monitoring

Monitoring blood glucose during pregnancy is a cornerstone of glycemic control (ADA, 2009). It is primarily accomplished by daily self-monitoring of blood glucose (SMBG) by the patient and Hb A1c tests every 4 to 6 weeks to confirm glycemic control of the previous 120 days. Periodic laboratory measurements of plasma glucose are used only to supplement or test the accuracy of SMBG (ADA, 2009).

SMBG should be done 3 to 10 times a day (ADA, 2008), depending on difficulty of glycemic control, but postprandial levels must be assessed. The capillary blood glucose samples are taken before meals and snacks, 60 to 90 minutes after meals (Yogev and Hod, 2007), at bedtime, and occasionally between 2 AM and 4 AM (Kitzmiller and others, 2008).

Glucose monitoring should begin before conception. If this is not possible, it should begin as soon as pregnancy is suspected or determined. A portable blood glucose reflectance meter is readily available to rent or buy. The meter is used to read chemical test strips. The results should be recorded in a logbook and brought to each prenatal visit. For correct interpretation of blood glucose, it is critical to know whether the home monitor and strips provide whole blood or plasma results. The laboratory blood glucose test uses plasma, and many home capillary monitors measure whole blood glucose. Whole blood glucose values are about 15% lower than plasma; this is related to dilution (Chernecky and Berger, 2001). (See Self-Monitoring of Blood Glucose under Nursing Interventions for Diabetes and Pregnancy.)

Continuous glucose monitoring can be beneficial for unexplained elevations in Hb A1c, or unexplained hypoglycemia and hyperglycemia (ADA, 2008). Two new continuous glucose monitoring systems are currently available: Gluco Watch G2 Biographer (GW2B) and the Continuous Glucose Monitor system by Medtronic MiniMed. The GW2B is a noninvasive device worn as a wristwatch with a disposable autosensor that pulls glucose through the skin. (For additional information, go to *http://www.glucowatch.com*.) The Continuous Glucose Monitor system uses a subcutaneous sensor to perform ongoing glucose measurements throughout the day. The device is worn for 3 days, and the information obtained is then downloaded into a computer, which graphically prints out the blood glucose levels. Both devices can be helpful in determining at what time during the day the blood sugars are abnormal (Yogev and Hod, 2007).

Urine Testing

Ketones

If the patient becomes ill or blood glucose levels are greater than 200 mg/dl, urine testing for ketones should be done. In pregnancy, ketonuria may be caused by dietary insufficiencies such as low carbohydrate intake, low calorie intake, or skipped meals or snacks; it can also occur when ketoacidosis is present.

Sugar

Because of the lowered renal threshold for glucose, glucosuria is not used as a means of determining management.

Table 10-5   Changes in Insulin Need During Pregnancy

Trimester	Insulin Need	Common Problems
First	Decrease 10%–25% to avoid hypoglycemia	Blood sugar very unstable; nocturnal hypoglycemia common
Second	Daily insulin requirement increases gradually. Typically, over pregnancy baseline: • Type 1 increase 10%–20% • Type 2 increase 30%–90%	Mother switches from a glucose-based to a lipid-based energy to spare glucose for fetal growth
Third	0.9–1.2 U/kg/day	Related to diminished responsiveness to insulin
35th Week of gestation	Insulin levels plateau and may slightly decrease	
Labor and delivery	In active labor may decrease to 0	
Postpartum	Decrease markedly related to loss of placental hormones	Hypoglycemia

Insulin Management

Normal insulin needs change during pregnancy related to insulin-antagonistic placental hormones and increased inflammatory mediators. Table 10-5 outlines the normal changes in insulin need during pregnancy. Early in pregnancy, insulin requirements may decrease slightly. At about 15 weeks of gestation, the insulin requirements begin to gradually increase until approximately 35 weeks of gestation, when insulin requirements usually level off. Around 38 weeks of gestation, requirements may slightly decrease. A rapid decrease may indicate placental compromise (see Insulin Administration, under Nursing Management).

Types of insulin

The usual type of insulin used for the pregnant woman with diabetes is a biosynthetic human insulin (Humulin), made by genetically programming *Escherichia coli* bacteria to produce insulin. Adverse reactions to insulin, which include hypersensitivity or allergic skin reactions, lipodystrophy, and tissue resistance, rarely occur with biosynthetic human insulin as compared with the animal-based insulins (Beaser and Joslin Diabetes Center, 2008).

Insulin classifications

The current classifications of insulin today are rapid-acting insulins such as lispro (Humalog) and aspart (NovoLog), short-acting regular (Humulin R), and intermediate acting neutral protamine Hagedorn (NPH; Humulin N).

The two rapid-acting insulins, lispro and aspart, can be substituted for regular insulin at a 1:1 rate and are preferred during pregnancy and lactation (Singh and Jovanovic, 2007). The advantages of the rapid-acting insulins are they work faster (within 10 to 15 minutes) and have a shorter duration (lasting only 3 to 5 hours) than regular insulin.

Table 10-6   Comparison Chart for Human Insulins

Type	Appearance	Onset	Peak (hr)	Duration (hr)
Rapid-acting	Clear solution	10–15 min	1½	3–5
Short-acting	Clear solution	0.5 hr	3–4	6–8
Intermediate-acting	Cloudy suspension	2–4 hr	4–12	12–24

Table 10-7   Calculation Guidelines for Insulin During Pregnancy

Trimester	Insulin Dosage (Unit/kg Body Weight)
Prepregnant	0.6
First trimester	0.7
Second trimester	0.8
Third trimester until 36 weeks	0.9
Third trimester from 36 to 40 weeks	1.0
Postpartum	0.6

Data from American College of Obstetricians and Gynecologists (ACOG): *Pregestational diabetes mellitus, clinical management guidelines for obstetrician-gynecologists*, No. 60, 2005, ACOG and Sweet Success.

In contrast, the onset of regular insulin is slower, taking 30 minutes or longer, and it has a longer duration time of 6 to 8 hours, which lasts past the mealtime. Therefore the rapid-acting insulins cause less postprandial hyperglycemia, decrease the rate of hypoglycemia, and significantly reduce Hb A1c levels. However, the patient must eat as soon as she takes her injection unless she is lowering high blood glucose. High glycemic index foods such as bread, rice, potatoes, and sucrose products are covered much better with the rapid-acting insulins than with regular insulin, but with slow glycemic foods they may cause hypoglycemia. When regular insulin is used, snacks are essential in the morning, the afternoon, and at bedtime to prevent premeal hypoglycemia because it peaks at 4 hours. See Table 10-6 for onset, peak, and duration of insulins.

Newer insulins are available, such as the delayed-absorption peakless basal insulin glargine (Lantus) and detemir (Levemir). Research needs to be done to direct the use of these newer insulins for the pregnant or lactating woman with diabetes. Both of these insulins are considered Pregnancy Category C (Prescriber's Letter, 2007).

Insulin dosage

Insulin doses must be constantly adjusted as the pregnancy progresses. The patient's 24-hour insulin dosage is usually calculated according to trimester. Table 10-7 provides calculation guidelines for insulin dosage during the three trimesters. Table 10-8 presents common causes and treatment for early morning hyperglycemia. Individualized modifications of insulin need depend on various factors. For women with GDM or class B diabetes that had been controlled with oral agents, the 24-hour insulin dosage is usually calculated according to the patient's present weight and weeks of gestation. If the patient is thin, her need is lower than normal. However, if

Table 10-8 Early Morning Hyperglycemia

Cause	Definition	2 AM–4 AM Blood Sugar	Treatment
Somogyi effect	Nocturnal hypoglycemia causes a surge of counterregulatory hormones that increase the morning blood glucose	Low	Decrease evening NPH or increase kilocalories of bedtime snack OR Change the evening NPH from predinner to prebedtime snack
Dawn phenomenon	Exaggerated growth hormone effect between 5 AM and 8 AM in conjunction with the waking process	Normal	Change the evening NPH from predinner to prebedtime snack Cautious use of early morning regular insulin (3 AM–6 AM)
Waning insulin	Inadequate insulin coverage relative to evening caloric intake	Elevated	Increase evening NPH dose Change evening NPH dose from predinner to prebedtime snack

NPH, Neutral protamine Hagedorn (insulin).

she is extremely overweight, her need is increased from the norm. For pregestational women with diabetes already on insulin, the insulin dosage is evaluated and adjusted based on current control and weeks of gestation.

Dosage distribution

The 24-hour insulin requirement is divided into two components:

- Basal (long-acting) that takes care of the glucose produced by the liver of approximately 5 gram of glucose per hour
- Bolus (rapid- or short-acting) insulin that takes care of the glucose eaten during a meal.

Of the total 24-hour insulin dose during pregnancy, 45% of the total daily dose should be provided as basal insulin and 55% as bolus insulin related to increase insulin resistance. For the nonpregnant patient it is usually 50:50.

The 24-hour insulin requirement is further divided into two to four injections each day, to be given 20 to 30 minutes before a meal if regular insulin is used or just before the meal if rapid-acting insulin is used. Patients with type 1 diabetes most likely need three or more injections per day.

Conventional insulin therapy usually uses two to three daily injections. For a *two-dose regimen*, the morning dose is usually two thirds of the woman's 24-hour dose, of which one third is regular insulin and two thirds is NPH. Her predinner dose is the remaining one third of her 24-hour dose, of which one half is rapid- or short-acting insulin and one half is NPH. The greatest risk with this type of dosing is the evening intermediate-acting insulin peaking during the middle of the night. A *three-dose regimen* is similar to the two-dose regimen, but the evening intermediate-acting insulin (NPH) is held to bedtime to decrease nocturnal hypoglycemia

Intensive insulin therapy is provided by way of *multiple daily injections or the insulin pump.* The insulin dosage is based on premeal blood glucose levels and grams of carbohydrate in the meal to be eaten. This provides for more dietary flexibility. With the multiple-dose injections method, a basal dose of insulin of approximately 50% of the day's total insulin requirement is given as intermediate-acting insulin, in the morning and evening. The morning dose is one third of the long-acting dose, and the predinner dose is two thirds of the long-acting dose. The patient then gives herself rapid- or short-acting insulin before each meal, based on the number of carbohydrate grams in the planned meal and her premeal blood glucose level. The equation used is 1.5 units of rapid- or short-acting insulin per 10 carbohydrate grams at breakfast and one unit of rapid- or short-acting insulin per 10 carbohydrate grams at lunch and dinner. No additional insulin is given if the blood glucose is in the normal range (70 to 100 mg/dl). If the blood glucose is lower than 70 mg/dl, the dose is decreased by two units of insulin.

Insulin pump

It is a small, battery-operated device (the size of a cell phone) worn around the waist with a belt that contains a reservoir that is filled with rapid-acting insulin to provide a continuous insulin infusion. Indications for its use include erratic blood glucose levels, need for flexibility in meal and sleep schedules, or difficulty controlling postprandial or early morning blood glucose level (Mensing, 2006). To promote the success of the insulin pump, understanding of the following is paramount:

- Frequent SMBG
- Carbohydrate counting
- Calculating bolus insulin
- Problem solving through interpretation of blood glucose pattern
- Adjusting insulin based on the preceding results

Dosage adjustments

Adjustments in insulin may need to be made every 5 to 10 days during pregnancy to achieve target glucose control, based on SMBG. Insulin need is increased by stress, the presence of infection, and steroids. Always start by fixing the fasting blood sugar first. Usually adjust by one to two units or 10% of dosage, not to exceed four units, in response to a pattern of blood glucose levels. However, if early morning hyperglycemia occurs, refer to Table 10-8 for common causes and treatment. Nocturnal hypoglycemia is more common during pregnancy. Symptoms such as night sweating, nightmares, difficulty sleeping, or morning headaches may indicate nocturnal hypoglycemia.

To treat a temporary loss of control, a premeal correction bolus is recommended rather than using a sliding scale. The current insulin dose of rapid- or short-acting insulin is adjusted using an insulin sensitivity factor formula to determine the amount the blood sugar will be lowered by one unit of insulin. This is determined by using the rule of 1500 if regular insulin is used and the rule of 1700 if rapid-acting insulin is used. According to these rules, either divide the total daily insulin dosage the patient is taking by 1500 or 1700. This equals the amount the glucose level will drop with one unit of insulin.

Insulin Therapy for Gestational Diabetes Mellitus

When medical nutritional therapy (MNT) with exercise does not keep the fasting plasma glucose lower than 95 mg/dl or the 2-hour postprandial lower than 120 mg/dl, insulin should be initiated (ADA, 2004b).

Oral glucose-lowering agents

Oral glucose-lowering agents have not been recommended during pregnancy because of the risk for fetal anomalies and reactive hypoglycemia. However, several studies have compared glyburide, a type of sulfonylurea drug, with insulin in women with GDM who were unable to meet glycemic control on MNT. The gestational diabetic patients on glyburide achieved glycemic control when compared to insulin therapy (Langer and others, 2000; Durnwald and Landon, 2005; Jacobson and others, 2005). This particular sulfonylurea does not cross the placenta to the fetus. Glyburide has not been FDA approved for use during pregnancy; therefore its use is restricted to investigational research. It should not be concluded that other sulfonylurea drugs are safe to be used during pregnancy.

Metformin is an effective treatment of anovulation in women with polycystic ovary syndrome. Its continued used during pregnancy has been shown in preliminary trials to reduce the risk of spontaneous abortion and lower fasting insulin levels in these patients (Lord, Flight, and Norman, 2003; Checa and others, 2005; Hawthorne, 2006). Metformin has not been FDA-approved for use during pregnancy; therefore its use is restricted to investigational research.

Diet Management

Diet is another cornerstone of therapy in the management of diabetes. The current diabetic diet is less restrictive and encourages individualization (ADA, 2008). Consideration must be given to prepregnancy weight, general health status, dietary habits, activity level, and insulin therapy. Folic acid supplements of 400 mcg/day are recommended before conception and throughout the first trimester to decrease the risk for neural tube defects. (See Medical Nutrition Therapy, under Nursing Management, for in-depth diabetic dietary guidelines.)

Exercise Recommendations

Exercise is an important component in establishing and maintaining glucose control; improved insulin sensitivity is evident after 4 weeks of exercise (Kitzmiller and others, 2008). (See Activity and Exercise Functional Health Pattern, under Nursing Management, for specifics on exercise during pregnancy.) However, in the presence of such diabetic complications as uncontrolled hypertension, advanced retinopathy, and severe autonomic or peripheral neuropathy or in the presence of urine ketones, a regular exercise program may be contraindicated (ADA, 2009).

Maternal Surveillance with Preexisting Diabetes

Frequent laboratory tests to be done during pregnancy to monitor the patient's diabetes status follow:

- Hb A1c test every 4 to 6 weeks
- Blood glucose fingerstick each prenatal visit to evaluate accuracy of SMBG

- Urine for protein, sugar, ketones, nitrate, and leukocyte esterase at each prenatal visit. (Positive for nitrates and leukocyte esterase indicates possible UTI and should be followed up with a urine culture and sensitivity. Positive for protein indicates further evaluation for preeclampsia. Positive for ketone indicates further dietary workup to evaluate eating habits.)
- Kidney function with a 24-hour creatinine clearance and total protein to be done each trimester
- Retinal examination in the first trimester and then as indicated
- Thyroid panel for women with type 1 diabetes in the first trimester to include free thyroxine (T_4), thyroid-stimulating hormone, and antimicrosomal antibodies and then as indicated

In the presence of cardiovascular disease, a cardiologist should be a part of the health care team.

Antepartum Fetal Surveillance

Antepartum monitoring is essential to evaluate early and periodic fetal condition and help time the delivery to coincide with optimal outcome.

Ultrasound

Ultrasound examinations are usually done at intervals throughout the pregnancy. They are done to help accurately predict gestational age and provide reassurance about fetal organ development. They also give information about fetal growth rate, activity quality, amniotic fluid volume, and biophysical profile evaluation.

Alpha-fetoprotein (MSAFP)

Alpha-fetoprotein helps detect open fetal defects such as open neural tube or ventral wall defects of omphalocele or gastroschisis. The fetus of a woman with type 1 diabetes is at increased risk for these defects.

Fetal biophysical tests

A variety of fetal biophysical tests are used to monitor fetal well-being starting around 28 weeks' gestation. They include fetal movement counting, biophysical profile, non-stress test, amniotic fluid volume assessment, and fetal Doppler studies. In the presence of elevated maternal serum glucose, biophysical profile and amniotic fluid volume may not be reliable indicators of fetal wellbeing (Vintzileos, 2007) (see Chapters 3 and 4).

Amniocentesis

Amniocentesis is usually used to ascertain the lecithin/sphingomyelin (L/S) ratio. An L/S ratio of 2.0 or greater when PG is present is sufficient to expect that surfactant levels are high enough in the fetus to prevent the development of respiratory distress syndrome (RDS). Amniocentesis is generally done if elective delivery is planned in a patient before 39 weeks with suboptimal dating (ACOG, 2008b).

Management of Diabetic Ketoacidosis

DKA is caused by ineffective insulin combined with an elevation of counter-regulatory hormones such as glucagon, catecholamines, cortisol, and growth hormone to move glucose into cells, leading to hyperglycemia (diabetes). The liver tries to compensate by increasing its production of glucose, only to further raise blood glucose levels. The lack of glucose for cell use causes the body to break down fat for energy, which results in ketone (acetone) release, ketosis (serum acetone at a 1:2 dilution or greater). The respiratory system attempts to compensate by increasing the respiratory rate and depth (Kussmaul respirations), blowing off carbon dioxide. A decline in pH (less than 7.3), a drop in serum bicarbonate (less than 15 mg/dl), and an abnormal elevated anion gap (greater than 12) results.

When the woman's buffering system is unable to compensate, metabolic acidosis develops. The excessive glucose and ketone bodies result in osmotic diuresis and ketonuria with subsequent fluid and electrolyte loss, volume depletion, and cellular dehydration. Infections of urine, skin, lungs, or amniotic fluid; noncompliance with insulin administration; or dietary indiscretion are precipitating factors.

Category II fetal heart rate tracings are very common. In deciding the plan of care, keep in mind that the fetal heart rate usually improves as the maternal DKA is corrected (Foley, 2004).

The critical care management protocols for ketoacidosis are summarized in Critical Care Intervention for Perinatal Ketoacidosis, under Nursing Management.

Preterm Labor Management

According to a Cochrane Systematic Review (Roberts and Dalziel, 2006) and American College of Obstetricians and Gynecologists (ACOG, 2008a), a single course of corticosteroids is recommended for all pregnant women at risk for preterm delivery between 24 and 34 weeks' gestation. In the diabetic patient, nifedipine is the preferred tocolytic drug as to effectiveness and safety (Weiner and Buhimschi, 2009). Magnesium sulfate or indomethacin may also be used to allow for the administration of corticosteroids. Because beta-sympathomimetics can stimulate hyperglycemia and even cause ketoacidosis, their use is not recommended for the patient with diabetes.

Intrapartum Management

The woman with well-controlled diabetes who has no complications does not need to deliver before term if the fetus is not macrosomic and the biophysical profile is reassuring. Early delivery may be necessary if the woman has not had good glucose control, has a history of a stillbirth, has developed complications such as a hypertensive disorder of pregnancy or vasculopathy, or if the fetal estimated weight is LGA to decrease the risk of shoulder dystocia or there is an indication of fetal compromise (AHRQ, 2008b). In any of these cases, an induction or cesarean birth may be scheduled. Documentation of fetal lung maturity is appropriate if gestational age is uncertain or for elective induction before 39 weeks (ACOG, 2008b).

During an induction or spontaneous labor, intermittent subcutaneous insulin or a continuous insulin infusion is required. Most women with GDM do not require insulin during labor (see Intrapartum Management, under Nursing Management).

Insulin Infusion

Continuous insulin infusion

If a continuous insulin infusion is needed, regular insulin is satisfactory and cost effective. Usually 25 units of regular insulin are added to 250 mg of normal saline (NS) (ACOG, 2005). Piggyback insulin is infused to the main IV line of D_5 LR or D_5 1/2 NS. The IV rate and supplemental insulin vary based on hourly capillary blood glucose value (see Potential Complication: Hypoglycemia, Intrapartum).

Intermittent subcutaneous insulin

If intermittent subcutaneous injections are used, one third to one half of the patient's prepregnancy dosage of insulin may be given the morning of the induction. An intermediate-acting insulin most likely is not used because of the drop in insulin requirement after delivery. A continuous 5% glucose infusion is started at approximately 100 ml/hr. Supplemental regular insulin is given based on glucose values obtained every 1 to 2 hours to maintain plasma glucose between 80 and 120 mg/dl or capillary whole blood glucose between 70 and 110 mg/dl.

Cesarean Birth

In the event a cesarean birth is planned, fetal lung maturity is usually predetermined. The cesarean is scheduled for early morning. The woman should drink nothing after midnight and hold her evening and morning dosages of insulin. Her capillary glucose level should be checked before and immediately following the delivery. Glucose is administered via IV.

Postpartum Management

At delivery there is an abrupt loss of the antagonistic placental hormones and suppression of the anterior pituitary growth hormone. Therefore there is a significant decrease in insulin need during the immediate postpartum period. Insulin requirements for the patient with GDM disappear in most women (ADA, 2007). For the woman with type 2 diabetes, the insulin dose is typically minimal for 1 to 3 days. The woman with type 1 diabetes may require small doses, which are determined by the blood glucose levels. By the third or fourth postpartum day, insulin requirements usually increase to about two thirds of the prepregnancy dosage.

Frequent blood glucose monitoring may be necessary for the first 48 hours postpartum to determine the individual patient's insulin need. Women who were not insulin-dependent before pregnancy most likely do not need insulin. During the early postpartum period, the importance of ongoing glycemic control should be stressed. The Diabetes Control and Complications Trial Research Group (1996) showed that keeping blood glucose levels within normal limits reduced the risk for diabetic complications such as retinopathy by 76%, nephropathy by 50%, neuropathy by 60%, and cardiac problems by 35%.

To maintain normal blood glucose levels after delivery, ongoing SMBG, comprehensive meal planning as outlined for pregnancy, and regular exercise along with possible oral hypoglycemic agents or insulin regimen are required.

All women, following a pregnancy complicated with GDM, must understand the need for ongoing, long-term follow-up. Women who have had GDM have a 35% to 60% risk for developing type 2 diabetes mellitus within the next 20 years (Kitzmiller, Dang-Kilduff, and Taslimi, 2007). Maintaining a normal weight and exercising regularly have been shown to decrease the risk to 25% (Care Management Institute, 2005; Kitzmiller, Dang-Kilduff, and Taslimi, 2007). (See Postpartum Nursing Interventions for appropriate postpartum teaching.)

NURSING MANAGEMENT

Prevention

The two major goals of care for pregnant women with diabetes are to promote a healthy, normally developed newborn and prevent complications of diabetes from adversely affecting the pregnant woman. Counseling before conception is aimed at planning a pregnancy rather than simply allowing it to occur. Euglycemia should be attained and maintained for a minimum of 1 to 2 months before conception to reduce the risks of birth defects and congenital abnormalities to no more than the general population.

Education about diet, glucose monitoring, exercise, and insulin adjustments is necessary for the woman to self-manage diabetes during pregnancy. Education and referrals should be aimed at promoting as much independence as the woman is willing and cognitively able to assume.

Preconception Nursing Interventions for Diabetes[*]

Goals

- Achieve euglycemia for 1 to 2 months before conception to prevent fetal anomalies. Determine glucose control by reviewing the patient's home SMBG record and Hb A1c. Achieve Hb A1c test of less than 6%. Obtain health history of the following:
  - Determine the type and duration of diabetes.
  - Assess the current diabetes management, including insulin usage, prior or current use of oral glucose-lowering agents, SMBG pattern and results, medical nutrition therapy (MNT), and physical exercise pattern. Medication change may be needed if the patient is using oral agents.
  - Review the known chronic complications of diabetes such as retinopathy, autonomic neuropathy (gastroparesis, urinary retention, hypoglycemic unawareness, or orthostatic hypotension), peripheral neuropathy, and nephropathy and macrovascular changes such as hypertension or atherosclerotic vascular disease. Note: Angiotensin-converting enzyme inhibitor hypertensive agent is contraindicated during pregnancy. Avoid beta blockers and diuretics as well.
  - Determine whether the patient has a recent history of severe ketoacidosis or hypoglycemic episodes.
  - Determine any history of recent infections.
  - Ask about other medications being taken, such as antihypertensive agents, lipid-lowering agents, or aspirin therapy. Also ask whether alternative therapy practices are being used.
  - Inquire about the patient's patterns of using health screenings such as physical, dental, and eye checkups, Pap smears, and immunizations (especially rubella).
  - Assess for negative health behaviors such as substance abuse, smoking, subclinical food issues, and alcohol intake. Encourage lifestyle changes as indicated.

---

[*]Foley, 2004; ACOG, 2005; Moore and Catalano, 2009.

Physical Examination

- **General.** Determine age, weight, body mass index, and height to attain or maintain reasonable body weight to enhance glycemic control.
- **Vital signs.** Determine temperature, pulse, respiration, and blood pressure (BP) (hypertension), including orthostatic BP changes (autonomic neuropathy). The BP goal for the patient with diabetes is lower than 130/80 mm Hg.
- **Skin.** Observe visible rashes or lesions, and select injection sites.
- **Eyes.** Refer to ophthalmologist for a dilated eye examination to rule out retinopathy.
- **Oral examination.** Evaluate oral and dental health, and emphasize importance of biannual dental checkup with cleaning.
- **Thyroid palpation.** Rule out hypothyroidism or hyperthyroidism.
- **Cardiovascular disease.** Evaluate for angina, claudication, decreased pulses, vascular bruits, and ECG abnormalities to rule out coronary heart disease. If found, refer for screening tests for coronary artery disease such as exercise stress testing, stress perfusion imaging, stress echocardiography, or catheterization.
- **Abdomen.** Rule out abnormal pulsations and organomegaly, especially of the liver.
- **Genital.** Perform a pelvic examination and Pap smear to rule out vaginal infection.
- **Neurologic.** Assess for signs of peripheral neuropathy; include ankle and knee reflexes, vibratory sensation below knee with tuning fork, light touch and pinprick sensation, and foot screening. Foot screening includes history of foot problems, deformity, muscle atrophy, calluses, swelling, blisters, ingrown or thick toenails, and use of appropriate footwear. Check protective foot sensation with monofilament testing instrument. Refer to podiatrist as indicated using the five-step LEAP Program.
- **Autonomic neuropathy.** Evaluate gastrointestinal and genitourinary functions.
- **Peripheral vascular disease.** Screen for intermittent claudication (intermittent pain or cramps in legs), loss of heat sensitivity in feet, dorsalis pedis and posterior tibial pulses by palpation and auscultation, hair growth on legs and big toes, and tingling or numbness in feet.

Psychosocial Assessment

- Determine any psychosocial stressors such as affect/mood, quality of life related to diabetes and compliance issues such as medical management, and resources.
- Screen for psychiatric history, depression, anxiety/stress, and eating disorders.

Laboratory Evaluation

- Fasting plasma glucose level
- Hb A1c
- Serum creatinine
- Fasting lipid profile: total cholesterol, LDL, HDL, triglycerides to rule out dyslipidemia; goals: LDL lower than 100 mg/dl; triglycerides lower than 200 mg/dl; HDL higher than 55

- Thyroid panel: T_4 thyroid-stimulating hormone, antimicrosomal antibodies (antithyroid) because of a 5% to 10% chance of concurrent hyperthyroidism or hypothyroidism with type 1 diabetes
- Rubella titer to check for immune status
- Microalbuminuria with a 24-hour albumin excretion with creatinine clearance or a random spot collection for albumin/creatinine ratio to evaluate for nephropathy
- Urinalysis for culture if sediment is abnormal or if symptoms are present
- Electrocardiogram (ECG)
- Treadmill test if diabetes mellitus has persisted for more than 10 years or signs and symptoms of cardiac disease are present

Education Regarding Interaction of Family Planning, Diabetes, and Pregnancy

- Importance of effective contraception until tight glycemic control is achieved
- Risk and prevention of congenital anomalies and spontaneous abortion by tight glycemic control and avoidance of substance use
- Tight glycemic control increases risk for hypoglycemia, especially in type 1 diabetes
- Effects of pregnancy on maternal diabetic complications: pregnancy may accelerate retinopathy; in the presence of incipient renal failure, pregnancy may worsen the disease process; untreated coronary artery disease may cause maternal death during pregnancy
- Increased risks of obstetrical complications such as pregnancy-induced hypertension
- Risks to fetus and neonate
- Referral to diabetes educator, counselor, and social worker as indicated

Education in Self-Management

- Significance of tight glycemic control
- Five keys to tight control: diet, exercise, SMBG, stress control, and insulin administration and regulation to be adjusted based on SMBG
- SMBG before meals, 60 to 90 minutes after meals, and occasionally between 2 AM and 4 AM.
- Use the Hb A1c test every 4 to 6 weeks to determine stable glycemic control
- Effect of stress and illness on glycemic control
- Use of record-keeping system to include blood glucose values with times, insulin dosages with times, foods eaten, activity with time and duration, and urine testing when needed

Nursing Interventions for Diabetes During Pregnancy

Health Perception Functional Health Pattern

- **Confirmation.** Confirm pregnancy as early as possible.
- **Interventions.** Reevaluate or initiate preconceptual interventions as stated earlier.

- **Testing.** Do Hb A1c test routinely every 2 to 3 months to determine ongoing glycemic control. Use a laboratory that uses glycosylated hemoglobin assay methods that have passed certification testing by the National Glycohemoglobin Standardization program so that the results are traceable to the Diabetes Control and Complications Trial reference method. The glycated hemoglobin assay method uses whole blood specimens in addition to lyophilized specimens.

Nutrition Functional Health Pattern—Medical Nutritional Therapy (ADA, 2008)

- **Goal.** Maintain normal glycemic control, reach a reasonable body weight, and achieve optimal serum lipid levels while obtaining adequate calories and nutrients for increased metabolic needs during pregnancy.
- **Key dietary points**
  - There is no diabetic diet; there is just good nutrition. Promote eating a wholesome, balanced diet consistent with ethnic, cultural, and financial considerations (Kitzmiller and others, 2008).
  - Total carbohydrates are more important than type of carbohydrates.
  - Consistent carbohydrate intake from day to day and at each meal and snack is essential.
  - Emphasize importance of 28 g/day of fiber by including whole grains, fruits, and vegetables.
  - Saturated fat and sugary foods must be limited.
  - Reasonable body weight should be achieved and maintained; moderate weight loss (10 to 20 pounds), regardless of starting weight, has been shown to reduce hyperglycemia, dyslipidemia, and hypertension.
  - Eat at about the same time each day.
  - Eat foods from all food groups.
  - Use portion control.
  - Eat healthy snacks to prevent low blood sugar.
- **Ideal body weight (IBW).** The following formula determines the IBW: 100 pounds for first 5 feet of height + 5 pounds per inch for each 1 inch over 5 feet (+10% for large frame) (–10% for small frame).
- **Percentage of body fat.** Calculating the body mass index, waist-to-hip ratio, and the percentage of body fat by underwater weighing, skinfold measurements, or bioelectric impedance determines the percentage of body fat.
- **Detailed dietary history.** The following formula calculates caloric needs:
  - Baseline calories = IBW × 10
  - Activity calories
  - Sedentary = IBW × 3
  - Moderate = IBW × 5
  - Strenuous = (IBW × 7) – 10
  - Obesity –500 calories
  - Pregnant +300 calories
  - Kcal = baseline calories + activity calories – obesity + pregnancy
- **Calorie distribution** (ACOG, 2005)
  - 10% to 20% at breakfast
  - 5% to 10% at midmorning snack

- 20% to 30% at lunch
- 5% to 10% at midafternoon snack
- 30% to 40% at dinner
- 5% to 10% at bedtime snack
- **Division of calories from protein.** Protein should be 15% to 20% of total calories unless kidney disease exists; if this is the case, then restrict to 0.8 g/kg/day normal recommended dietary allowance (RDA).
- **Division of calories from lipids.** Lipids should be 30% to 40% of total calories; individualized on the basis of weight, blood sugar level, and blood lipid level. Emphasize lipids from monounsaturated fats, such as avocados, olives, peanuts, and canola oils. Saturated fats are to be less than 7%, and avoid trans fats.
- **Division of calories from carbohydrates.** The percentage of carbohydrates ranges from 40% to 50%, depending on weight, lipid profile, and type of diabetes. For example, if triglyceride and very low density lipoprotein (VLDL) levels are high, decrease carbohydrate and increase monounsaturated fat intake, unless triglyceride levels are greater than or equal to 1000. If this is the case, reduce dietary fat to less than 10% to reduce the risk for pancreatitis. Emphasize low glycemic index carbohydrates and soluble fiber foods such as whole grains, fruits, vegetables, and legumes. Limit simple sugars to less than 10% of the total calories. Consistent carbohydrate intake from day to day and at each meal and snack is important for glucose control. Postprandial blood glucose level is dependent on the carbohydrate content of the meal and contributes most to neonatal macrosomia. Preconception and during the first trimester the woman need 130 grams of carbohydrates a day. During the second and third trimesters, the carbohydrate intake needs to increase to at least 175 gram per day.
- **GDM dietary guidelines.** Women with gestational diabetes are sensitive to carbohydrates, especially at breakfast, and should limit sugary and concentrated sweets, as well as processed convenience foods. Better control is achieved if total carbohydrates are around 40%, protein around 20%, and fat around 40%, and monounsaturated and polyunsaturated fat intake is increased (ADA, 2004b). Eating a small breakfast (less than 10% of the daily total calories) made up of whole grains and protein-rich foods might help control blood sugar because the morning blood glucose level is likely to be high. "Free foods" such as cabbage, cucumbers, green onions, mushrooms, zucchini, spinach, celery, green beans, radishes, and lettuce may be eaten as desired.
- **Water.** One glass of water is to be consumed every waking hour until 2 hours before bedtime. This is important because it keeps the kidneys healthy and decreases preterm labor contractions.
- **Vitamin and minerals**
  - Without a deficiency, there is no clear evidence of benefit from vitamin and mineral supplementation (ADA, 2008).
  - Folate in dosages of 600 mcg/day is needed to decrease the incidence of small-for-gestational-age babies and neural tube defects.
- **Fiber.** Soluble fiber such as legumes, fruit, and oat bran form gels that delay the absorption of nutrients from the intestine. This helps control diabetes by preventing dramatic swings in blood glucose levels. Insoluble fiber, such as wheat

Table 10-9   American Diabetes Association and American Dietetic Association: New Exchange List* for Meal Planning

Group	Carbohydrates	Protein	Fat	Calories/Serving
Carbohydrates				
Starch	15	3	1 or less	80
Fruit	15	0	0	60
Vegetables	5	2	0	25
Other carbohydrates	15	Varies	Varies	Varies
Milk				
Skim	12	8	0–3	90
Low fat	12	8	5	120
Whole	12	8	8	150
Meat and Meat Substitutes				
Very lean	0	7	0–1	35
Lean	0	7	3	55
Medium fat	0	7	5	75
High fat	0	7	8	100
Fat group	0	0	5	4

*In grams.

bran, cannot be digested and speeds the movement of food through the intestines, decreasing the risk for constipation. If carbohydrate counting is being used for meal planning, subtract fiber from total carbohydrate grams if a food contains 5 g or more of dietary fiber.

- **Sodium.** A normal intake of sodium is 2400 to 3000 mg each day unless the woman with diabetes has chronic hypertension. In this situation, the sodium should be limited to less than 2400 mg.
- **Meal plan.** Translate all of this information into a meal plan using the exchange list, carbohydrate counting, food pyramid, or plate method.
- **Exchange system.** The exchange system divides foods into seven categories: starch and bread, fruit, vegetables, meat, fat, and other carbohydrates that are the simple sugary foods. Each food within a category provides similar amounts of carbohydrate, protein, fat, and calories; therefore any food within a group can be exchanged for any other food in the same group. See Table 10-9 for meal planning guidelines and Table 10-10 for a sample exchange plan summary.
  - By noting the proper serving size within a group, the patient can choose different foods within a group and still consume the same division of foods and similar calories each day. A dietitian usually initiates the number of servings in each group. The other carbohydrate group was added in 1995. When a patient decides to have a dessert, she notes the number of grams of carbohydrate and then decreases other carbohydrate servings by that amount. In this way, carbohydrate consistency is maintained from day to day.
- **Carbohydrate counting.** There are three levels of carbohydrate counting. Level 1 focuses on carbohydrate consistency only. Level 2 focuses on the relationships

Table 10-10   Exchange Plan Summary

Food Exchange Groups	Nutrients Provided	Calories per Serving	Serving Sizes
Starch (bread, cereals, grains, starchy vegetables)	15 g carbohydrate 3 g protein 3 g fiber	80	½ cup cereal, grain, or pasta 1 slice bread
Fruits	15 g carbohydrate 3 g fiber	60	½ cup fresh fruit ½ cup fruit juice ½ cup dried fruit
Vegetables	5 g carbohydrate 2 g protein 2–3 g fiber	25	½ cup cooked vegetables ½ cup vegetable juice 1 cup raw vegetables
Other carbohydrates: snack foods and sweet desserts	15 g carbohydrates Protein varies Fat varies	Varies	2 small cookies ½ cup ice cream
Milk			
Skim; very low fat	12 g carbohydrate 8 g protein Trace grams of fat	90	1 cup skim milk 8 oz plain nonfat yogurt
Low fat	12 g carbohydrate 8 g protein 5 g fat	120	1 cup 2% milk 8 oz plain low-fat yogurt
Whole	12 g carbohydrates 8 g protein 8 g fat	150	1 cup whole milk 8 oz whole plain yogurt
Meat and substitutes			
Very lean	7 g protein 0–1 g fat	35	1 oz chicken: white meat, no skin ¼ cup nonfat cottage cheese 2 egg whites
Lean	7 g protein 3 g fat	55	¼ cup 4.5% fat cottage cheese 1 oz lean pork or beef 1 oz chicken: white meat with skin
Medium fat	7 g protein 5 g fat	75	1 egg 4 oz tofu

Continued

Table 10-10   Exchange Plan Summary—cont'd

Food Exchange Groups	Nutrients Provided	Calories per Serving	Serving Sizes
High fat	7 g protein 8 g fat	45	1 oz roast beef, pork, or lamb 1 oz processed sandwich meats 1 oz American, cheddar, or Swiss cheese 2 Tbsp peanut butter
Fat	5 g fat	100	Varies

Developed from American Dietetic Association: *Exchange lists to meal planning*, Chicago, 1995, ADA.

among food, diabetes medications, physical activity, and blood glucose levels and takes appropriate action by adjusting the appropriate diabetes management. Level 3 adds the component of matching short-acting bolus insulin dosing to the carbohydrate amount of that meal. There is a consistent basal dose of long-acting insulin given daily, usually 50% of the total daily insulin requirement given in divided doses: one third in the morning and two thirds before dinner. Then the short-acting insulin is given before each meal based on the number of carbohydrates in the meal: usually, 1.5 units per 10 grams of carbohydrate eaten at breakfast and 1 unit per 10 grams eaten at lunch and dinner. The reason more insulin is required in the morning is that the body is more insulin-resistant at that time. If carbohydrates are being counted, subtract fiber from total carbohydrate grams if a food contains 5 g or more dietary fiber. If the premeal blood sugar is above or below normal, add or subtract insulin as outlined under insulin dosage distribution earlier in this chapter. It might be necessary to check blood sugar in 2 hours to evaluate the plan.

- **Food pyramid.** Individuals with diabetes may use the new food pyramid as a meal plan (*http://MyPyramid.gov*). Whole grains, fresh fruits and vegetables, and low-fat dairy products and meat are emphasized. Starchy vegetables such as corn, potatoes, and peas are treated as bread, and grains and cheese are considered protein. Special attention is needed to keep the number of servings of carbohydrates consistent from day to day, limiting fat and simple sugar.
- **Plate method.** To use this method, imagine that the plate is divided into three sections to determine similar serving sizes of protein, a starch food, and a vegetable. Then add a fruit or a beverage to the meal. If the diet allows more carbohydrates for the meal, add a bread or starch serving.
- **Referral.** Refer the patient to a registered dietitian or nutritionist for development of an individualized dietary plan. Discuss problems associated with strict adherence to the prescribed diet.

Elimination Functional Health Pattern

- **UTI.** Prevent infection by drinking 8 to 10 glasses of water a day and emptying the bladder every 2 hours.

Sleep and Rest Functional Health Pattern

- **Fatigue.** Obtain enough rest and sleep to prevent fatigue.

Activity and Exercise Functional Health Pattern[*]

- **Amount and type of exercise.** If patient is older than 35 years of age or shows signs of cardiovascular disease, a stress ECG can be used to evaluate cardiovascular status to prevent silent myocardial infarction.
- **Regular exercise program.** Increasing the uptake of glucose into the cells and decreasing central obesity, hypertension, and dyslipidemia decrease insulin requirements.
- **Water consumption.** Ingesting water before, during, and after exercising prevents dehydration.
- **Abdominal injection site.** Exercising the area of insulin injection increases absorption of insulin from that area.
- **Postexercise hypoglycemia.** Exercise-induced hypoglycemia may be exacerbated in pregnancy. It can be reduced by exercising after a meal or carbohydrate snack.
- **Low blood sugar level.** The patient should be encouraged to carry glucose tablets or a snack designed to treat low blood sugar.
- **Aerobic and resistance exercise.** Aerobic exercise with resistance training for a minimum of 30 minutes most days of the week is the best type of exercise.
- **Exercise.** Exercise must not cause maternal or fetal stress, or uterine contractions. The patient should be taught to palpate the uterus for contractions during exercise and stop if any occur.
- **Protecting the feet.** Wearing properly fitted shoes with silica gel or air midsoles and wearing cotton and polyester socks to prevent blisters and keep the feet dry helps to protect the feet from injury.
- **Diabetic identification bracelet.** Encourage the patient to wear a diabetic identification bracelet.
- **Limited activity.** If hypertension, ketonuria, or vascular disease is present, limit activity to decrease metabolic needs.

Self-Perception Functional Health Pattern

- **GDM.** Assess feelings about diagnosis of GDM.
- **DM.** Assess feelings about managing a pregnancy complicated with DM.
- **Family response.** Assess family and partner responses.

Role Relationship Functional Health Pattern

- **Relationship responsibilities.** Assess how pregnancy and the management of DM will affect relationship responsibilities.
- **Work absences.** Assess ability to interrupt occupation, such as accommodations for job absences.
- **Economic considerations.** Assess economic considerations, such as insurance coverage.

ADA, 2009; Kitzmiller and others, 2008.

Sexuality Functional Health Pattern

- **Assessment.** Assess for sexuality problems.
- **Obstetric history.** Assess for preeclampsia, preterm labor, cesarean birth, congenital anomalies, macrosomia, birth injury, and neonatal metabolic abnormalities.

Coping Functional Health Pattern

- **Life stresses.** Ask patient about perceived life stresses, such as adjusting to GDM; managing DM; and juggling family, job, and financial concerns. Good questions include, "Is there anything in particular that is worrying you about yourself, your significant other, or your baby?" and "How do you feel about being pregnant and having DM?"
- **Patient concerns.** Discuss issues that cause worry, such as the baby's health, need for ongoing insulin, and emotional peer support.
- **Patient support.** Provide emotional support.
- **Physical stresses.** Assess for domestic violence, inflammation, infection, and psychologic stress.
- **Patient understanding.** Assess understanding of the effects of stress on blood glucose levels. Stress increases blood glucose level via contrainsular hormones.
- **Patient fears.** Allay the fear that increased insulin needs equals worsening diabetes and educate that increased insulin needs really means a healthy, growing placenta.
- **Support referrals.** Make needed referrals to diabetes support groups, Sidelines National Network (a high-risk pregnancy support group), and social services (American Diabetes Association). Advise of the importance of carrying a diabetic identification card and wearing a Medic-Alert bracelet or necklace.
- **Resource referrals.** Provide referrals to Lifescan telelibrary for information regarding diabetes (800-847-7226); American Diabetic Association (800-342-2382); and National Institutes of Health (*http://diabetes.niddk.nih.gov*).

Cognitive Functional Health Pattern

- **Visits.** Suggest more frequent prenatal visits.
- **Disease process.** Assess patient and family knowledge of the disease process and treatment, including the relationships among diet, exercise, insulin, illness, and stress. Determine patient and family understanding of the effects of diabetes on pregnancy and the effects of pregnancy on diabetes.
- **Complications.** Prevent complications with tight glycemic control using MNT, insulin administration, exercise plan, SMBG, urine test for ketones, early recognition and treatment for signs of hypoglycemia, and sick-day management.
- **Fetal evaluation.** Evaluate the fetus with periodic ultrasound scans to monitor for gestational age, structural growth, and fetal growth; take maternal-serum alpha fetoprotein (MSAFP) measurements, take daily fetal movement count after 24 weeks of gestation, take fetal echocardiogram between 20 and 23 weeks of gestation to rule out congenital heart disease; make a biophysical profile

with NST and amniotic fluid volume (AFV) for fetal surveillance; and possibly perform amniocentesis to determine fetal lung maturity.

Breastfeeding Effects on Insulin

- Hypoglycemia is common.
- Nocturnal hypoglycemia is particularly common.
- Caloric intake is increased from 500 to 800 kcal.
- Insulin requirements are adjusted on the basis of SMBG.

Self-Monitoring of Blood Glucose

- **Self-monitoring.** Teach importance of self-monitoring. Explain or review the importance of SMBG using a reflectance meter and enzyme strips.
- **Goals.** Fasting, premeal, and bedtime blood glucose goals during pregnancy are 60 to 99 mg/dl. Peak postprandial blood glucose goals are 100 to 129 mg/dl. Mean daily blood glucose goal of less than 110 mg/dl (Kitzmiller and others, 2008).
- **Technique.** Demonstrate proper technique, and observe a return demonstration. The U.S. Food and Drug Administration (2005) general guidelines for proper technique include the following:
  - Wash hands with soap and water and dry completely.
  - Prick the fingertip with a lancet.
  - Hold the end down until a small drop of blood appears.
  - Use a small drop of blood to cover the reaction area of the strip.
  - Follow the manufacturer's instructions for inserting the test trip and using the SMBG meter.
  - Read the record.
  - The device should be calibrated and cleaned as outlined in the manual.

Hypoglycemia Management

- **Significance.** The significance of hypoglycemia on the patient and fetus should be taught.
  - Teach symptoms such as sweating, irritability, tremulousness, headache, fatigue, tachycardia, hunger, bad dreams, and circumoral numbness.
  - Teach rule of 15:15 management: if blood sugar is low, take 15 g of fast sugar (carbohydrate), wait 15 minutes, then check blood sugar. If greater than 60%, eat a meal to stabilize sugar. If less than 60%, repeat the 15:15 rule.
  - The best choices of 15 g of carbohydrate are commercial glucose tablets, or 1 cup skim milk to prevent rebound hyperglycemia (Kitzmiller and others, 2008). One cup of orange juice may be used if the blood glucose is below 50 mg/dl.
  - In the presence of hypoglycemia-induced nausea, 0.15 mg subcutaneous glucagon may elevate the blood sugar sufficiently to allow the patient to eat.
  - Teach a family member or friend how to inject glucagon in case the patient loses consciousness because of hypoglycemia. The usual dose is 1 mg injected subcutaneously. If there are no signs of improvement in 15 to 20 minutes, contact emergency medical services.

Sick-Day Rule

Teaching points

- If she is unable to eat, she should continue to take insulin, check blood sugar levels, and check urine for ketones. Notify the health care provider.
- The stress of illness can cause blood glucose to rise related to counter hormones.
- A plan that outlines when to call a health care provider should be provided.
- The patient should continue to take insulin even when she is unable to eat, because the liver continues to make glucose.
- Blood glucose should be checked.
- A supplemental short-acting insulin plan based on blood glucose levels is normally used during illness.
- The urine is tested for ketones.
- The insulin dose is normally doubled if urine ketones are present.
- An easily digestible liquid diet containing fluids, carbohydrates, and salt is initiated. Carbohydrate food choices are cola, lemon-lime soda, or orange juice. Replace sodium and potassium with foods such as broth, tea, or saltine crackers. Take fluids in small amounts every hour.
- Vomiting episodes must be immediately reported to the health care provider.

Critical Care Intervention for Perinatal Ketoacidosis (DKA)[*]

- **Correct volume depletion.** A dose of 1 L of NS is administered over the first hour. Then 200 to 500 ml/hr is given until 80% fluid deficit is corrected in approximately 24 hours. If hypernatremia develops, 0.45% saline is used to hydrate. Note: NS is the preferred fluid initially because the hypotonic solutions such as Ringer's lactate or 0.45% NS can cause a rapid decline in plasma osmolarity, which may lead to cellular swelling and resultant cerebral edema (Foley, 2004).
- **Reduce blood glucose levels with insulin.** An IV bolus is administered with 0.1 unit of regular insulin per kg. Then a continuous infusion of insulin is started to give 0.1 unit of regular insulin per kg per hour (50 units regular insulin in 500 ml of NS). If serum glucose is not dropping by 20% in 2 hours, the insulin rate should be doubled. The IV insulin should be continued until anion gap is normal (less than 12) and HCO_3^- is 18 to 31 mEq/L. To decrease risk for hyperglycemia, subcutaneous insulin is given before discontinuing IV drip.
- **Blood glucose levels.** Serum blood glucose testing is performed every 1 to 2 hours. The goal is to decrease blood glucose by 50 to 70 mg/dl/hr.
- **Ketones with glucose.** When serum glucose level is 250 mg/dl or less, insulin infusion is decreased by 50% and the IV line is changed to 5% dextrose. To give 5 to 10 g of glucose per hour, piggyback administration at approximately 100 ml/hr is provided. Once serum glucose is less than 150 mg/dl, patient is fed appropriate food.
- **Potassium (K⁺) balance.** After the initial liter of fluid and urine output of at least 30 ml/hr, K⁺ is added to each liter of fluid to prevent hypokalemia with the correction of the metabolic acidosis. When K⁺ level is 4 to 5.5 mEq,

---

[*]Foley 2004; ACOG, 2005; Moore & Catalano, 2009.

10 to 20 mEq/hr is given. If K⁺ is less than 4 mEq, 30 to 40 mEq/hr is given. When K⁺ level is low on admission, K⁺ is immediately added to IV infusion to avoid arrhythmias or cardiac arrest and respiratory muscle weakness.
- **Bicarbonate (HCO).** If arterial pH is less than 7.1, 44 mEq is given every 2 hours until pH is greater than 7.1. If arterial pH is greater than 7.1 mEq, sodium bicarbonate is not given.
- **Monitoring.** Ongoing monitoring is provided every 2 to 4 hours until stable.
  - Arterial blood gases (pH, PO_2, $PaCO_2$, O_2 saturation)
  - Serum electrolytes and anion gap (electrolytes panel). Goal: HCO 18 to 31 mEq/L; Na⁺ above 150 mEq/L; K⁺ 3.5 to 5.5 mEq/L; anion gap less than 12 mEq/L
  - Serum ketones (acetone)
- **General supportive measures:**
  - Establish two IV access lines immediately.
  - Give oxygen by mask at 10 to 12 L/min.
  - Anticipate insertion of an arterial line for arterial blood gases.
  - Perform continuous peripheral pulse oximetry for noninvasive arterial blood oxygen saturation.
  - Insert Foley catheter for strict hourly output.
  - Evaluate kidney function with a serum BUN and creatinine to decrease risk for fluid overload.
  - Use invasive hemodynamic monitoring in the presence of renal compromise.
  - Initiate continuous ECG and monitor for ST segment depression, for inverted T waves, or for the appearance of U waves following the T wave.
  - Continuously monitor fetal heart rate and prepare for delivery if a Category III fetal heart rate tracing persists after initial stabilization.
  - Keep the mother positioned to avoid vena cava syndrome.
- **Treat predisposing factors.** Predisposing factors include noncompliance with insulin administration; dietary indiscretion; UTIs and infections of the skin, lungs, or amniotic fluid; vomiting and dehydration; diabetic gastroparesis; and use of steroids. Urinalysis is performed for culture and sensitivity to rule out URI; CBC with differential, chest radiograph, and amniocentesis may be considered.
- **Evaluation.** The condition is evaluated with ongoing physical assessment.
  - Provide neurologic checks every hour for signs of cerebral edema that include deteriorating mental status, sluggish pupillary light reflex, or headache.
  - Evaluate vital signs.
  - Assess for signs of pulmonary edema, including dyspnea, tachypnea, tachycardia, wheezing, or crackles on auscultation.
  - Assess for hypovolemia, including urine output less than 30 ml/hr, hypotension, or tachycardia.

Intrapartum Nursing Interventions for Diabetes
- **Preterm labor.** Preterm labor is treated with magnesium sulfate or indomethacin because beta-sympathomimetic agents can interfere with glucose control.
- **Corticosteroids.** If corticosteroids are needed to enhance fetal lung maturity, two doses of 12 mg betamethasone are administered intramuscularly

Table 10-11   Use an Infusion Pump and Adjust Rate Based on Blood Glucose Levels

Plasma/Capillary Blood Glucose (mg/dl)	Insulin Dosage (U/hr)
<90	0.0 except for Type 1 DM, then 0.5
90–110	1.0
111–130	2.0
131–150	3.0
151–170	4.0
171–190	5.0

Reference: Moore T, Catalano P: Diabetes in pregnancy. In Creasy R, Resnik R, Iams J, Lockwood C, Moore T, editors: *Creasy & Resnik's maternal-fetal medicine: principles and practice,* ed 6, Philadelphia, 2009, Saunders.

24 hours apart or dexamethasone, 6 mg, is given intramuscularly every 12 hours for four doses. Insulin need will increase and IV insulin may be the route of choice.

- **Goal of insulin management during labor.** Maintain glucose levels between 80 and 110 mg/dl to decrease neonatal hypoglycemia and perinatal asphyxia (Hawkins and Casey, 2007; Moore and Catalano, 2009).
- **Insulin and glucose requirements:**
  - Insulin requirements typically decrease with onset of labor; at onset of active labor, insulin is decreased to zero.
  - Glucose requirements in active labor are 5 to 7 grams per hour.
  - Determine last insulin dose to ascertain insulin peak.
  - Withhold usual morning insulin dosage and breakfast.
  - Give nothing by mouth except ice chips.
  - Obtain baseline blood glucose every 1 to 2 hours.
  - Start continuous IV infusion of D_5LR or D_5 1/2 NS at 100 to 125 ml/hr
  - Set up insulin solution by diluting 25 units of aspart or lispro insulin in 250 ml of NS and flush line with 25 ml to decrease insulin-binding capacity of insulin to plastic surfaces.
  - Piggyback insulin infusion to mainline IV at connection closest to insertion site. Use an infusion pump and adjust rate based on blood glucose levels as outlined in Table 10-11.
  - Adjust the IV rate and supplemental short-acting insulin according to the blood glucose values every 1 to 2 hours.
  - Keep 50% dextrose at the bedside to treat profound hypoglycemia.
  - Usually dextrose intravenous fluids are not needed to maintain glucose control in diet-controlled GDM patients.
- **Intermittent subcutaneous insulin method.** If used instead of the insulin infusion method, perform the following:
  - Be prepared to give one third to one half of the patient's pregnancy insulin dosage in the morning.
  - Start a continuous infusion based on glucose levels.
  - Administer regular insulin in 2 to 5 units per dose to maintain the blood sugar.

- **Continuous fetal monitoring.** Observe continuous fetal monitoring for baseline fetal heart rate, variability, and periodic or episodic patterns that develop in response to labor (Macones and others, 2008).
- **Labor progress:**
  - Evaluate labor progress and ultrasound results for potential problems with dystocia, arrest of descent, or failure to progress (see Chapter 29).
  - Monitor and record vital signs every 15 minutes to every 1 hour; take temperature every 1 to 4 hours.
  - Maintain hourly input-output measurements.
  - Assess urine for ketones at every void or every 4 hours with indwelling catheter.
  - Assess for complications such as hypoglycemia, ketoacidosis, UTI, upper respiratory infection, polyhydramnios, which increases risk for fetal cord prolapse with rupture of membranes, and fetal macrosomia, which increases risk for shoulder dystocia.
- **Cesarean delivery:**
  - Schedule for early morning.
  - Give nothing by mouth and hold morning insulin dose.
  - Monitor blood glucose levels every hour and administer short-acting insulin and glucose based on blood sugar levels.
  - After delivery, administer IV D_5W at a rate of 100 to 125 ml/hr.
  - Check blood glucose every 2 to 4 hours.
  - No insulin may be needed related to the sudden drop of the placental hormone, human placenta lactogen (HPL), after delivery of the placenta.

Postpartum Nursing Interventions for Types 1 and 2 Diabetes

- **Insulin.** Insulin is administered based on blood glucose level. The initial goal is to prevent hypoglycemia and severe hyperglycemia rather than achieve euglycemia (80 to 150 mg/dl). If the fasting or postprandial blood sugar is greater than 150 mg/dl, the dosage of insulin is recalculated at 0.6 U/kg/24 hr based on postpartum weight. When repeated rapid- or short-acting insulin is needed, the routine schedule of insulin or oral agents is resumed. New insulin dose is usually 50% to 60% of end-pregnancy dose. Tighter control is gradually resumed. The final goal is preprandial blood sugar level of 70 to 120 mg/dl.
- **Education:**
  - Teach the importance of ongoing tight glycemic control with MNT, exercise plan, SMBG, glucose-lowering medications, and early detection of diabetic complications.
  - Teach the need for family planning to ensure optimal glycemic control before the start of any subsequent pregnancy. According to the AHRQ (2008b) systematic review, when selecting a contraceptive method for the patient with diabetes, the same criteria are to be used as with any other patient. Low-dose estrogen-progestin oral contraceptives and IUDs are not contraindicated unless other comorbidity factors exist (Dunlop and others, 2008).
- **Breastfeeding.** Breastfeeding should be encouraged. Breastfeeding decreases fasting and postprandial blood glucose levels and increases HDL cholesterol

levels (AHRQ, 2008b). Therefore during breastfeeding, the insulin requirement is usually considerably less, and protein and carbohydrate snacks are necessary. The woman's dietary needs will increase usually 500 to 800 calories. Teach the patient to expect fluctuations in her glucose levels during weaning and to continue close glucose monitoring. Reassure the mother that insulin does not cross into breast milk. However, elevated glucose levels are present in the breast milk if her blood glucose is high. Monitor for mastitis and nipple infections because of the increased risk they present. Sore nipples that do not respond to the usual nonspecific treatment are treated with nystatin ointment to the nipples and nystatin suspension for the infant as well.

Postpartum Nursing Interventions for Gestational Diabetes Mellitus

- **Monitoring.** For the patient with GDM, monitor blood sugar after delivery.
- **Education.** Recurrence risk for GDM in the next pregnancy is 35% to 75% (Bottalico, 2007). The woman with GDM has a 50% to 60% increased risk for developing type 2 DM (Kjos, 2007). The importance of the screening program for early detection of development of diabetes is advised. This includes a 75-g, 2-hour oral glucose tolerance test at the 6-week postpartum checkup and a random or fasting blood glucose annually (Box 10-1). Share the National Diabetes Education Program *Small Steps Big Rewards* resource at *http://www.ndep.nih.gov*.
- **Lifestyle modifications.** There is a relationship between maintaining optimal weight and the decreased risk for later development of type 2 diabetes. If the woman stays lean and fit, her risk decreases to 25%. If the woman is or becomes obese, the risk for diabetes increases to 75% (Kitzmilller and others, 2007). If the woman is obese, especially with increased abdominal fat, a weight loss of 5 to 10 pounds will make a difference in the amount of insulin the pancreas must produce. For example, an active thin person's pancreas may produce only 35 to 40 U/day as compared with a person who is overweight, whose pancreas may be required to produce 150 U/day to clear the same amount of glucose. Encourage the woman to follow a nutritional diet and exercise regularly to decrease risk. A gradual weight loss of 0.5 to 1 pound per week is recommended.
- **Family planning.** Low-dose estrogen-progestin oral contraceptives and IUD may need to be considered. There has been some concern related to the use of progesterone-only contraception. One study indicated a twofold increased risk of developing type 2 diabetes when a progesterone-only oral contraceptive (Minipill) is used following a pregnancy complicated with GDM. However, another study did not find this to be true with the use of depomedroxyprogesterone acetate (AHRQ, 2008b).

CONCLUSION

The ultimate goal of nursing care for a pregnant woman with diabetes is to minimize the effects of risks and complications. This is accomplished by educating the woman and her family to recognize early signs and symptoms of management failures and identify and solve management issues that they are capable of solving.

Box 10-1   Nurse Practitioner Protocol for Postpartum Testing After Gestational Diabetes Mellitus

Glucose Tolerance Test
- Perform a 75-g glucose tolerance test at the first postpartum checkup between 6 and 8 weeks after delivery or shortly after the woman stops breastfeeding.

Test Preparation
- Instruct the patient to eat an additional 150 g of complex carbohydrates (e.g., 10 additional slices of bread each day) for 3 days before the test.
- Instruct the patient to abstain from eating, drinking (except water), and smoking for 8 hours before the test.
- Have the patient rest in the office for 30 minutes just before the test.
- Draw a fasting plasma glucose level.
- Administer 75 g of oral glucose drink.
- Draw plasma glucose at 2 hours.
- Interpret and reclassify gestational diabetes mellitus after pregnancy according to new criteria for the diagnosis of diabetes mellitus (Expert Committee, 2001).

Normal Results
- Medical diagnosis: previous abnormality of glucose tolerance
- Fasting plasma glucose, less than 110 mg/dl
- 2-hour postprandial, less than 140 mg/dl

Impaired Glucose Tolerance Results
- Fasting plasma glucose, 110 to 125 mg/dl
- 2-hour postprandial, 140 to 199 mg/dl

Type 2 Diabetes Mellitus Results
- Fasting plasma glucose, equal to or greater than 126 mg/dl
- 2-hour postprandial, greater than 200 mg/dl
- Random plasma glucose, equal to or greater than 200 mg/dl with symptoms (polyuria, polydipsia, and unexplained weight loss)

Follow-Up
- If results indicate impaired glucose tolerance, the annual well-woman examination should include a fasting blood glucose following a 3-hour fast. If the results of this test are 110 mg/dl or greater, further testing is needed.
- If the glucose levels are normal, glycemia should be reassessed annually.

It is also accomplished by promoting a relationship that encourages mutual work among the patient, her family, and members of the health care team.

The outcome of the pregnancy should be a mother without additional diabetic complications, a healthy newborn, and a family who is ready and able to integrate the new baby into their world. An added side benefit of educating the pregnant woman who is already insulin dependent is that she commonly learns useful skills that aid in her self-management of diabetes for the remainder of her life.

BIBLIOGRAPHY

Agency for Healthcare Research and Quality (AHRQ): *Screening for gestational diabetes mellitus,* Evidence Synthesis No 60, 2008a, AHRQ.

Agency for Healthcare Research and Quality (AHRQ): *Therapeutic management, delivery, and postpartum risk assessment and screening in gestational diabetes,* Evidence Report/Technology Assessment No. 162, 2008b, AHRQ.

American Association of Clinical Endocrinologists (AACE) Diabetes Mellitus Clinical Practice Guideline Task Force: AACE Diabetes mellitus guidelines: screening and diagnosis, *Endocr Pract* 13(Suppl 1):12–22, 2007.

American College of Obstetricians and Gynecologists (ACOG): *Antenatal corticosteroid therapy for fetal maturation,* Committee Opinion No. 402, 2008a, ACOG.

American College of Obstetricians and Gynecologists (ACOG): *Fetal lung maturity,* Practice Bulletin No. 97, 2008b, ACOG.

American College of Obstetricians and Gynecologists (ACOG): *Pregestational diabetes mellitus: clinical management guidelines for obstetricians-gynecologists,* No. 60, 2005, ACOG.

American Diabetes Association (ADA): Position statement: gestational diabetes mellitus, *Diabetes Care* 27(Suppl 1):S88, 2004a.

American Diabetes Association (ADA): Position statement: aspirin therapy in diabetes, *Diabetes Care* 27(Suppl 1):S72–S73, 2004b.

American Diabetes Association (ADA): Position statement: gestational diabetes mellitus, *Diabetes Care* 27(Suppl 1):S88–S90, 2004c.

American Diabetes Association (ADA): Position statement: nutrition recommendations and interventions for diabetes, *Diabetes Care* 30(Suppl 1):S61, 2007.

American Diabetes Association (ADA): Position statement: diagnosis and classification of diabetes mellitus, *Diabetes Care* 31(Suppl 1):S62, 2008.

American Diabetes Association (ADA): Position statement: standards of medical care in diabetes-2009, *Diabetes Care* 32(Suppl 1):S13, 2009.

Barclay L, Murata P: Treating gestational diabetes may reduce childhood obesity, *Diabetes Care* 30:2287–2292, 2007.

Barclay L, Murata P: Breastfeeding may reduce the risk for obesity in children of women with gestational diabetes, *Diabetes Care* 29:1105–1109, 2006.

Beaser R, Joslin Diabetes Center: *Joslin's insulin deskbook: designing and initiating insulin treatment programs,* Boston, 2008, Joslin Diabetes Center.

Bottalico JN: Recurrent gestation diabetes: risk factors, diagnosis, management, and implications, *Semin Perinatol* 31(3):176–184, 2007.

Care Management Institute, Kaiser Permanente: *Adult diabetes clinical practice guidelines,* Oakland, CA, Kaiser Permanente, Care Management Institute, Dec. p. 206, 2005. Retrieved from www.guideline.gov.

Carroll M, Yeomans E: Diabetic Ketoacidosis in pregnancy, *Crit Care Med* 33:S347–S353, 2005.

Center for Disease Control and Prevention (CDC): Guidelines for vaccinating pregnant women, *MMWR* 56(RR6), Retrieved from, 2007 www.cdc.gov/vaccines/pubs/downloads/b_preg_guide.pdf.

Centers for Disease Control and Prevention (CDC): State incidence of diabetes among adults: selected U.S. States, 2005-2007, *MMWR* 57(43):1169–1173, 2008.

Checa M, Requena A, Salvador C, and others: Insulin-sensitizing agents: use in pregnancy and as therapy in polycystic ovary syndrome, *Human Reprod Update* 11:375–390, 2005.

Chernecky C, Berger B: *Laboratory tests and diagnostic procedures,* ed 3, Philadelphia, 2001, Saunders.

Dabelea D: The predisposition of obesity and diabetes in offspring of diabetic mothers, *Diabetes Care* 30(suppl 2):S169, 2007.

Dabelea D, Knowler W, Pettitt D: Effect of diabetes in pregnancy on offspring: follow-up research in Pima Indians, *J Matern Fetal Med* 9(1):83–88, 2000.

Daitchman J, Vermeulen M, Ray J: Acanthosis nigricans among women with gestational diabetes mellitus and risk of adverse pregnancy outcomes, *Diabetes Care* 31(5):e30, 2008.

Diabetes Control and Complications Trial Research Group: The effect of intensive treatment of diabetes on the development and progression of long-term complications in insulin-dependent diabetes mellitus, *N Engl J Med* 329(14):977–986, 1993.

Diabetes Control and Complications Trial Research Group: Effect of pregnancy on microvascular complications in the diabetes control and complications trial, *Diabetes Care* 23(8):1084–1091, 2000.

Diabetes Control and Complications Trial Research Group: Pregnancy outcomes in the Diabetes Control and Complications Trial, *Am J Obstet Gynecol* 174(4):1343–1353, 1996.

Doyle E, and others: A randomized, prospective trial comparing the efficacy of continuous subcutaneous insulin infusion with multiple daily injections using insulin glargine, *Diabetes Care* 27(7):1554–1558, 2004.

Dudley D: Diabetic-associated stillbirth: incidence, pathophysiology, and prevention, *Obstet Gynecol Clin North Am* 34:293–307, 2007.

Dunlop A, Jack B, Bottalico J, Lu M, and others: The clinical content of preconception care: women with chronic medical conditions, *Am J Obstet Gynecol* 199(6):S310–S327, 2008.

Durnwald C, Landon M: Glyburide: a new alternative for treating gestational diabetes? *Am J Obstet Gynecol* 193:1–2, 2005.

European Practice in Gynaecology and Obstetrics (EPGO): *Diabetes and pregnancy*, Amsterdam, 2004, Elsevier.

Expert Committee on the Diagnosis and Classification of Diabetes Mellitus: Report of the Expert Committee on the Diagnosis and Classification of Diabetes Mellitus, *Diabetes Care* 24(Suppl 1):S5, 2001.

Foley M: Diabetic ketoacidosis in pregnancy. In Foley M, Strong T, Garite T, editors: *Obstetric intensive care: a practical manual*, ed 2, New York, 2004, McGraw-Hill.

Hawkins J, Casey B: Labor and delivery management for women with diabetes, *Obstet Gynecol Clin North Am* 34:323–334, 2007.

Hawthorne G: Metformin use and diabetic pregnancy: has its time come? *Diabet Med* 23:223–227, 2006.

Hinton A, Sibai B: Hypertensive disorders in pregnancy. In Reece E, Coustan D, Gabbe S, editors: *Diabetes in women: adolescence, pregnancy, menopause*, ed 3, Philadelphia, 2004, Lippincott Williams & Wilkins.

Jacobson G, Ramos G, Ching J, and others: Comparison of glyburide and insulin for the management of gestational diabetes in a large managed care organization, *Am J Obstet Gynecol* 193:118–124, 2005.

Kahn R, and others: The metabolic syndrome: time for a critical appraisal, *Diabetes Care* 28(9):2289–2304, 2005.

Kendrick J, and others: Reliability of reporting of self-monitoring of blood glucose in pregnant women, *J Obstet Gynecol Neonatal Nurs* 34(3):329–334, 2005.

Kitzmiller J, Dang-Kilduff L, Taslimi M: Gestational diabetes after delivery, *Diabetes Care* 30(Suppl 2): S225, 2007.

Kitzmiller J, and others: Managing preexisting diabetes for pregnancy: summary of evidence and consensus recommendation for care, *Diabetes Care* 31(5):1060–1080, 2008.

Kjos S: After pregnancy complicated by diabetes: postpartum care and education, *Obstet Gynecol Clin North Am* 34:335–349, 2007.

Langer O: Oral anti-hyperglycemic agents for the management of gestational diabetes mellitus, *Obstet Gynecol Clin North Am* 34:255–274, 2007.

Langer L, and others: A comparison of glyburide and insulin in women with gestational diabetes mellitus, *N Engl J Med* 343(16):1134–1138, 2000.

Leguizamon G, Igarzabal M, Reece E: Periconceptional care of women with diabetes mellitus, *Obstet Gynecol Clin North Am* 34:225–239, 2007.

Lord J, Flight I, Norman R: Metformin in polycystic ovary syndrome: systematic review and meta-analysis, *BMJ* 327:951–953, 2003.

Macones G, Hankins G, Spong C, and others: The 2008 National Institute of Child Health and Human Development workshop report on electric fetal monitoring: update on definitions, interpretation, and research guidelines, *J Obstet Gynecol Neonatal Nurs* 37(5):510–515, 2008.

Mensing C: *The art and science of diabetes self-management education: a desk reference for healthcare professionals*, Chicago, 2006, American Association of Diabetes Education.

Moore T, Catalano P: Diabetes in pregnancy. In Creasy R, Resnik R, Iams J, Lockwood C, Moore T, editors: *Creasy and Resnik's maternal-fetal medicine: principles and practice*, ed 6, Philadelphia, 2009, Saunders.

Mulholland E, Njoroge T, Mersereau P, Williams J: Comparison of guidelines available in the United States for diagnosis and management of diabetes before, during, and after pregnancy, *J Womens Health* 16(6):790–801, 2007.

Nathanielsz P, Poston L, Taylor P: In utero exposure to maternal obesity and diabetes: animal models that identify and characterize implications for future health, *Obstet Gynecol Clin North Am* 34: 201–212, 2007.

Prescriber's Letter: *Treatment of diabetes in women who are pregnant* 23(230913), 2007.

Richardson A, Carpenter M: Inflammatory mediators in gestational diabetes mellitus, *Obstet Gynecol Clin North Am* 34:213–224, 2007.

Roberts D, Dalziel S: Antenatal corticosteroids for acceleration fetal lung maturation for women at risk of preterm birth, *Cochrane Database Syst Rev* (Issue 3), 2006.

Singh C, Jovanovic L: Insulin analogues in the treatment of diabetes in pregnancy, *Obstet Gynecol Clin North Am* 34:275–291, 2007.

Takoudes T, and others: Risk of cesarean wound complications in diabetic gestations, *Am J Obstet Gynecol* 191(3):958–963, 2004.

Vintzileos A: antepartum fetal surveillance in pregnancies complicated by diabetes mellitus, *Female Patient* 32(4):50–53, 2007.

U.S. Food and Drug Administration (FDA): Glucose meters and diabetes management, 2005. Retrieved from www.fda.gov/Diabetes/glucose.html#5.

U.S. Department of Health and Human Services (USDHHS): *Lower Extremity Amputation Prevention (LEAP): the five step LEAP Program.* Retrieved from www.hrsa.gov/leap/fivestep.htm.

United States Preventive Services Task Force (USPSTF): *Screening for gestational diabetes mellitus: Recommendation statement,* 2008, AHRQ. Retrieved from www.ahrq.gov/clinic/uspstf08/gestdiab/gdrs.htm.

Walkinshaw S: Type 1 and type 2 diabetes and pregnancy, *Curr Obstet Gynaecol* 14:375, 2004.

Weiner C, Buhimschi C: *Drugs for pregnant and lactating women,* ed 2, Philadelphia, 2009, Saunders.

World Health Organization: *Medical eligibility criteria for contraceptive use,* ed 3, Geneva, 2004, WHO.

Yogev Y, Hod M: Use of new technologies for monitoring and treating diabetes in pregnancy, *Obstet Gynecol Clin North Am* 34:241–253, 2007.

11

Cardiac Disease

Pregnancy complicated with cardiac disease is potentially dangerous to maternal well-being. The understanding of normal and abnormal cardiovascular physiology in pregnancy can help enormously in anticipating problems and preventing complications.

INCIDENCE

The incidence of cardiac disease in the pregnant population complicates less than 1% of all pregnancies (Hameed and Foley, 2004). Rheumatic fever, once responsible for 88% of cardiac disease cases in pregnancy, is now on the decline. Congenital disease now plays a more prominent role. Mitral stenosis is still the most frequently seen cardiac condition in pregnant women (Klein and Galan, 2004; Tan, 2004). However, because of better childhood management of congenital heart disease, pregnancy outcomes are generally positive. Nonetheless, cardiac disease accounts for 15% of maternal mortality during pregnancy (Chang and others, 2003). Cardiac lesions are referred to as congenital or acquired and can be further classified as cyanotic or acyanotic (Hameed and Foley, 2004). Pregnancy is contraindicated in patients with cyanotic heart disease (right to left shunt) because of increased maternal mortality (Hameed and Foley, 2004). Pregnancy is contraindicated in the presence of the following cardiac conditions (Hameed and Foley, 2004; Tan, 2004; Blanchard and Shabetai, 2009) related to the CV danger:
- Severe left ventricular dysfunction
- Complex cyanotic congenital heart disease
- Pulmonary hypertension
- Dilated cardiomyopathy
- Marfan syndrome with aortic involvement
- Eisenmenger's syndrome

ETIOLOGY

Cardiac disease in pregnancy takes a variety of forms and varies in functional severity. Some of the specific forms follow (Hameed and Foley, 2004; Klein and Galan, 2004; Tan, 2004):
- Rheumatic heart disease
- Congenital heart disease

- Congestive cardiomyopathies
- Cardiac dysrhythmias
- Infective endocarditis
- Ischemic heart disease
- Valve deformities

NORMAL PHYSIOLOGY

Antepartum

Cardiac Output

In the antepartum period, *cardiac output* (the amount of blood pumped by the left ventricle into the aorta) rises significantly as early as the first trimester of pregnancy. It continues to rise and reaches a plateau between 28 and 34 weeks of gestation. It rises in response to the plasma volume increase, hormonal influences, and autonomic nervous system (ANS) influences. This increase in cardiac output can cause patients to report signs and symptoms that mimic, to some degree, those of cardiac disease (Klein and Galan, 2004; Tan, 2004), including the following:

- Dyspnea
- Orthopnea
- Dyspnea with exertion
- Edema
- Syncope
- Palpitations

Blood Volume

Blood volume increases by plasma volume expansion and red blood cell multiplication. The systemic vascular resistance decreases by 20% (Hameed and Foley, 2004). The mean plasma volume increase is 50% over the prepregnant volume, and red cell multiplication is in proportion to volume expansion if nutritional requirements are met. In early pregnancy, the increased volume with each heart stroke increases cardiac output. As pregnancy continues, the heart rate increases to offset increased stroke volume. Increased volume maintains a dilated systemic vasculature.

Hormonal Influences

Hormonal influences affect resistance to blood flow and contractility of the myocardium. Increased estrogen leads to systemic vasodilation. Vasodilation increases cardiac output because of lowered peripheral resistance. Prolactin increases myocardial contractility (Blanchard and Shabetai, 2009; Tomlinson, 2005).

Autonomic Nervous System

During pregnancy, ANS influences on blood flow become more prominent. In the nonpregnant state, when the ANS is blocked, there is little effect on blood pressure. However, in pregnancy, when the ANS is activated or blocked, dramatic changes in the maternal blood pressure can result. The cardiovascular system is hyperfilled from increased blood volume and hyperdynamic because of the predominance of the ANS (see Chapter 1).

Venous Pressure

Increased venous pressure, especially in the lower extremities, occurs in pregnancy. This can lead to a normal finding of an accentuated jugular pulse.

Heart

A slightly enlarged heart sometimes occurs in pregnancy because of the upward and leftward anatomic displacement of the heart. Benign dysrhythmias can occur, presumably because of the normal influences on myocardial contractility.

Inferior Vena Cava

When the weight of the gravid uterus lies against the inferior vena cava, partial or total occlusion reduces return volume to the heart and subsequent output.

Intrapartum

Hemodynamic responses to labor are also important; labor can be a critical period in the care of a pregnant woman with cardiac disease. Uterine contractions normally increase cardiac output 20% to 30% and stroke volume because of increased intravascular volume, which leads to an increase in the workload of the heart. During the contraction, an additional 300-500 ml of blood is forced out of the uterus into the maternal circulation (Hameed and Foley, 2004). The workload can be relieved by positioning the patient laterally and by administering pain relief, especially with epidural anesthesia (Hameed and Foley, 2004; Klein and Galan, 2004).

Postpartum

In the immediate postpartum period, there is a high risk for fluid volume overload caused by remobilization of fluid into vascular compartments. It is important to be cautious with administration of intravenous fluids and oxytocin after birth, both of which may further complicate the risk.

Pathophysiology

To understand the pathophysiology of cardiac disease in pregnancy, one must understand what functional lesion is present. It is also necessary to understand various terms describing cardiac function.

Stroke Volume

Stroke volume is the amount of blood ejected with each contraction of the left ventricle. It is affected by four interrelated factors:
- Diastolic filling pressure (preload)
- Distensibility of the ventricle
- Myocardial contractility
- Aortic pressure, which is the amount of pressure the ventricle, must overcome to push blood into the aorta (afterload)

Contractility

There is a direct relationship between diastolic volume and the amount of blood pumped during systole. The greater the diastolic filling pressure, the more the fibers of the left ventricle stretch during diastole and the harder they contract during systole, increasing stroke volume and cardiac output. However, if the muscle fibers are stretched beyond a certain point, there is a loss of distensibility. This loss decreases the force of contractions and therefore decreases cardiac output.

Preload

Preload is the force responsible for stretching the ventricular muscles. It is also called *diastolic filling pressure*. If the preload is low, the ventricular muscle will not stretch enough for effective contractility. This leads to decreased stroke volume. If preload is too high, the muscle fibers will be overstretched. This also results in decreased contractility, leading in turn to decreased stroke volume.

Afterload

Afterload is the amount of pressure resistance in the aorta to the emptying of the left ventricle. It is the volume in the ventricles at the end of diastole and is also called *systemic vascular resistance*. Systemic vascular resistance (or afterload) is measured by taking blood pressure readings. The higher the afterload, the greater the force required by the left ventricle to overcome aortic pressure with systolic pressure to force the aortic valve to open. A high afterload decreases stroke volume and cardiac output if the pressure cannot be effectively overcome. Right heart failure may result from persisting high afterload.

Signs and Symptoms

With cardiac disease in pregnancy, the actual lesion is responsible for the specific symptoms. Basically, cardiac disease causes problems with preload or afterload. The usual signs that the cardiac condition is deteriorating in a patient with preexisting cardiac disease are as follows:

- Dyspnea severe enough to limit usual activity
- Progressive orthopnea
- Paroxysmal nocturnal dyspnea
- Syncope during or immediately following exertion
- Chest pain associated with activity

In addition, a pregnancy with preexisting cardiac disease can increase predisposition to thromboembolic changes, palpitations, and fluid retention. These complications sometimes require prophylactic treatment or increases in dosage of current drug therapy. Other conditions of the cardiovascular system, such as chronic hypertension, can also rapidly deteriorate. Patients with chronic hypertension may develop cardiac functional compromise during pregnancy because of the increased volume expansion (see Chapter 22).

Symptoms of cardiac disease in general are classified by the functional incapacity. The classification does not change in pregnancy, although symptoms may worsen. The New York Heart Association classifications of cardiac disease (Klein and Galan, 2004) follow:

- *Class I*: asymptomatic at all degrees of activity; uncompromised
- *Class II*: symptomatic with increased activity; slightly compromised
- *Class III*: symptomatic with ordinary activity; markedly compromised
- *Class IV*: symptomatic at rest; incapacitated

These are prognostic indicators of maternal and fetal complications (Hameed and Foley, 2004; Klein and Galan, 2004; Blanchard and Shabetai, 2009). Box 11-1 outlines the three maternal risk subgroups.

Box 11-1   Maternal Risk Subgroups

Group 1: Mortality Less than 1%
- Atrial or ventricular septal defect
- Bioprosthetic Valve
- Pulmonic/Tricuspid valve disease
- Patent ductus arteriosus
- Mitral valve prolapse with regurgitation
- Tetralogy of Fallot (corrected with good repair)
- Mitral stenosis or aortic regurgitation NYHA class I and II

Group 2: Mortality 5% to 20%
- Mitral stenosis NYHA class III and IV or with atrial fibrillation
- Aortic stenosis
- Coarctation of aorta without valve involvement
- Uncorrected tetralogy of Fallot
- Previous myocardial infarction
- Marfan syndrome with normal aorta
- Artificial heart valve

Group 3: Mortality Approximately 50%
- Pulmonary hypertension
- Endocarditis
- Marfan syndrome with aortic involvement
- Eisenmenger's syndrome
- Coarctation of aorta with valvular involvement
- Peripartum cardiomyopathy with persistent left ventricular dysfunction

NYHA, New York Heart Association.

MATERNAL EFFECTS

Sudden, severe pulmonary edema occurs if afterload is high. If pulmonary hypertension is present in cardiac lesions such as mitral stenosis or tetralogy of Fallot, right cardiac failure occurs with a resultant increase in preload and decreased stroke volume.

Quite independent of hemodynamic changes, systemic emboli can occur. Patients with atrial fibrillation or mitral valve problems causing atrial fibrillation are particularly susceptible to embolic episodes if not treated adequately with anticoagulants.

Cyanotic heart disease generally does not decrease the pregnant woman's ability to oxygenate her blood unless there is pulmonary hypertension. In atrial or ventricular septal defects, pulmonary hypertension may progress and reverse existing shunts. The rate of maternal mortality is 50% if this occurs (Klein and Galan, 2004).

A dissecting aneurysm, either with coarctation of the aorta or in Marfan syndrome, is associated with a 50% maternal mortality. A dissecting aneurysm can develop suddenly as the pregnancy advances and fluid volume increases.

Pregnant patients with a mechanical heart valve need close monitoring related to the risk for thrombosis, despite anticoagulation (Chan, Anand, and Ginsberg, 2000;

Ginsberg and others, 2003; Nassar and others, 2004). Warfarin is most effective in preventing valve thrombosis; however, it is teratogenic especially between 6 and 12 weeks of gestation, may cause CNS defects during the second and third trimester related to subtle bleeding episodes, and can cause cerebral hemorrhage if given too close to delivery. Unfractionated heparin (UH) or low-molecular-weight heparin (LMWH) does not cross the placenta and is very safe for the fetus but not as effective in preventing valve thrombosis. Therefore the safest medication for the fetus is not the best for the pregnant woman. Thus the treatment plan should always be decided in collaboration with the pregnant woman (Emery, 2004; Klein and Galan, 2004; Tan, 2004).

FETAL AND NEONATAL EFFECTS

Fetal effects are the result of decreased systemic circulation or decreased oxygenation. If maternal circulation is compromised because of cardiac functional incapacities, uterine blood flow may be reduced severely. In early pregnancy, this can result in spontaneous abortion. If the uterine blood flow reduction occurs with advancing pregnancy, the fetus can experience effects of deprivation ranging from growth retardation to central nervous system hypoxia. Preterm delivery may be necessary if maternal life is threatened, and the resultant neonatal morbidity associated with prematurity is high.

If maternal oxygenation is impaired, as in cyanotic heart disease or acute pulmonary edema, fetal oxygenation is also impaired. Depending on the severity and length of time of decreased oxygenation, fetal central nervous system hypoxia can result in degrees of mental retardation, fetal distress, or even fetal death (Klein and Galan, 2004).

If either parent has a congenital cardiac defect, the fetus has an increased risk of 3.4% to 14.3% for having a congenital cardiac defect (Hameed and Foley, 2004). This could be devastating to the neonate already compromised by hypoxia or prematurity.

DIAGNOSTIC TESTING

Diagnosis of cardiac disease is made by the presentation of symptoms. If type of cardiac disease is unknown, the definition of the cardiac lesion is usually made by a cardiologist. An electrocardiogram (ECG), an echocardiogram, a series of laboratory tests including cardiac enzymes and electrolytes, and a chest radiograph are the usual means, during pregnancy, to define the lesion or assess current status. When the pregnant woman is given anticoagulant therapy, coagulation studies are done. If the woman is taking digitalis, therapeutic blood levels are measured.

USUAL MEDICAL MANAGEMENT AND PROTOCOLS FOR NURSE PRACTITIONERS

General Management

Usual medical management is accomplished with a team approach. The obstetrician, maternal fetal medicine specialist, anesthesiologist, intensive care specialist, and cardiologist work as a team involving the pregnant cardiac patient in the management of her prenatal care (Hameed and Foley, 2004). Cardiac medications are usually adjusted to be compatible with pregnancy, and dosages are adjusted when symptoms first present or worsen.

Early ultrasound of the fetus helps in accurate dating. Later, near 28 weeks of gestation, ultrasound can be used serially to document continued fetal growth and well-being. Fetal heart rate monitoring or biophysical profiles (BPPs) may be started by 24 weeks of gestation.

Bedrest, or at least restricted activity, is necessary throughout the last trimester for women with class III heart disease. If symptoms present in women with class I or II heart disease, limitations may be necessary for maternal comfort and well-being and also for adequate fetal oxygenation. The time of presentation of symptoms of cardiac decompensation is usually when maternal fluid volume expansion is greatest. This occurs during the pregnancy near 28 weeks of gestation or in the postpartum period as the then unneeded volume is remobilized.

When cardiac disease is caused by rheumatic fever, the patient has a prosthetic valve, or a history of previous endocarditis, prophylactic antibiotic therapy should be instituted during labor and continued into the postpartum period. Ampicillin, gentamicin, and amoxicillin are the antibiotics usually used (Hameed and Foley, 2004).

Throughout pregnancy and labor, care is aimed at reducing cardiac workload, especially the effects of tachycardia. During labor, pain relief is provided by regional anesthesia. Assistance with the delivery through the use of forceps in the second stage is often necessary. Vaginal delivery is preferred, if possible, because there are fewer hemodynamic disturbances. Sometime after 36 weeks of gestation a plan for labor induction is made after amniocentesis shows lung maturity.

In addition to other monitoring, an invasive line for hemodynamic monitoring of the mother is necessary during labor and during the unstable postpartum period. Central venous pressure and pulmonary wedge pressure readings aid in management of preload and afterload pressures. Careful titration of fluid volume can aid in preventing pulmonary edema and cardiac overload. Oxygen at 5 to 6 L/min may be needed if cyanotic cardiac disease is present. When decompensation of the cardiac disease occurs, placing the mother's life in jeopardy, termination of the pregnancy might be necessary. This procedure can occur before fetal viability or can result in extreme prematurity of the neonate. Consideration is first given to the safety of the mother.

Issues in the intrapartum period include advance planning of the route of delivery, thromboprophylaxis, hemodynamic monitoring, analgesia-anesthesia options, and antibiotic prophylaxis. Those issues are best addressed with the team, including representatives from maternal fetal medicine, neonatology, cardiology, and anesthesiology (Hameed and Foley, 2004; Tan, 2004).

Drug Therapy

The drug therapy chosen depends on the cardiac lesion. Consideration should be given to maternal benefits and fetal risks. Common anticoagulant drugs used in cardiac disease and pregnancy are low-molecular-weight heparin (LMWH) and unfractionated heparin (UFH). For some, warfarin sodium (Coumadin), low-dose aspirin, furosemide (Lasix), digitalis, beta-blockers such as propranolol (Inderal), antidysrhythmics such as quinidine, or disopyramide phosphate (Norpace) may be used. Drugs from newer classifications maybe continued from the prepregnant state if it is difficult to stabilize the mother when she is taking the drugs just mentioned.

Heparin

Heparin is the most common anticoagulant recommended during pregnancy. It does not cross the placenta and has no teratogenic risk associated with its use. Warfarin crosses the placenta and may have teratogenic effects. Therefore its use is not recommended during pregnancy except for one exception. In pregnant patients with a mechanical heart valve, warfarin may be considered because of the increased risk of venous thromboembolism with the use of heparin. According to the American College of Chest Physicians' evidence-based clinical practice guidelines (Bates and others, 2008), warfarin may be considered after the thirteenth week of gestation until close to delivery, if the risk assessments indicate a high risk of VTE.

Two types of heparin are used: low-molecular-weight heparin (LMWH) and unfractionated heparin (UFH). According to the American College of Obstetricians and Gynecologists (ACOG) and the American College of Chest Physicians (Bates and others, 2008), low-molecular-weight heparin and unfractionated heparin are safe for both mother and fetus and can be used for prophylactic or therapeutic anticoagulation in pregnancy. Because of the longer half-life and increased bioavailability of LMWH, it is a more efficient anticoagulant except for acute management of pulmonary embolism and in women with mechanical heart valves. It also has fewer side effects and a more favorable dosing schedule (daily versus twice daily). LMWH requires less monitoring, and control can be achieved rather quickly as an outpatient in comparison with unfractionated heparin. However, LMWH costs more, and because its half-life is longer than UFH, it must be stopped more than 24 hours before delivery and intravenous heparin instituted to lessen the risk for hemorrhage, hematoma, or wound dehiscence at the time of delivery (Marik and Plantz, 2008). See Chapter 14 for more complete information on the use of anticoagulants in pregnancy.

Furosemide

Furosemide (Lasix) is a commonly used diuretic in pregnancy. Dosage can vary from 40 to 80 mg one or two times daily subcutaneously. Intravenous dosage is usually ordered by the single dose and is also 40 to 80 mg, depending on the severity of fluid overload. Thiazides are rarely used because severe potassium deficiency can result. Diuretics reduce amniotic fluid volume and cross the placenta to the fetus.

Digitalis

Digitalis is a glycoside commonly used in cardiac disease because it increases contractility and decreases heart rate. Although it does cross the placental barrier, it does not affect fetal cardiac function. However, this crossing can decrease maternal concentrations and require the dosage to be adjusted.

Tocolytics

The drug terbutaline is contraindicated for treatment of preterm labor in women with cardiac disease. Beta-sympathomimetics increase cardiac rate and workload, as well as the potential for pulmonary edema. Magnesium sulfate decreases calcium levels and has a direct effect on myocardial contractility. If magnesium sulfate is used to treat preterm labor, magnesium and calcium levels must be monitored frequently because magnesium may upset the delicate balance of cardiac electrolytes, cause vasodilation, and lead to decreased blood pressure and thus decreased cardiac output.

Beta-Blockers

Propranolol, labetalol, and other beta-blockers may be used to treat hypertension because they have a decreased pulsating effect on the aorta, or they may be used as antidysrhythmics. Beta-blockers can increase uterine tone and lead to preterm labor. They may also decrease cardiac output and therefore reduce uterine blood flow. Other antidysrhythmics used during pregnancy include quinidine and disopyramide phosphate. Most antidysrhythmics have not been well studied for their fetal effects. However, quinidine, verapamil, and beta-blockers have been used without evidence of teratogenic effects (Lopez-Sendon and others, 2004).

Quinidine

Quinidine is used as an antidysrhythmic because it depresses myocardial excitability, conductive velocity, and contractility. It has never been studied in animals for effects on the fetus. Therefore as with most antidysrhythmics, it is given when the benefits outweigh the risks. Because quinidine has been used for many years, there is clinical experience with it in pregnancy.

Disopyramide Phosphate

Disopyramide phosphate is an antidysrhythmic drug with effects similar to those of quinidine. However, it is chemically unrelated to any other antidysrhythmics. It decreases the sinus node recovery period and lengthens the response time in the atrium. It has no effect on alpha- or beta-adrenergic receptors, but it has been reported to cause increased uterine contractility. Its use in pregnancy has been studied in animals, and no fetal anomalies have been found.

NURSING MANAGEMENT

Tertiary Prevention

Nursing measures must be directed toward prevention of complications. Nutrition must be adequate in iron and folic acid to prevent anemia, which would increase cardiac workload. Sodium restriction may be necessary, but intake should not fall below 2.5 g/day during pregnancy. Increased dietary fiber can decrease the risk for constipation and thereby reduce heart workload. If the patient is taking a diuretic, she should be instructed in the dietary restriction of sodium and the increase of dietary sources of potassium to decrease the risk for potassium deficiency. This is particularly important when digitalis and diuretics are used together as part of the pharmacologic regimen.

A referral should be made to a registered dietitian for management of the dietary modifications with complex pharmacologic treatment. It is difficult to totally replace lost potassium dietarily or to take in high-fiber foods when bedrest complicates the management. Foods high in potassium (such as bananas, whole grains, and citrus fruits) should be included, but they may not provide the total therapeutic replacement. Supplementary iron and foods high in iron may be restrictively expensive for some patients, necessitating referral to the governmental supplementation program WIC (Women, Infants, and Children).

It is important to differentiate symptoms associated with blood volume increases in normal pregnancies from early signs of volume overload in the pregnant cardiac patient. The patient should be instructed to report any signs of infection and the potential need for antibiotics to prevent bacterial endocarditis. This is particularly important for patients with valve replacements.

Plans should be made early in the pregnancy for restriction of activities and possible prolonged bedrest. Relief from emotional stress can be facilitated if family care can be prearranged. During the pregnancy, attention must be directed at reducing and eliminating anxiety. The patient's anxieties regarding her own well-being, fetal well-being, and her family's care in her absence are likely to increase cardiac workload. Sedation provides only a partial solution. Realistic information about risks and benefits for mother and fetus facilitate adequate coping and reduce anxiety over uncertainties.

When pregnancy termination must occur for the mother's safety and well-being, consideration of potential future pregnancy is very important. Contraceptive means may be limited. Permanent surgical intervention is often not a safe procedure for a woman with class III or IV cardiac disease. Birth control pills also are often contraindicated because they have thromboembolic potential. For the sexually active couple, consistent use of a diaphragm, condoms, or foam might be a problem. Careful counseling in the area of contraception must include a realistic examination of the hazards of subsequent pregnancy to the health of the woman. Her sexual partner should be included in the counseling.

Nursing Interventions for Prevention of Cardiac Decompensation

- When taking the initial history, determine which drugs the patient is taking. (The nurse should be aware of specific drugs commonly used in cardiac disease that are contraindicated in pregnancy and note the dosage, which may need to be changed. Women are usually very aware of potential fetal harm from any drug therapy and often have numerous questions that the nurse should be prepared to answer.)
- At each prenatal visit, assess blood pressure, apical/radial pulses, lung sounds, weight gain, edema, Homans' sign, and chest pain.
- Diagnose and treat such contributing factors of cardiac decompensation as dysrhythmias, hypertension, anemia, or infection.
- Determine the patient's and her family's understanding of the effects of her heart disease on pregnancy and the effects of pregnancy on her heart disease.
- Assess for factors that increase stress.
- Report any signs of arrhythmia such as palpitations, irregular heart rate, apical and radial differences, and progressive edema.

- Report any signs of pulmonary edema such as crackles, abnormal heart sounds, a cough, and dyspnea.
- Report signs of thromboembolism such as pain, redness, tenderness, or swelling in the extremities or chest pain.
- Emphasize the importance of more frequent prenatal visits. During the first half of pregnancy, the patient is usually seen every 2 weeks. During the last half of pregnancy, she is usually seen weekly.
- Emphasize the importance of monitoring and immediate reporting of any signs of cardiac decompensation or congestive heart failure. Such signs are generalized edema, distention of neck veins, dyspnea, pulmonary crackles, frequent moist cough, or heart palpitations.
- Instruct the patient about the importance of daily weighing. A sudden weight gain indicates fluid retention.
- Provide the patient with information on the importance of avoiding constipation and straining during a bowel movement.
- Teach the importance of limiting activity (depending on the classification of heart disease). Patients with class I or II cardiac disease need 10 hours of sleep every night and 30 minutes of rest after meals in a semi-Fowler position. Patients with class III or IV cardiac disease usually need bedrest for most of each day.
- Refer to home health care or nurse specialists as indicated.
- Refer to a high risk pregnancy support group.

Nursing Interventions for Early Detection of Preterm Labor

- Assess the home situation for adequate help and support for modified bedrest.
- Evaluate for signs and symptoms of preterm labor through questioning on a routine basis.
- Educate the patient regarding recognition of signs and symptoms of preterm labor because most of the cardiac medications used in pregnancy are reported to increase uterine contractility.
- Teach the benefits of bedrest in reducing uterine irritability and improving uterine blood flow.
- Provide instructions as to what a contraction feels like, warning signs of preterm labor, and the importance of immediately reporting any of these signs.
- Assess the patient's risk for fear.

Nursing Interventions for Anticipatory Grieving

- Discuss loss- and grief-related issues in the antepartum period as appropriate.
- Include family members in the decisions made for medical management.
- Provide support and follow-up as indicated in Chapter 7.
- Take family and mother, if able, for a tour of the level III nursery.
- Discuss the couple's desires in the birth plan and explain any alterations such as epidural, episiotomy, and outlet forceps to decrease the workload on the heart.

Critical Care Nursing Interventions

- Potential complications that require critical care nursing interventions are dysrhythmias, congestive heart failure, thromboembolism, pulmonary edema, electrolyte and fluid imbalance, hypertension, disseminated intravascular coagulation, and superimposed pregnancy complications. These problems are related to increased circulating volume, increased workload during labor, and postpartum remobilization of fluid superimposed on an already compromised cardiac state (Hameed and Foley, 2004; Anthony, 2005; Tomlinson, 2005; Blanchard and Shabetai, 2009).

- The complications are minimized or managed as indicated by a normal sinus rhythm without S_3 or S_4 heart sounds; no signs of congestive heart failure; normal pulmonary artery pressure, pulmonary arterial wedge pressure, and central venous pressure; absence of chest pain, frothy or bloody sputum, and pain or redness in lower extremity vascular beds; clear lung fields; and normal fluid balance and serum electrolytes.
- Continuous ECG monitoring of the mother is essential during any evaluation phase and during labor.
- Monitor vital signs every 15 minutes to 1 hour as indicated by the stability of the mother's condition.
- During labor, assess maternal temperature every 2 to 4 hours.
- Auscultate lung fields every 1 to 4 hours as indicated by the severity and stability of her condition. Report any signs of lung fluid immediately.
- Continuously monitor the FHR, after 24 weeks of gestation, during an acute phase of evaluation. In addition, monitor FHR during labor.
- Weigh the patient daily and assess her for peripheral edema.
- Assess the patient for fear and anxiety.
- At the first signs of fluid overload, be prepared to insert invasive monitoring lines to evaluate the degree of fluid overload and determine treatment.
- During insertion of monitoring lines, observe for dysrhythmias (especially premature ventricular contractions), for wave form changes indicating specific passage through the right atrium (low amplitude waves), for right ventricular wall (tall amplitude) waves, and for pulmonary wedge (smaller, lower pressures with diastolic and systolic) waves. Report abnormalities immediately to the provider (usually anesthesiologist) inserting the catheter.
- Following catheter insertion, continuous ECG monitoring for the cardiac rate is usual.
- Report S_3 and S_4 heart sounds, increased central venous pressure, pulmonary artery pressure, and pulmonary arterial wedge pressure or dysrhythmias, especially premature ventricular contractions. Evaluate every 15 minutes in the initial acute phase, then every 1 to 4 hours as appropriate to measure the degree of stabilization. (Table 11-1 outlines normal readings for each and the significance of low or high readings.)
- Inspect the site of arterial catheter insertion at least once each shift for signs of infection such as redness or drainage.
- Insert a Foley catheter and monitor intake and output hourly. (Urinary output of at least 30 ml/hour is a sensitive measure of adequacy of circulating volume to other vital areas of the body.)
- Administer cardiac glycosides, diuretics, vasodilators, anticoagulants, and antibiotics as ordered.

Table 11-1   Hemodynamic Pressure Readings

	Normal Pregnancy (mm Hg)	Low	High
CVP (measures right ventricular end-diastolic pressure when tricuspid valve is open and therefore right atrium and ventricle are common chambers)	1-10	Reflects inadequate circulatory volume from: Hemorrhage Third spacing Extreme vasodilation	Reflects: Increased preload High pulmonary resistance Poor cardiac contractility
Systolic PAP (reflects pressure in pulmonary artery when right ventricle is contracting and pulmonary valve is open)	15-22	Reflects a decreased venous return to heart from: Hemorrhage Third spacing Extreme vasodilation	Reflects: Increased blood volume Pulmonary arteriole constriction in response to increased P_{CO_2} and decreased P_{O_2} Increased blood pressure with pulmonary disease such as embolus or edema
Diastolic PAP (reflects left heart when pulmonary valve is closed and left valves are open)	8-10		
PAWP (reflects only pressure from left side of heart)	3-10	Results from: A low circulating volume Extreme vasodilation	Reflects: Increased preload Poor contractility Increased afterload Increased P_{CO_2}

CVP, central venous pressure; *PAP*, pulmonary artery pressure; *PAWP*, pulmonary arterial wedge pressure.

- Administer oxygen as ordered.
- Administer salt-poor intravenous fluids as ordered for maternal hydration to run only at a specifically ordered rate via infusion pump.
- Prepare for delivery. If vaginal birth is to be attempted, prepare for epidural anesthesia and shorten second-stage labor with forceps. If cesarean birth is planned, prepare for epidural anesthesia.
- Notify the level III nursery.

Postpartum Nursing Interventions

- Continue postpartum hemodynamic monitoring for a minimum of 24 to 72 hours.
- Assess blood pressure and apical and radial pulses after central invasive monitoring is discontinued.
- Auscultate lung fields every 1 to 4 hours as indicated by status of recovery and stabilization. The first several hours are critical as fluid shifts during remobilization of the increased pregnancy volume.
- Assess for presence of chest pain, shortness of breath, general anxiety, and edema.
- Provide adequate pain relief to prevent increased cardiac workload.
- Reevaluate feeding method for infant, especially if breastfeeding was strongly desired and fatigue during recovery phase and after discharge may become a risk to the mother.
- Provide photographs of delivered infant to mother; encourage early family contact.
- Refer to nursing specialists for critical care assistance.
- Refer to social service representative or chaplain for psychosocial or spiritual assistance.
- Encourage family participation in newborn visits and care.
- Facilitate and encourage exploration of feelings regarding maternal and newborn outcomes.
- Refer to intensive care nursery parent support group.
- Refer to social services for assistance with home care.
- Refer to and assist with follow-up with physician specialists.
- Provide education for medication and medical follow-up.
- Provide counseling to the woman and her partner about contraception because choices may be limited and risks and hazards of more common methods may need to be explored. Oral contraceptives are contraindicated if she is on anticoagulation because of thromboembolic potential (Auerbach and Lockwood, 2004). If the sexual partnership is not stable, an IUD may not be a good choice because of the risk for infection, sepsis, and bacterial endocarditis if the mother has a prosthetic valve (Hameed and Foley, 2004; Blanchard and Shabetai, 2009).

CONCLUSION

The primary goal of nursing care for the pregnant woman and her family when cardiac disease complicates the pregnancy is to reduce potential risks for complications. This is accomplished by education of the woman and her partner; routine assessment of all systems involved; referral to appropriate nursing, nutritional, social, and medical experts; and facilitation of patient participation in decisions. Identification of fears and solutions helps the family to maintain desired control of care. Anticipatory guidance assists in preliminary planning for potential problems and their solutions. The nurse is often in the best position to advocate for the family and coordinate the multidisciplinary team.

BIBLIOGRAPHY

Anthony J: Critical care of the obstetric patient. In James D, and others, editors: *High risk pregnancy: management options*, ed 3, Philadelphia, 2005, Saunders.

Auerbach R, Lockwood C: The diagnosis and treatment of thromboembolic disease in pregnancy. In Foley M, Strong T, Garite T, editors: *Obstetric intensive care*, ed 2, New York, 2004, McGraw-Hill.

Bates S, Greer I, Pabinger I, Sofaer S, Hirsh J, American College of Chest Physicians: Venous thromboembolism, thrombophilia, antithrombotic therapy, and pregnancy: American College of Chest Physicians evidence-based clinical practice, *Chest* 133(6 Suppl):844S-886S, 2008.

Blanchard D, Shabetai R: Cardiac diseases. In Creasy R, Resnik R, Iams J, Lockwood C, Moore T, editors: *Creasy and Resnik's maternal-fetal medicine: principles and practice*, ed 6, Philadelphia, 2009, Saunders.

Chan W, Anand S, Ginsberg J: Anticoagulation of pregnant women with mechanical heart valves: a systematic review of the literature, *Arch Intern Med* 160(2):191–196, 2000.

Chang J, and others: Pregnancy-related mortality surveillance-United States 1990-1999, *MMWR Morb Mortal Wkly Rep* 52(SS02):1, 2003.

Emery S: Anticoagulation in pregnancy: Q&A on low molecular weight heparin, *OBG Management Online*, 2004. Retrieved from http://www.obgmanagement.com/PastIssues.asp

Ginsberg J, and others: Anticoagulation of pregnant women with mechanical heart valves, *Arch Intern Med* 163(6):694–698, 2003.

Hameed A, Foley M: Cardiac disease in pregnancy. In Foley M, Strong T, Garite T, editors: *Obstetric intensive care manual*, ed 2, New York, 2004, McGraw-Hill.

Klein L, Galan H: Cardiac disease in pregnancy, *Obstet Gynecol Clin North Am* 31:429, 2004.

Lopez-Sendon J, Swedberg K, McMurray J, and others: Expert consensus document on beta-adrenergic receptor blockers, *Eur Heart J* 25(15):1341–1362, 2004. Retrieved from http://www.guideline.gov.

Marik P, Plante L: Venous thromboembolic disease and pregnancy, *N Engl J Med* 359(19):2015–2033, 2008.

Nassar A, and others: Pregnancy outcome in women with prosthetic heart valves, *Am J Obstet Gynecol* 191(3):1009–1013, 2004.

Tan J: Cardiovascular disease in pregnancy, *Curr Obstet Gynaecol* 14(3):155, 2004.

Tomlinson M: Cardiac disease. In James D, and others, editor: *High risk pregnancy: management options*, ed 3, Philadelphia, 2005, Saunders.

12

Renal Disease

O f the various physiologic alterations in pregnancy, those affecting the kidney and urinary tract are the most striking. Improvements in our knowledge related to pregnancy care have meant better care for pregnant women with renal disease. This chapter focuses on urinary tract infection (UTI) and kidney infections, urethral and renal calculi, chronic kidney disease (CKD), and acute renal failure (ARF) in pregnancy.

Chronic kidney disease precedes pregnancy and is classed by stages. Stages 1 and 2 indicate mild renal impairment, stage 3 moderate, stage 4 severe, and stage 5 indicates kidney failure. As a rule ARF is divided into three categories: prerenal, intrinsic renal, or postrenal, based on the precipitating insult.

INCIDENCE

Infection

Symptomatic bacteriuria occurs in 1% to 1.5% of pregnancies. Asymptomatic bacteriuria complicates another 2% to 10% of all pregnancies (Williams and Davison, 2009). If the asymptomatic bacteriuria is left untreated, 40% of these women will develop symptoms of UTI. Approximately 30% to 40% of women with untreated asymptomatic bladder infections will develop pyelonephritis during pregnancy (Finnish Medical Society Duodecim, 2007; Williams and Davison, 2009).

Urethral and Renal Calculi

Calculi rarely occur in pregnancy (0.03% to 0.35% prevalence) (Williams and Davison, 2009). Urethral stones occur twice as often as renal stones.

Acute Renal Failure

Acute renal failure rarely occurs during pregnancy (1 per 10,000 pregnancies) (Asrat and Nageotte, 2004).

Chronic Kidney Disease

CKD occurs in approximately 6 to 12 cases per 10,000 pregnancies (Dunlop and others, 2008).

ETIOLOGY

Infection

The cause of bacteriuria is often bacteria from the gastrointestinal tract contaminating the perineal area. Often, the organism implicated is *Escherichia coli*. It is common when contaminants from the rectal area are brought forward across the urethral meatus during perineal hygiene. It can also occur from trauma to the meatus during sexual intercourse, forcing perineal contaminants into the urethra. Bacteria may migrate from the urethra into the bladder and proliferate before the next urination. Bacteria may also pass into the dilated ureters during pregnancy and migrate into the kidney itself, causing inflammation of the tubules. Occasionally, other perineal organisms, such as yeast, are introduced into the bladder and cause infection.

Urethral and Renal Calculi

Calculi may form because of pregnancy induced urinary status, related to decreased peristalsis of the ureters, mechanical obstruction related to increased intraureteral pressure especially on the right side, or smooth muscle relaxation of the ureters related to placental hormones. There is also increased calcium excretion in the urine and urinary excretion rate of calcium stone inhibitors (citrate and magnesium) is increased in pregnancy.

Acute Renal Failure

ARF results from a precipitating insult. The precipitating insult of *prerenal failure* is usually severe hypovolemia and decreased perfusion to the kidneys as the result of severe hemorrhage, dehydration, or septic shock. *Intrinsic renal failure,* in the form of acute tubular necrosis, is usually secondary to a severe pregnancy complication that progresses to hemodynamic instability or severe disseminated intravascular coagulation. Such severe pregnancy complications are preeclampsia/HELLP, acute fatty liver of pregnancy, amniotic fluid embolism, pyelonephritis, and prolonged intrauterine fetal demise. *Postrenal failure* is usually secondary to a renal tract obstruction (Asrat and Nageotte, 2004). ARF causes the retention of nitrogenous waste products such as blood urea nitrogen and creatinine and the inability to maintain normal fluid and electrolyte balance.

Chronic Kidney Disease

Chronic kidney disease precedes pregnancy and may result from any of the causes of renal disease in premenopausal women such as glomerulonephritis, systemic lupus erythematosus (SLE), polycystic kidney disease, and diabetes.

NORMAL PHYSIOLOGY

The kidneys fulfill several functions essential for the body. They excrete water, electrolytes, and nitrogenous waste products. They perform a major function in acid-base balance and are active in the renin-angiotensin-aldosterone system. The kidney also produces erythropoietin, which aids in stimulating red blood cell production.

The kidneys have the largest blood supply of any organ in the body. Renal blood flow accounts for 20% to 25% of the cardiac output. The blood to each kidney is supplied by a renal artery, which branches finally into the afferent arteriole, leading into the glomerulus. From the glomerulus, the efferent arteriole leads out via branches into the renal vein.

Filtration of the blood through the glomerulus is the result of four forces acting on the capillaries: the permeability of the capillary walls, the hydrostatic pressure in the glomerular capillaries, the hydrostatic pressure in the glomerular capsule, and the osmotic pressure of the circulating plasma proteins. It is the pressure within the glomerular capillaries that determines the filtration rate. Glomerular filtration produces a protein-free filtrate of plasma. The glomeruli act as ultrafilters with microscopic pores. The microscopic pores do not normally allow the larger protein or glucose molecules through but rather send them along the circulatory route to the tubules. The major excretory product into urine is sodium. The tubules act on the glomerular filtrate to produce urine. Substances are reabsorbed from the glomerular filtrate either actively or passively. Substances such as water passively follow sodium that is actively reabsorbed into the urine. Urea, a nitrogenous waste product, diffuses passively. Glucose is actively reabsorbed against the concentration gradient after being freely filtered in the glomerulus.

The tubule cells also secrete a number of substances, such as potassium, hydrogen, ammonium (NH_4^+), and organic anions and cations. As the glomerular filtrate flows through the proximal tubule, sodium is actively reabsorbed and chloride follows passively. Water follows with the change in osmotic pressure. As it reaches the loop of Henle in the tubule, the fluid volume is reduced by 80%. As the fluid flows through the thin, descending loop of Henle, water is removed passively because of the hypertonicity of the interstitial tissues. As the fluid enters the distal convoluted tubules, it becomes hypotonic.

If circulating antidiuretic hormone is elevated, the distal tubule is permeable to water and the urinary fluid then becomes isotonic to the interstitial fluid. Chloride, sodium, and passive osmotic diffusion of water further reduce the urinary fluid volume as it enters the collecting duct, where it changes from an isotonic to a hypertonic fluid. The urinary fluid and sodium removed in the loop of Henle return to the general circulation.

If the antidiuretic hormone level is low, the distal tubule is not permeable to water and the urinary fluid remains hypotonic. It loses its solutes and increases its hypotonicity. The ultimate outcome is that the urine is both dilute and increased in volume.

The kidney regulates acid-base balance by maintaining plasma bicarbonate between 26 and 28 mEq/L in response to the respiratory system's maintenance of carbonic acid at 1.3 to 1.4 mEq/L. Organic anions in the urine accept hydrogen ions, producing carbonic acid, which is in turn broken down into water and carbon dioxide. Ammonia (a combination of nitrogen and three hydrogen ions) takes on another hydrogen ion and becomes NH_4^+ and then is excreted in the urine. In this way, the kidney serves as an efficient buffering mechanism.

During pregnancy, the kidney size increases and a number of alterations occur in renal function. Secondary to prostaglandin E_2, renal blood flow increases, vascular resistance decreases, and glomerular filtration rate increases 30% to 50% over that in the nonpregnant state. Because of this increased filtration rate, nitrogenous waste products such as creatinine, urea, and uric acid are cleared in greater quantities. Therefore urine clearance levels are higher and serum levels are lower than in nonpregnant women.

As the filtrate enters the tubules, considerable changes in the mechanisms controlling salt and water excretion occur. Progesterone normally causes increased salt loss. In pregnancy, this is countered by a rise in aldosterone to two to three times the nonpregnant levels. As a result, sodium is actually retained in the tissues in larger amounts, thus aiding in the necessary volume expansion of pregnancy.

The healthy pregnant woman also excretes larger amounts of sugar in her urine. This is not related to the blood glucose levels but rather to an intermittent tubular failure to reabsorb glucose.

Amino acid excretion is known to be increased in pregnancy. This is thought to be caused by a partial failure of the normal reabsorptive mechanisms. The increased excretion of amino acids is related to high levels of cortisol in pregnancy. Plasma albumin levels are normally lower.

Water-soluble vitamins, such as ascorbic acid, nicotinic acid, and folates, are also excreted at higher levels in the urine during pregnancy. This increased excretion is caused by failure of the tubules to reabsorb and can be serious when folate and protein intake are marginal.

Another important consideration of the high nutrient content of the urine is acknowledging its value as a culture medium for bacteria. Progesterone and prostaglandin E2 (PGE_2) enhances the potential for UTI by relaxing the musculature of the bladder and inhibits urethral peristalsis. The dilation of the ureters, especially on the right side, is further compromised by the obstruction of the gravid uterus. All these factors contribute to the likelihood of urinary stasis of a fluid rich in nutrients, which substantially increases the potential for ascending UTI.

During pregnancy, the kidneys produce increased amounts of erythropoietin and renin. Erythropoietin increases the RBC mass; however, with the increased plasma volume greater than the increased RBC mass, hemoglobin normally is lower. Renin acts to form angiotensin, which in turn increases the production of aldosterone. The aldosterone increase preserves sodium and facilitates blood volume expansion. The sensitivity to the pressor effects of renin-angiotensin is low during pregnancy, and normally the blood pressure does not rise.

SIGNS AND SYMPTOMS

Infection
Common signs of acute bladder infection are frequency, dysuria, and urgency of urination or strangury (the urge to pass urine having just done so). Urine may have an offensive smell. Pyelonephritis is usually present when fever, chills, nausea, vomiting, malaise, back pain, and costovertebral angle (CVA) tenderness occur.

Calculi
Frequent presenting symptoms of calculi are hematuria, sudden onset severe colicky radiating pain from the back to the abdomen, nausea, vomiting, and fever.

Acute Renal Failure

Abrupt onset of oliguria or anuria, flank pain, hematuria, and proteinuria can indicate acute tubular necrosis–type renal failure. Acute renal failure causes the retention of nitrogenous waste products and the inability to maintain normal fluid and electrolyte balance.

Nitrogenous Waste Buildup

Symptoms of increased nitrogenous waste products in the bloodstream include mental confusion, apathy, and itchy skin. Urinary output may be diminished, and the specific gravity is low.

Electrolyte Imbalance

- Potassium excess occurs when the plasma potassium is higher than 5.6 mEq/L. Signs include tachycardia and later bradycardia, electrocardiogram changes with a high T wave and depressed ST segment, and oliguria, abdominal distention, or diarrhea.
- Sodium excess occurs when the plasma sodium is greater than 147 mEq/L. Signs include a urine specific gravity above 1.03; restlessness; dry, sticky mucous membranes; oliguria; hypertension; tachycardia; and edema. Severe hypernatremia can cause convulsions.
- Sodium deficit does not occur.
- Calcium deficit occurs when plasma calcium levels are lower than 4.5 mEq/L. Signs include irritability, twitching around the mouth, numbness, muscle spasms, hypotension, dysrhythmias, and diarrhea. Severe hypocalcemia may cause convulsions.
- Primary base bicarbonate deficit can occur because of the inability of the tubules to secrete buffers. Metabolic acidosis may develop. Signs include urine pH below 6.0, plasma pH below 7.35, disorientation, and shortness of breath or deep, rapid breathing.

Fluid Imbalance

If renal tissues are severely damaged from hypertensive lesions, diabetic nephropathic lesions, or infectious processes, the loss of intravascular osmotic pressure can produce systemic and pulmonary edema. Signs and symptoms of pulmonary edema are sudden in onset and include shortness of breath, crackles, frothy sputum, and decreased Po_2.

Chronic Kidney Disease

Symptoms are rare until the glomerular filtration rate is less than 25% of normal and renal function is less than 50% of normal. Symptoms are the result of accumulation of waste products in the blood, electrolyte abnormalities, and anemia. Other signs of chronic renal disease can be associated with generalized edema and proteinuria, increased blood pressure, and decreased urinary volume. These symptoms rarely worsen during pregnancy unless hypertensive disorders of pregnancy are superimposed on an impaired renal function. The development of preeclampsia before 30 weeks of gestation if accompanied with heavy proteinuria may indicate unrecognized CKD (Williams and Davison, 2009).

MATERNAL EFFECTS

Infections
Infection in the urinary tract may predispose a woman to preterm labor (Williams and Davison, 2009). With pyelonephritis, 15% to 20% will develop bacteremia and in rare cases septic shock and capillary leakage leading to pulmonary edema.

Acute Renal Failure
If dialysis becomes necessary, pregnancy outcome is problematic.

Chronic Kidney Disease
Kidney disease with preserved renal function usually causes minimal kidney deterioration and most often leads to a positive pregnancy outcome. Overall the outcome is positive when the serum creatinine is less than 1.5 mg/dL and blood pressure levels are within normal limits. The more impaired the renal function and the more associated complications, the greater the likelihood of renal deterioration and an adverse pregnancy outcome such as anemia, preeclampsia, and chronic hypertension (Dunlop and others, 2008; Williams and Davison, 2009). Pregnancy is rare in women with stage 5 kidney disease on dialysis because of infertility. Fertility often returns following a successful renal transplant.

After renal transplant in the past, pregnancy was extremely rare, not only because of the woman's renal status but also because of her age by the time of transplant. Today greater than 50% of pregnancies progress to term in the face of a 30% incidence of preeclampsia. The greatest loss is in the first trimester (Williams and Davison, 2009). Immunosuppressive drug therapy must be considered antenatally and postpartum (Williams and Davison, 2009).

FETAL AND NEONATAL EFFECTS

Because of the loss of water from the plasma volume, circulation to the uterus can be diminished. The fetus can suffer nutritionally from the resultant deficiency. Intrauterine growth restriction is common in the fetus of a woman with renal disease as well as preterm birth. If hypertension is also present, arterial resistance to blood flow into the intervillous space can cause chronic hypoxemia of the fetus. Depending on the severity and chronicity of hypoxia, the fetus can suffer central nervous system damage and face potential demise.

DIAGNOSTIC TESTING

Infection
Obtain a clean-voided urine specimen. If the urine is cloudy and positive for nitrite and leukocyte esterase with the dipstick test, then a UTI is likely. Urine microscopy and culture is necessary during the first trimester to diagnose the presence of an asymptomatic UTI or at any time to determine causative organism and antibiotic sensitivities.

Significant bacteriuria may represent either bladder or kidney infection. The differentiation is made by the symptoms presented. However, asymptomatic pyelonephritis can occur, just as bladder infection can be asymptomatic. Asymptomatic pyelonephritis should be suspected when urine cultures detect recurrent or persistent infection despite antibiotic therapy. For this reason, urine cultures should be repeated after a course of antibiotic therapy and then every 4 to 6 weeks for the remainder of the pregnancy.

Calculi

If clinical suspicion is high for urethral or renal calculi, 90% can be identified by abdominal radiograph or intravenous urogram (IVU).

Acute Renal Failure

The diagnosis of intrinsic renal failure can usually be established by kidney ultrasonography or CT scan that demonstrate hypodense areas in the renal cortex. Renal function studies are usually done to ascertain the precipitating insult and the degree of impairment. Such laboratory studies include serum creatinine, blood urea nitrogen (BUN), 24-hour urine collection for creatinine clearance, and total urinary protein. Laboratory values differ in pregnancy beginning as early as 8 to 10 weeks of gestation. This should be considered when interpreting the results (Asrat and Nageotte, 2005; Williams and Davison, 2009). Table 12-1 describes differences between nonpregnant and pregnant normal values. Laboratory findings also differ based on the precipitating insult. Table 12-2 describes differences between prerenal and renal failure.

Renal biopsy to diagnose a specific renal lesion is contraindicated during pregnancy because of the increased blood flow to the kidney. Increases in capillary pressures predispose the kidney to greater potential for hemorrhage, which can lead to further kidney damage.

Table 12-1   Renal Function Studies

Diagnostic Laboratory Test	Nonpregnant Normal Value	Pregnant Normal Value
Blood Urea Nitrogen	7–20 mg/dl	5–12 mg/dl
Creatinine, serum	<1.5 mg/dl	<0.8 mg/dl
Uric acid, serum	1.5–6 mg/dl	1.2–4.5 mg/dl
Urinary creatinine clearance	90–130 ml/min	120–160 ml/min
24-hr urinary protein	<150 mg/24 hr	<260 mg/24 hr

Table 12-2   Diagnostics in Differentiating Renal Failure

Diagnostic Laboratory Test	Prerenal	Renal
Blood urea nitrogen	Elevated	Elevated
Creatinine, serum	Normal	Elevated
Renal failure index	<1	>1
(urine x serum creatinine/urine creatinine)		
Response to fluid	Good	None
Need for dialysis	No	Maybe

Chronic Kidney Disease

Chronic kidney disease usually results in an accumulation of waste products in the blood, electrolyte abnormalities, and anemia. Renal function studies such as blood urea nitrogen, serum creatinine, and urine creatinine clearance are elevated. Electrolytes, potassium, and phosphorus, are elevated and bicarbonate level and calcium are decreased. A complete blood count (CBC) may indicate anemia related to decreased erythropoietin production or hemoconcentration.

USUAL MEDICAL MANAGEMENT AND PROTOCOLS FOR NURSE PRACTITIONERS

General Management

Treatment of renal disease in pregnancy depends on the nature of the disease.

Infection

The most common causative organism of UTI during pregnancy is *Enterobacteriaceae*. Asymptomatic bacteriuria and symptomatic bacteriuria are treated primarily with nitrofurantoin (Macrobid). After the first trimester trimethoprim with or without sulfamethoxazole can be used. It should not be given during the first trimester. There is an increased neural tube defect risk because it is a folic acid antagonist. Other antibiotics used during pregnancy are cefazolin, cephalexin, ceftriaxone, and gentamicin (Williams and Davison, 2009). Antibiotic therapy must be continued in maximum doses for 7 to 10 days. High doses are required during pregnancy because of increased excretion caused by greater renal blood flow. If reculture demonstrates continued bacterial growth, the course of antibiotics must be reinstituted for 6 weeks. Reculture is again done, and if it is positive, an antimicrobial such as nitrofurantoin can be continued for the duration of the pregnancy (Williams and Davison, 2009). If a fever develops, the patient should be hospitalized to receive parenteral antibiotic therapy. Cephalosporins are the drug of choice while awaiting culture and sensitivity results.

Urethral and Renal Calculi

Sixty percent of stones pass with conservative treatment of hydration, bedrest, pain relief with analgesics such as morphine, butorphanol, or Tylenol, and infection prevention with antibiotic therapy. Surgical intervention is necessary in approximately 30% of the cases occurring during pregnancy. Temporary placement of a urethral stent or percutaneous nephrostomy tube is usually done.

Acute Renal Failure

Treatment of ARF starts with early identification and treatment of the precipitating insult. The aim of treatment is to retard the development of uremic symptoms and restore acid-base balance, electrolyte balance, and volume homeostasis. Prerenal ARF is rapidly reversed by restoration of renal perfusion by restoring normal fluid and electrolytes. The source of the loss of fluids determines the composition of fluid replacement. Hypovolemia, caused by hemorrhage, is best treated with a crystalloid solution such as normal saline and colloid solutions such as albumin or packed red blood cells.

Any fluid replacement should be guided by laboratory values of electrolytes and acid base. Intrinsic renal ARF fluid management is even more complex and may need to be carefully monitored with hemodynamic monitoring such as pulmonary artery wedge pressure to prevent fluid overload that can lead to pulmonary edema. In the presence of volume overload, a diuretic such as furosemide (Lasix) is indicated as well as dopamine to dilate the renal vasculature. Short-term dialysis is indicated when BUN rises above 50 to 70 mg/dL or creatinine rises above 6 to 7 mg/dL (Asrat and Nageotte, 2004). Postrenal ARF is treated by removal of the obstruction.

Chronic Kidney Disease

The treatment for chronic kidney disease is complicated. The hypertension that is frequently associated with the disease requires control with an antihypertensive drug. The common antihypertensive agents used because they preserve kidney function, angiotensin-converting enzyme (ACE) inhibitors or angiotensin II receptor blockers, are fetotoxic drugs and should not be given during pregnancy (Williams and Davison, 2009). Low dose aspirin (81 mg/day) should be started early in pregnancy to decrease the risk of preeclampsia (Duley and others, 2007). The urinary output and fluid intake must be closely monitored to prevent fluid overload. Salt solutions must be administered with great caution because of the inability to excrete large quantities of salt and the potential for overwhelming edema, especially in the lungs. Diuretics can be used to aid in excretion of retained fluid, and electrolyte balance must then be closely monitored. If acidosis occurs, lack of an adequate buffering system in the kidneys can create further problems when salt solutions must be administered for their alkalinizing effects. Because the production of erythropoietin is suppressed in chronic renal failure, it is not uncommon to find an associated anemia in pregnancy. Coupled with the tendency for hemodilution on hemoglobin measurement, the anemia can be quite severe, causing shortness of breath, easy fatigue, and failure of fetal growth. These signs may be initially overlooked and attributed to other causes. Increased folic acid and iron supplementation assist normal physiology and counteract some pathologic findings.

The effects of hypertension, loss of protein, and retention of sodium and water can create a life-threatening situation for the mother. If the fetus has little chance of surviving, the choice for termination of the pregnancy should be offered to the mother. If the maternal condition is likely to deteriorate, the risks and benefits of continuing the pregnancy should be discussed with the woman and her family. For the pregnancy that continues, fetal evaluation is ordered. Ultrasound examinations may be done every 2 weeks from 24 weeks of gestation on. Nonstress tests (NSTs) are usually done weekly after 26 weeks of gestation. Daily fetal activity charts are also kept.

End-Stage Renal Disease

Most patients with end-stage renal disease who become pregnant do so accidentally and without the advantage of preconceptual management considerations. Therefore both surgical termination of pregnancy and spontaneous fetal loss probably cause fetal loss rates to be artificially high. Attempts at managing pregnancy complicated by end-stage renal disease with hemodialysis or peritoneal dialysis have provided improved success in pregnancy outcome (Williams and Davison, 2009). However, these patients must be monitored closely for anemia, hemorrhage, infection, and preterm labor. Iron and erythropoietin should be given as serum iron and hemoglobin levels indicate.

Drug Therapy

Antimicrobials

Antimicrobials are prescribed for UTIs. It is important, for maintenance of blood levels, to administer them at evenly spaced intervals. The woman should be instructed to drink more fluids and to take the entire prescription. In the hospital setting, when antimicrobials are given intravenously, the site should be inspected for an inflammatory reaction. The site should also be changed every 48 hours to prevent phlebitis (see Chapter 26).

Tetracyclines are contraindicated for use in pregnancy because of rare maternal acute fatty liver necrosis. In addition, they bind with calcium orthophosphates and cause a permanent yellow staining of the fetal dentition. Chloramphenicol is not used in pregnancy because of the fatal gray syndrome that occurs in infants born of mothers receiving the drug. Sulfonamides and nitrofurantoin are contraindicated somewhat in the last trimester because of their potential for increasing levels of fetal bilirubin.

Antihypertensive Agents

Perinatal outcomes are improved by controlling hypertension in the pregnant woman with renal disease (see Chapter 22).

Diuretics

Diuretics are often used if fluid retention is contributing to hypertension. They also help to prevent pulmonary edema. Any diuretic can cause electrolyte imbalance. The pregnant woman especially should be instructed to report signs of potassium deficit and to help prevent this condition with an increased dietary intake of potassium. Bananas and citrus fruits are high in potassium.

NURSING MANAGEMENT

Prevention

Prevention of symptomatic UTIs is greatly aided by nursing interventions. Pregnant women should be educated to practice correct perineal hygiene and to report any indication of vaginitis or UTI. Routine evaluation of the urine should be carried out at each office visit. The voided specimen should be fresh, not saved from home, and should be evaluated for protein, nitrites, or leukocyte esterase, which are produced in increased amounts when bacterial growth is significant. If the protein level is 1 or more in the absence of pregnancy-induced hypertension or if nitrites are evident, a clean-catch specimen should be obtained for urinalysis, culture, and sensitivity studies. The pregnant woman should be encouraged to drink at least 3000 ml of fluid every 24 hours.

Tertiary prevention of complications from existing renal disease is also important. A careful history should include questions regarding repeated bacteriurias, hypertension when not pregnant, and renal function studies if hypertension, diabetes, or connective tissue disorders have been previously diagnosed. This information helps in screening those women at risk for complications such as preeclampsia, pulmonary edema, uteroplacental insufficiency, and progression of existing renal disease.

Nursing Interventions for Renal Disease

- Assess for risk for fluid overload and renal function using the identified diagnostic test.
- In the presence of renal failure, fluid intake should be carefully monitored and intake should equal output unless the patient is febrile. If the patient is febrile, 100 ml of additional fluid is needed for every degree Celsius of elevation from 38° C.
- Evaluate the degree of edema.
- When drug therapy is prescribed, teach the patient about the purpose, dosage schedule, and potential side effects.
- Discuss the importance of nutritional modifications and make referrals to a registered dietitian when necessary. This is especially relevant if sodium or protein intake is decreased or there is a need for increased protein, iron, or potassium.
- Teach the patient or family to do home blood pressure monitoring.
- Instruct the patient and family about the importance of recognizing and reporting signs of fluid or electrolyte imbalance, medicine-induced side effects, and superimposed preeclampsia or HELLP (*h*emolysis, *e*levated *l*iver enzymes, and *l*ow *p*latelet count) syndrome.
- Modify home activities to reduce onset of dangerous hypertension and avoid added fatigue factors.
- Teach the patient how to avoid infections.
- Teach the patient the signs and symptoms of preterm labor and when to report it if it becomes regular (four painless contractions per hour unrelieved by 1 hour of rest).
- Avoid using urinary catheters in the presence of renal disorders to prevent introduction of new bacteria into the urinary tract. Avoid indwelling catheters without triple lumen because they are intended for irrigation with antibacterial agents.
- Always obtain a clean catch urine specimen to run a 48-hour culture and sensitivity before beginning the first dose of antimicrobial therapy. (It is not necessary to have results first, but they should be reviewed within 3 days of sending the specimen to select the appropriate antimicrobial.)
- Perform dipstick urine test for protein, nitrites, and leukocyte esterase at each antepartum office visit and at least weekly for hospitalized patients.
- Ask the patient at each visit whether she has symptoms of burning, frequency, and flank pain and assess whether she presents with signs of preterm labor.
- Educate the patient about the importance of drinking a variety of fluids (avoid high acid, carbonated, or caffeinated beverages), at least 8 to 10 ounces every waking hour.

- Instruct the patient to empty her bladder at least every 2 hours while awake and to void after intercourse.
- Tell the patient to perform perineal hygiene front to back.
- Educate the patient about the importance of reporting signs of kidney or bladder infections immediately.
- Educate the patient regarding prophylactic antibiotic therapy if she has a history of pyelonephritis.
- Start fetal surveillance with electronic fetal monitoring, biophysical profile (BPP), NSTs, AFV, or some combination of testing by 28 to 32 weeks of gestation.
- After 24 weeks of gestation, evaluate for fetal intrauterine growth restriction every 4 to 6 weeks by ultrasound.

Critical Care for Acute Renal Failure*
- Carefully evaluate intake and output of any high risk patient.
- Assess for hypertensive disorders of pregnancy or disseminated intravascular coagulation.
- Evaluate laboratory and diagnostic data such as BUN and serum creatinine levels. (These are frequently the earliest signs of acute kidney failure.)
- Assess for signs of superimposed preeclampsia by evaluating blood pressure at each antepartum visit or daily if hospitalized.
- Assess for signs of hemorrhage and coagulopathy.
- Assess respirations and breath sounds for early detection of pulmonary edema if there is a possibility of renal compromise.
- Assess for signs of fluid, electrolyte, and acid-base imbalances.
- Prevent acute renal failure by assisting in replacement of blood and fluids in the event of massive hemorrhage.
- Report early signs of an infection.
- If acute renal failure develops be prepared to use invasive hemodynamic monitoring to assess intravascular volume (see Chapter 11) and kidney dialysis.
- Report any signs of preeclampsia or fluid, electrolyte, or acid-base imbalances to the attending physician.
- Report abnormal blood chemistries to the attending physician.
- Perform dialysis as ordered.
- Weigh the patient at each dialysis exchange.
- Report any signs of abnormal fluid retention if the patient is on dialysis.
- Administer appropriate salt-poor intravenous fluids if pyelonephritis or signs of renal failure are present.
- Refer the patient to a nurse clinician or specialist for education regarding dialysis.

CONCLUSION

The primary aim for care of the pregnant woman with bacteriuria is prevention of symptomatic UTI and preterm labor. Prophylactic administration of antibiotics with instructions for increased oral fluids and proper perineal hygiene are most effective.

---

*Asrat and Nageotte, 2005; Maresh and others, 2005; Martin and Foley, 2009.

Prompt treatment of renal tract infection and medical response to maternal renal failure can prevent life-threatening events for the mother and intrauterine growth restriction or intrauterine fetal death. In the presence of mild renal impairment, pregnancy does not affect renal function. In the presence of moderate-to-severe renal impairment, pregnancy outcomes can be significantly affected (Williams and Davison, 2009). Pregnancy after renal transplant has been quite successful if the original medical condition is stabilized and carefully monitored.

BIBLIOGRAPHY

Asrat T, Nageotte M: Acute renal failure in pregnancy. In Foley M, Strong T, Garite T, editors: *Obstetric intensive care manual*, ed 2, New York, 2004, McGraw-Hill.

Asrat T, Nageotte P: Renal disease. In James D, and others, editors: *High risk pregnancy: management options*, ed 3, Philadelphia, 2005, Saunders.

Duley L, Henderson-Smart DJ, Meher S, King JF: Antiplatelet agents for preventing pre-eclampsia and its complications, *Cochrane Database Syst Rev*, (Issue 2), Art. No.: CD004659, 2007.

Dunlop A, Jack B, Bottalico J, Lu M, and others: The clinical content of preconception care: women with chronic medical conditions, *Am J Obstet Gyncol* 199(6 Suppl 2):S310–327, 2008.

Finnish Medical Society Duodecim: Systematic diseases in pregnancy, *EBM guidelines: Evidence-based medicine(Internet)*. Helsinki, Finland, 2007, Wiley Interscience.

Maresh M, James D, Neales K: Critical care of the obstetric patient. In James D, and others, editors: *High risk pregnancy: management options*, ed 3, Philadelphia, 2005, Saunders.

Martin S, Foley M: Intensive care monitoring of the critically ill pregnant patient. In Creasy R, Resnik R, Iams J, Lockwood C, Moore T, editors: *Creasy and Resnik's maternal-fetal medicine: principles and practice*, ed 6, Philadelphia, 2009, Saunders.

Williams D, Davison J: Renal disorders. In Creasy R, Resnik R, Iams J, Lockwood C, Moore T, editors: *Creasy and Resnik's maternal-fetal medicine: principles and practice*, ed 6, Philadelphia, 2009, Saunders.

13

Autoimmune Rheumatic Diseases

utoimmune rheumatic diseases can occur during pregnancy because a large percentage of patients with an autoimmune disease are women of childbearing age. These diseases result from the body's immune system inability to distinguish "self" from "nonself." When this inability occurs, the body manufactures T cells and antibodies directed against its own cells. This immunologic defect may be cellular or humoral in nature. Examples of cell-mediated autoimmune diseases are rheumatoid arthritis (RA) and multiple sclerosis. Frequently, pregnancy has no effect or may improve these diseases. Humoral autoimmune diseases result from abnormal antibody formation. Examples of these disorders are systemic lupus erythematosus (SLE) and acquired thrombophilias such as antiphospholipid syndrome (APS). These autoimmune diseases worsen or are associated with pregnancy loss or placental insufficiency. This chapter focuses on SLE and APS, two autoimmune disorders most frequently encountered that have serious consequences for pregnancy.

Two components of venous thromboembolic disease are deep vein thrombosis (DVT) and pulmonary embolism.

INCIDENCE

Systemic Lupus Erythematosus

According to some sources (Dunlop and others, 2008), the incidence of SLE in United States women from their late 20s to early 40s is 14.6 to 50.8 per 100,000 in the general population with a greater increase in the African American population. The predictions in the 1970s and early 1980s of an incidence of 6:100,000 have been changed dramatically because of the improved ability to diagnose SLE by radioimmune assays. Women are affected 10 times more often than men.

Whether a woman is pregnant or not, SLE may be characterized by exacerbations and remissions. Survival after exacerbation is 90% in the first 5 years and 80% after 10 years. Survival generally depends on the degree of cardiac and renal involvement and the extent of multisystem insult.

Antiphospholipid Syndrome

The incidence of patients with antiphospholipid antibodies is 2% to 8% of the general population. Of patients with SLE, 30% are positive for antiphospholipid antibodies.

271

ETIOLOGY

The exact causes of SLE and APS are unknown. Evidence indicates that causes may be interrelated with immunologic, environmental, hormonal, and genetic factors (Warren and Silver, 2004; Porter and Branch, 2005). Predisposing factors include viral infections, physical or psychologic stress, sunlight, immunization, and pregnancy.

NORMAL PHYSIOLOGY

See discussion of normal physiologic adaptations in pregnancy described by systems and functions in Chapter 1 and by the coagulation cascade in Chapter 20.

PATHOPHYSIOLOGY

In SLE and APS, the body is unable to distinguish "self" from "nonself." An immunologic deficit allows antibodies to be formed that attack the body's own cells and proteins. More than 50 autoantibodies and antigen-antibody complexes collectively have been identified in the serum of affected individuals.

Systemic Lupus Erythematosus

The autoimmune responses in SLE cause suppression of the body's normal immunity and damage to body tissue. The autoimmune response may initially involve one organ system or every organ system. The most common organ systems are skin, joints, kidneys, lung, cardiac, and nervous system. In pregnancy, inflammation of the connective tissue of the decidua can result in problems of placental implantation and functioning.

Antiphospholipid Syndrome

The antiphospholipid antibodies that are characteristic of APS are formed against normal plasma proteins that are involved in the coagulation cascade and disrupt the phospholipids-dependent anticoagulant process leading to a procoagulant state. These same antibodies can have a direct toxic effect on the trophoblast tissue impeding uteroplacental blood flow. They also interfere with the prostacyclin thromboxane balance by interfering with prostacyclin production.

SIGNS AND SYMPTOMS

Systemic Lupus Erythematosus

Clinical manifestations depend on the system(s) being attacked by the autoantibodies. The most common symptoms are fever, malaise, fatigue, weight loss, skin rashes, and polyarthralgia. Table 13-1 gives clinical manifestations specific to various systems involved in SLE.

Antiphospholipid Syndrome

The presence of antiphospholipid antibodies does not produce symptoms until a clot is precipitated. Therefore the common secondary signs and symptoms are:
- Superficial thrombophlebitis
- Deep vein thrombophlebitis

Table 13-1   Clinical Manifestations of Systemic Lupus Erythematosus

System	Clinical Manifestations
General	Malaise
	Fatigue
	Fever
	Weight loss
Integumentary	Skin rashes, butterfly rash
	Mucous membrane ulcers
Musculoskeletal	Arthralgia
Cardiovascular	Pericarditis
	Myocarditis
	Endocarditis
	Tachycardia
Respiratory	Pleuritis
	Dyspnea
	Pneumonitis
Renal	Urinary tract infection
	Nephrotic syndrome characterized by:
	• Hematuria
	• Proteinuria
	• Urine sediment and cellular casts
	Glomerular nephritis
	May progress to total kidney failure
Central nervous system	Emotional instability
	Seizure disorders
	Psychosis
	Headaches
	Irritability
	Depression
Gastrointestinal	Mucosal ulcers of mouth
	Anorexia
	Nausea and vomiting
	Diarrhea
	Constipation
Hematologic	Chronic anemia
	Thrombocytopenia
	Leukocytopenia
	Lupus anticoagulant
Ocular	Conjunctivitis
	Photosensitivity

- Thrombosis (arterial or venous)
- Pulmonary embolism
- Septic pelvic thrombophlebitis

APS may be suspected when a patient gives a strong family history, has an unproven suspicious personal history, or has repeated spontaneous abortions when other underlying conditions have been ruled out.

MATERNAL EFFECTS

Systemic Lupus Erythematosus

If the SLE has been in remission for at least 6 months before conception and renal function is normal, optimal pregnancy outcome is high (Dunlop and others, 2008). If SLE is active at the time of conception, exacerbation of the disease is common, especially involving the renal and central nervous systems (Warren and Silver, 2004). Disease flares are common during pregnancy. It is unknown if pregnancy increases the number of flares (Dunlop and others, 2008).

Complications such as preeclampsia, HELLP (*h*emolysis, *e*levated *l*iver enzymes, and *l*ow *p*latelet count) syndrome in association with preeclampsia (see Chapter 22), and preterm labor are the most common. The risk for disease deterioration during pregnancy or postpartum is high if the patient has severe renal insufficiency before becoming pregnant.

Antiphospholipid Syndrome

APS may lead to a life-threatening event for the mother, especially venous and arterial thrombosis, pulmonary emboli, or stroke. During pregnancy and the postpartum period, 5% to 12% of patients will develop a venous or arterial thrombosis (ACOG, 2005). A pregnant woman with an acquired thrombophilia such as APS is at greater risk for abruption, severe preeclampsia before 34 weeks of gestation, iatrogenic preterm labor, antenatal or postpartum deep vein thrombophlebitis, and pulmonary embolism (ACOG, 2005). These patients should be screened for anemia, thrombocytopenia, and underlying renal disease.

FETAL AND NEONATAL EFFECTS

Systemic Lupus Erythematosus

SLE affects pregnancy by increasing the risk for spontaneous abortion by 8% to 40% (Warren and Silver, 2004), depending on the severity of exacerbations and the length of remission before conception. The risk for a spontaneous abortion is directly related to maternal renal involvement.

After spontaneous abortion risk, early intrauterine growth restriction with a high risk for stillbirth remains the next major risk to the fetus/newborn. The risk is primarily the result of the malformation of the placenta and placental insufficiency in serving the nutritional and respiratory functions for the fetus. The placenta has connective tissue as part of its makeup. Microangiopathic changes take place in the placenta, resulting in disruption of normal functioning. Premature labor and potential preterm birth presents a third major risk to the newborn (see Chapter 23). In addition, if the mother is positive for anti-Ro or anti-La antibodies or both, the neonate is at risk for neonatal lupus syndrome (Lockshin, Salmon, and Erkan, 2009). Fifty percent of neonates with neonatal lupus will manifest skin lesions that appear as erythematous, scaling plaques. These are usually seen on the face or scalp and typically disappear after a few months. Other transient manifestations are thrombocytopenia, hepatitis, and hemolytic anemia. However, if the neonate develops cardiac lesions as the result of neonatal lupus syndrome, permanent congenital heart block can result.

Antiphospholipid Syndrome

APS significantly increases pregnancy loss. It is estimated that 80% of women with APS experience at least one fetal loss (ACOG, 2005). The high loss rate of pregnancy through recurrent spontaneous abortions and unexplained second or third trimester fetal death may be related to an incompletely diagnosed acquired thrombophilia problem in the mother or failure to understand family history factors that may have been related to undiagnosed thrombophilia in family members (Porter and Branch, 2005). In viable fetuses, the risks of intrauterine growth restriction related to uteroplacental insufficiency, chronic abruption, chronic abruption oligohydramnios (CAOS), preterm labor, and preterm delivery are increased. There also appears to be an increased risk for cardiac or neurologic anomalies in the fetus of a mother with methylene tetrahydrofolate reductose (MTHFR) mutation or low homocysteine levels. When these factors are correctly and more completely diagnosed, a management plan can be developed and significantly decrease the loss rate and improve prognosis for outcomes.

MEDICAL DIAGNOSIS

Systemic Lupus Erythematosus

The American College of Rheumatology has identified the following 11 criteria for the classification of SLE, 4 or more of which must be present to confirm the diagnosis:
- Malar rash (butterfly rash)
- Discoid rash (erythematous, scaly rash on the face, scalp, ears, arms or chest)
- Photosensitivity
- Oral ulcers (usually painless)
- Arthritis (involving two or more joints)
- Serositis (pleuritis or pericarditis)
- Renal disorder (persistent proteinuria over 0.5 g/day; cellular casts)
- Neurologic disorder (seizure or psychosis)
- Hematologic disorder (hemolytic anemia, leucopenia, lymphopenia, or thrombocytopenia)
- Immunologic disorder (anti-DNA positive)
- Antinuclear antibody (ANA-positive titer)

Patients who present with fewer than 4 criteria are referred to as having *lupus-like disease.*

During pregnancy, if the fetus is diagnosed with congenital heart block and the mother has not previously been diagnosed with lupus, she should have a complete SLE workup. In addition, certain clinical manifestations indicate a need to investigate a pregnant woman's predisposition for SLE and the lupus anticoagulant:
- Recurrent fetal losses
- Thrombotic events
- Prolonged coagulation studies
- Positive autoantibody tests
- Thrombocytopenia

Antiphospholipid Syndrome

According to the American College of Obstetricians and Gynecologists (ACOG, 2005), APS is defined by certain laboratory and clinical criteria. One clinical and one laboratory criterion must be present to confirm the diagnosis.

Clinical Criteria

- Vascular thrombosis
- Venous
- Arterial
- Fetal loss
- One or more unexplained fetal deaths beyond 10 weeks of gestation
- One or more premature births before 34 weeks of gestation
- Three or more unexplained consecutive spontaneous abortions without hormonal or chromosomal abnormalities

Laboratory Criteria

- Anticardiolipin antibody (aCL)
- Lupus anticoagulant (LA)

USUAL MEDICAL MANAGEMENT AND PROTOCOLS FOR NURSE PRACTITIONERS

Autoimmune rheumatic diseases are chronic diseases that are likely to exacerbate. Therefore, pregnancy planning must include consideration of the patient's current medical management.

Systemic Lupus Erythematosus

General Management

Women with SLE should be counseled about:
- Medical and obstetric risks of miscarriage, fetal death, fetal growth restriction, preeclampsia, preterm labor, and neonatal lupus
- Planning pregnancy
- Importance of being at least 6 months in remission before conception

After conception, a pregnancy complicated with SLE or other autoimmune disease requires close supervision of both the woman and the fetus. These patients will need frequent visits to assess SLE status and to screen for obstetric risks. They should be evaluated for evidence of anemia, thrombocytopenia, renal disease, and thrombophilias.

Other Management

Other methods of treatment and management depend on clinical manifestations. For example, if the major threat to maternal health stems from cardiac problems related to valvular problems, a cardiology consultation may be sought. Medical management is directed at treatment and stabilization. If the primary clinical characteristics are arthritic in nature, a rheumatologist may be consulted. If pulmonary problems, hypertension, coagulation defects, or renal problems are the presenting complications, a pulmonologist, cardiologist, hematologist, or nephrologist should be consulted (see Chapters 11 through 15 and 22).

Drug Therapy for Systemic Lupus Erythematosus

The four most common categories of drugs used in the general treatment of SLE are NSAIDs and aspirin, corticosteroids, antimalarials, and cytotoxic agents such as azathioprine, methotrexate, cyclosporine A, and cyclophosphamide (Cytoxan).

During pregnancy in the patient with SLE, the goal is to keep drug therapy to a minimum. Patients who have a mild form of the disease or who are experiencing a remission require minimal to no medication. The usual drug therapy, when indicated, includes an antiinflammatory drug, especially a corticosteroid or low-dose aspirin. The corticosteroid of choice is prednisone or methylprednisolone because they are inactivated by the placenta and do not reach the fetus in any significant amount. Fluorinated corticosteroids such as betamethasone or dexamethasone are not inactivated by the placenta and are used when the intent is to treat the fetus (Lockshin, Salmon, and Erkan, 2009). NSAIDs (except low-dose aspirin) and cytotoxic agents should be discontinued before pregnancy. Long-term use of NSAIDs during pregnancy is associated with decreased fetal urine output, oligohydramnios, premature closure of the ductus, fetal pulmonary hypertension, necrotizing enterocolitis, and neonatal renal insufficiency. An antimalarial drug, hydroxychloroquine, is currently being considered as first-line therapy for SLE in pregnancy. This drug appears to be safe (Silver, 2004; Warren and Silver, 2004; Porter and Branch, 2005; Lockshin, Salmon, and Erkan, 2009).

When corticosteroids and hydroxychloroquine are inadequate in managing severe exacerbations, a cytotoxic agent, such as cyclosporine A or azathioprine, is sometimes considered when the benefits outweigh the risks. Cyclophosphamide or methotrexate should never be used during pregnancy related to their teratogenic properties.

Antiphospholipid Syndrome

General Management

The three goals of current medical treatment for APS are as follows:
- Thrombosis prevention with low-dose aspirin (81 mg) plus heparin (currently the most common treatment); throughout pregnancy and for 6 to 8 weeks postpartum, use prophylactic doses of heparin if no thrombotic history, or full anticoagulation doses of heparin if there is a history of a thrombotic event. See Chapter 14 for management of heparin.
- Improvement of placental blood flow by decreasing thromboxane to prostacyclin ratio with low-dose aspirin
- Immune system suppression with prednisone and intravenous immunoglobulin (IVIG) (used less frequently today because of the side effects of steroids)

NURSING MANAGEMENT

Secondary and Tertiary Prevention

Preventive nursing care focuses on early recognition and reporting of signs of SLE flare, recognition and evaluation for any of the thrombophilias, and avoidance of the common pregnancy complications precipitated by SLE and the thrombophilias. In an effort to do that, the family members and the pregnant woman need adequate information for her care. Collaboration with the medical management plan includes reinforcing preconceptual counseling, interpreting clinical information in lay terms, and being vigilant in physical and psychosocial assessments for the family and the pregnant woman.

Prenatal Nursing Interventions for Systemic Lupus Erythematosus

- Discuss the importance of having good control over SLE before the woman becomes pregnant.
- Discuss the possible effects of SLE or the thrombophilias on pregnancy and the possible risk for exacerbations of SLE during pregnancy.
- Assess for evidence of anemia, thrombocytopenia, and thrombophilias.
- Be prepared to assess for thrombophilia by doing a complete thrombophilia workup as described in standard medical management and nurse practitioner protocols. This assessment is needed to determine whether anticoagulation is necessary and whether prophylactic or therapeutic dosing is needed. If needed, instruct the patient in administration.
- Assess for underlying renal disease by checking urine for protein and specific gravity that measures retention of urea solutes, serum creatinine, and 24-hour urine for total protein and creatinine clearance.
- Monitor for signs or symptoms of SLE flare.
- Emphasize the importance of frequent prenatal visits to detect early preeclampsia, preterm labor, and SLE exacerbations.
- Discuss implications of all drug therapies. Teach the patient and family about the self-administration of all prescribed medications.
- Assess for signs of infection at each prenatal visit, especially urinary tract and upper respiratory infections because prednisone drug management can mask signs of infection and lower resistance.
- Assess weight gain.
- Measure the blood pressure in the same arm and in the same position each visit; determine the mean arterial pressure.
- Emphasize the importance of a balance between activity and adequate rest as well as adequate nutrition.
- Teach prevention and recognition of preterm labor.
- Provide emotional support as needed.
- Instruct regarding skin care such as washing with a mild soap, avoiding sun exposure, using sunscreens, and avoiding products that cause side effects.
- Assess fetal surveillance with some combination of nonstress tests, biophysical profiles, or placental Doppler flow studies.
- Evaluate fetal growth by ultrasound every 3 to 4 weeks after 24 weeks of gestation. Measure fundal height between ultrasound evaluations.
- Instruct in the importance of counting fetal movements beginning at 24 weeks of gestation.
- Refer to the Lupus Foundation of America and to a high risk pregnancy support group such as Sidelines.
- Assess family coping styles and ability to cope with the effects of chronic illness. Refer for psychosocial evaluation and support as needed.

Postpartum Nursing Interventions for Systemic Lupus Erythematosus

- Assess for early signs of maternal infection by checking temperature every 4 hours.
- Assess breath sounds for early evidence of pneumonia.
- Assess for hematoma formation and lack of wound healing (episiotomy or cesarean incision).
- Monitor for SLE exacerbation.
- Be prepared to restart maintenance therapy.
- Provide adequate information about true chances for survival of fetus or newborn.
- Make appropriate grief referrals (see Chapter 7).
- Discuss the importance of birth control and the effects of various birth control methods on the disease. Oral contraceptives containing estrogen may increase the risk of thromboembolism especially in the patient who is positive for antiphospholipid antibodies. An IUD may increase the risk for an infection. Therefore the progestin only or barrier methods carry the least risk to the patient.

Prenatal Nursing Interventions for Antiphospholipid Syndrome

- Discuss medical and pregnancy risks associated with this condition such as fetal loss, thrombosis or stroke, preeclampsia, intrauterine growth restriction, and preterm labor.
- Assess for evidence of anemia, thrombocytopenia, and underlying renal disease.
- Emphasize the importance of frequent prenatal visits.
- Screen for preeclampsia and preterm labor.
- Discuss implications of all drug therapies. Teach the patient and family about the self-administration of all prescribed medications.
- If heparin is used in thromboprophylaxis, discuss the importance of 1000 mg of calcium daily, vitamin D, and weight-bearing exercises to decrease the risk for osteoporosis.
- Prepare patients for the importance of serial ultrasounds every 3 to 4 weeks starting around 17 to 18 weeks of gestation to monitor fetal growth impairment and oligohydramnios and to evaluate uteroplacental perfusion. Around 32 weeks of gestation or earlier if there are signs of IUGR, daily fetal movement counts, biophysical profiles or nonstress test with amniotic fluid volume measurements are usually added.
- Teach prevention and recognition of preterm labor.
- Refer to a high risk pregnancy support group such as Sidelines.

Intrapartum Nursing Interventions for Antiphospholipid Syndrome

- Monitor closely for preeclampsia and uteroplacental insufficiency with continuous electronic fetal monitoring.
- Monitor closely for bleeding. Be prepared to hold or adjust the anticoagulant during labor as ordered.
- If patient has been on an anticoagulant, spinal and epidural blocks increase the risk for spinal hematoma. According to the American Society of Regional Anesthesia (ASRA), regional anesthesia should not be used until 24 hours after the last injection for patients on full-dose anticoagulation dosing, or 12 hours if the patient is on unfractionated heparin thromboprophylaxis dosing, or 24 hours if the patient is on LMWH thromboprophylaxis dosing.

Postpartum Nursing Interventions for Antiphospholipid Syndrome

- Provide adequate information about true chances for survival of fetus or newborn.
- Make appropriate grief referrals (see Chapter 7).
- Be prepared to resume anticoagulant therapy and continue for 6 to 8 weeks (refer to Intrapartum and Postpartum Management of Patients on Heparin above).
- Discuss the importance of birth control and the effects of various birth control methods on the disease. Oral contraceptives containing estrogen is contraindicated related to the increased risk of thromboembolism. An IUD may increase the risk for an infection. Therefore progestin only and barrier methods carry the least risk to the patient (Dunlop and others, 2008).

Intrapartum Critical Care Interventions for Systemic Lupus Erythematosus or Antiphospholipid Syndrome

- Evaluate cardiac function by assessing for signs of congestive heart failure, blood pressure, and pulse rate for dysrhythmias; ECG monitoring and invasive monitoring may become necessary.
- Evaluate renal function by assessing urinary output, specific gravity, and proteinuria every 4 hours in the presence of hypertension (see Chapter 12).
- Evaluate pulmonary function by assessing breath sounds every 4 hours and determining whether chest pain develops. If tocolytics are used or if the patient has a positive history of pulmonary, cardiac, or renal involvement, the pulmonary assessment should be done more often (see relevant chapters for cardiac, renal, and hypertension critical care).
- Evaluate the hematologic function by assessing for signs of venous thromboembolism and initiate prophylactic treatment with heparin as appropriate (see Chapter 14).
- Observe closely for late-onset preeclampsia.
- If there is a positive history of central nervous system involvement, evaluate the central nervous system function by assessing for seizure activity, unexpected mood swings, or transient changes in level of consciousness.
- If either cardiac or renal complications are severe or if preeclampsia is superimposed, prepare for invasive hemodynamic monitoring.
- If noninvasive monitoring is ordered instead, use ECG and conventional blood pressure monitoring to assess the hemodynamic status (see Chapters 11 and 22).
- Initiate prompt treatment of early pulmonary problems with antibiotics, bronchodilators, or diuretics as appropriate (see Chapter 15).

CONCLUSION

Autoimmune disease greatly complicates management of both the disease and the pregnancy. The complications, although not insurmountable, require close supervision. The keys to a successful outcome for mother and baby include the following:
- Accurate diagnosis of the specific disease, the systems involved, or the thrombophilic abnormalities identified
- Preconceptual counseling to attempt pregnancy only after at least 6 months of remission

- Vigilance during the pregnancy for progression of the disease, effects on the fetus, and development of pregnancy-related maternal complications

With better, more accurate diagnostic laboratory evaluations available through radio-immune assays and a greater number of coagulopathies being identified through laboratory testing for various factors, closer and more adequate follow-up can now be provided. Nursing care must be directed at early detection of signs and symptoms, education of the mother and involved family members, and careful evaluation of the fetal status. If the pregnancy fails despite good care, grief support and referrals can aid the family affected by maternal connective tissue disorders and thrombophilias. Because autoimmune diseases, including SLE and APS, are multisystem disorders, see the relevant chapters for specific nursing care related to effects on each system.

BIBLIOGRAPHY

American College of Obstetricians and Gynecologists (ACOG): Antiphospholipid syndrome. ACOG Practice Bulletin No. 68, *Obstet Gynecol* 106(5):1113–1121, 2005.

Dunlop A, Jack B, Bottalico J, and others: The clinical content of preconception care: women with chronic medical conditions, *Am J Obstet Gyncol* 199(6 Suppl 2):S310–327, 2008.

Lockshin M, Salmon J, Erkan D: Pregnancy and rheumatic diseases. In Creasy R, Resnik R, Iams J, Lockwood C, Moore T, editors: *Creasy & Resnik's maternal-fetal medicine: principles and practice,* ed 6, Philadelphia, 2009, Saunders.

Lockwood C: Thromboembolic disease in pregnancy. In Creasy R, Resnik R, Iams J, Lockwood C, Moore T, editors: *Creasy & Resnik's maternal-fetal medicine: principles and practice,* ed 6, Philadelphia, 2009, Saunders.

Porter T, Branch D: Autoimmune diseases. In James D, and others, editors: *High risk pregnancy: management options,* ed 3, Philadelphia, 2005, Saunders.

Silver B: Systemic lupus erythematosus in the pregnant patient. In Foley M, Strong T, Garite T, editors: *Obstetric intensive care manual,* ed 2, New York, 2004, McGraw-Hill.

Warren J, Silver R: Autoimmune disease in pregnancy: systemic lupus erythematosus and antiphospholipid syndrome, *Obstet Gynecol Clin North Am* 31(2):345–372, 2004.

Weiner C, Buhimschi C: *Drugs for pregnant and lactating women,* ed 2, Philadelphia, 2009, Saunders.

14

Venous Thromboembolic Disease

Deep vein thrombosis (DVT) and pulmonary embolism (PE) are two components of venous thromboembolic disease.

INCIDENCE

The risk of venous thromboembolism occurring during pregnancy is 0.1% to 1.8% (James and others, 2006; Marik and Plante, 2008). About 15% of Americans of European ancestry carry one or more of the genes for thrombophilia (Marik and Plante, 2008).

ETIOLOGY

About one half of the cases of venous thromboembolism during pregnancy are associated with a common risk factor for thrombophilia (Zotz, Gerhardt, and Scharf, 2003). Thrombophilia, an inheritable hypercoagulable condition, is most commonly the result of activated protein C resistance caused by mutations of the Factor V Leiden (FVL) gene, prothrombin gene *(G20210A)*, protein C or S deficiency, antithrombin III, or hyperhomocysteinemia (*MTHFR C677T*, the gene causing folate deficiency) (Krivak and Zorn, 2007).

Other risk factors for the development of venous thromboembolism during a pregnancy are as follows:

- Bedrest or immobility for 4 days or more
- Obesity (defined as a body mass index greater than 20)
- Smoking
- Medical conditions such as diabetes, congestive heart failure, nephritic syndrome or a severe infection
- Severe varicose veins
- Hyperemesis and dehydration
- Trauma
- Cesarean delivery (64% of VTE occurs following cesarean delivery [Blanco-Molina and others, 2007])
- Previous history of thrombosis
- Acquired antiphospholipid syndrome (See Chapter 13)

NORMAL PHYSIOLOGY

Pregnancy is normally a hypercoagulable state with increased fibrin generation; increased coagulation factors II, VII, VIII, and X; decreased fibrinolytic activity; and decreased free protein S levels. Venous stasis in the lower extremities resulting from compression of the inferior vena cava and pelvic veins, coupled with hypercoagulopathy, develops around 25 weeks of gestation and lasts for approximately 6 weeks postpartum.

SIGNS AND SYMPTOMS

Classic signs of DVT and PE are similar to some of the discomforts of pregnancy such as dependent edema, tachycardia, tachypnea, and dyspnea. Unilateral leg pain, erythema, low grade fever, or edema are typical symptoms of a DVT (RCOG, 2007). Pain with foot dorsiflexion, referred to as positive Homans' sign, may indicate a deep vein thrombosis in the lower extremity during pregnancy (Urbano, 2001). A PE may present with tachypnea, tachycardia, dyspnea, and pleuritic chest pain. With a massive PE other symptoms are lightheadedness, syncope, or collapse.

MATERNAL EFFECTS

If venous thromboembolism occurs during pregnancy a pulmonary embolism can result. Pulmonary embolism is the leading cause of maternal death related to childbirth (James and others, 2006; Dresang and others, 2008). Common adverse pregnancy outcomes in patients with some form of thrombophilia are venous thromboembolism, arterial thrombosis, severe preeclampsia, and abruptio placentae (Stella, Ghulmiyyah, and Sibai, 2006).

FETAL AND NEONATAL EFFECTS

Thrombophilia increases the risk of early and late pregnancy loss and intrauterine growth restriction (Robertson and others, 2006).

DIAGNOSTIC TESTING

Universal screening for inherited thrombophilia is not cost effective. However, thrombophilia screening is recommended during pregnancy in patients with a personal or family history of thromboembolism. The most common inherited thrombophilias are Factor V Leiden heterozygous gene, prothrombin gene mutation *G20210A*, protein C deficiency, protein S deficiency, antithrombin-III deficiency and methylene tetrahydrofolate reductase (MTHFR) homozygous gene (Kyrle and Eichinger, 2005).

All pregnant women with signs and symptoms of venous thromboembolism should be evaluated by objective tests such as venous compression Doppler ultrasonography, magnetic resonance venography, and pulsed Doppler study. Multidetector-row (spiral) computed tomography, electrocardiography, and/or chest x-ray are tests used to diagnosis pulmonary embolism. The D-dimer test is not a reliable test during pregnancy (RCOG, 2007).

USUAL MEDICAL MANAGEMENT AND PROTOCOLS FOR NURSE PRACTITIONERS

Thromboprophylaxis

Two nonpharmacologic prophylactic methods used to reduce DVT formation are graduated compression stockings and intermittent pneumatic compression devices. Both reduce the risk of venous stasis by preventing blood from pooling in the calves of the legs. According to two different Cochrane reviews of randomized, controlled trials, DVT was reduced with their use (Amaragiri and Lees, 2003; Kakkos and others, 2008). Intermittent pneumatic compression devices may further promote thromboprophylaxis by stimulating the production of fibrinolysis (Kohro and others, 2005).

The two most recommended pharmacologic prophylactic methods to reduce DVT formation are low-dose unfractionated heparin (UFH) and low molecular weight heparin (LMWH). According two Cochrane systematic reviews, LMWH is considered the heparin of choice for prophylaxis because of fewer side effects and mortality risk (Magee and others, 2003; van Dongen and others, 2004). Side effects of heparin are bleeding, allergic reactions, osteoporosis, and heparin-induced thrombocytopenia (Greer and Nelson-Piercy, 2005). Combining nonpharmacologic with a pharmacologic prophylactic modality was found to be even more effective in lowering the incidence of DVT according to a Cochrane review (Kakkos and others, 2008).

Warfarin has known teratogenic effects if taken during pregnancy. In extremely rare cases, warfarin has been used in the second trimester and the beginning part of the third trimester in patients with artificial heart valves (Bates and others, 2008; Chen, Anand, and Ginsberg, 2000; Krivak and Zorn, 2007). This is because these patients have developed valvular thrombi while on heparin. Warfarin is compatible with breastfeeding (Weiner and Buhimschi, 2009).

Acute Venous Thromboembolism (VTE)

Anticoagulation therapy is required for patients experiencing a DVT during pregnancy. Therapeutic doses of heparin will be given for the duration of the pregnancy. Anticoagulation therapy is recommended for 6 months following the pregnancy for the first VTE and for life if it is a recurrent VTE. Warfarin is usually the anticoagulant used following delivery. A temporary inferior vena caval (IVC) filter may be placed to decrease the risk of a pulmonary embolism.

Heparin Therapy

Heparin is the anticoagulant of choice during pregnancy. The dosing of heparin depends on whether the patient is at risk for or has an acute thromboembolism. The therapeutic anticoagulation dosing is used if the patient has an acute venous thromboembolism. The thromboprophylaxis dosing is used if the patient has a positive prior history of DVT during pregnancy or associated with hormonal contraceptives; a known thrombophilia and history of DVT or a positive family history of DVT; or is positive for antiphospholipid syndrome (APS). Reference the American College of Chest Physicians evidence-based clinical practice guidelines for specific recommendations (Bates and others, 2008). Table 14-1 provides an outline for heparin dosing.

Table 14-1   Heparin Dosing for APS During Pregnancy

Heparin Type	Dosing
Thromboprophylaxis Dosing Protocols	
Unfractionated heparin (UFH)	First trimester: 5000 units twice a day
	Second trimester: 7500 units twice a day
	Third trimester: 10,000 units twice a day
Low-molecular-weight heparin (LMWH)	Enoxaparin (Lovenox): 40 mg once a day or 30–80 mg every 12 hours (to achieve a level of antifactor Xa of 0.2–0.4 U/ml 4 hours postinjection)
Therapeutic Anticoagulation Dosing Protocols	
Unfractionated heparin (UFH)	Subcutaneous injections every 8-12 hours or continuous heparin pump to achieve an activated partial thromboplastin time (aPTT) level of 1.5–2 baseline except in the presence of lupus anticoagulants, then antifactor Xa of 0.4–0.7 U/ml)
Low-molecular-weight heparin (LMWH)	Weight adjusted: Enoxaparin: 1–1.5 mg/kg every 12 hours or Tinzaparin: 175 U/kg once daily (to achieve a level of antifactor Xa of 0.4–0.7 U/ml)

Data from Lockwood C: Thromboembolic disease in pregnancy. In Creasy R, Resnik R, Iams J, Lockwood C, Moore T, editors: *Creasy & Resnik's maternal-fetal medicine: principles and practice*, ed 6, Philadelphia, 2009, Saunders; Weiner C, Buhimschi C: *Drugs for pregnant and lactating women*, ed 2, Philadelphia, 2009, Saunders.

There are two types of heparin: low molecular-weight heparins (LMWHs) and unfractionated heparin (UFH). Both forms of heparin do not cross the placenta and are considered acceptable during pregnancy. UFH is less expensive. LMWHs have the advantage of a longer half-life and reduced risk of heparin-induced thrombocytopenia (ACOG, 2007; Weiner and Buhimschi, 2009). Because of its longer half-life compared with unfractionated heparin, it is not the preferred heparin to be used just prior to the intrapartum period, especially if an epidural or spinal regional anesthetic is planned for pain relief or cesarean birth. Unfractionated heparin is also more effectively reversed with protamine, whereas LMWH is more resistant to reversal (Lockwood, 2009).

There are some risks associated with heparin therapy, which must be addressed with patients. Long-term therapy carries a risk for contributing to loss of bone density. Therefore additional calcium should be supplemented daily. When given in multiple dose subcutaneous injections, it must be given using an atraumatic technique. Using ice before and after the injection helps alleviate bruising.

Pregnant women are advised to use the abdomen for injection because the absorption rate is less likely to be affected and because the abdomen has a large fatty "apron" providing good subcutaneous tissue. The concentration of heparin also affects the amount of bruising. Whenever possible, the most concentrated form should be used to deliver no more than 0.5 ml per injection.

Low-molecular-weight heparin

LMWH is given subcutaneously or intravenously once or twice daily. Because of the increased drug clearance during pregnancy, twice a day dosing may be necessary to obtain therapeutic levels. Some recommend following plasma antifactor Xa levels during pregnancy to ensure a therapeutic level (Fox, Laughon, Bender, Saltzman, and Rebarber, 2008).

Unfractionated heparin

Heparin maybe delivered intravenously, subcutaneously by pump, or two or three times a day with subcutaneous injections. When delivered through a pump, it is given at continuous levels. When the drug is given in multiple injections, it is important to give it at regular intervals. Activity of UFH is measured by activated partial thromboplastin time except in the presence of lupus anticoagulants. In these patients, protamine sulfate or an antifactor Xa should be used (Lockwood, 2009).

Treatment of Pulmonary Embolism

In the event of a life-threatening pulmonary embolism, the first priority is to stabilize the airway, breathing, and circulation, initiate intravenous unfractionated heparin, and then transfer to the intensive care unit. Thrombolytic therapy, percutaneous catheter thrombus fragmentation, or surgical embolectomy may be used after consideration of the risks (Dresang, Fontaine, Leeman, and King, 2008; RCOG, 2007).

NURSING MANAGEMENT

Nursing Interventions for Antepartum Anticoagulation Therapy

In the event that anticoagulants become necessary, if injections are subcutaneous, be prepared to teach or reinforce heparin administration as follows (Auerbach and Lockwood, 2004):

- The sites should be rotated in the fatty tissue of the thighs, hips, and abdomen.
- The area should be cleansed with alcohol in a circular motion and then iced for 1 minute with an ice cube to reduce bruising.
- The injection should be given in one motion without aspiration. A syringe with a short, 25-gauge needle should be used.
- The area should not be rubbed after the injection. Ice may be used following the injection.
- A return demonstration of the technique can be provided with normal saline.
- At least three correctly executed injections should be demonstrated by the woman and also by one family member.
- Instruct the woman to report side effects, such as bleeding gums, nose-bleeds, and easy bruising or excessive tissue trauma at injection sites.
- A pump designed for home use can also infuse heparin continuously subcutaneously.

Home nursing care personnel should be involved in the setup and administration of heparin with this unit.

Intrapartum and Postpartum Management of Patients on Heparin

- For patients on full-dose anticoagulation heparin for an acute thromboembolic diagnosis, artificial heart valve, or chronic atrial fibrillation, change to intravenous heparin to take advantage of its short half-life (1½ hours).
- Other patients requiring full-dose anticoagulation may be managed with prophylactic doses of heparin during the labor and delivery period.
- Patients on prophylactic heparin anticoagulation should be instructed to withhold their heparin injections at the onset of labor.
- To minimize epidural and spinal hematoma risk, LMWH is best stopped 24 hours before regional anesthesia if on twice daily therapeutic doses and 24 hours prior on once daily prophylactic dosing (ACOG, 2007). Therefore it is preferred to switch the patient to unfractionated heparin at around 36 weeks of gestation. LMWH should not be restarted until 12 hours following removal of the epidural or spinal catheter (Weiner and Buhimschi, 2009).
- Epidural anesthesia appears to be safe in women taking unfractionated, prophylactic heparin if the partial thromboplastin time (PTT) is normal. If necessary, unfractionated heparin is effectively reversed with protamine.
- Unfractionated heparin can be resumed following a vaginal delivery within 4 to 6 hours and 12 hours after a cesarean. If the patient is switched to Coumadin, there must be an overlap with heparin for the first 4 to 5 days. Coumadin creates a rapid decrease in protein C. Therefore overlapping with heparin is important to prevent paradoxical thromboembolism. An International Normalized Ratio (INR) measures therapeutic or prophylactic levels. For therapeutic dosing, an INR of 2 to 3 is desired. For prophylactic dosing, an INR of 1 to 2 is desired. Anticoagulants should be continued for at least 6 weeks following delivery related to the increased risk for embolic formation. With a history of any thrombolic event, lifelong anticoagulation is indicated (Bates and others, 2008).
- Warfarin is safe during breastfeeding.

CONCLUSION

One of the primary goals of care of the pregnant woman is to prevent venous thromboembolism. Early recognition of conditions that predispose a woman to thromboembolism can help prevent maternal death as well as promote a healthy newborn outcome. When a pregnant woman presents with signs of a venous thromboembolism, it is important to treat appropriately with anticoagulation. In the presence of a life-threatening pulmonary embolism, stabilization is the first priority. Thrombolytic therapy, percutaneous catheter thrombus fragmentation, or surgical embolectomy may be used (Dresang, Fontaine, Leeman, and King, 2008).

BIBLIOGRAPHY

Amaragiri SV, Lees T: Elastic compression stockings for prevention of deep vein thrombosis, *Cochrane Database Syst Rev* (Issue 3), Art. No.: CD001484, 2003.

American College of Obstetricians and Gynecologists (ACOG): Prevention of deep vein thrombosis and pulmonary embolism, *Clinical Management Guidelines for Obstetricians - Gynecologists*, No. 84, Washington, DC, 2007, ACOG.

Auerbach R, Lockwood C: The diagnosis and treatment of thromboembolic disease in pregnancy. In Foley M, Strong T, Garite T, editors: *Obstetric intensive care*, ed 2, New York, 2004, McGraw-Hill.

Bates S, Greer I, Pabinger I, and others: Venous thromboembolism, thrombophilia, antithrombotic therapy, and pregnancy: American college of chest physicians evidence-based clinical practice guidelines, ed 8, *Chest* 133(6 Suppl):844S–886S, 2008. Retrieved from http://www.guidelines.gov.

Blanco-Molina A, Trujillo-Santos J, Criado J, and others: Venous thromboembolism during pregnancy or postpartum: findings for the RIETE Registry, *Thromb Haemost* 97(2):186–190, 2007.

Chen W, Anand S, Ginsberg J: Anticoagulation of pregnant women with mechanical heart valves: a systematic review of the literature, *Arch Intern Med* 160:191–196, 2000.

Dresang L, Fontaine P, Leeman L, King V: Venous thromboembolism during pregnancy, *Am Fam Physician* 77(12):1709–1716, 2008.

Fox N, Laughon K, Bender S, Saltzman D, Rebarber A: Anti-factor Xa plasma levels in pregnant women receiving low molecular weight heparin thromboprophylaxis, *Obstet Gynecol* 112(4):884–889, 2008.

Greer I, Nelson-Piercy C: Low-molecular-weight heparins for thromboprophylaxis and treatment of venous thromboembolism in pregnancy: a systematic review of safety and efficacy, *Blood* 106(2): 401–407, 2005.

James A, Jamison M, Brancazio L, Myers M: Venous thromboembolism during pregnancy and the postpartum period: incidence, risk factors, and mortality, *Am J Obstet Gynecol* 194:1311–1315, 2006.

Kakkos SK, Caprini JA, Geroulakos G, and others: Combined intermittent pneumatic leg compression and pharmacological prophylaxis for prevention of venous thromboembolism in high-risk patients, *Cochrane Database Syst Rev* (Issue 4), Art. No.: CD005258, 2008.

Kohro S, Yamakage M, Sato K, and others: Intermittent pneumatic foot compression can activate blood fibrinolysis without changes in blood coagulability and platelet activation, *Acta Anaesthesiol Scand* 49:660–664, 2005.

Krivak T, Zorn K: Venous thromboembolism in obstetrics and gynecology, *Obstet Gynecol* 109(3): 761–777, 2007.

Kyrle P, Eichinger S: Deep vein thrombosis, *Lancet* 365:1163–1174, 2005.

Lockwood C: Thromboembolic disease in pregnancy. In Creasy R, Resnik R, Iams J, Lockwood C, Moore T, editors: *Creasy & Resnik's maternal-fetal medicine: principles and practice*, ed 6, Philadelphia, 2009, Saunders.

Magee K, Sevcik WW, Moher D, Rowe BH: Low molecular weight heparins versus unfractionated heparin for acute coronary syndromes, *Cochrane Database Syst Rev* (Issue 1), Art. No.: CD002132, 2003.

Marik P, Plante L: Current concepts: venous thromboembolic disease and pregnancy, *N Eng J Med* 359(19):2025–2033, 2008.

Robertson L, Wu O, Langhorne P, and others (for the Thrombosis Risk and Economic Assessment of Thrombophilia Screening (TREATS) Study): Thrombophilia in pregnancy: a systematic review, *Br J Haematol* 132(2):171–196, 2006.

Royal College of Obstetricians and Gynaecologists (RCOG): Guidelines and Audit Committee of the RCOG: *Thromboembolic disease in pregnancy and the puerperium: acute management*, Green-top Guideline No. 28, London, 2007, RCOG. Retrieved from http://www.rcog.org.uk.

Segal J, Steiff M, Hofmann L, and others: Management of venous thromboembolism: a systematic review for a practice guideline, *Ann Intern Med* 146(3):211–222, 2007.

Stella C, Ghulmiyyah L, Sibai B: Thrombophilia and adverse maternal-perinatal outcomes, *Female Patient* 31:42–48, 2006.

Urbano F: Homans' sign in the diagnosis of deep venous thrombosis, *Hosp Physician* (3):22–24, 2001. Retrieved from http://www.jcomjournal.com/pdf/hp_mar01_homan.pdf.

van Dongen CJ, van den Belt AGM, Prins MH, Lensing A: Fixed dose subcutaneous low molecular weight heparins versus adjusted dose unfractionated heparin for venous thromboembolism, *Cochrane Database Syst Rev* (Issue 3), Art. No.: CD001100, 2004.

Weiner C, Buhimschi C: *Drugs for pregnant and lactating women*, ed 2, Philadelphia, 2009, Saunders.

Zotz R, Gerhardt A, Scharf R: Prediction, prevention, and treatment of venous thromboembolic disease in pregnancy, *Semin Thromb Hemost* 29(2):143–154, 2003.

15

Pulmonary Disease and Respiratory Distress

regnancy complicated by pulmonary disease can be dangerous to both maternal well-being and fetal outcome. Understanding alterations in pulmonary physiology and the additional changes in immune responses that occur during pregnancy can help the health care provider anticipate problems and prevent complications in patients with chronic and acute pulmonary disease. This chapter reviews the management of cystic fibrosis, asthma, respiratory infections, and respiratory emergencies such as acute respiratory distress syndrome (ARDS), pulmonary embolism, and anaphylactoid syndrome of pregnancy in the pregnant patient.

INCIDENCE

Pulmonary diseases have become more prevalent in the general population and in pregnant women.

Cystic Fibrosis

Thick, viscid secretions that lead to multisystem dysfunctions such as chronic pulmonary disease, malabsorption, insufficient pancreatic enzymes, nasal polyps, sinusitis, and elevated sweat electrolyte concentrations characterize cystic fibrosis, an autosomal recessive disease. This disease is caused by mutations in the cystic fibrosis transmembrane regulator (*CFTR*) gene localized on chromosome 7. It occurs most often (1:3200) in the white European and Ashkenazi Jewish ethnic groups, with a carrier rate of 4%. In addition, when the paternal parent is also a known carrier, the risk to the fetus is a 1:2 chance. Because women with cystic fibrosis now live longer and have improved quality of life, they face the new complication of pregnancy. The median age of survival of women with cystic fibrosis is about 37 years, and the disease occurs in 1 of 2000 births. Because of abnormally dense cervical mucus, women with cystic fibrosis are thought to have lower fertility rates (Whitty and Dombrowski, 2009).

Asthma

Reversible airway obstruction and bronchial hyperresponsiveness characterize asthma, a chronic inflammatory disorder of the tracheobronchial airways. Asthma is the most common serious medical condition to complicate pregnancy (Whitty and

Dombrowski, 2009), occurring in 4% to 8% of the general population and occurring in pregnancy at the same rate (Kwon, Belanger, and Bracken, 2003; Dombrowski and others, 2004; Dunlop and others, 2008).

Respiratory Infections

Respiratory infections that may have a significant effect on pregnancy outcome include bronchitis, pneumonia, and tuberculosis. Bronchitis progressing to pneumonia complicates 0.1% to 1% of all pregnancies. It is important to distinguish bronchitis from pneumonia because pneumonia is more dangerous. Tuberculosis, once considered rare in the United States, is now increasing in women of childbearing years. In endemic areas around the world, tuberculosis may occur in 0.1% of pregnancies. Endemic areas include countries with high tuberculosis prevalence or long-term facilities, such as prisons or mental health facilities. The risk of tuberculosis is increased among health care workers and immigrants, and in patients with a positive history for human immunodeficiency virus (HIV), alcohol addition, and intravenous drug use.

Respiratory Emergencies

Respiratory emergencies are rare in pregnancy and include pulmonary embolism, anaphylactoid syndrome of pregnancy (formerly called *amniotic fluid embolism*), and ARDS. Respiratory emergencies are generally secondary to other physiologic complications. Patients may have acute asthmatic exacerbation or, through drug exposure, be at risk for respiratory alkalosis, acidosis, or infections. Pulmonary embolism may occur in as many as 60% to 80% of patients with untreated or inadequately treated deep vein thromboses (DVTs) (Sharma, 2006). It is the leading cause (46%) of pregnancy-related deaths (Cox, Kilpatrick, and Geller, 2004).

Anaphylactoid syndrome of pregnancy is a rare but extremely dangerous obstetric complication; the exact incidence is unknown; the complication is unpreventable and unpredictable. It is currently thought that the entry of amniotic fluid and fetal cells into the maternal circulation in certain patients triggers an anaphylactic reaction, causing an acute onset of maternal dyspnea and hypotension, followed shortly by cardiopulmonary collapse; of clients who survive the acute event, 40% develop ARDS, left-sided heart failure, as well as severe disseminated intravascular coagulation (DIC) and multisystem organ failure. When it does occur, there is a reported 60% to 80% maternal mortality and of the 20% to 40% that survive, 85% will have resulting neurologic damage (Clark and Dildy, 2004; Moore, 2008).

ARDS in pregnancy is also very rare. The outcome for mother and fetus is variable and depends on the underlying cause and the extent of other organ or system involvement.

ETIOLOGY

Infections are frequently identified as being caused by viruses, influenza, *Streptococcus pneumoniae, Haemophilus influenzae, Mycoplasma, Chlamydia,* or tuberculosis. These infections may also cause respiratory complications in women already compromised by asthma or cystic fibrosis. The etiology of pulmonary emboli is usually DVT, whereas the etiology of anaphylactoid syndrome of pregnancy is unknown. ARDS is often preceded by respiratory sepsis, infections such as varicella or herpes simplex virus, severe preeclampsia/eclampsia, severe hemorrhage, or severe trauma/injury (Martin and Foley, 2009).

NORMAL PHYSIOLOGY

In pregnancy, the following alterations in respiratory anatomy and physiology occur:
- The lower ribs flare out, and the subcostal angle and transverse diameter of the chest increase.
- The diaphragm rises by approximately 4 cm.
- Progesterone stimulates the respiratory centers to produce hyperventilation and a sensation of dyspnea.
- Because of hyperventilation, there is a decrease in alveolar tension and PCO_2 relative to respiratory alkalosis; compensation for decreased plasma bicarbonate.

To understand respiratory function as it relates to pregnancy, it is important to understand some of the following basic terminology:
- *Functional residual capacity.* The most important parameter for the health care provider to understand. It is the volume of the lungs at the end of a normal exhalation. It is affected by several factors:
  - Supine position
  - Obesity
  - Pregnancy
  - Impaired chest wall mechanics
  - Thoracoabdominal splinting
  - Ascent of the diaphragm (as with abdominal distention)
  - Increased airway resistance
  - Atelectasis
  - Decreased removal of secretions
  - General anesthesia
  - Pulmonary edema
- *Vital capacity.* The volume of air expired with maximal inspiration. It is the effective working volume of the lungs and correlates well with deep breathing and effective coughing. It decreases in patients with restrictive lung diseases such as asthma, cystic and pulmonary fibrosis, massive ascites, pneumothorax, and pleural effusion. During a normal pregnancy it does not change.
- *Tidal volume.* The volume of gas that moves in and out of the lungs during normal, quiet breathing. It decreases with weaker lung compliance, lessened respiratory muscle strength, and anesthesia; it increases in pregnancy by 50%.
- *Closing capacity.* The lung volume at which small airways begin to close. Normally, functional residual capacity is greater than closing capacity.
- *Dead space.* The anatomic area where gas exchange does not occur. In pulmonary embolism there is dead space.

PATHOPHYSIOLOGY

Infections of the respiratory system, asthma, and cystic fibrosis can all lead to obstruction of the airway and alveoli. Obstruction causes an inability to clear CO_2 and results in hypercarbia. Patients with obstructive pulmonary disease may also be unable to breathe in sufficient amounts of oxygen. Hypoxia is the major threat to the fetus because the maternal-fetal placental unit depends on a passive system of oxygen uptake and the fetus grows in a lower PO_2 than its host, the mother.

SIGNS AND SYMPTOMS
General Signs of Respiratory Distress

Dyspnea

Most women experience dyspnea at some time during a normal pregnancy. It may be a normal response to the anatomic pressure of the gravid uterus against the diaphragm and the conscious awareness of an increase in respiratory rate. Dyspnea is also a classic symptom of respiratory disease and distress, especially when coupled with prolonged expiratory phase hypoxemia.

Because respiratory physiology in a normal pregnancy tends toward respiratory alkalosis, hypoxemia is initially not accompanied by a corresponding increase in CO_2 (hypercarbia). Hypercarbia generally occurs in severe hypoxemia.

Leukocytosis

The complete blood cell count may show an increase in leukocytes, with a left shift on differential if there is a bacterial infection. If mycoplasmal pneumonia is present, an increase in the sedimentation rate is common also. Hemoconcentration also may be seen.

Cough

A productive cough may be seen in cystic fibrosis as a normal part of the disease. If it produces thick, dark, bloody, or rusty-colored sputum, infection is probably superimposed. Productive cough in an asthmatic pregnant woman should be treated as an infection in the respiratory tract. Any thick or colored mucus that is produced with coughing is presumed to be a sign of infection.

Other Signs

Other signs and symptoms of respiratory distress include the following:
- Fever
- Sudden onset of chills
- Chest pain, pleuritic pain
- Bronchial breath sounds
- Purulent sputum
- Chest dullness
- Decreased breath sounds
- Rales, crackles
- Egophony, whispered pectoriloquy

A chest radiographic film may show infiltration and either segmental or lobar consolidation.

Asthma Exacerbations Signs

Clinical manifestations of asthma exacerbation are progressively worsening symptoms of cough, wheezing, shortness of breath, chest tightness, and sputum production (NAEPP, 2005). These symptoms occur on a continuum ranging from mild persistent to severe life-threatening.

Anaphylactoid Syndrome of Pregnancy Signs

Anaphylactoid syndrome of pregnancy presents as sudden combined cardiovascular and respiratory collapse during labor, delivery, or within the first 30 minutes postpartum. Classic signs are:

- Acute onset of respiratory distress, often during labor, delivery, or within 30 minutes following delivery
  - Unexpected, rapid onset dyspnea
  - Facial erythema
  - Cough
  - Cyanosis
  - Chest pain
  - Seizures
  - Restlessness
  - Pulmonary edema
- Acute onset of circulatory collapse
  - Severe hypoxia
  - Severe hypotension

If the patient does not die from the initial respiratory insult, she needs to overcome the severe hemorrhage and coagulation that follow.

- Acute onset of coagulation
  - Uterine bleeding at delivery is not easily controlled.
  - Oozing may begin from puncture sites.

MATERNAL EFFECTS

Cystic Fibrosis

The physiologic changes of pregnancy are not tolerated as well by the patient with cystic fibrosis, which increases the risk for respiratory decompensation and therefore increases maternal mortality. If the patient has malnutrition, liver disease, pancreatic failure, or severe lung disease such as hypoxemia or pulmonary hypertension, maternal mortality is significantly increased. Labor is an especially vulnerable time, with risk for possible heart failure.

Asthma

Asthma seems to have no consistent effect on pregnancy. The severity of the disease is unchanged in 33% of pregnant women with asthma, is improved in 33%, and is worsened in 33% (Revan, Sun, and McMorris, 2002). If it worsens, the more severe symptoms usually occur during gestational weeks 17 to 24. A pregnancy factor that may promote asthma improvement is the fact that pregnancy hormones—progesterone and prostaglandins—have a natural bronchodilator effect. Factors that may exacerbate asthma during pregnancy are:

- Pulmonary refractoriness to cortisol
- Increased susceptibility to respiratory infection related to immune system changes
- Increased risk for gastroesophageal reflex disease (GERD)

In women with adequately controlled asthma during pregnancy, their risk of complications is no greater than nonasthmatic women (ACOG, 2008; Dunlop and others, 2008). However, uncontrolled asthma during pregnancy increases the risk for preeclampsia, hypertension, and hyperemesis gravidarum. In women with adequately controlled asthma during pregnancy, their risk of complications is not greater than nonasthmatic women (ACOG, 2008; Dunlop and others, 2008).

Respiratory Infections

Bronchitis poses little threat to pregnant women except that it may more readily progress to pneumonia. Pneumonia is the most common non-obstetric infection to cause maternal mortality during pregnancy (Whitty and Dombrowski, 2009). Pneumonia frequently is accompanied by a productive cough. Because of the anatomic accommodations to the respiratory system in pregnancy, forceful coughing to raise sputum may be more difficult. It is also more likely to cause painful separation of the cartilage between ribs and occasionally a spontaneous pneumothorax (Whitty and Dombrowski, 2009).

Respiratory Emergencies

Pulmonary embolism is the leading cause of maternal mortality with an approximately 15% risk for maternal death in the presence of a pulmonary emboli (Gates, Brocklehurst, and Davis, 2002).

ARDS can be the final result of several different obstetric complications, including inhalation of gastric contents during anesthesia and disseminated intravascular coagulation, as seen in preeclampsia, eclampsia, abruptio placentae, dead fetus syndrome, anaphylactoid syndrome of pregnancy, sepsis, infections associated with varicella or herpes simplex virus, severe hemorrhage, and acute exacerbation of asthma. All of these can be fatal to the mother.

FETAL EFFECTS

The greatest fetal threat is hypoxemia secondary to any condition that leads to acute respiratory emergencies. Chronic respiratory disease, such as asthma and cystic fibrosis (CF), can result in uteroplacental insufficiency, intrauterine growth restriction, and prematurity. A true respiratory emergency, such as pulmonary embolism or anaphylactoid syndrome of pregnancy, may necessitate emergency cesarean delivery at the same time that maternal resuscitation is being attempted. If maternal hypoxia and respiratory acidosis occur, the fetal brain is vulnerable to the resultant fetal hypoxia. Depending on the degree of hypoxia and the timing of the event in fetal gestational age, the fetus may suffer some degree of irreversible brain damage or death.

DIAGNOSTIC TESTING

Cystic Fibrosis

In 2001, the American College of Obstetricians and Gynecologists (ACOG), the American College of Medical Genetics (ACMG), and the National Institutes of Health (NIH) initiated carrier screening protocols for cystic fibrosis (Shulman and Elias, 2001) for the following individuals:

- Adults with a positive family history of CF
- Partners of individuals with CF
- White couples of European and Ashkenazi Jewish heritage planning a pregnancy or seeking prenatal care

The 25 ACMG/ACOG (25-mutation testing panel) is used (The Reference Laboratory at the Cleveland Clinic, 2004).

Asthma

People with asthma have airways that are hyperresponsive to stimuli such as allergens, viruses, air pollutants, exercise, and cold air. The hyperactivity is manifested by bronchospasm, mucosal edema, and mucus plugging in the airways, with hyperinflation of the lungs. Because of the inflammation in airway mucosa, forced expiratory volume (FEV_1) measured with a spirometer or peak expiratory flow rate (PEFR) measured with a peak flow meter (Table 15-1) can help to objectively quantify the degree of obstruction. Measurement of these two values is also useful in monitoring the effectiveness of treatment (NAEPP, 2005; ACOG, 2008).

Diagnostic Testing for Respiratory Compromise

Diagnostic testing is the same for pregnant women as for nonpregnant women. The following tests are routine when respiratory compromise is evident:

- Complete blood cell count
- Sputum culture
- Oxygenation by pulse oximetry
- Chest radiograph with abdominal shield
- Oxygenation by pulse oximetry
- Arterial blood gases when oxygen saturation remains less than 95% (Table 15-1)
- Pulmonary function tests (Table 15-2)

Table 15-1   Arterial Blood Gas Values in Pregnant and Nonpregnant Women

	pH	Po_2 (mm Hg)	Pco_2 (mm Hg)	HCO_3 (mEq/L)
Pregnant	7.40–7.46	80–106	26–32	18–22
Nonpregnant	7.35–7.45	75–100	35–45	22–26

Data from Bolorowski R: Maternal-fetal blood gas physiology. In Dildy G, and others, editors: *Critical care obstetrics*, ed 4, New York, 2004, Blackwell; Epocrates, 2009.

Table 15-2   Comparison of Pulmonary Values in Pregnant and Nonpregnant Women

Definition of Terms	Nonpregnant	Pregnant	Clinical Significance
Tidal Volume (V_T) = amount of air moved in one normal respiratory cycle	450 ml	600 ml	
RR = number of respirations per min	16/min	Slight increase	
Minute ventilation = volume of air moved per min; $V_T \times RR$	7.2 L	9.6 L	Increased O_2 available to fetus
FEV_1	80%–85% of vital capacity	Unchanged	Valuable to measure because there is no change
PEFR		Unchanged	Valuable to measure because there is no change
FVC = maximum amount of air that can be moved from maximum inspiration to maximum expiration	3.5 L	Unchanged	If over 1 L, pregnancy usually tolerated well
RV = amount of air that remains in lung at end of a maximal expiration	1000 ml	Decreases to approximately 800 ml	Improves gas transfer from alveoli to blood

FEV_1, Forced expiratory volume in 1 second; $PEFR$, peak expiratory flow rate; FVC, forced vital capacity; RR, respiratory rate; RV, residual volume; V_T, tidal volume.

In addition, if DVT is suggested, compression ultrasonography is the preferred test. When pulmonary embolism is suspected, chest x-ray with lead apron fetal shielding, spiral computed axial tomography, and a D-dimer assay may be obtained (Farquharson and Greaves, 2005). If an anaphylactoid syndrome of pregnancy is suggested, coagulation blood studies are ordered during the critical care recovery, after initial resuscitation (Anthony, 2005).

Blood Gas Interpretation

Interpretation of blood gases should be done in a systematic fashion, beginning with the pH. Normal adult pH is 7.35 to 7.45. A pH of less than 7.35 indicates acidemia. Next, it is important to understand whether the pH is primarily respiratory or metabolic (i.e., from respiratory failure or from kidney failure) or whether it is mixed, stemming from both problems.

To sort out the blood gases, both the pH and the pulmonary arterial carbon dioxide ($PaCO_2$) must be evaluated in relationship to the relative change in the pH.

If the following three scenarios are examined, it is possible to determine the degree of acidosis:

- $PaCO_2$ is high, but pH is relatively low: *simple respiratory acidosis*
- $PaCO_2$ is high, but pH is lower than expected: *mixed metabolic and respiratory acidosis*
- $PaCO_2$ and pH are both low: *simple metabolic acidosis*

A pH of greater than 7.45 indicates alkalemia. To sort out whether the cause is respiratory, metabolic, or mixed, consider the following (Gei and Suarez, 2004):

- $PaCO_2$ is high, and pH is also relatively high: *simple metabolic alkalosis*
- $PaCO_2$ is low, but pH is higher than expected: *mixed respiratory and metabolic alkalosis*
- $PaCO_2$ is low, but pH is high: *simple respiratory alkalosis*

Anaphylactoid Syndrome of Pregnancy

The diagnosis of anaphylactoid syndrome of pregnancy must be made from the clinical picture.

A definitive diagnosis is made only by ruling out other possible diagnoses such as septic shock, pulmonary embolism, eclampsia, placental abruption, uterine rupture, uterine atony, myocardial infarction, aortic dissection, or anaphylactic reaction to local anesthetic.

USUAL MEDICAL MANAGEMENT AND PROTOCOLS FOR NURSE PRACTITIONERS

Cystic Fibrosis

- Provide preconceptual counseling to enable the patient to be in optimal physical condition.
- Provide genetic counseling and carrier testing of the father.
- Perform pregnancy screen for such risk factors as severe lung disease, pulmonary hypertension using echocardiogram, poor nutritional status, or liver/pancreatic diseases.
- Consult with a pulmonary specialist or, ideally, a specialist in cystic fibrosis.
- Obtain a baseline and ongoing pulmonary function using forced vital capacity, FEV_1, lung volumes, and pulse oximetry.
- Assess for pulmonary hypertension with echocardiogram.
- Closely monitor nutritional status with ongoing diagnostic screens of total protein, serum albumin, prothrombin time related to vitamin K deficiency, and fat-soluble vitamins A and E.
- Provide dietary consultation; an increased caloric intake (20% to 50% above normal recommendation) is necessary because of decreased digestive enzymes.
- Closely monitor weight gain.
- Closely monitor for pulmonary infection.
- Treat pulmonary infections promptly and vigorously with antibiotics, fluids, and respiratory therapy to include physical therapy and bronchial drainage.
- Provide early screening for diabetes because it frequently occurs in women with cystic fibrosis.
- Assess fetal well-being and intrauterine growth pattern (refer to Chapter 3).

- During labor, monitor closely for right-sided heart failure. Be prepared to treat with diuretics and oxygen.
- Manage pain effectively to decrease pulmonary and cardiac workload.

Asthma

Asthma must be as aggressively treated during pregnancy as at any other time because the benefits of asthma control far outweigh the risks associated with the medications. Almost all common asthma medications are considered safe during pregnancy and lactation (NAEPP, 2005; ACOG, 2008). According to the NAEPP (2005), the following four management components are recommended for managing asthma during pregnancy:

- Ongoing monitoring of the disease, noting signs and symptoms, pulmonary function studies with a spirometer and peak expiratory meter, and history of asthma exacerbation
- Avoidance of triggers such as allergens, tobacco smoke, and pollutants/irritants
- Pharmacologic therapy using the stepwise approach (Table 15-3). Table 15-4 provides a summary of the most commonly used asthma medications during pregnancy.
- Education to promote self-management in collaboration with health care provider, correct use of inhalers, and management plan of acute exacerbations using the NAEPP (2005) algorithm

Respiratory Infections

Viral Bronchitis or Upper Respiratory Infection

The most common respiratory infections during pregnancy are viral bronchitis and the common cold. These should never be treated with antibiotics. The best care is supportive: keep track of fever, contact health care provider if fever is higher than 102° F, increase fluids, use nasal saline spray, use humidifiers at bedtime, and occasionally use a nasal corticosteroid (no more than twice daily).

Nasal congestion is often more pronounced during pregnancy because of the hormonal influences on mucosal swelling. Treating nasal congestion also treats the cough, frequently because the cough is caused by postnasal discharge. This symptom is generally worse at night. Avoid the use of an antitussive or expectorant such as guaifenesin during pregnancy and lactation unless the benefit justifies the potential perinatal risk (Weiner and Buhimschi, 2009).

If an antihistamine is necessary, chlorpheniramine and tripelennamine are the antihistamines of choice during pregnancy even though they are more sedating than the second-generation antihistamines, according to ACOG and the American College of Allergy, Asthma, and Immunology (2000). Whenever possible, avoid all oral decongestants during the first trimester.

Pneumonia

Pneumonia is an inflammation of the lower respiratory tract, including the alveoli and bronchioles. It may be caused by bacterial or viral invasion or chemical contact with the respiratory tract. Coinfection with HIV or tuberculosis may worsen the prognosis for mother and fetus.

Table 15-3 Stepwise Treatment Approach to Asthma During Pregnancy

	Step 1: Mild Intermittent	Step 2: Mild Persistent	Step 3: Moderate Persistent	Step 4: Severe Persistent
Peak expiratory flow	80%-100% of personal best	≤80% of personal best	60%-80% of personal best	<60% of personal best
Signs and symptoms	≤2 times/week	>2 time/wk but <1 time/day	Daily	Frequently
Exercise tolerance	Good	May not be affected	Diminished	Poor
Nocturnal waking	≤2 times/mo	>2 times/mo but <1 time/wk	>1 time/wk	Nightly
Work attendance	Good	May not be affected	Diminished	Poor
Treatment	Quick relief: Short-acting inhaled beta$_2$-agonist (Albuterol) Daily long-term control, none	Quick relief: Short-acting beta$_2$-agonist (Albuterol) Daily long-term control preferred treatment: low-dose inhaled corticosteroid (budesonide) Daily long-term control alternative treatment: Leukotriene mediator (montelukast or zafirlukast), mast cell stabilizer (cromolyn), or sustained-release (theophylline)	Quick relief: Short-acting beta$_2$-agonist (Albuterol) Daily long-term control low or medium-dose inhaled corticosteroid (budesonide and salmeterol) *or* inhaled corticosteroid (low or medium dose) and add either leukotriene receptor antagonist or sustained-release (theophylline)	Quick relief: Short-acting beta$_2$-agonist (Albuterol) Daily long-term control: high-dose inhaled corticosteroid (budesonide) *and* salmeterol *and if needed* oral corticosteroid tablets or syrup while making repeated attempts to reduce systemic steroids and maintain control with high-dose inhaled steroids

Data from National Asthma Education and Prevention Program (NAEPP): Managing asthma during pregnancy: recommendations for pharmacologic treatment — 2004 update, *J Allergy Clin Immunol* 115(1):34–46, 2005. Retrieved from http://www.nhlbi.nih.gov/halth/prof/lung/asthma/practgde.htm; American College of Obstetricians and Gynecologists (ACOG): Asthma in pregnancy, ACOG Practice Bulletin No. 90, *Obstet Gynecol* 111(2):457-464, 2008.

Table 15-4   Summary of Common Medications for Asthma During Pregnancy

Drug Class	Drug Action	Medication	Dose
Quick-Relief Medications			
Short-acting beta₂-agonists	Bronchodilators; relax smooth muscle of the bronchioles	Albuterol (Proventil)	MDI: 2–4 puffs q20min up to 4h; then q1–4h, then prn Use spacer
Long-Term Control Medications			
Inhaled corticosteroids	Antiinflammatory agents decrease edema and mucus secretions in the bronchioles by inhibiting the synthesis of leukotrienes and activation of inflammatory cells; use with a bronchodilator	Budesonide (Pulmicort)	Dry powder inhaler 200 mcg/inhalation Low daily dose: 200-600 mcg Medium daily dose: 600-1200 mcg High dose: more than 1200 mcg
Mast-cell stabilizers	Mild-to-moderate antiinflammatory agent that inhibits the degranulation of mast cells, blocking eosinophil chemotaxis and activation, improving asthma trigger control	Cromolyn sodium	MDI: 2–4 puffs tid/qid

Leukotriene mediators	Decreases bronchospasm, mucus secretion, and vascular permeability	Montelukast (Singulair) 10 mg po q PM Zafirlukast (Accolate) 20 mg po bid
Sustained-release theophylline	Mild-to-moderate bronchodilator used primarily with inhaled corticosteroids to prevent nocturnal asthma symptoms	Methylxanthines and various generic drugs (Theo-Dur, Slo-bid); theophylline blood levels may be followed with the use of this drug 100, 200, 300, or 450 mg bid
Oral (systemic corticosteroids)	Use of systemic steroids during pregnancy increases the risks for congenital malformation, preeclampsia, and preterm delivery; however, for severe asthma, the benefits still outweigh the risks	

Data from National Asthma Education and Prevention Program (NAEPP): Managing asthma during pregnancy: recommendations for pharmacologic treatment—2004 update, *J Allergy Clin Immunol* 115(1):34-46, 2005. Retrieved from *www.nhlbi.nih.gov/halth/prof/lung/asthma/asthma/practgde.htm*, National Asthma Education and Prevention Program (NAEPP): *Expert Panel Report 3 guidelines for the diagnosis and management of asthma*, Publication No. 08-5846, Bethesda, MD, 2007, National Heart, Lung, and Blood Institute, Nationals Institute of Health. Retrieved from *www.nhlbi.nih.gov/guidelines/asthma/asthsumm.pdf*.
MDI, Metered-dose inhaler.

Careful consideration should be given to such possible differential diagnoses as pulmonary embolism, asthma, and pulmonary edema prior to diagnosing pneumonia in pregnancy. A chest radiograph, arterial blood gases, arterial saturation with pulse oximetry, and both blood and sputum cultures are usually obtained to diagnose the extent of infection and identify the organism(s) responsible. If atypical bacterial infection is suspected, cold agglutinins are used to test for mycoplasma pneumonia (Whitty and Dombrowski, 2009).

Usually, therapy is started with a broad-spectrum antibiotic; then, once the specific causative organism or organisms are detected and reported with sensitivity, more specifically directed antibiotic therapy is used. For gram-negative and *Staphylococcus aureus* infection, a combination third-generation cephalosporin is usually used. Antibiotic therapies in pregnancy usually require high doses and continue for 10 to 14 days because of increased blood volume and dilution. Oxygen therapy should be provided as well.

For viral pneumonias, the course may be complicated by a secondary bacterial infection. Although broad-spectrum antibiotics such as cephalosporins may work for the secondary infection, antivirals such as amantadine are not used in pregnancy except in fulminant respiratory failure. Amantadine is both embryotoxic and teratogenic in animal studies and is therefore reserved for life-threatening disease in the pregnant woman. Acyclovir is currently recommended for varicella pneumonia in pregnant women.

According to the recently revised CDC guidelines, prepregnancy care should include advice about routine influenza vaccination with the inactivated vaccine if the pregnancy occurs during the influenza season (CDC, 2007). Pneumococcal vaccine is recommended before, but not during, pregnancy for high risk patients with conditions such as asthma, chronic pulmonary or cardiac disease, diabetes mellitus, or immune compromise disease (CDC, 2009).

Tuberculosis

Treatment regimens for tuberculosis include the following:
- Absence of active disease with less than 2 years converted PPD (purified protein derivative [tuberculin]) status is treated with 300 mg/day of isoniazid, starting after the first trimester and continuing for 6 to 9 months.
- Women younger than 35 years with an unknown duration of positive PPD result should receive 300 mg/day of isoniazid for 6 to 9 months postpartum.
- Women older than 35 years do not receive isoniazid unless they have active disease.
- Women with active disease in pregnancy are treated immediately with isoniazid (INH), 300 mg, combined with rifampin (RIF), 600 mg and ethambutol 1 grams daily for 2 months; then followed by INH and RIF for an additional 7 months.
- Pyridoxine (vitamin B_6), 50 mg/day, is an essential supplement for all patients taking INH to decrease hepatotoxicity.

Although isoniazid, ethambutol, and rifampin have been used in pregnancy with no adverse fetal effects, antituberculous agents that may not be used include streptomycin, kanamycin, ethionamide, capreomycin, cycloserine, and amikacin

(American Thoracic Society, CDC, and Infectious Diseases Society of America, 2003; CDC, 2009). There is minimal information about the safety of pyrazinamide (PZA) in pregnancy. However, it has been used if the benefit outweighs the potential risk (American Thoracic Society, CDC, and Infectious Diseases Society of America, 2003).

Breastfeeding is not contraindicated when antituberculous drugs are being used by the mother. A small amount of these drugs cross into breast milk but the amount does not produce toxicity in the nursing newborn according to the American Thoracic Society, CDC, and Infectious Diseases Society of America (2003; CDC, 2009).

NURSING MANAGEMENT

Prevention

Pregnant women with chronic diseases, such as cystic fibrosis and asthma, should be counseled before becoming pregnant about the importance of having their disease under good control, continuing good management, and avoiding exposure to environmental agents that may exacerbate or trigger disease response.

Pregnant women should be counseled during early pregnancy to avoid exposure to crowds of people during influenza season and during other acute respiratory disease outbreaks and to avoid exposure to people infected with HIV and tuberculosis. Because of the depressed immune response in normal, healthy pregnant women, they are more susceptible to contracting infections than are nonpregnant women.

Nursing Interventions for Respiratory Infections

- Discuss the risks of exposure to respiratory infections with the woman and her family.
- Encourage early treatment of upper respiratory signs and symptoms.
- Encourage health-promoting behaviors such as the following:
  - Avoid crowds during high infection incidence.
  - Use a cool mist humidifier at night to help the respiratory tract stay healthy.
  - Drink at least 8 oz of nutritious liquid or water each hour of the day while awake.
- Respond to detected or reported signs and symptoms, chest radiograph, and sputum and blood cultures, as warranted.
- Treat with appropriate oral or intravenous antibiotics, when necessary.
- Have baseline function studies in early pregnancy available for comparison of disease states.
- Seek and keep referrals and collaborate with pulmonary specialists.
- Use small volume nebulizers (SVNs) as needed in the acute phase if the woman is hospitalized; otherwise, an inhaler with spacer should be used with beta-agonists, antiinflammatories, and corticosteroids, as needed. There are actually two categories of medications to use:
  - *Rescuers.* These are beta-agonists such as albuterol and should be used only on an outpatient basis in conjunction with controllers (described next). If rescuers are used on an outpatient basis more than four times a day or more than

three times a week, several areas need to be evaluated: the patient's usage technique, the appropriate dosage of controllers, and any acute illness in the patient that would benefit from inpatient care.

- *Controllers.* These are corticosteroids, which may be taken orally or in inhaler form, and antihistamines, which are generally taken orally. Both may be used during pregnancy and in combination with each other, especially when there is an allergic component to the disease and resultant infection (see Tables 15-2, 15-3, and 15-4).
- Teach women with chronic respiratory tract disease how to self-detect and prevent preterm labor.

Antepartum Nursing Interventions for Pregnancy Complicated with Asthma

- Discuss the importance of maintaining asthma control during pregnancy. Inadequate asthma management increases the risk for adverse maternal and fetal outcomes. Systematic review of various asthma medications indicates the safety (with no increase in congenital abnormalities) of the following drugs: albuterol; Pulmicort Turbuhaler (budesonide inhalation powder), an inhaled corticosteroid; cromolyn; and leukotriene modifiers (montelukast and zafirlukast) (NAEPP, 2005; ACOG, 2008). Oral corticosteroids are associated with an increased risk for isolated cleft lip if taken during the first trimester, as well as an increased risk for preeclampsia and preterm delivery. However, for severe asthma, the benefits of oral corticosteroids still outweigh the risks.
- Assess for complementary alternative medicine use and advise accordingly. Emphasize that alternative healing methods are no substitute for prescribed pharmacologic therapy (Perlman and Serbin, 2001; NAEPP, 2005).
- Encourage management collaboration with the obstetric team and asthma and allergy specialists.
- Explain the difference between asthmatic and normal airways and what happens during an asthma attack.
- Reinforce the importance of not smoking, because smoking contributes to asthma.
- Teach the importance of avoiding environmental triggers, which include the following: inhalant allergens such as pollens and molds; dust mites; cockroach antigens; irritants such as cigarette smoke, spray cleaners, and colognes; nonspecific stimuli such as infections; foods such as wine, shellfish, wheat, eggs, nuts, or dairy products; and medicines such as aspirin and some nonsteroidal antiinflammatory drugs (NAEPP, 2005).
- Teach the importance of continuing all needed medications to control asthma without exacerbation or activity limitation. The benefits of medication have been shown to far outweigh the risks. Uncontrolled asthma is a more dangerous risk to both mother and baby than medication-controlled asthma.
- Teach correct use of inhalers with a spacer.
- Instruct the patient in the use of a peak flow meter; provide parameters for concern and increased use of rescuers, based on the patient's weight and height.

- Instruct the patient in the use of controllers and rescuers.
- Develop and explain the individualized asthma action plan for when and how to take rescue actions based on the stepwise treatment approach to asthma outlined in Table 15-3.
- Demonstrate how to use the peak flow meter and explain that it should be used with moderate and severe persistent asthma or to help regulate medicine changes.
- Emphasize the importance of having an ultrasound during the first trimester to confirm the accuracy of the due date and having repeat ultrasounds during the second and third trimesters to follow fetal growth.
- Be prepared to implement fetal surveillance tests such as fetal movement counts and biophysical profiles with nonstress tests by 32 weeks of gestation.
- Teach to self-detect signs of preterm contractions.
- Teach the importance of adequate calories and nutrients. Make appropriate referrals to a dietitian, the WIC (Women, Infants, and Children) program, and specialists in high risk pregnancy.
- Access educational materials from the following Internet sites:
  - American College of Allergy, Asthma, & Immunology Patient Education: *Managing Asthma and Allergies during Pregnancy*. Available at http://www.acaai.org/public/advice/pregnasth.htm
  - National Heart, Lung, and Blood Institute: *Practical Guide for the Diagnosis and Management of Asthma*. Available at http://www.niehs.nih.gov/health/docs/asthma-plan.pdf

Intrapartum Nursing Interventions for Asthmatics

- Instruct the patient to continue her routine asthma medications.
- Assess PEFR at time of admission and every 4 to 12 hours dependent on severity of the asthma.
- Maintain adequate maternal oxygenation. A pulse oximetry may be used to evaluate maternal oxygenation status. Normal is greater than 95%.
- Maintain adequate hydration during labor.
- Monitor fetal well-being according to institutional protocol.
- Preferred analgesic to manage pain is fentanyl; avoid the use of histamine-releasing narcotics such as meperidine (Demerol) or morphine.
- If labor induction or augmentation is medically indicated, prostaglandin E_2 and oxytocin are safe (Whitty and Dombrowski, 2009).
- If the patient was on chronic oral corticosteroid therapy during pregnancy for more than 1 month, parenteral steroids (100 mg of hydrocortisone every 8 hours) are used during labor to prevent adrenal suppression.
- If cesarean delivery is indicated, lumbar anesthesia is the preferred method because it decreases oxygen consumption and minute ventilation; general anesthesia should be used only as a last resort (ACOG, 2008).
- Avoid carboprost (PGF_{2a}), ergotamine, and methergine for the treatment of postpartum hemorrhage because these drugs increase the risk of bronchospasms (Whitty and Dombrowski, 2009).

Postpartum Nursing Interventions for Asthmatics

- Assess the patient carefully for hemorrhage and respiratory distress.
- Discuss the importance of continuing the same asthma medications during breastfeeding. Only small amounts of asthma medications enter the breast milk (NAEPP, 2005). To decrease the medication in breast milk, instruct the patient to take asthma medications 15 minutes after breastfeeding.

Nursing Interventions for Acute Exacerbation of Asthma

- The goal is to prevent hypoxia.
- Be prepared to provide resuscitation as required.
- Position in semi-Fowler to improve ventilation.
- Administer oxygen per nonrebreather face mask or with CPAP as indicated and ordered.
- Establish IV access.
- Obtain a good history, if possible, of similar attacks and effective therapy.
- Ascertain how the patient is using a peak flow meter to monitor signs before initiating rescue medication because it is easy to confuse the shortness of breath that is normal during pregnancy with the shortness of breath that signals exacerbation of asthma.
- Evaluate patient understanding of how to use inhalers with a spacer. Perform an objective physical examination that includes auscultation of breath signs and addresses the following questions:
  - General appearance: Is the patient cyanotic?
  - Can she complete sentences without shortness of breath?
  - Can she walk across a room?
  - Is she using accessory muscles?
- Obtain some or all of the following additional data:
  - Temperature, pulse, and respiratory rate
  - Laboratory values for forced expiratory volume or peak expiratory flow rate (repeat after bronchial dilation treatment)
  - Pulse oximetry monitoring
  - Breath sounds with auscultation of all lung fields; mental status, skin color and for respiratory secretions.
  - Chest radiograph
  - Arterial blood gas levels (see Table 15-1), cardiac monitoring, and electronic fetal monitoring after point of viability
  - Monitor intake and output.
- Treat an acute exacerbation based on lung function (FEV_1 or PEF), oxygen saturation, and symptoms following the NAEPP algorithm: *Management of asthma exacerbation during pregnancy and lactation: home* and *Management of asthma exacerbation during pregnancy and lactation: emergency department and hospital-based care* (NAEPP, 2005). Albuterol, a short-acting inhaled beta$_2$ agonist, via nebulizer or MDI, is the initial treatment medication. Be prepared to give corticosteroids as well. If MDI or nebulized treatment is not effective, be prepared to administer terbutaline (0.25 mg) subcutaneously every 15 minutes for 3 doses.

- If infection is present, treat infection (see actual respiratory infection assessment and interventions).
- If the weeks of gestation are equal to or greater than 24 weeks, monitor the fetus during the acute phases, initially by 12 to 24 hours of electronic fetal monitoring and then by nonstress tests twice weekly or biophysical profiles when stable after 28 to 32 weeks of gestation. The fetus is also evaluated by ultrasound for growth rate every 3 to 4 weeks and the woman is taught how to assess fetal activity.

Critical Care Interventions for Respiratory Emergencies

- The goal is to prevent hypoxia.
- Be prepared to provide resuscitation as required.
- Be prepared to provide ventilation and oxygenation as indicated; administer oxygen per nonrebreather face mask or with CPAP.
- Position in semi-Fowler to improve ventilation.
- Establish IV access.
- Assess vital signs, breath sounds, mental status, skin color and respiratory secretion.
- Pulse oximetry monitoring
- Chest radiograph
- Arterial blood gas levels (see Table 15-1), and cardiac monitoring
- Drug screen and alcohol level
- Assess fetal status.
- Indications for endotracheal intubation according to Gei and Suarez (2004)
  - Gastropulmonary reflux and aspiration
  - Airway obstruction
  - Respiratory arrest
  - Depressed mental status
  - Difficulty managing secretions
- Indications for mechanical ventilation according to Gei and Suarez (2004)
  - Severe respiratory or combined respiratory and metabolic acidosis
  - Sustained respiratory rate of 40/min
  - Abnormal breathing pattern suggestive of increased respiratory workload and/or respiratory muscle fatigue
  - Depressed mental status
  - Severe hypoxemia

Critical Care Interventions of Acute Pulmonary Edema and Pulmonary Embolism

- Chest radiograph
- Magnetic resonance image or computed tomographic scan
- Contrast dye studies, if embolism suspected
- Elevation of head of bed
- Oxygen therapy via nonrebreather at 10 L/min or continuous positive airway pressure
- Establish IV access
- Nitroglycerine
- Continuous pulse oximetry and cardiac monitoring

- Furosemide
- Fetal heart and maternal blood pressure monitoring
- Digoxin as clinically indicated
- Anticoagulant therapy with heparin for therapeutic levels for embolism (see related Chapter 14); therapeutic levels will be necessary for the remainder of the pregnancy or for a minimum of 3 to 6 months after the pregnancy
- Cardioversion as clinically indicated
- Continuous electronic fetal heart rate monitoring
- In the presence of anaphylactoid syndrome of pregnancy, resuscitation is usually required. Cardiac output is increased with crystalloid fluids to replenish intravascular volume, and a vasopressor such as dopamine, norepinephrine, or epinephrine to treat acute hypotension (Clark and Dildy, 2004; Martin and Foley, 2009)

Critical Care Interventions of Anaphylactoid Syndrome of Pregnancy

- Recognize this life-threatening diagnosis.
- Provide supportive therapies of oxygen, maintaining cardiac output and organ perfusion, and correct DIC.
- Ensure IV access; if client does not have an IV line, start one immediately because a delay of even a few minutes may result in circulatory collapse and make IV access more difficult; consider having two IV lines in place.
- Initiate cardiopulmonary resuscitation (CPR) if indicated. If fetus is undelivered, be prepared for a perimortem cesarean delivery after 5 minutes of unsuccessful CPR.
- Administer oxygen to maintain normal saturation.
- Prepare for and assist with intubation and ventilation with 100% of the fractions of inspired oxygen (FiO_2) if patient loses consciousness.
- Administer crystalloid IV fluids rapidly if patient is hypotensive; if blood pressure is maintained, do not overload with fluids because it can result in pulmonary edema resulting from developing ARDS.
- Monitor vital signs, pulse oximetry, skin color, temperature, and moisture frequently.
- Have emergency medications to assist in patient stabilization, according to Moore (2008).
    - Dopamine (Intropin) to maintain perfusion by increasing myocardial contractility, increase systolic blood pressure, dilate renal vasculature, increase renal blood flow, and increase GFR
    - Digoxin (Lanoxin) to improve myocardial contractility
    - Hydrocortisone (Hydrocort, Cortef) to treat the immune response
    - Uterotonics postdelivery to enhance myometrial contractility to decrease uterine atony such as:
        - Oxytocin (Pitocin) to enhance myometrial contractions and decrease capillary permeability
        - Methylergonovine (Methergine) to promote stronger myometrial contractions by acting directly on the uterine smooth muscle
        - Carboprost tromethamine (Hemabate), a prostaglandin that promotes longer-lasting myometrial contractions

- Chest radiograph and 12-lead ECG to assist in hemodynamic management
- Observe for signs and symptoms of shock.
- Observe for signs and symptoms of coagulopathy (inability to control intra-partum or immediate postpartum vaginal bleeding or bleeding from IV site or puncture or trauma sites).
- Send laboratory work
  - Arterial blood gases
  - CBC
  - Platelet count
  - Fibrinogen
  - Fibrin degradation products
  - Partial thromboplastin time
  - Tryptase
- Prepare for and assist with placement of central line (a pulmonary artery catheter may be useful for further hemodynamic management).
- Administer blood; blood products such as packed RBCs, platelets, fresh-frozen plasma, and cryoprecipitate; or volume expanders as ordered.
- Prevent hypothermia by using warmed blankets and intravenous fluids.
- If fetus is undelivered, continuously monitor fetal heart rate and position mother to prevent vena cava syndrome.
- Inform and reassure patient and family as much as possible during crisis.

CONCLUSION

Respiratory disease can complicate a pregnancy, and pregnancy can complicate the management of acute or chronic respiratory disease. These complications require early health-promoting activities, prompt response and supervision, and close collaboration with pulmonary specialists.

BIBLIOGRAPHY

American College of Obstetricians and Gynecologists (ACOG) and American College of Allergy, Asthma, and Immunology: The use of newer asthma and allergy medications during pregnancy, *Ann Allergy Asthma Immunol* 84(5):475–480, 2000.

American College of Obstetricians and Gynecologists (ACOG): Asthma in pregnancy, ACOG practice Bulletin No. 90, *Obstet Gynecol* 111(2):457–464, 2008.

American Thoracic Society, Centers for Disease Control and Prevention (CDC), and Infectious Diseases society of America: Treatment of tuberculosis, *Am J Resp Crit Care Med* 167:603–662, 2003. Retrieved from http://www.cdc.gov/mmwr/preview/mmwrhtml/rr5211a1.htm#tab2

Anthony J: Critical care of the obstetric patient. In James D, and others, editors: *High risk pregnancy: management options*, ed 3, Philadelphia, 2005, Saunders.

Centers for Disease Control and Prevention (CDC): *Guidelines for vaccinating pregnant women*, Atlanta, 2007, Centers for Disease Control and Prevention. Retrieved from http://www.cdc.gov/vaccines/pubs/downloads/b_preg_guide.pdf.

Centers for Disease Control and Prevention (CDC): *Elimination: tuberculosis and pregnancy*, Atlanta, 2009, Centers for Disease Control and Prevention. Retrieved from http://www.michigan.gov/documents/mdch/pregnancy_193894_7.pdf.

Centers for Disease Control and Prevention (CDC): *Pneumococcal polysaccharide vaccine: what you need to know*, Atlanta, 2009, Centers for Disease Control and Prevention. Retrieved from http://www.cdc.gov/vaccines/pubs/vis/downloads/vis-ppv.pdf.

Clark S, Dildy G: Amniotic fluid embolism. In Foley M, Strong T, Garite T, editors: *Obstetric intensive care manual*, ed 2, New York, 2004, McGraw-Hill.

Cox S, Kilpatrick S, Geller S: Preventing maternal deaths, *Contemp Ob Gyn*, Sept 1, 2004.

Dombrowski M, and others: Asthma during pregnancy, *Obstet Gynecol* 103(1):5–12, 2004.

Dunlop A, and others: The clinical content of preconception care: women with chronic medical conditions, *Am J Obstet Gynecol* 199(6):S310–S327, 2008.

Farquharson R, Greaves M: Thromboembolic disease. In James D, and others, editors: *High risk pregnancy: management options*, ed 3, Philadelphia, 2005, Saunders.

Gates S, Brocklehurst P, Davis L: Prophylaxis for venous thromboembolic disease in pregnancy: the early postnatal period, *Cochrane Database Syst Rev* 2, CD001689, 2002.

Gei A, Suarez V: Respiratory emergencies during pregnancy. In Foley M, Strong T, Garite T, editors: *Obstetric intensive care manual*, ed 2, New York, 2004, McGraw-Hill.

Gilmore D, Wakim J, Secrest J, Rawson R: Anaphylactoid syndrome of pregnancy: a review of the literature with latest management and outcome data, *AANA J* 71(2):120–126, 2003.

Kwon H, Belanger K, Bracken M: Asthma prevalence among pregnant and childbearing-aged women in the United States: estimates from national health surveys, *Ann Epidemiol* 13(5):317–324, 2003.

Martin S, Foley M: Intensive care monitoring of the critically ill pregnant patient. In Creasy R, Resnik R, Iams J, Lockwood C, Moore T, editors: *Creasy & Resnik's Maternal-fetal medicine: principles and practice*, ed 6, Philadelphia, 2009, Saunders.

Moore L: Amniotic fluid embolism. *eMed Obstet Gynecol* August 12:1-13, 2008. Retrieved from http://emedicine.medscape.com/article/253068-overview.

National Asthma Education and Prevention Program (NAEPP): *Expert Panel Report 3 guidelines for the diagnosis and management of asthma*, Publication No. 08-5846, Bethesda, Md, Oct., 2007, National Heart, Lung, and Blood Institute, National Institutes of Health. Retrieved from http://www.nhlbi.nih.gov/guidelines/asthma/asthsumm.pdf.

National Asthma Education and Prevention Program (NAEPP): Managing asthma during pregnancy: recommendations for pharmacologic treatment—2004 update, *J Allergy Clin Immunol* 115(1):34-46, 2005. Retrieved from http://www.nhlbi.nih.gov/health/prof/lung/asthma/astpreg/astpreg_full.pdf.

Perlman A, Serbin J: Complementary and alternative medicine: does it have a role in treating asthma? *Womens Health Prim Care* 4:282, 2001.

Revan V, Sun E, McMorris M: Management of asthma in pregnancy, *Female Patient* 27(9):18, 2002.

Sharma S: Pulmonary embolism, *eMedicine*, 2006. Retrieved from http://emedicine.medscape.com/article/300901.

Shulman L, Elias S: Cystic fibrosis, *Clinics in Perinatol* 28(2):383-393, 2001.

The Reference Laboratory at the Cleveland Clinic: *Cystic fibrosis carrier screen for pregnant or pre-pregnant couples*, 2004. Retrieved from https://my.clevelandclinic.org/Documents/Pathology/TechnicalBriefs-Oct2004-CF.pdf.

Weiner C, Buhimschi C: *Drugs for pregnant and lactating women*, ed 2, Philadelphia, 2009, Saunders.

Whitty J, Dombrowski M: Respiratory diseases in pregnancy. In Creasy R, Resnik R, Iams J, Lockwood C, Moore T, editors: *Creasy & Resnik's maternal-fetal medicine: principles and practice*, ed 6, Philadelphia, 2009, Saunders.

16

Spontaneous Abortion

S pontaneous abortion (SAB) is a natural termination of pregnancy before the fetus has reached viability. A fetus of less than 20 weeks of gestation and weighing less than 500 g is not considered viable. SAB is further divided into early and late. An *early abortion* occurs before 12 weeks of gestation, and a *midtrimester* or *late abortion* occurs between 12 and 20 weeks of gestation. An SAB is commonly referred to as a *miscarriage* or *spontaneous pregnancy loss*. This term is preferred in talking with patients because the word *abortion* is frequently associated with induced abortions.

INCIDENCE

SAB occurs in approximately 10% to 30% of all clinically apparent pregnancies, with a recurrence loss of 25% to 47% (ACOG, 2001; Dawood, Farquharson, and Quenby, 2004).

ETIOLOGY

Sporadic Abortions

Nonrecurring Genetic Abnormality

Early abortions are likely to be caused by a nonrecurring genetic abnormality of the embryo (Cunningham and others, 2010). Studies substantiate the fact that approximately 50% of most early abortions (before 12 weeks of gestation) have a chromosomal abnormality (Goddijn, Leschot, 2000; Valley, Jackson-Williams, and Fly, 2006). The majority of these chromosomal abnormalities are related to numeric error occurring during meiotic cell division of the ovum or sperm or early mitotic cell division of the zygote or blastocyst.

Teratogenic Agents

Exposure to various teratogenic agents, such as high-dose radiation (Cunningham and others, 2010), chemicals, cytotoxic drugs (Baste and others, 2009), cocaine (Brent and Beckman, 1994), second-hand cigarette smoke (Meeker and others, 2007), alcohol (Pietrantoni and Knuppel, 1991), smoking (Brent and Beckman, 1994; Floyd

311

and others, 1999), moderate-to-heavy caffeine consumption (Cnattingius and others, 2000), and heavy decaffeinated coffee consumption (Fenster and others, 1997), can cause placental vascular compromise and embryonic damage, leading to an SAB. These teratogenic agents act in a dose-dependent manner (ACOG, 2001).

Systemic Infections

Any severe viral, bacterial, parasitic, or fungal infection that causes viremia or bacteremia can cause congenital malformations and stimulate abortions. There is an increased risk for a spontaneous abortion with a first-trimester varicella infection (AAP and ACOG, 2007). However, rubella, cytomegalovirus, coxsackievirus, herpesvirus, toxoplasmosis, and *Listeria* do not cause a severe enough infection to cause a sporadic SAB (RCOG, 2003; Matovina and others, 2004).

Uncontrolled Systemic Diseases

Systemic diseases that are not well controlled, such as diabetes, systemic lupus erythematosus, sickle cell anemia, hypertensive cardiovascular disease, phenylketonuria, and thyroid imbalance can cause an SAB.

Obesity

Obesity has been associated with increased risk for a sporadic abortion (Lashen, Fear, and Sturdee, 2004).

Environmental Factors

A relationship has been shown between stressful life events and working the night shift with an increased risk for SAB (Axelsson, Ahlborg, and Bodin, 1996; Neugebauer and others, 1996). Exposure to certain organic solvents has been linked to an increased SAB risk (Sharara, Seifer, and Flaws, 1998).

Recurrent Abortions

Chromosomal Disorders

Parental structural chromosome abnormalities account for approximately 2% to 5% of recurrent abortions (ACOG, 2001; RCOG, 2003).

Maternal Age

There appears to be a significantly increased risk for SAB in women older than 36 years (Nybo and others, 2000).

Uterine Anomalies

Structural uterine defects that interfere with the growth and development of the embryo or fetus may elicit an abortion. The uterine defect may be the result of a congenital defect or an acquired defect secondary to diethylstilbestrol (DES) exposure.

Antiphospholipid Syndrome

Antiphospholipid syndrome is one example of an autoimmune-mediated pregnancy loss. This disorder is characterized by presence of antiphospholipid antibodies. Two of the most common of these antibodies are lupus anticoagulant and anticardiolipin antibody. They both cause vascular endothelium damage and block the release of prostacyclin. Placental thrombosis and vascular insufficiency occur, causing subsequent fetal death (Meroni and others, 2004).

Inherited Thrombophilic Defect

Thrombophilia, an inheritable hypercoagulable condition, is most commonly the result of activated protein C resistance caused by mutations of the Factor V Leiden (FVL) gene, prothrombin gene (G20210A), protein C or S deficiency, antithrombin III, or hyperhomocysteinemia (MTHFR C677T, the gene causing folate deficiency) (RCOG, 2003; Kovalevsky and others, 2004; Sheiner and others, 2005). The hypercoagulable state causes systemic thrombosis and uteroplacental insufficiency, which result in recurrent abortions (see Chapter 14).

Incompetent Cervix

An incompetent cervix is a weak, structurally defective cervix that spontaneously dilates around 16 weeks of gestation.

NORMAL PHYSIOLOGY

Embryo and Placenta Development

The gametes (sperm and ovum) undergo developmental changes before fertilization. During the gamete maturation process, the number of chromosomes is reduced to 23, which is half the original number. This process is called *meiosis.*

When fertilization takes place and a mature sperm enters the mature ovum, the 23 chromosomes from each gamete pair up to form a new cell with 46 chromosomes called the *zygote.* This new cell begins mitotic cell division. When the zygote has developed into a solid ball of cells, it is called a *morula.* As maturation continues, the morula develops into a *blastocyst.* At this stage, an outer layer of cells called the *trophoblast,* which will form the placenta and fetal membranes, and an inner cluster of cells called the *embryoblast,* which will form the embryo, are present.

On approximately the sixth day after fertilization, the blastocyst is ready to implant into the endometrium of the uterus. This is accomplished as the trophoblast cells begin to secrete a proteolytic enzyme that digests an opening a few cells wide and burrows its way into the uterine lining. A small amount of blood may be lost at this time, which can cause mild vaginal spotting. The opening is closed by a blood clot at first and later by regenerated epithelium.

After the blastocyst is implanted into the endometrium of the uterus, the endometrium is called the *decidua.* The decidua is usually divided into three parts. The part of the decidua lying directly beneath the implanted blastocyst is called the *decidua basalis.* This is where the placenta primarily grows. The part of the decidua that covers the buried blastocyst is called *decidua capsularis,* and the remainder of the decidua that is not in direct contact with the blastocyst is called *decidua vera.*

After ovulation, when the mature ovum is released from the ovary, the ovary enters its luteal phase. During this time it excretes high levels of progesterone and some estrogen to prepare and maintain the endometrium for the fertilized ovum. Both hormones stimulate the glandular cells of the endometrium to secrete mucus and glycogen and increase the blood supply to the endometrium to facilitate an adequate nutritional environment for the implanted blastocyst, embryo, or fetus. Progesterone also facilitates the maintenance of pregnancy by keeping the myometrium quiet so that implantation can take place. For the corpus luteum to continue its production of progesterone and estrogen, the trophoblastic tissue must secrete human chorionic gonadotropin (hCG) until the placenta is mature enough to take over the production of hormones. This hormone maintains the corpus luteum for about the first 8 weeks of gestation.

Placental Immunology

The mother's body does not reject the blastocyst, which remains a mystery. On the surface of all body cells are structural antigens. The lymphocyte white blood cells are able to identify these antigens as either familiar or unfamiliar (foreign), and these white blood cells manufacture antibodies to destroy the antigens if they are identified as foreign. Because the antigens are determined genetically, half the antigens on fetal cells come from each parent. Therefore half the antigens should be foreign to the mother's body.

Currently, it is unknown what mechanism or mechanisms prevent the rejection of the fetus. Some recent research suggests that the immunologic interaction between mother and fetus appears to be beneficial for fetal and placental growth and development and limits trophoblast invasion. This is the result of immunotolerance and immunosuppression. First, the placental tissue (syncytiotrophoblast) that contacts with maternal tissue lacks the ability to activate the immune system. Second, the placenta tissue (cytotrophoblast) does not stimulate major histocompatibility complex (MHC) antigen formation because of the presence of human leukocyte antigen G (HLA-G). Therefore the mother creating immunotolerance (Mor and Abrahams, 2009) does not normally produce harmful antipaternal antibodies. Certain cytokines (transforming growth factor-beta [TGF-ß] and interleukin 10), prostaglandin E_2, hCG, and steroid hormones appear to have immunosuppressive activity in normal gestational tissue. Progesterone is also important in maintaining the pregnancy throughout the nine months by inhibiting myometrial activity and preventing T cell–mediated rejection (Ragusa and others, 2004).

Cervical Changes

An important structure that facilitates pregnancy continuation is the cervix. The cervix must resist the forces of gravity and intrauterine pressure for 9 months and then become soft and distensible, allowing the fetus to pass through to the vagina. The pregnancy is maintained primarily because of the formation of a sphincterlike structure that forms at the internal cervical os (Iams, 2009). This develops because of the distending muscular isthmus above and the cervix below, which is composed primarily of connective tissue (ground substance) plus collagen with scattered smooth muscle fibers (Huszar and Walsh, 1991).

During pregnancy, collagen fibers are laid down in an orderly fashion among the connective tissue, which gives the cervix strength to remain firm and closed. At the end of pregnancy, rearrangement of the collagen fibers takes place so that the fibers become more separable, promoting softening of the cervix (Iams, 2009). Numerous cervical glands line the cervical canal. During pregnancy, hypertrophy and hyperplasia of the cervical glands occur as well, forming the mucus plug.

PATHOPHYSIOLOGY

Embryo, Fetal, Placental Effect

Death of the embryo or failure of the embryo or placenta to develop normally is usually the first step in the sequence of events that lead to an SAB. Hemorrhage into the decidua basalis results, which causes necrotic changes at the site of implantation. Infiltration of leukocytes follows. Because of the absence of functioning fetal circulation, the chorionic villi often become edematous and resemble a hydatidiform mole. At the same time, hormonal levels of progesterone and estrogen drop, causing decidual sloughing, which results in vaginal bleeding. The uterus becomes irritable, and uterine contractions result.

Cervical Incompetence

An incompetent cervix contains more smooth muscle than a normal cervix (Iams, 2009); the collagen concentration is also less than normal. Cervical resistance is lowered because collagen fibers give the cervix strength to remain firm and closed. This is usually caused by one of three factors: a congenital defect, past cervical trauma, or hormonal factors.

Congenital Defect

With a congenital defect, the lower genital tract is structurally abnormal. A genetically inherited short cervical length can increase the risk for cervical incompetence. Exposure to DES can affect the lower uterine segment, increasing the risk as well (Kaufman and others, 2000).

Cervical Trauma

Cervical trauma is usually the result of mechanical trauma such as excessive dilation for curettage, cervical biopsy, or cervical lacerations acquired during a previous delivery.

Hormonal Factors

Increased amounts of relaxin, the effects of exogenous estrogen and progesterone, and multiple gestations all increase the risk for cervical incompetence. *Relaxin*, a hormone secreted by the corpus luteum, causes connective tissue remodeling, which affects the collagen concentration. Levels of relaxin are increased in multiple gestations.

SIGNS AND SYMPTOMS

Vaginal Bleeding

The classic sign of an SAB is vaginal bleeding. At first, the bleeding usually appears as dark spotting related to the decreased hormonal levels of progesterone and estrogen that cause the decidua (endometrium) to begin to slough. It may progress to frank, bright red bleeding as the products of conception begin to separate, opening up uterine blood vessels.

Abdominal Pain

Pain may be manifested in different ways. It may be rhythmic or persistent, and it may present as a low backache or as pelvic pressure or tenderness over the uterus.

Incompetent Cervix

A woman with an incompetent cervix commonly presents with complaints of pelvic pressure, increased vaginal discharge, or light spotting. Spontaneous cervical dilation is painless and unaccompanied by contractions, amniotic fluid leakage, or signs of infection.

CLASSIFICATION

SABs are classified into seven clinical types: threatened, inevitable, complete, incomplete, missed, septic, and recurrent (Fig. 16-1). Table 16-1 lists signs and symptoms manifested by each type.

MATERNAL EFFECTS

The major contributions to maternal death surrounding an SAB are related to two potential complications that rarely occur today: hemorrhage and infection. Hemorrhage may be related to a delay in seeking medical treatment or to perforation of the uterus during surgical treatment. Infection may be related to a delay in diagnosing a septic abortion or to inappropriate use of antibiotics.

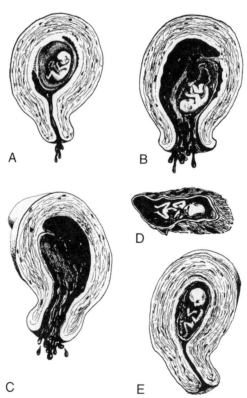

Figure 16-1 Types of spontaneous abortions. **A,** Threatened. **B,** Inevitable. **C,** Incomplete. **D,** Complete. **E,** Missed. (From Lowdermilk D, Perry S: *Maternity & women's health care,* ed 9, St. Louis, 2007, Mosby.)

Table 16-1   Clinical Classification of Spontaneous Abortions

Classification	Definition	Manifestations
Threatened	Condition in which continuation of pregnancy is in doubt	Vaginal bleeding or spotting, which may be associated with mild cramps of back and lower abdomen Closed cervix Uterus that is soft, nontender, and enlarged appropriate to gestational age
Inevitable	Condition in which termination of pregnancy is in progress	Cervical dilation Membranes may be ruptured Vaginal bleeding Mild-to-painful uterine contractions
Complete	Condition in which products of conception are totally expelled from uterus	
Incomplete	Condition in which fragments of products of conception are expelled and part is retained in uterus	Profuse bleeding because retained tissue parts interfere with myometrial contractions
Missed	Condition in which embryo or fetus dies during first 20 weeks of gestation but is retained in uterus for 4 weeks or more afterward	Amenorrhea or intermittent vaginal bleeding, spotting, or brownish discharge No uterine growth No fetal movement felt Regression of breast changes
Septic	Condition in which products of conception become infected during abortion process	Foul-smelling vaginal discharge
Recurrent	Condition in which two or more successive pregnancies have ended in spontaneous abortion	

FETAL EFFECTS

Death of the fetus always occurs as the result of an SAB. In fact, it may be the actual cause of the abortion.

DIAGNOSTIC TESTING

Spontaneous Abortion

When vaginal bleeding occurs during the first 20 weeks of pregnancy, careful evaluation must be made to determine whether the bleeding is a threatened abortion or is related to another cause. About 20% of all patients experience some vaginal bleeding during the first trimester, and only about half of these women actually have SABs

(Cunningham and others, 2010). Therefore consideration must be given to other possible causes of vaginal bleeding, which may be related to one of the following:

- Normal implantation of the blastocyst into the endometrium
- Lesions of the cervix or vagina or cervical polyps that bleed because of increased vascularity of the vagina and cervix during pregnancy
- Cervicitis or vaginitis
- Hydatidiform mole
- Ectopic pregnancy
- Carcinoma of the cervix

The evaluation to differentiate among the various possible causes of vaginal bleeding usually includes inspecting the vagina and cervix by a speculum examination to rule out vaginal or cervical lesions or cervical polyps, along with a Pap smear to rule out carcinoma. Vaginal ultrasound is usually done to determine whether there is an intrauterine gestational sac. This rules out an ectopic pregnancy. A gestational sac, if present, should be identifiable with ultrasound by 6 weeks after the last menstrual period. Real time ultrasound can be used to document lack of heart movement, which indicates fetal death. Quantitative beta-hCG assays and progesterone levels are helpful in determining the state of the fetus. Serial doubling of quantitative beta-hCG assays every 36 to 48 hours between gestational weeks 3 and 10 and progesterone levels greater than 15 ng/ml strongly indicates a healthy pregnancy. See Table 17-3 for a summary of diagnostic tests.

If the patient presents with signs of an inevitable abortion, tests are not usually necessary to make the diagnosis. Any patient with a history of cervical trauma or painless second trimester abortion should be examined weekly during the second trimester for an incompetent cervix.

Box 16-1 provides a nurse practitioner workup summary.

Incompetent Cervix

In an incompetent cervix, a vaginal examination indicates cervical softening, but dilation of the cervix typically occurs later. Transvaginal ultrasound measuring of the length of the cervix is the best diagnostic tool to detect early cervical changes. Incompetent cervix is diagnosed if the cervix shortens below 20 to 25 mm or below 25 to 30 mm in the presence of a funnel or beak (effacement at the internal os moving to the external os). Zilianti and others (1995) suggested a useful acronym to describe the presence of effacement seen on transvaginal ultrasound: TYVU. A normal cervix without any funneling is a T. As the cervix begins to efface at the internal os moving to the external os, it first looks like a Y, with further shortening toward the external os as a V, and finally to a fully effaced cervix as a U.

USUAL MEDICAL MANAGEMENT AND PROTOCOLS FOR NURSE PRACTITIONERS

Most often, when vaginal bleeding is definitely related to an SAB, treatment centers on determining the cause (if possible), keeping the couple informed, and providing emotional support instead of attempting to sustain the pregnancy. This protocol is based on the following factors:

- In an early threatened abortion, the embryo or fetus is usually dead before the bleeding begins.

Box 16-1   Nurse Practitioner Workup Summary

- **Evaluation of amount of blood loss**
  - **Subjective report**
  - **Vital signs**
  - **Orthostatic blood pressure.** Check orthostatic blood pressure if condition permits. To do this, take the patient's blood pressure and pulse while she is supine. Retake these vital signs after the patient has been standing for 5 minutes. A decrease in systolic blood pressure of 10 mm Hg or an increase in the pulse rate of 10 beats per min or more is interpreted as an indication of significant blood loss.
  - **Pulse pressure.** The *diastolic blood pressure* reflects the amount of systemic vasoconstriction present; the *pulse pressure* (difference between systolic and diastolic pressure) indicates stroke volume; the *systolic blood pressure* denotes the interrelationship between the level of vasoconstriction and the stroke volume. A narrowing of the pulse pressure (normal 30 to 40 mm Hg) is an early sign of hypovolemia.
  - **Hypothenar refilling.** Squeeze the hypothenar area of the hand (the fleshy elevation of the ulnar side of the palm) for 1 to 2 seconds. Normal blood volume is indicated by initial blanching with return to the normal pink coloration within 1 to 2 seconds. A blood volume deficit of 15% to 25% is indicated by delayed refilling.
- **Menstrual history.** Last normal menstrual period, frequency, duration, and flow.
- **Gynecologic history**
  - **Contraceptive history**
  - **Sexually transmitted disease**
- **Obstetric history**
- **Coagulation disorder history**
- **Physical examination**
  - **Abdominal examination**
  - **Auscultation**
  - **Percussion**
  - **Palpation (tender area last)**
  - **Rebound tenderness**
  - **McBurney point**
  - **Iliopsoas**
  - **Obturator test**
  - **Murphy sign**
- **Vaginal speculum examination** to determine the following:
  - **Source of the bleeding.** Rule out cervical or vaginal causes such as polyps, cervical or vaginal lesions, vaginal infection, vaginal trauma, cervical pregnancy, cervical cancer, or pelvic inflammatory disease.
  - **Amount of vaginal bleeding**
  - **Cervical status: opened or closed**
  - **Presence of tissue at the cervix**
- **Bimanual vaginal examination**
- **Uterine examination.** Determine uterine size, and determine the presence of an adnexal mass or tenderness.

Continued

| **Box 16-1** | Nurse Practitioner Workup Summary—cont'd |

- **Diagnostic data**
  - **Quantitative serum human chorionic gonadotropin (hCG)**
  - **Progesterone levels**
  - **Hemoglobin and hematocrit with complete blood cell count**
  - **Blood type, platelet count, and antibody screen**
  - **Vaginal ultrasound**
  - **Urine for culture and sensitivity**

- Approximately 50% of all early abortions are associated with chromosomal anomalies and are nature's way of preventing the birth of a genetically defective child.
- In late abortions, after 12 weeks of gestation, maternal factors are usually the cause, and death does not usually precede the vaginal bleeding. However, if the pregnancy is maintained, the bleeding itself can increase perinatal mortality or the risk for developing congenital abnormalities.
- Controlled studies have also failed to prove that bedrest, hormones such as progesterone, or sedatives have any effect on the outcome of a threatened abortion.
- Administration of medications during organogenesis (weeks 3 to 8) exposes the embryo to possible teratogenic effects.

Threatened Abortion

When a threatened abortion is diagnosed, an assessment is done to determine the probable outcome. Prompt evacuation of the uterus must be carried out if any of the following findings are present:

- Bleeding has become excessive.
- Any part of the products of conception has been lost.
- The cervix shows signs of dilation.
- Signs and symptoms of an intrauterine infection are present.
- Definite diagnosis of a dead fetus is made with ultrasound.

To assess for the presence of one of these negative findings, a medical workup is done that usually includes the following:

- Pelvic examination to determine signs of dilation
- Blood count for red blood cells, hemoglobin, and hematocrit to aid in the determination of the amount of blood lost and the presence or absence of anemia
- Blood count for white blood cells to determine whether an infection is present
- Vaginal ultrasound, serial serum quantitative beta-hCG assays, and serum progesterone values to determine whether the fetus is alive. (Indicators of fetal well-being include a well-formed gestational ring with central echoes from the embryo, serum progesterone greater than 10-15 ng/ml, and serial doubling of quantitative beta-hCG assays.)

If the assessment does not reveal a negative finding, the patient is usually managed as an outpatient. She has frequent physician's visits and is instructed to limit her activity, abstain from intercourse, and save any passed tissue. If an IUD is in place and the string is visible, it is usually removed. Further treatment depends on the signs and symptoms that develop.

Inevitable, Complete, or Incomplete Abortion

Once the cervix begins to dilate, there is no hope for pregnancy continuation and an abortion becomes inevitable. If part of the products of conception is lost, the abortion becomes incomplete; if all of the products of conception are lost, the abortion is complete.

From the time an abortion becomes inevitable until it becomes complete, naturally or with surgical intervention, there is a high risk for complications such as hemorrhage or an infection. The risk for hemorrhage usually correlates with the gestational age of the pregnancy. For the first 6 weeks, the placenta is very tentatively attached to the decidua of the uterus. Therefore if an SAB occurs before 6 weeks of gestation, the bleeding usually takes the form of a heavy menstrual period.

Between 6 and 12 weeks of gestation, the chorionic villi of the placenta begin to grow into the decidua of the uterus, and by week 12 or shortly after, the chorionic villi have deeply penetrated into the decidua. If an SAB occurs after the placenta has completed its penetration process (week 12), the fetus is usually expelled before placental separation. Bleeding is usually held in check by the placenta until it separates from the uterus and then by uterine contractions if the separation is complete. Therefore the most severe bleeding is seen between 6 and 12 weeks of gestation because the placenta can detach before expulsion of the fetus. Severe bleeding can result after 12 weeks of gestation if the placenta does not separate completely and parts are retained. If the gestational age is known, the risk for bleeding can be more easily estimated.

The risk for infection usually depends on many factors, such as the nutritional state of the patient, perineal hygiene, and whether anything other than a sterile speculum entered the vagina after dilation began.

If all the embryonic or fetal and placental tissue can be identified and there are no signs of bleeding or infection, the abortion is complete and no surgical intervention is necessary. If the abortion is incomplete, systematic reviews provide an A level of evidence that expectant management to allow spontaneous resolution was found to be just as safe a treatment plan as immediate surgery and has a 82% to 96% success rate (Griebel, Halvorsen, Golemon, and Day, 2005). Complications were similar between the two treatment groups with less incidence of pelvic inflammatory disease in the expectant management group.

However, prompt evacuation of the uterus may be indicated in the presence of excessive cramping, heavy bleeding, or evidence of sepsis. According to the Cochrane Review (Forna and Gülmezoglu, 2002), vacuum aspiration is preferred over sharp curettage. It is safe, quick, and less painful than sharp curettage. *Vacuum aspiration* is the removal of the products of conception with a vacuum aspirator suction curet that is inserted through the dilated cervix after the patient is anesthetized. The vacuum aspirator is moved gently over the surface of the uterine wall in a systematic pattern to cover all the uterine cavity and the products of conception are collected in a vacuum container.

This procedure is done primarily in an outpatient setting. The woman is hospitalized only if severe bleeding or signs of infection are present. If time permits, a history and physical examination are usually performed and a complete blood count is done.

A tube of blood is usually held for typing and cross-matching in case a transfusion becomes necessary. A dilute solution of intravenous (IV) oxytocin is often started before the surgery to reduce blood loss and to decrease the risk for uterine perforation by causing the uterus to contract and thicken. A preoperative medication of 5 to 10 mg of diazepam (Valium) may be ordered. The procedure can be done with a paracervical block, especially if the procedure is performed on an outpatient basis, or with the patient under a light general anesthesia. If the procedure is done with the patient under local anesthesia, the patient may experience some cramping sensations during the procedure.

If the bleeding is severe, the patient's vital signs must be stabilized before surgery. This is usually accomplished by infusing 1 to 2 L of a crystalloid solution such as IV lactated Ringer's solution with 30 units of oxytocin per 1000 ml. If lactated Ringer's solution with oxytocin is used, the infusion rate is usually set at 200 ml/hr or more. This large dose of oxytocin is needed during the first half of pregnancy because the uterus is less sensitive to oxytocin at this time because of the low levels of estrogen present to potentiate its effect. If oxytocin is not effective, an erythrocyte infusion or another appropriate blood component may be used. If signs of infection are present or develop, antibiotic therapy is usually initiated.

If the cervix is not partially dilated, dilation is usually accomplished slowly by placing *Laminaria* dilators or a prostaglandin suppository or gel in the cervix before the evacuation procedure. *Laminaria* tents, such as *Laminaria digitata* or *Laminaria japonica*, are natural cervical dilators made from seaweed, the stems of which have been peeled, dried, and sterilized. Synthetic alternatives are being used more frequently. Dilapan, a hygroscopic cervical dilator, and Lamicel, an alcohol polymer sponge impregnated with 450 mg of magnesium sulfate and compressed into a tent, are two commonly used synthetic dilators.

Inserted into the full length of the cervical canal, the dilators absorb cervical fluids and swell, dilating the cervix slowly (Fig. 16-2). The patient may experience cramping, which is easily controlled with a mild analgesic. Then, at the time of surgery or before the evacuation procedure, the *Laminaria* dilators are removed. Serial applications of prostaglandin gel or vaginal suppositories placed in the cervix can accomplish the same result. Because both methods dilate the cervix slowly, they decrease the risk for cervical trauma, which can occur with mechanical dilators.

Missed Abortion

Most missed abortions terminate spontaneously. However, if there are no signs of an SAB at the time a missed abortion is diagnosed, it was once thought that immediate evacuation of the uterus was necessary to prevent sepsis, disseminated intravascular coagulation or psychologic stress related to carrying a dead fetus. Currently, patients are being given an option of expectant management or medical therapy with intravaginal misoprostol. Expectant management has a general success rate of 16% to 76% (Sairam and others, 2001; Luise and others, 2002; Wood and Brain, 2002). One randomized clinical trial found that patients had an 80% success rate after using 800 mcg misoprostol intravaginally and repeated after four hours if needed (Wood and Brain, 2002).

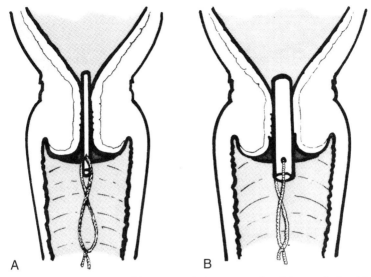

Figure 16-2 A, Properly inserted laminaria. **B,** Laminaria after 8 hours of absorbing cervical fluid, causing it to swell and dilate cervix gradually. (Illustration by Vincenza Genovese, Phoenix, Ariz.)

Recurrent Spontaneous Abortion

Some recurrent abortions occur by chance; others are related to a maternal or paternal cause. Treatment should focus on identifying the cause and treating it accordingly. The current suggested screening and treatment methods after a recurrent SAB are outlined next. According to the American College of Obstetrics and Gynecology (2001), it is not necessary to routinely screen for endocervical bacteria or viruses or to test for glucose intolerance, thyroid abnormalities, paternal human leukocyte antigen status, or maternal antipaternal antibodies after recurrent pregnancy loss. After unexplained recurrent SAB, the couple should be encouraged by the 35% to 85% successful pregnancy rate without treatment (ACOG, 2001).

Chromosomal Disorder

When a couple repeatedly loses an embryo or fetus early in gestation, a chromosomal disorder of the father or mother may be the cause. A genetic history should be taken, karyotyping is recommended, and genetic counseling should follow as indicated.

Uterine Anomalies

Uterine defects are occasionally the cause of late recurrent SABs. During vacuum aspiration for an SAB, the uterine cavity should be closely examined for any abnormalities. If a double uterus is noted, a hysterosalpingography or hysteroscopic evaluation and reparative surgery have been shown to be therapeutic (ACOG, 2001).

Endocrine Factors

A luteal phase defect (LPD) occurs in approximately 35% of recurrent spontaneous abortions. However, there is no reliable method to diagnose LPD (Bukulmez and Arici, 2004). The benefits of supplemental natural progesterone suppositories are unproved (ACOG, 2001). It is used for patients undergoing ovulation induction and IVF. When used in these cases, the usual dose is 1 applicator 8% PV per day. To be most effective, the progesterone should be started at the time of ovulation and continued until 10 to 12 weeks of gestation (Weiner and Buhimschi, 2009).

In patients with polycystic ovary syndrome (PCOS), a hyperandrogenic disorder, metformin therapy throughout the pregnancy is being studied (Glueck and others, 2001; Ramidi and others, 2009). Hypothyroidism is treated with thyroid replacement medication. The dosage is titrated to maintain normal TSH levels.

Immunologic Factors: Antiphospholipid Syndrome

A patient who tests positive for a lupus anticoagulant or an anticardiolipin antibody on two different occasions, 6 weeks apart, should be placed on thromboprophylaxis during the next pregnancy. Therapeutic recommendations are aspirin, 81 mg/day, followed by unfractionated or low-molecular-weight heparin (LMWH). Refer to Table 14-1 for heparin dosing guidelines. Weight-bearing exercise and calcium and vitamin D supplementation are encouraged to lower the risk for osteoporosis. According to the American College of Obstetrics and Gynecology (2001), mononuclear cell immunization and intravenous immunoglobulin (IVIG) are not effective in preventing a recurrent SAB (see Chapter 13). According to the HepASA Trial, aspirin alone is just as effective as the combination therapy of aspirin and LMWH (Laskin and others, 2009).

Incompetent Cervix

Treatment for recurrent abortions caused by an incompetent cervix is usually cerclage, a surgical procedure in which a purse-string suture is placed around the cervix to reinforce it. Preoperative vaginal cultures are obtained and appropriate treatment instituted for group B streptococcus, *Neisseria gonorrhoeae*, and *Chlamydia*. This surgical procedure is considered in three different circumstances, described in the following paragraphs.

Prophylactic Cerclage

The prophylactic cerclage is usually performed based on a positive obstetric history around 10 to 14 weeks of gestation, before cervical dilation, effacement, or shortening takes place and before any bleeding or cramping is present. After the procedure, prophylactic antibiotics, such as penicillin for 5 days, are given. Instruct the patient to abstain from intercourse, not to stand for prolonged periods of more than 90 minutes, and not to lift anything heavy.

Therapeutic Cerclage

The therapeutic cerclage is placed when transvaginal ultrasound reveals signs of funneling or beaking (beginning effacement at the internal os moving to the external os) and shortened cervical length, in the absence of other discernible causes. After the procedure, prophylactic antibiotics, such as penicillin for 5 days, are given. Instruct the patient to abstain from intercourse, not to stand for prolonged periods of more than 90 minutes, and not to lift anything heavy. If the transvaginal cervix length is less than 25 mm, the patient is encouraged to stop working. If the cervix length is less than 20 mm the patient is told to limit her activity.

Rescue Cerclage

The rescue cerclage is placed when the transvaginal ultrasound reveals advanced cervical dilation, shortened cervical length, or bulging or hourglass membranes. Amniocentesis may be performed to reduce the bulging and obtain cultures. After the procedure, prophylactic antibiotics and indomethacin are usually prescribed. These patients are on bedrest with bathroom privileges only until stabilized with no further evidence of preterm labor changes.

NURSING MANAGEMENT

Prevention

Because teratogenic agents increase the risk for an SAB, preventive measures should be taken to avoid this area of risk. These measures should be instituted before pregnancy. The woman should maintain a healthful lifestyle, including eating a nutritious diet, not smoking, not drinking alcoholic beverages, and receiving available immunizations against infectious diseases. When pregnancy is diagnosed, instructions given to the expectant mother include ways she can decrease her chance of contracting infections, such as by eating nutritiously, avoiding fatigue, and avoiding people with infections. She is also instructed that if she eats meat, to cook it well; if she has a pet cat or bird, to leave the cleaning of the litter area to someone else; and if she works in the yard, to use gloves to avoid contact with the toxoplasmosis virus. She is instructed to avoid radiographs and medications, especially nonprescription ones, unless they are ordered by her obstetrician.

Nursing Interventions for Hemorrhage Management

- Obtain a history of onset, duration, amount, color, and consistency of bleeding.
- Obtain a history of associated symptoms, prior bleeding episodes, and physical activity at onset of bleeding.
- Record visual blood loss in cubic centimeters of blood stained on pad in a certain period of time, or weigh saturated pads, linen protectors, or linen (1 g × 1 ml).
- Record blood pressure, pulse, and respirations as indicated (depends on severity).
- Observe for passage of tissue or clots.
- Observe for signs of shock.
- Keep an accurate record of intake and output.
- Refer to laboratory data such as hemoglobin level, hematocrit level, and red blood cell count.
- Determine gestational age by estimated date of delivery.
- Save all expelled tissue and clots for examination.
- If bleeding is severe or the hemoglobin or hematocrit level is low, start an IV line with a 14-gauge intracatheter and normal saline to be prepared for blood component therapy or blood administration as ordered. Start another IV line to administer a crystalloid solution such as lactated Ringer's solution as ordered, usually 1.5 to 2 liters given through a warming device (Anthony, 2006). Prepare

for type and cross-match, and have oxytocin available. Usual dose of oxytocin is 10 to 40 units in 1000 ml of 0.9% (normal) saline or D5W solution to infuse at a rate to control uterine atony (Weiner and Buhimschi, 2009).
- Notify physician if the blood pressure drops, pulse or respirations increase, more than one pad is saturated with blood in 1 hour, urinary output drops below 30 ml/hr or 120 ml/4 hr, or the hematocrit level is less than 30% or hemoglobin level less than 11 g. Be prepared to intervene based on percentage of blood loss. See Table 19-3 for guidelines for blood component replacement.
- Assist with expectant management, medical therapy, or surgical management based on diagnosis and patient choice.

If no signs of an inevitable, incomplete, or missed abortion are found, the following interventions apply:
- Provide discharge instructions that include the importance of limiting activity, abstaining from intercourse, and returning for a reevaluation appointment.
- Instruct as to the importance of notifying the physician immediately if bleeding becomes heavier than a period or persists, if cramps develop, or if a fever develops.
- Encourage the patient to continue to take prenatal vitamins and eat foods high in protein, iron, and fiber.

If signs of an inevitable, incomplete, or missed abortion are present, the following interventions apply:
- Assist with a transvaginal ultrasound to confirm intrauterine products of conception in the presence of an incomplete abortion.
- Facilitate the discussion as to the benefits and risks of expectant management, medical therapy, and surgical management. There is research evidence that indicates when patients are provided an opportunity to participate in the treatment decision they have better subsequent mental health (Wieringa-DeWaard and others, 2002).
- Prepare for surgical or medical intervention as applicable.
- Provide comfort measures and grief support (reference nursing interventions for anticipatory grieving below).

Postsurgical Nursing Interventions to Prevent Complications or to Provide Early Detection of Signs of Hemorrhage, Infection, and Anemia
- Be prepared to give methylergonovine maleate (Methergine), 200 mg orally every 6 hours for six doses if bleeding is heavy.
- Check the vital signs according to protocol.
- Check vaginal discharge according to protocol.
- Refer to laboratory data such as white blood cell count.
- Teach the importance of perineal care after each voiding, and encourage changing perineal pads often.
- If signs of an infection develop, be prepared to administer antibiotics as ordered.
- Discharge instructions include appropriate perineal care: shower (no baths) for first 2 weeks; no using tampons, douching, or having sexual intercourse for 2 weeks; and notify physician if an elevated temperature or a foul-smelling vaginal discharge develops.

- Determine the mother's blood type and Rh factor.
- If the mother is RhD-negative be prepared to administer Rh_o (D) immune globulin. The usual dose is Rh_o (D) immune globulin standard dose (Rho-GAM; HypRho-D) IM 300 micrograms if the gestational age is greater than 12 weeks or Rh_o (D) globulin microdose (HypRho-D MiniDose, MicRho-GAM) IM 50 micrograms for a gestation of 12 weeks or less.
- Refer to laboratory data, such as hemoglobin, to rule out anemia.
- Provide discharge instructions as to the importance of eating foods high in iron and protein to promote tissue repair and red blood cell replacement. Foods high in iron include meat, legumes, dried fruits, whole grains, and green, leafy vegetables. Iron from plant-based foods is less well absorbed by the body, but absorption can be improved by eating these foods along with a food high in vitamin C.

Nursing Interventions for Anticipatory Grieving

- Assess the significance of the loss to all family members.
- Acknowledge, permit, and help individual family members identify feelings of relief, sadness, distress, or neutrality toward the loss.
- Encourage the patient and her family to express their individual levels of satisfaction and control regarding the actual miscarriage experience.
- Give the parents choices and opportunities for decision making.
- Provide physical care such as back rubs or nourishment as needed.
- Consider any significant cultural beliefs or values. Refer to a pastor, priest, or chaplain based on family's request for spiritual assistance to work through their grief.
- Refer to a support group such as Resolve Through Sharing, Compassionate Friends *(http://www.compassionatefriends.org)*, or SHARE Pregnancy and Infant Loss Support, Inc *http://www.nationalshareoffice.com*
- Refer to psychologic support or counseling if indicated.
- Provide family with a list of helpful publications, including the following:
  - Understanding Miscarriage: Coping With the Loss (Krames Communication, 800-333-3032)
  - When Pregnancy Fails (Susan Borg and Judith Lasker)
  - Death of a Dream (Donna and Rodger Ewy)
  - After a Loss in Pregnancy (Nancy Barezin)
  - Ended Beginnings (Claudia Panuthos and Catherine Romeo)
  - Empty Arms: Coping After Miscarriage, Stillbirth and Infant Death (Ilse Sherokee and Arlene Appelbaum)
  - Stillbirth, Miscarriage and Infant Death (Compassionate Friends support group) (http://www.compassionatefriends.org/Resources/Available_Brochures.aspx)

See Chapter 7 for more information about this topic.

- Warn about the *"anniversary phenomenon."*
- Discuss with the family the importance of grieving the loss before becoming pregnant again. Many parents try to lessen their grief by quickly planning and becoming pregnant. According to Frost and Condon (1996), another pregnancy too soon inhibits mourning and delays resolution.

Nursing Interventions to Decrease Risk for Recurrence

- Discuss with the couple the cause, if known, or otherwise explain possible reasons for an SAB.
- If this is a second or third SAB, the couple should be encouraged to have a diagnostic and genetic workup to attempt to determine the cause. This might include the following:
  - Karyotyping of abortus
  - Karyotyping of parents
  - Pelvic ultrasound to rule out uterine anomaly
  - Ruling out autoimmune disease with tests for lupus anticoagulant or anticardiolipin (aCL) antibodies
  - Thyroid panel and fasting blood sugar, only if symptoms indicate
- Teach the couple the importance of using contraception except for Depomedroxyprogesterone acetate (Depo-Provera) for at least 3 to 6 months to allow time for the woman's body to recover. After an abortion, the woman usually ovulates during the next cycle, but there is a significantly increased risk for endometrial abnormalities for a minimum of the next two cycles.
- Develop and consistently use a self-administered, matter-of-fact, nonjudgmental questionnaire to ascertain lifestyle behaviors such as patterns of smoking, alcohol consumption, caffeine intake, recreational drug use, non-prescription medication use, and occupation.
- Analyze the responses for potential risk.
- Motivate the family to make lifestyle changes to improve health-related behaviors by providing them with information about health risks and possible effects on pregnancy outcome.
- Provide supportive counseling to aid the family in making changes and help them to build self-esteem and overcome feelings of guilt. Avoid using threatening statements that make them feel guilty.
- Assess the patient's immunization record and encourage immunization for rubella if rubella titer is less than 1:10.
- Provide instructions regarding ways to decrease the chance of contracting an infection, such as eating nutritiously, preventing fatigue, avoiding people with infections, cooking meat well, and leaving the cleaning of the litter area of any pet cats or birds to someone else to avoid contact with the toxoplasmosis virus.
- Instruct the pregnant woman to avoid radiographs and medications, especially nonprescription drugs, unless ordered by her obstetrician.
- Make appropriate community referrals to resources that enable implementation of family's goals.

CONCLUSION

Many times, an SAB is nature's way of eliminating a fetus with chromosomal defects. These defects can be caused by an unpreventable, nonrecurring genetic abnormality or by a preventable teratogenic agent. The nurse can lower the incidence of SAB by implementing an education program. This program should include educating about the effects of alcohol, smoking, infections, radiographs, cocaine, and other teratogenic agents on the developing fetus. In these cases and in cases in which the cause is unpreventable, the nurse provides emotional support so that the parents are not left with emotional scars because of anxiety or guilt over their failure to maintain the pregnancy to term.

In some cases, the cause is related to a maternal defect. The nurse should work with the health care team to recognize these cases and then make appropriate referrals to facilitate treatment so that a recurrent abortion does not occur.

BIBLIOGRAPHY

American Academy of Pediatrics (AAP) and American College of Obstetricians and Gynecologists (ACOG): *Guidelines for perinatal care*, ed 6, Washington, DC, 2007, Author.

American College of Obstetricians and Gynecologists (ACOG): *Management of recurrent early pregnancy loss, ACOG Practice Bulletin,* No. 24, Washington, DC, 2001, Author.

Anthony J: Major obstetric hemorrhage disseminated intravascular coagulation. In James D, and others, editors: *High risk pregnancy: management options,* ed 3, Philadelphia, 2006, Saunders.

Axelsson G, Ahlborg G Jr, Bodin L: Shift work, nitrous oxide exposure and spontaneous abortion among Swedish midwives, *Occup Environ Med* 53(6):374–378, 1996.

Baste V, Moen B, Riise T, and others: Infertility and spontaneous abortion among female hairdressers; the Hordaland Health Study, *J Occup Environ Med* 50(12): 1371-1377, 2009.

Brent R, Beckman D: The contribution of environmental teratogens to embryonic and fetal loss, *Clin Obstet Gynecol* 37(3):646–670, 1994.

Bukulmez O, Arici A: Luteal phase defect: myth or reality, *Obstet Gynecol Clin North Am* 31(4):727–744, 2004.

Cnattingius S, and others: Caffeine intake and the risk of first-trimester spontaneous abortion, *N Engl J Med* 343(25):1839–1845, 2000.

Cunningham F, Leveno K, Bloom S, Hauth J, Rouse D, and Spong C: *Williams' obstetrics*, ed 23, New York, 2010, McGraw-Hill Medical.

Dawood F, Farquharson R, Quenby S: Recurrent miscarriage, *Curr Obstet Gynaecol* 14:247, 2004.

Fenster L, and others: Caffeinated beverages, decaffeinated coffee, and spontaneous abortion, *Epidemiology* 8(5):515–523, 1997.

Floyd R, Decoufle P, Hungerford D: Alcohol use prior to pregnancy recognition, *Am J Prev Med* 17(2):101–117, 1999.

Forna F, Gülmezoglu AM: Surgical procedures to evacuate incomplete miscarriage, *Cochrane Database Syst Rev* (Issue 4), Art. No.: CD001993, 2002.

Frost M, Condon J: The psychological sequelae of miscarriage: a critical review of the literature, *Aust N Z J Psychiatry* 30(1):54–62, 1996.

Glueck C, and others: Continuing metformin throughout pregnancy in women with polycystic ovary syndrome appears to safely reduce first trimester spontaneous abortion: a pilot study, *Fertil Steril* 75(1):46–52, 2001.

Goddijn M, Leschot N: Genetic aspects of miscarriage, *Clin Obstet Gynecol* 14:855–865, 2000.

Griebel C, Halvorsen J, Golemon T, Day A: Management of spontaneous abortion, *AAFP* 72(7): 1243–1250, 2005.

Huszar G, Walsh M: Relationship between myometrial and cervical functions in pregnancy and labor, *Semin Perinatol* 15(2):97–117, 1991.

Iams J: Cervical insufficiency. In Creasy R, Resnik R, Iams J, Lockwood C, Moore T, editors: *Creasy & Resnik's maternal-fetal medicine: principles and practice*, ed 6, Philadelphia, 2009, Saunders.

Kaufman R, and others: Continued follow-up of pregnancy outcomes in diethylstilbestrol-exposed offspring, *Obstet Gynecol* 96(4):483–489, 2000.

Kovalevsky G, and others: Evaluation of the association between hereditary thrombophilias and recurrent pregnancy loss, *Arch Intern Med* 164(5):558–563, 2004.

Lashen H, Fear K, Sturdee D: Obesity is associated with increased risk of first trimester and recurrent miscarriage: matched case control study, *Hum Reprod* 19(7):1644–1646, 2004.

Laskin C, Spitzer K, Clark C, and others: Low molecular weight heparin and aspirin for recurrent pregnancy loss: results from the randomized, controlled HepASA trial, *J Rheumatol* 36(2):279–287, 2009.

Luise C, Jermy K, Collons W, Bourne T: Expectant management of incomplete, spontaneous first-trimester: outcome according to initial ultrasound criteria and value of follow-up visits, *Ultrasound Obstet Gynecol* 19:580–582, 2002.

Matovina M, and others: Possible role of bacterial and viral infections in miscarriages, *Fertil Steril* 81(3):662–669, 2004.

Meeker J, Missmer S, Vitonis A, and others: Risk of spontaneous abortion in women with childhood exposure to parental cigarette smoke, *Am J Epidemiol* 166(5):571–575, 2007.

Meroni P, and others: Antiphospholipid antibodies as cause of pregnancy loss, *Lupus* 13(9):649–652, 2004.

Mor G, Abrahams V: The immunology of pregnancy. In Creasy R, Resnik R, Iams J, Lockwood C, Moore T, editors: *Creasy & Resnik's maternal-fetal medicine: principles and practice*, ed 6, Philadelphia, 2009, Saunders.

Neugebauer R, and others: Association of stressful life events with chromosomally normal spontaneous abortion, *Am J Epidemiol* 143(6):588–596, 1996.

Nybo, Andersen A, and others: Maternal age and fetal loss: population based register linkage study, *BMJ* 320(7251):1708–1712, 2000.

Pietrantoni M, Knuppel R: Alcohol use in pregnancy, *Clin Perinatol* 18(1):93–111, 1991.

Ragusa A, and others: Progesterone supplement in pregnancy: an immunologic therapy? *Lupus* 13(9):639–642, 2004.

Ramidi G, Khan N, Glueck C, and others: Enoxaparin-metformin and enoxaparin alone may safely reduce pregnancy loss, *Transl Res* 153(1):33–43, 2009.

Royal College of Obstetricians and Gynaecologists (RCOG). *The investigation and treatment of couples with recurrent miscarriage*, London (UK): RCOG. Retrieved from http://www.guideline.gov, May, 2003.

Sairam S, Khare M, Michailidia G, Thilaganathan B: The role of ultrasound in the expectant management of early pregnancy loss, *Ultrasound Obstet Gynecol* 17:506–509, 2001.

Sharara F, Seifer D, Flaws J: Environmental toxicants and female reproduction, *Fertil Steril* 70(4): 613–622, 1998.

Sheiner E, and others: Pregnancy outcome following recurrent spontaneous abortions, *Eur J Obstet Gynecol Reprod Biol* 118(1):61–65, 2005.

Valley V, Jackson-Williams L, Fly C: Abortion inevitable, *eMedicine*, 2006. Retrieved from http://emedicine.medscape.com.

Weiner C, Buhimschi C: *Drugs for pregnant and lactating women*, ed 2, Philadelphia, 2009, Saunders.

Wieringa-DeWaard M, Hartmann E, Ankum W, and others: Expectant management versus surgical evacuation in first trimester miscarriage: health-related quality of life in randomized and non-randomized patients, *Hum Reprod* 17:1638–1642, 2002.

Wood S, Brain P: Medical management of missed abortion: A randomized clinical trial [published correction appears in *Obstet Gynecol* 100:175, 2002], *Obstet Gynecol* 99:563–566, 2002.

Zilianti M, and others: Monitoring the effacement of the uterine cervix by transperineal sonography: a new perspective, *J Ultrasound Med* 14(10):719–724, 1995.

17

Ectopic Pregnancy

An ectopic pregnancy develops as the result of the blastocyst implanting somewhere other than in the endometrium of the uterus. Sites of an ectopic pregnancy (Fig. 17-1) are the fallopian tube, ovary, cervix, or abdominal cavity. The majority of ectopic pregnancies (97%) are located in the fallopian tube, with 0.5% located on an ovary, 0.3% on the cervix, and 1.5% in the abdominal cavity (Attar, 2004; ACOG, 2008).

Of all tubal ectopic pregnancies, 55% are located in the *ampulla*, or largest portion of the tube. The next most common site is the *isthmus*, or the narrow part of the tube that connects the interstitium to the ampullar portion. Three percent of ectopic pregnancies are located in the *interstitium*, which is the muscular portion of the tube adjacent to the uterine cavity. Rarely does the ectopic pregnancy locate in the *fimbria* or terminal end of the tube (Lozeau and Potter, 2005; Cunningham and others, 2010). The outcome and gestational length of the tubal ectopic pregnancy are influenced by its location in the fallopian tube.

INCIDENCE

The incidence of ectopic pregnancy in the general population is approximately 2% of all pregnancies (Molinaro and Barnhart, 2007; Lin, Bhatt and Dogra, 2008). The incidence is increased following the use of assisted reproductive technologies (Kulp and Barnhart, 2008).

ETIOLOGY

Previous Tubal Infections
Previous pelvic infections caused by certain sexually transmitted diseases such as chlamydia or gonorrhea, postpartum endometritis, and postabortal uterine infections can predispose a woman to tubal infection (CDC, 2007; ACOG, 2008). A tubal infection can damage the mucosal surface of the fallopian tube, causing intraluminal adhesions and scarring that interfere with tubal motility.

Previous Tubal or Pelvic Surgery
During surgery, if blood is allowed to enter the fallopian tubes, tubal adhesions can result from the irritation of the mucosal surface. Therefore previous tubal surgery and previous pelvic surgery can cause tubal pregnancies.

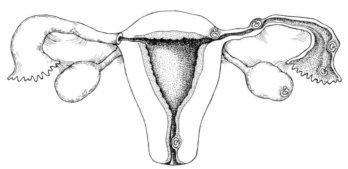

Figure 17-1 Common sites for an ectopic pregnancy.

Hormonal Factors

Altered estrogen and progesterone levels or inappropriate levels of prostaglandins, oxytocin, or catecholamines can interfere with normal tubal motility of the fertilized ovum.

Contraceptive Failure

Intrauterine devices (IUDs) are 99% effective in decreasing the risk for all pregnancies, including ectopic pregnancies. However, in the event of a pregnancy occurring while an IUD device is in place, there is an increased risk for an ectopic pregnancy. The cause is unknown but may be related to altered tubal motility or a tubal infection.

There does not seem to be an increased risk for ectopic pregnancy with the use of progestin-only contraceptives. However, any pregnancy that occurs due to contraceptive failure is more likely to be ectopic (Hatcher and others, 2007). When the morning-after pill is used and fails, there is an increased risk for ectopic pregnancy because the pill has a high estrogen level, which interferes with tubal motility (Cunningham and others, 2010). Of women who become pregnant after tubal ligation, 60% experience an ectopic pregnancy (Marchiano, 2004).

Assisted Reproduction

There is an increased incidence of ectopic pregnancy associated with ovulation-stimulating drugs such as human menopausal gonadotropin and clomiphene citrate. These drugs alter the estrogen and progesterone levels in the woman's body, which can affect tubal motility. There is an increased risk, as well, of an ectopic pregnancy with in vitro fertilization or gamete intrafallopian transfer because underlying tubal damage is frequently one of the factors predisposing a woman to require this type of infertility treatment.

Behavioral Factors

Maternal cigarette smoking at the time of conception (thought to affect tubal motility) has an independent and dose-related effect on the risk for ectopic pregnancy (Attar, 2004). It is thought to affect the ciliary action in the fallopian tubes.

Transmigration of Ovum

Migration of the ovum from one ovary to the opposite fallopian tube can occur by an extrauterine or intrauterine route. This can delay transportation of the fertilized ovum to the uterus. In this case, trophoblastic tissue is present on the blastocyst before it reaches the uterine cavity; therefore the trophoblastic tissue implants itself on the wall of the fallopian tube.

NORMAL PHYSIOLOGY

The fallopian tube wall is muscular and narrow and contains few ciliated cells at the interstitial area. In the ampullar area, the fallopian tube becomes less muscular, the luminal size increases, and the ciliated cells are more abundant.

The fimbriated end of the fallopian tube serves to pick up the ovum when it is released from the ovary. Then the fallopian tube has the unique function of moving the ovum and sperm in opposite directions almost simultaneously, by *peristaltic* (muscular) contractions and ciliated activity. Two or more adjacent pacemakers in the ampullar and isthmic areas of the fallopian tube initiate this tubal activity by sending out myoelectrical activity in either direction.

The net directional movement in the fallopian tubes varies during the menstrual cycle. During menstruation, the net directional force is toward the uterus starting from the ampullar area to prevent menstrual blood reflux into the tubes (Pulkkinen and Talo, 1987). This is stimulated primarily by estrogen-induced prostaglandins. Just before ovulation, the directional force from the ampullar area is inward, to pick up the released ovum from the ovary and move it into the ampullar area of the fallopian tube. At the same time, the directional force from the uterine area is the opposite, to facilitate sperm mobility toward the ovum (Pulkkinen and Talo, 1987). This is influenced by estrogen primarily. After fertilization, the directional force varies in the ampullar area, which delays ovum transport. Approximately 5 days after ovulation, the net directional force from the middle of the ampullar area is inward through the isthmus, to transport the ovum to the uterus. This is influenced by increasing progesterone and prostaglandin E_2. Approximately 7 days after ovulation, the myoelectrical activity becomes variable again, moving in both directions from each of the pacemakers (Pulkkinen and Talo, 1987).

The fertilized ovum reaches the uterine cavity in 6 to 7 days—just about the time the trophoblast cells begin to secrete the proteolytic enzyme and start to develop the threadlike projections called *chorionic villi*, which initiate the implantation process.

The uterus is normally prepared by estrogen and progesterone to accept the fertilized ovum, now called a *blastocyst*. As the chorionic villi invade the endometrium, the villi are held in check by a fibrinoid zone. The uterus is also supplied with an increased blood supply capable of nourishing the products of conception.

PATHOPHYSIOLOGY

Tubal Ectopic Pregnancy

Because most ectopic pregnancies initially implant in a fallopian tube, the pathophysiology focuses on tubal ectopic pregnancies. The blastocyst burrows into the epithelium of the tubal wall, tapping blood vessels, by the same process as normal implantation into the uterine endometrium.

Table 17-1   Tubal Pregnancy

Type	Duration (Weeks)	Usual Method of Termination
Ampullar	6-12	Tubal abortion
Fimbriated	6-12	Tubal abortion
Isthmic	6-8	Tubal rupture
Interstitial	12-14	Tubal rupture startle response

The environment of the tube, however, is quite different because of the following factors:

- Resistance to the invading trophoblastic tissue by the fallopian tube is decreased.
- Muscle mass lining the fallopian tubes is decreased; therefore their distensibility is greatly limited.
- The blood pressure is much higher in the tubal arteries than in the uterine arteries.
- Decidual reaction is limited; therefore human chorionic gonadotropin (hCG) is decreased and the signs and symptoms of pregnancy are limited.

It is because of these characteristic factors that termination of a tubal pregnancy occurs gestationally early by an abortion, spontaneous regression, or rupture, depending on the gestational age and the location of the implantation (Table 17-1). If the embryo dies early in gestation, spontaneous regression often occurs. If spontaneous regression fails to occur, usually an ampullar or fimbriated tubal pregnancy ends in an abortion and an isthmic or interstitial pregnancy ends in a rupture (Cunningham and others, 2010).

A tubal abortion (Fig. 17-2) occurs primarily because of separation of all or part of the placenta. This separation is caused by the pressure exerted by the tapped blood vessels or tubal contractions. With complete separation, the products of conception are expelled into the abdominal cavity by way of the fimbriated end of the fallopian tube, and unless there is an injured blood vessel, the bleeding stops. With an incomplete separation, bleeding continues until complete separation takes place, and the blood flows into the abdominal cavity, collecting in the rectouterine cul-de-sac of Douglas.

Tubal rupture (Fig. 17-3) results from the uninterrupted invasion of the trophoblastic tissue or tearing of the extremely stretched tissue. In either case, the products of conception are completely or incompletely expelled into the abdominal cavity or between the folds of the broad ligaments by way of the torn tube.

The duration of the tubal pregnancy depends on the location of the implanted embryo or fetus and the distensibility of that part of the fallopian tube. For instance, if the implantation is located in the narrow isthmic portion of the tube, it ruptures early, within 6 to 8 weeks; the distensible interstitial portion may be able to retain the pregnancy up to 14 weeks. An ampullar or fimbriated tubal pregnancy is usually lost between 6 and 12 weeks of gestation.

The outcome of the pregnancy at the time of the interruption depends on the age of the embryo or fetus and whether the rupture is complete or incomplete. In rare cases, when the abortion occurs very early in the pregnancy and the placenta is initially separated completely from the tubal wall, the trophoblastic tissue reimplants

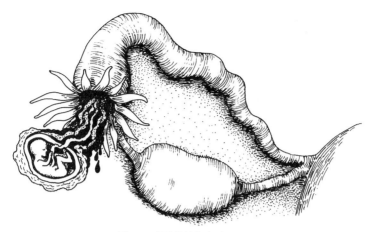

Figure 17-2 Tubal abortion.

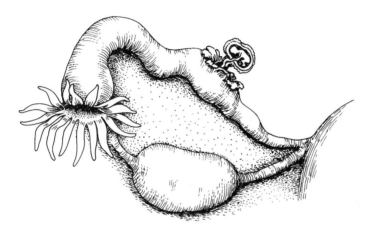

Figure 17-3 Tubal rupture.

in the abdominal cavity and the placenta and embryo or fetus will continue to grow. This leads to the development of a secondary abdominal pregnancy. Usually only a small amount of blood is lost at this time.

If the rupture is incomplete, in rare cases, the ruptured part of the placenta reattaches to some surrounding abdominal tissue. This leads to the development of a tuboabdominal, tuboovarian, or broad ligament pregnancy. In most instances, however, the embryo or fetus dies at the time of the abortion or rupture. If not surgically removed, it can be absorbed if small or, if too large to be absorbed, it can mummify or calcify. When the bleeding is slight, no problems result. However, in most cases blood vessels are torn open and bleeding is profuse. This blood and the lost products of conception collect in the cul-de-sac of Douglas, causing severe pain and hypovolemia. A real emergency is present, which can end in maternal death if the bleeding is not quickly stopped.

Abdominal Ectopic Pregnancy

An abdominal pregnancy almost always results from an implantation secondary to a tubal rupture or abortion through the fimbriated end of the fallopian tube. In these cases, the placenta continues to grow after attachment to some abdominal structure, usually the surface of the uterus, broad ligaments, or ovaries. However, it can be any abdominal structure, including the liver, spleen, or intestines. Because the invading trophoblastic tissue is not held in check, it can erode major blood vessels at any time and cause severe bleeding. Fetal movements are also painful because they are not cushioned by the myometrium.

Cervical Ectopic Pregnancy

In very rare cases, the fertilized ovum bypasses the uterine endometrium and implants itself in the cervical mucus. Accelerated migration of the blastocyst through the uterus caused by an intrauterine device or changes in the endometrial lining as the result of prior curettage or endometrial inflammation are possible contributing factors (Molinaro and Barnhart, 2007). Because the uterine artery gains entry to the uterus by way of the cervix, there is an abundant blood supply to a cervical ectopic pregnancy and tremendous bleeding can ensue when removal is attempted.

SIGNS AND SYMPTOMS

Before Rupture

Currently, most ectopic pregnancies are diagnosed before rupture based on the three most classic symptoms: abdominal pain, delayed menses, and abnormal vaginal bleeding (spotting) that occurs 6 to 8 weeks after the last normal menstrual period.

Abdominal Pain

Abdominal pain occurs nearly 100% of the time if allowed to progress. It is usually first manifested by a dull, lower quadrant, unilateral pain caused by tubal stretching followed by a sharp, colicky tubal pain caused by further tubal stretching and stimulated contractions. It progresses to a diffuse, constant, severe pain generalized throughout the lower abdomen (Lipscomb, Stovall, and Ling, 2000).

Delayed Menses

A history of a period that is delayed approximately 1 to 2 weeks or a lighter than usual or irregular period is reported by 75% to 90% of the patients (Della-Giustina and Denny, 2003).

Abnormal Vaginal Bleeding

Mild to intermittent dark red or brown vaginal discharge occurs in 79% of the cases related to uterine decidual shedding secondary to decreased hormones such as progesterone and hCG (Tay and others, 2000).

Absence of Common Signs of Pregnancy

Absence of common signs of pregnancy, secondary to decreased pregnancy hormonal levels, frequently occurs (Cahill and Wardle, 2006).

Abdominal Tenderness

Abdominal tenderness occurs in more than 91% of the cases (Tay and others, 2000).

Tubal Rupture

Exacerbation of the pain occurs during tubal rupture in an ectopic pregnancy.

After Tubal Rupture

Generalized, Unilateral, or Deep Lower Quadrant Acute Abdominal Pain

Abdominal pain is caused by blood irritating the peritoneum.

Referred Shoulder Pain

Referred shoulder pain is related to diaphragmatic irritation from blood in the peritoneal cavity.

Faintness and Dizziness

Faintness and dizziness occur in the presence of significant bleeding.

Signs of Shock

Shock is related to the severity of the bleeding into the abdomen.

Afebrile State

In the beginning, usually no signs of an infection are present.

MATERNAL EFFECTS

Ectopic pregnancies account for 9% of all pregnancy-related maternal deaths (CDC, 2009) and are the leading cause of maternal mortality (Minino, Heron, Murphy, and Kochanek, 2007). Hemorrhage is the major cause of death and occurs most frequently with a cervical or abdominal ectopic pregnancy.

FETAL AND NEONATAL EFFECTS

Death is almost certain for the fetus in an ectopic pregnancy. About 5% of abdominal ectopic pregnancies reach viability (Tasnim and Mahmud, 2005). However, it is not recommended to continue an abdominal pregnancy if it is diagnosed early because of the extreme risk for hemorrhage at any time during the pregnancy. The risk for fetal deformity is also high related to pressure deformities caused by oligohydramnios.

DIAGNOSTIC TESTING

Diagnosis before extrauterine rupture or abortion can minimize tubal damage, decrease maternal mortality from hemorrhage, and simplify management of an ectopic pregnancy. However, because this condition mimics other diseases (Table 17-2) and no one diagnostic tool is specific for detecting an early ectopic gestation, early diagnosis is difficult.

Table 17-2   Pelvic Pain: Differential Diagnosis

	Appendicitis	Cholelithiasis During Pregnancy	Ectopic (Unruptured or Ruptured)*	Ovarian Cyst	Pelvic Inflammatory Disease	Spontaneous Abortion
Chief complaint	Abdominal pain	Abdominal pain Associated flatulence	Abdominal pain	Lower abdominal or pelvic pain	Lower abdominal and pelvic pain	Cramping with or without vaginal bleeding
Workup of Associated Symptoms						
P: Provocation What causes the symptoms? What makes symptoms better or worse?		Pain associated with high-fat meal	Sex and activity increase symptoms	Increased with movement, especially when standing or stooping		
Q: Quality or Quantity How does the pain feel?	Steady ache or colicky	Lancinating, cramping, colicky, or steady up to 1 hr	Dull pain/*deep acute abdominal pain*	Dull	Tender	Crampy
R: Region or Radiation Where are the symptoms? Do symptoms spread?	Usually generalized or unilateral RLQ	Originating in midportion of epigastrium, radiating to back, chest, shoulders	Unilateral or bilateral lower quadrant/ *generalized deep/ referred shoulder pain related to diaphragmatic irritation*	Unilateral	Lower bilateral abdominal or pelvic pain radiating to lower back or down one or both legs	Pressure pain, generalized or localized in the lower abdomen

S: Severity scale How severe are the symptoms?	Severe	Severe	Mild to severe; Vague, cramping/severe	Mild to severe	Mild to severe	Mild to severe
T: Timing When did the symptoms begin? Associated with menses?	Sudden onset	Abrupt onset pain	Continuous or intermittent	Frequently after onset or cessation of menses		
Review of symptoms (ROS)	Anorexia N/V preceded by pain Low-grade fever (100.2°-100.6° F)	Flatulence, bloating/indigestion Anorexia N/V Pain associated with high-fat meals	Delayed menses/amenorrhea Absence of common signs of pregnancy Urinary frequency After rupture: vertigo/fainting *Decreased BP and increased pulse, if bleeding is continuous and rapid*	N/V Amenorrhea Possible fever	Possible vaginal discharge, dysuria, dyspareunia, menstrual abnormality Anorexia N/V Possible high fever Positive signs of high risk sexual behaviors	Vaginal bleeding Any sign of shock equal to obvious bleeding

Continued

Table 17-2 Pelvic Pain: Differential Diagnosis—cont'd

	Appendicitis	Cholelithiasis During Pregnancy	Ectopic (Unruptured or Ruptured)*	Ovarian Cyst	Pelvic Inflammatory Disease	Spontaneous Abortion
Complete physical examination	RLQ tenderness at McBurney's point Abdominal guarding/muscular rigidity on palpation Rebound tenderness Positive iliopsoas and obturator test	Localized abdominal tenderness on palpation Positive Murphy sign	Lower abdominal tenderness on palpation After rupture: severe generalized abdominal tenderness		↑Lower abdominal bilateral tenderness with deep and light palpation	No abdominal tenderness
Pelvic examination	No vaginal discharge Rectal examination may increase pain		Dark red or brown vaginal discharge Cervix and uterus slightly soft to palpation Positive CMT Positive adnexal mass	Tenderness with pelvic examination Enlarged ovaries palpated 50% of the time Unilateral adnexal mass with tenderness	Positive BUS Purulent vaginal discharge Cultures may be increased for gonorrhea/Chlamydia ↑Positive CMT ↑Positive adnexal tenderness Palpable adnexal if abscess is present	Cervix closed or dilated Vaginal bleeding mild to severe Negative CMT Negative adnexal mass

Diagnostic data	CBC may show polymorphonuclear leukocytosis	Amylase, alkaline phosphates elevated	Transvaginal ultrasound to reveal ectopic mass or a uterine sac	Pelvic or transvaginal ultrasound should demonstrate the cyst	Elevated ESR	Transvaginal ultrasound
					C-reactive protein elevated	Quantitative hCG
	May use high resolution, real-time ultrasonography	Abdominal ultrasound may indicate stones	Positive hCG levels that do not double in 48 hr		WBC elevated with left shift	
			Progesterone levels less than 8 mg/ml		Pelvic or transvaginal ultrasound	
					CT scan may indicate a thickened fluid-filled tube	
					Endometrial biopsy	
					Laparoscopy	

*Signs and symptoms of ruptured ectopic pregnancy are in *italics*.

†Minimum criteria for diagnosis.

BP, Blood pressure; *BUS*, Bartholin, urethral, scene glands; *CBC*, complete blood count; *CMT*, cervical motion tenderness; *ERS*, erythrocyte; *N/V*, nausea and vomiting; *RLQ*, right lower quadrant; *RUQ*, right upper quadrant; *WBC*, white blood cells.

A pertinent history and physical examination are the foundations for initiating an appropriate diagnostic workup that results in the accurate and timely diagnosis of an ectopic pregnancy. Physical findings can include a normal or slightly enlarged uterus, palpable adnexal mass in 50% of tubal ectopic pregnancies, and cervical motion tenderness 50% of the time as well. The most important diagnostic tools are serial hCG levels, and transvaginal ultrasound (TVU). For a summary of the diagnostic test results and interpretation, see Table 17-3.

Serial Serum Beta-Human Chorionic Gonadotropin Levels

The fertilized ovum and the chorionic villi produce hCG, which maintains the corpus luteum to produce progesterone and estrogen. This maintains the pregnancy until the placenta is mature enough to assume that role at around 10 weeks of gestation. In a normal pregnancy, hCG is present in detectable levels (greater than 2 mIU/ml) in the maternal serum 8 to 10 days after fertilization. Levels normally double every 48 hours for the first 5 to 8 weeks after conception, rising well above 100,000 mIU/ml and then gradually decreasing after 10 weeks. In an ectopic or spontaneous abortion, hCG levels rise slower than normal and usually plateau at about 6 weeks below 6000 mIU/ml (Lipscomb, Stovall, and Ling, 2000). A consistently decreasing hCG level indicates a nonviable pregnancy (ACOG, 2008). Thus serial hCG levels 48 hours apart aid in the differentiation between a normal and an abnormal pregnancy.

Transvaginal Ultrasound

The usefulness of ultrasound in the diagnosis of an ectopic pregnancy is increasing continuously. In the past, ultrasound was useful only in diagnosing an intrauterine pregnancy, which would rule out an ectopic pregnancy. One exception was in the case of an advanced abdominal pregnancy. In these cases, ultrasound would show a fetal head outside the uterus.

TVU is becoming an important diagnostic tool in diagnosing ectopic pregnancy before rupture because the probe can be placed closer to the pelvic structures. With the more sophisticated real-time equipment and an expert technician, all normal pregnancies should be seen by TVU by 3 to 4 weeks after fertilization. When hCG levels are 1500 to 2000 mIU/ml or greater, a normal intrauterine pregnancy should be visible with TVU (ACOG, 2008). Therefore when hCG levels are greater than 1500 mIU/ml with no visible intrauterine pregnancy, ectopic pregnancy is very likely (Lozeau and Potter, 2005). With TVU, the location of the gestational sac of an early ectopic pregnancy can be visualized only 20% of the time (Sherbahn, 2001). If an ectopic sac is identified, it is measured for size and attempts are made to determine any fetal cardiac activity. This determines which therapy is used.

In 10% to 20% of ectopic pregnancies, a "pseudosac" produced by decidual reaction in the uterus is seen and can be confused with an intrauterine gestation. A corpus luteum cyst can be confused as an adnexal mass indicating an ectopic pregnancy as well. Any mass seen on ultrasound must contain a yolk sac, fetal pole, or fetal cardiac activity to indicate a pregnancy (Seeber and Barnhart, 2006).

Table 17-3   Diagnostic Tests

Test	Results	Interpretations
Serum progesterone	Greater than 25 ng/ml	Normal intrauterine pregnancy (except after ovarian stimulation)
	Greater than 5 ng/ml but less than 25 ng/ml	Undetermined viability
	Less than 5 ng/ml	Nonviable; may indicate ectopic pregnancy or a spontaneous abortion
Beta-hCG	Detected in the serum 8–10 days after fertilization	Normal intrauterine pregnancy
	Levels normally double every 36–48 hours for the first 5–8 weeks after conception	
	Levels at about 4.5 weeks (50–250 mIU/ml)	
	Levels at about 6.5 weeks (10,000 mIU/ml)	
	Levels peak at 8–10 weeks (100,000–150,000 mIU/ml)	
	After 10-week start, decreases sharply	
	Prolonged doubling time of hCG levels may indicate an ectopic pregnancy or a spontaneous abortion	May indicate an ectopic pregnancy or a spontaneous abortion
	Levels plateau at around 6 weeks	Predictive of ectopic pregnancy
	Extremely high levels	Hydatidiform mole or multiple gestation
Transvaginal ultrasound	Visible intrauterine fetal sac after hCG levels are greater than 1500–2000 mIU/ml	Normal intrauterine pregnancy, 5–6 weeks of gestation
	Pulsating fetal heart within the intrauterine sac	Normal intrauterine pregnancy, 6.5–7 weeks of gestation
	No fetal heart action within the intrauterine sac after 7 weeks	Spontaneous abortion
	Absence of intrauterine sac with hCG greater than 1500–2000	Ectopic pregnancy
	Pseudogestational sac without fetus found in uterus or fetal sac found in tubes	Ectopic pregnancy

hCG, Human chorionic gonadotropin.

Serum Progesterone Levels

Serum progesterone levels are used in combination with hCG levels and TVU to determine who needs further testing. In a normal pregnancy, the corpus luteum produces an increased amount of progesterone for the first 8 to 10 weeks. Then the placenta takes over the production of progesterone. Serum progesterone levels above 20 ng/ml most often indicate a normal intrauterine pregnancy. In an ectopic pregnancy, progesterone levels are usually decreased to lower than 5 ng/ml (ACOG, 2008). Values between 5 and 20 ng/ml are not conclusive and indicate the need for further testing (ACOG, 2008). If the woman had medication-induced ovarian stimulation, these values may not be applicable.

USUAL MEDICAL MANAGEMENT

Tubal Ectopic Pregnancy before Rupture

Surgical Treatment

The type of surgical management depends on the location and cause of the ectopic pregnancy, the extent of tissue involvement, and the patient's wishes for future fertility. The choice of treatment for an unruptured tubal pregnancy is a laparoscopic salpingostomy, in which a longitudinal incision is made over the pregnancy site and the products of conception are gently and very carefully removed to prevent or control the bleeding (Hajenius and others, 2007).

To rule out persistent trophoblastic growth, follow-up treatment includes serial hCG levels. Usually, hCG is undetectable by the twelfth postsurgical day.

Nonsurgical Medical Treatment

A well-studied medical therapy in the treatment of an ectopic pregnancy is methotrexate. Methotrexate, a type of chemotherapy, is a folic acid antagonist that interferes with DNA synthesis and cell multiplication, causing dissolution of the ectopic mass (Lozeau and Potter, 2005). Criteria according to ACOG (2008) for its use follow:

- Hemodynamically stable with no signs of severe abdominal pain, weakness, dizziness, syncope, orthostatic hypotension, tachycardia, or falling hematocrit
- Ectopic sac smaller than 3.5 cm in diameter
- Fetus not alive as indicated by any cardiac activity
- Serum hCG levels lower than 5000 mIU/ml
- Liver function studies within normal limits
- Normal kidney function as indicated by normal serum creatinine
- No evidence of peptic ulcer disease, ulcerative colitis, or active pulmonary disease
- No evidence of leukopenia (blood leukocytes greater than 3500/mm^3)
- No evidence of thrombocytopenia (platelet count greater than 100,000/mm^3)
- No evidence of AIDS due to additive immunosuppressive effects

Protocols for methotrexate therapy include single-dose, two-dose, and multiple-dose regimens.

- Single-dose method: Methotrexate 50 mg per square meter of body surface intramuscularly. Repeat dose if beta-hCG levels have not dropped at least 15% between day 4 and day 7.

- Two-dose method: Methotrexate 50 mg per square meter of body surface intramuscularly day 0. Repeat Methotrexate on day 4.
- Multiple-dose method: Methotrexate, 1 mg/kg intramuscularly every other day (odd days) and folinic acid, a rescue drug to minimize side effects, intramuscularly every other day (even days), until beta-hCG levels drop at least 15% in a 48-hour period; or maximum of four doses each (Lozeau and Potter, 2005). Hajenius and others (2007) concluded, on the basis of a Cochrane Review, that medical treatment with systemic methotrexate is an effective alternative nonsurgical treatment option for a small, unruptured ectopic pregnancy. It can also be used if the ectopic pregnancy persists after surgical management.

Follow-up continues until β-hCG levels are nondetectable. Average resolution of the ectopic pregnancy is 7 weeks, but it can take anywhere from 35 to 109 days.

Surgical intervention may be necessary if any of the following occurs to the patient:
- Experiences worsening abdominal pain indicating tubal rupture
- Becomes hemodynamically unstable
- β-hCG levels increase, plateau, or fail to decline 15% by day 7

Tubal Ectopic Pregnancy after Rupture

After a ruptured tubal pregnancy, a *laparotomy salpingectomy* (removal of the affected fallopian tube) is the most common surgical treatment. Occasionally, a *salpingo-oophorectomy* (removal of the affected fallopian tube and adjacent ovary) is performed if the blood supply to the ovary is affected or if the ectopic pregnancy involved the ovary. Otherwise, preservation of the ovary is recommended. If the couple does not wish to have more children, a hysterectomy may be done if the woman's condition is stable.

Abdominal Ectopic Pregnancy

For an abdominal pregnancy, hemorrhage is a serious possibility because the placenta can separate from its attachment site at any time. Abdominal surgery to remove the embryo or fetus is usually done as soon as an abdominal pregnancy is diagnosed. Leaving the placenta in situ, which was a standard of practice, has a significant risk of ensuring infection, hemorrhage, and intestinal obstruction. Therefore an attempt to ligate the placental blood supply and remove the placenta is the current practice. If the placenta cannot be removed, methotrexate may be used to facilitate involution (Molinaro and Barnhart, 2007).

Cervical Ectopic Pregnancy

Because of the risks of uncontrollable hemorrhage and urinary tract injury, surgical management is the last alternative treatment for a cervical ectopic pregnancy. Methotrexate is being successfully used. The agent is injected directly into the gestational sac or given systematically as outlined earlier (Molinaro and Barnhart, 2007). If methotrexate is contraindicated and surgical management is necessary, several methods are used to diminish the risk for hemorrhage. Such treatments include a cerclage and local injection of vasopressin before evacuation, inflation of a 30-ml Foley catheter bulb in the cervix, and vaginal packing after curettage, or potassium chloride injection into the gestational sac (Molinaro and Barnhart, 2007).

NURSING MANAGEMENT

Prevention

An ectopic pregnancy is closely associated with tubal scarring. Preventing tubal scarring is the key to prevention of an ectopic pregnancy. Discussing safe sex practices that prevent sexually transmitted infection should be a routine part of well-woman care. Screening for chlamydia and gonorrhea should be included in the yearly gynecologic examination for at-risk women because they often have no symptoms. A sexually transmitted infection should be treated to prevent pelvic inflammatory disease (PID). If PID does develop, rapid treatment can decrease the chance of tubal scarring. When a woman chooses an IUD, descriptions of the signs of PID should be included in the teaching.

If pregnancy occurs while the woman has an IUD in place, ectopic pregnancy should be considered because it is more likely to occur. Because a correlation exists between cigarette smoking and an increased risk for an ectopic pregnancy, women during their childbearing years should be encouraged to avoid smoking. If an elective abortion is desired, only medically prepared professionals should perform it. These measures decrease the chance of tubal defects and thereby decrease the incidence of an ectopic pregnancy. Because of the increasing incidence of ectopic pregnancy, health professionals should consider the possibility in any woman who presents with any type of abdominal discomfort during her childbearing years.

Assessment

Because of the high maternal mortality associated with an ectopic pregnancy that goes undiagnosed until after rupture or tubal abortion, it is essential for nurses to be alert to signs and symptoms of this pregnancy complication. Therefore any woman in her childbearing years who experiences irregular vaginal spotting associated with a dull, aching pelvic pain, with or without signs of pregnancy, should be evaluated for a possible ectopic pregnancy. The following areas should be explored.

Risk Factors

A history of any PID, previous ectopic pregnancies, elective abortions, or prior infertility disorders is determined; these conditions can increase the patient's risk for a tubal defect.

Pain

If an ectopic pregnancy is suspected, a detailed history includes questions regarding the type of abdominal pain. The pain caused by an unruptured ectopic pregnancy can be a unilateral, cramplike pain related to tubal distention by the enlarging embryo or fetus. At the time of tubal rupture, many patients experience a sudden, sharp, stabbing pain in the lower abdomen. Blood in the peritoneum can cause a dull aching or severe, generalized pain. If the blood touches the diaphragm, it usually causes referred shoulder pain. Many times, movement of the body aggravates the pain.

Vaginal Bleeding

Assess for vaginal bleeding, and obtain a menstrual history. Vaginal bleeding is usually related to the sloughing of the endometrial lining related to decreasing progesterone and estrogen levels and can be continuous or intermittent in small or large quantities. It usually differs from the patient's normal period. Pad counts should be kept to determine the amount and type of vaginal bleeding.

Syncope

Assess for the presence of any signs of syncope. When an ectopic pregnancy ruptures or aborts, blood is lost into the peritoneal cavity. At this time, the patient can experience a feeling of faintness or weakness related to hypovolemia. If the bleeding is not continuous, the depleted blood volume is restored to near normal in 1 or 2 days by hemodilution, and the faint or weak feeling subsides. If the bleeding is profuse, the patient can go into shock quickly.

Vital Signs

To assess the amount of intraperitoneal blood loss, the patient's vital signs should be checked as frequently as the situation indicates.

Nursing Interventions to Allay Fear Regarding Possible Diagnosis

- Assess the family's anxiety over maternal well-being because 10% to 15% of pregnancy-related deaths are caused by ectopic pregnancy (Della-Giustina and Denny, 2003).
- Assess the family's level of guilt (e.g., their feeling as to what they did to cause this to happen).
- Assess the family's coping strategies and resources.
- Explain all diagnostic and treatment modalities and reasons for each in understandable terms.
- Prepare the patient for serial beta-hCG levels, progesterone levels, or TVU. If a TVU diagnostic procedure is ordered, have patient empty her bladder before the procedure.
- Prepare the patient for the medical or surgical procedure.

Postoperative Nursing Interventions

- Tell the patient that the incidence of persistent trophoblastic tissue growth following laparoscopic salpingostomy is 5% to 20% (ACOG, 2008).
- Prepare the patient for weekly hCG levels until results are negative. If levels increase or plateau, be prepared for methotrexate therapy.
- Validate with the couple that this is a loss of a pregnancy and it is acceptable to grieve over the loss.
- If the mother is RhD-negative and unsensitized, be prepared to administer Rh_o (D) immune globulin. The usual dose is Rh_o (D) immune globulin standard dose (RhoGAM; HypRho-D) IM 300 micrograms if the gestational age is greater than 12 weeks or gestation unknown; for a gestation of 12 weeks or less, the usual dose is Rh_o (D) globulin microdose (MicRhoGAM, HypRho-D MiniDose) IM 150 micrograms.

Nursing Interventions for Medical Management

- Review how the medication or medications work. Be prepared to discuss the risks and benefits of this type of management. Benefits include an 80% to 90% success rate (Weiner and Buhimschi, 2009), cost effectiveness, noninvasive outpatient management, and 83% preservation of tubal patency. Risks include long resolution time (average time 7 weeks, but range between 35 and 109 days), limitations in physical functioning, less energy, possible discomfort, and possible tubal rupture.

- Prepare the patient for possible increase in adnexal discomfort or pain related to tubal absorption or tubal distention caused by the formation of a hematoma, which usually lasts 4 to 12 hours, sometime between 5 and 10 days after initial dose of medication. Tubal rupture, however, must be considered and ruled out in the presence of severe or significant change in discomfort.
- Teach the patient appropriate pain management, such as ibuprofen 800 mg every 6 hours. Advise patients to avoid using aspirin and some antiinflammatory drugs such as ibuprofen (Motrin), naproxen (Aleve; Naprosyn), and indomethacin; they worsen the gastrointestinal side effects of the treatment.
- Explain that side effects such as nausea, vomiting, transient stomatitis, oral ulcers, and diarrhea occur in about 5% of cases.
- Provide emotional support for the patient and her family.
- Be prepared to obtain baseline levels such as a complete blood cell count and chemistry profile with liver enzymes and renal function studies including BUN and creatinine, platelet count, blood type, and Rh factor.
- Advise the patient as to the importance of follow-up that includes hCG titers until they reach zero because of continued inflammation of the ectopic site until resolution of the ectopic pregnancy is complete.
- Teach the patient the importance of refraining from alcohol consumption, vitamin supplements with folic acid (including prenatal vitamins), and sexual intercourse until the ectopic pregnancy is resolved to decrease the risk for medication side effects or exacerbating the rupture of the ectopic pregnancy.
- Teach the patient to report signs of ectopic rupture immediately, such as severe, sharp, stabbing, unilateral abdominal pain.
- Encourage the patient to avoid sun exposure related to the photosensitivity of the drug during treatment.
- Validate with the couple that this is a loss of a pregnancy and that it is acceptable to grieve over the loss.

Nursing Interventions for Anticipatory Grieving

- Assess the level of loss and desire for future childbearing.
- Encourage the patient and her family to express their feelings and concerns openly.
- Discuss with the patient and family the chances of recurrence (10%) and infertility problems (40% to 50%) (Seeber and Barnhart, 2006).
- Teach the couple the importance of using a contraceptive for at least three menstrual cycles to allow time for the woman's body to recover.
- Reassure regarding the safety of conception following methotrexate treatment without the increased risk of adverse pregnancy outcome (Svirsky and others, 2009).
- Refer to a support group, such as Resolve Through Sharing, if available (a comprehensive, passionate Internet resource can be found at *http://www.ectopicpregnancy. com*).
- Refer to a pastor, priest, or chaplain per family's request for spiritual assistance.
- See Chapter 7 for additional interventions.

CONCLUSION

The ultimate goal for nursing intervention is prevention of complications that can cause tubal or uterine defects. These complications set the stage for an ectopic pregnancy. If an ectopic pregnancy develops, the goal is to prevent complications during the treatment. Therefore efforts are best directed at prevention of future impairment of fertility through patient education. Education should include information for self-detection of signs of infections contributing to ectopic pregnancy. Efforts should also be directed at detecting and reporting early signs of an ectopic pregnancy so that diagnosis before a rupture or abortion can be made. Thus the complication of hemorrhage, which is the major cause of maternal death, can be prevented.

BIBLIOGRAPHY

American College of Obstetrics and Gynecology (ACOG): *Medical management of ectopic pregnancy,* Clinical Management Guidelines. No. 94, Washington, DC, 2008, Author.

Attar E: Endocrinology of ectopic pregnancy, *Obstet Gynecol Clin North Am* 31:779–794, 2004.

Cahill D, Wardle P: Bleeding and pain in early pregnancy. In James D, and others, editors: High risk pregnancy: management options, ed 3, Philadelphia, 2006, Saunders.

Centers for Disease Control and Prevention (CDC): *Fact sheet: pelvic inflammatory disease,* Washington, DC, 2007, CDC. Retrieved from http://www.cdc.gov/std/PID/pid-fact-sheet.pdf.

Centers for Disease Control and Prevention (CDC): *Female sterilization: Risk of ectopic pregnancy after tubal sterilization fact sheet,* Washington, DC, 2009, CDC. Retrieved from http://www.cdc.gov/reproductivehealth/unintendedPregnancy/EctopicPreg_factsheet.htm.

Cunningham F, Leveno K, Bloom S, Hauth J, Rouse D, Spong C: *Williams' obstetrics,* ed 23, New York, 2010, McGraw-Hill Medical.

Della-Giustina D, Denny M: Ectopic pregnancy, *Emerg Med Clin North Am* 21:565–584, 2003.

Hajenius P, Mol F, Mol B, and others: Interventions for tubal ectopic pregnancy, *Cochrane Database Syst Rev* (Issue 1), Art. No.: CD000324, 2007.

Hatcher R, and others: *Contraceptive technology,* ed 19, New York, 2007, Irvington Publishers.

Kulp J, Barnhart K: Ectopic pregnancy: diagnosis and management, *Womens Health* 4(1):79–87, 2008.

Lin E, Bhatt S, Dogra V: Diagnostic clues to ectopic pregnancy, *Radiographics* 28(6):1661–1671, 2008.

Lipscomb G, Stovall T, Ling F: Nonsurgical treatment of ectopic pregnancy, *N Engl J Med* 343(18):1325–1329, 2000.

Lozeau A, Potter B: Diagnosis and management of ectopic pregnancy, *Am Fam Physician* 72(9):1707–1714, 2005.

Marchiano D: Medical encyclopedia: ectopic pregnancy, *MedlinePlus,* Washington, DC, 2004, American Accreditation Health Care Commission.

Minino A, Heron M, Murphy S, Kochanek K for CDC Division of Vital Statistics. Deaths: final data for 2004, *National Vital Statistics reports* 55(19):1–120, 2007.

Molinaro T, Barnhart K: Ectopic pregnancies in unusual locations, *Semin Reprod Med* 25(2):123–130, 2007.

Pulkkinen M, Talo A: Tubal physiologic consideration in ectopic pregnancy, *Clin Obstet Gynecol* 30(1):164–172, 1987.

Royal College of Obstetricians and Gynaecologists (RCOG): *The management of tubal pregnancy,* Guideline No. 21, London, 2004, RCOG Press. Retrieved from http://www.rcog.org.uk/index.asp?PageID=1042.

Seeber B, Barnhart K: Suspected ectopic pregnancy, *Obstet Gynecol* 107(2):399–413, 2006.

Sherbahn R: *Ectopic pregnancy,* Gurnee, Ill, 2001, Advanced Fertility Center of Chicago. Retrieved from http://www.advancedfertility.com/ectopic.htm.

Svirsky R, Rozovski U, Vaknin Z, Pansky M, and others: The safety of conception occurring shortly after methotrexate treatment of an ectopic pregnancy, *Reprod Toxicol* 27(1):85–87, 2009.

Tasnim N, Mahmud G: Evidence based report: advanced abdominal pregnancy—a diagnostic management dilemma, *J Coll Physicians Surg Pak* 15(8):493–495, 2005.

Tay J, Moore J, Walker J: Ectopic pregnancy, *West J Med* 173(2):131–134, 2000.

Weiner C, Buhimschi C: *Drugs for pregnant and lactating women*, ed 2, Philadelphia, 2009, Saunders.

World Health Organization: Maternal mortality in 2005. Estimates developed by WHO, UNICEF, UNFPA< and the World Band, 2007.

18

Gestational Trophoblastic Disease

Gestational trophoblastic disease is a spectrum of pregnancy-related trophoblastic proliferative disorders without a viable fetus. The benign hydatidiform mole represents the beginning of the disease continuum, and metastatic gestational trophoblastic neoplasia (GTN) is at the end of the continuum. Malignant nonmetastatic (invasive) GTN is somewhere in the middle when the trophoblastic neoplasia invades the myometrium only.

HYDATIDIFORM MOLE

A hydatidiform mole is a benign proliferative growth of the trophoblast in which the chorionic villi develop into edematous, cystic, avascular, transparent vesicles that hang in a grapelike cluster (Fig. 18-1). There are two categories of hydatidiform moles: complete and partial.

Complete Moles
- Generalized areas of the chorionic villi become hyperplastic, edematous, and avascular.
- There is no embryo or fetus and amniotic sac.
- A diploid karyotype is present that is most often a 46,XX chromosomal pattern of paternal origin; a sperm with 23,X chromosomes duplicates itself because it fertilizes an ovum that contains no genetic material or the genetic material is inactive (ACOG, 2004). Occasionally (6% to 10% of the time) the karyotype is 46,XY. In these cases, two sperm have fertilized an ovum without genetic material (Bentley, 2003; ACOG, 2004). In either case the chromosomes are of paternal origin but the mitochondrial DNA has maternal origin (Berkowitz and Goldstein, 2009).

Partial Moles
- Localized areas of chorionic villi become hyperplastic, edematous, and avascular.
- There is an embryo or fetus and an amniotic sac, usually with multiple congenital anomalies.
- A triploid karyotype of 69,XXY, 69,XXX, or 69,XYY chromosomes is present in most of the cases: one set of chromosomes of maternal origin and two sets of paternal origin. In these cases, two sperm have fertilized an apparently normal ovum (Bentley, 2003; ACOG, 2004).

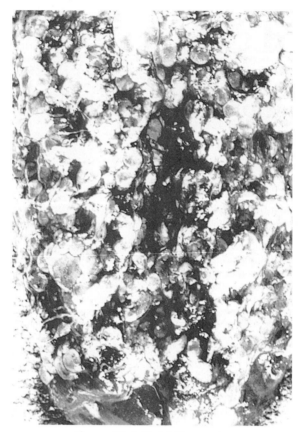

Figure 18-1 Hydatidiform mole.

Incidence

The incidence of hydatidiform mole in the United States is 1 per 1500 pregnancies (Berkowitz and Goldstein, 2005). In many other countries, especially in southeast Asia and the Far East, the incidence is 1 of every 120 pregnancies (Cohn and Herzog, 2000). There is a 1% to 2% increased risk for a repeat occurrence of hydatidiform mole (Hurteau, 2003).

Etiology

The cause of a hydatidiform mole is unknown, but it is theorized that an ovular defect, stress, or a nutritional deficiency (especially in carotene) may contribute to its development. Maternal age older than 35 years might be a factor as well because older oocytes are more susceptible to abnormal fertilization (Ngan, 2003). In rare cases a hydatidiform mole is related to an abnormal genetic predisposition (Fallahian, 2003).

Normal Physiology

Normally one sperm fertilizes one ovum and each contributes 23 chromosomes to form a new cell called a *zygote*. The zygote begins to grow immediately by undergoing a series of rapid mitotic cell divisions to form a solid mass of cells called a *morula*. As cellular activity continues, fluid begins to form in the center of the morula and causes the cells to rearrange until there is one single layer of cells lining the periphery and an inner cluster of cells. The single layer of cells, called the *trophoblast,* grows and develops into the placenta, and the inner cluster of cells, called the *embryoblast,* develops into a fetus. The umbilical cord eventually connects the two structures.

The trophoblast cells send out threadlike projections termed *chorionic villi* into the endometrium of the uterus primarily under the embryo to form the placenta. As the chorionic villi grow, they erode areas of the endometrium, forming intervillous spaces that fill with maternal blood. Invasion is normally held in check by the endometrium. Inside the chorionic villi, blood vessels and connective tissue begin to form. These blood vessels connect with the blood vessels inside the umbilical cord.

Pathophysiology

What actually causes the proliferation of the placenta is unknown. In any case, the trophoblastic tissue absorbs fluid from the maternal blood. Fluid then begins to accumulate in the chorionic villi because of inadequate or absent fetal circulation. As the pooling of fluid continues, vesicles are formed out of the chorionic villi.

Signs and Symptoms: Complete Mole

Characteristic symptoms of a complete hydatidiform mole are described in the following paragraphs.

Abnormal Uterine Bleeding

Abnormal uterine bleeding, which is intermittent or continuous (usually not profuse) and often brownish in color, occurs in approximately 75% of cases (Ngan, 2003). This is usually related to the lack of circulatory integrity of molar tissue. When the molar tissue starts separating from the uterus, bright red bleeding may result.

Variable Uterine Size

A uterus larger than expected for the estimated gestational age occurs in approximately 50% of the cases of complete mole (ACOG, 2004).

Ovarian Enlargement

Bilateral ovarian enlargement caused by theca lutein cysts occurs in 50% of patients with complete mole and may cause abdominal pain. This enlargement is usually related to the elevated levels of human chorionic gonadotropin (hCG) (Ngan, 2003).

Absence of Fetus

Inability to detect a fetal heart rate (FHR) after 10 to 12 weeks of gestation is an indication for ultrasound to be used to rule out a molar or other complication of pregnancy.

Other Signs and Symptoms

The following traditional signs and symptoms are rarely seen today because of the earlier diagnosis with ultrasound (Berkowitz and Goldstein, 2009):

- Hyperemesis gravidarum
- Anemia

- Preeclampsia signs such as proteinuria, hypertension, and edema before 24 weeks of gestation
- Hyperthyroidism
- Passage of vesicles or grapelike structures
- Respiratory distress related to a trophoblastic pulmonary embolus
- Coagulopathy

Signs and Symptoms: Partial Mole

A partial mole does not exhibit the preceding clinical symptoms as often. It may present with signs of an incomplete or missed abortion, which include irregular vaginal bleeding, no FHR, or a uterus that is small for the estimated delivery date.

Maternal Effects

Maternal effects of hydatidiform mole, if not diagnosed early, include the following:
- Preeclampsia
- Bleeding
- Anemia
- Hyperemesis gravidarum
- Intrauterine infection or sepsis
- Uterine rupture
- Rupture of ovarian cysts
- Trophoblastic embolism
- Emotional trauma
- GTN

After surgical evacuation of a complete mole, there is a 20% risk for developing a persistent GTN (Ngan, 2003). This risk increases 40% to 50% if there was marked trophoblastic proliferation before evacuation, as evidenced by a high serum hCG level, excessively enlarged uterus, or theca lutein cysts (Ngan, 2003). After a partial mole, there is only a 2% to 4% risk for developing a nonmetastatic GTN (Cohn and Herzog, 2000).

Fetal Effects

The embryoblastic tissue of the complete hydatidiform mole never develops into a fetus. The embryoblastic tissue of the partial hydatidiform mole is always abnormal and never matures. A living child can be delivered from a hydatidiform molar pregnancy. These are twin gestations, and only one of the gestational sacs is affected by the molar changes.

Diagnostic Testing

Diagnostic tests used to validate a hydatidiform mole include transvaginal ultrasound and serum hCG. Transvaginal ultrasound is the most accurate tool for diagnosing the presence of a mole. A characteristic pattern of multiple diffuse echogenic, intrauterine masses, or "snowstorm pattern" is shown in place of, or along with, an embryo or a fetus.

The trophoblast tissue starting at about the time of implantation secretes hCG hormone. In a normal pregnancy, hCG levels gradually increase until around 10 weeks of pregnancy; then the levels plateau at approximately 60,000 to 140,000 mIU/ml. Between 10 and 12 weeks of gestation, the levels begin to decline sharply. In a molar pregnancy, the hCG titers are persistently high or rising beyond the normal peak (Cunningham and others, 2010).

Usual Medical Management

Immediate Evacuation

The uterus is usually emptied by suction evacuation because sharp curettage increases the risk for uterine perforation (ACOG, 2004). If the patient is no longer interested in childbearing, however, an abdominal hysterectomy might be performed. Even if the ovaries are enlarged or cystic, they do not have to be removed; they usually regress spontaneously when the hCG levels decline.

The four primary complications of surgical evacuation of the uterine contents are hemorrhage, perforation of the uterus, infection, and respiratory insufficiency. Oxytocin infusion is started after evacuation has been completed to promote myometrial contractions, which will decrease bleeding. It is contraindicated except in the presence of hemorrhage to start the oxytocin or administer prostaglandins before surgery because of the increased risk for trophoblastic embolization with uterine contractions in the presence of a molar pregnancy (RCOG, 2004). Dilation of the cervix is usually accomplished while the patient is under general anesthesia unless the cervix is long and closed; then one of the cervical ripening methods may be used to dilate the cervix.

RhD-negative women may become sensitized after the evacuation of a hydatidiform mole. Therefore they should receive Rh_o (D) immune globulin within 72 hours after the surgery to prevent D isoimmunization.

Follow-up Assessment

Because of the existing risk for development of a GTN, these patients should be instructed regarding the importance of follow-up assessment. When the patient obtains this assessment, early detection of a tumor is possible and treatment is most effective. The follow-up assessment may include the following:

- Baseline hCG determination level 48 hours after evacuation, chest radiograph, and ultrasound scan of the abdomen; repeat hCG level in 48 hours
- Weekly serum hCG values until the hCG level drops to normal and remains normal for 3 consecutive weeks, then monthly for 6 months
- Regular pelvic examinations to assess uterine and ovarian regression and observe changes in the vagina that would indicate GTN
- Regular chest radiographs to detect pulmonary metastasis
- Assessments for symptoms such as dyspnea, cough, and pleuritic pain (may indicate pulmonary metastasis); dull headache, behavioral change, or dizzy spells (may indicate cerebral metastasis); right upper quadrant pain or jaundice (may indicate liver metastasis); and vaginal bleeding (may indicate vaginal metastasis)
- Recommendation that the patient use a contraceptive to avoid becoming pregnant during the follow-up assessment period, which usually lasts about 1 year, because the hCG of the GTN cannot be distinguished from the hCG level of pregnancy

Interpret the hCG levels according to the criteria standardized by the International Federation of Gynecologists and Obstetricians (FIGO) in consensus with the Society of Gynecologic Oncology, the International Society for the Study of Trophoblastic Disease, and the International Gynecologic Cancer Society (Kohorn, 2001):

- A plateau of the hCG level for 3 weeks or longer (days 1 to 21)
- Rise of hCG level over a 2-week period from days 1 to 14
- Persistence of detectable hCG level for 6 or more months

Prophylactic Chemotherapy

Some obstetricians recommend prophylactic chemotherapy, but its use is controversial. There is no evidence that such therapy improves long-term prognosis, and it may cause toxicity that occasionally leads to death. Gestational trophoblastic neoplasia may reoccur, requiring increasing amounts of chemotherapy (ACOG, 2004; Hernandez, 2008).

Coexisting Hydatidiform Mole with a Normal Fetus

An amniocentesis is usually performed to determine the fetal karyotype of a fetus that coexists with a hydatidiform mole. If the karyotype is normal and the woman's condition is stable, continuation of the pregnancy may be attempted. If the karyotype of the fetus is abnormal, uterine evacuation is recommended (Bruchim and others, 2000).

When continuation of the pregnancy is planned, the patient is usually placed on a regimen of limited activity to minimize vaginal bleeding and then closely monitored for pregnancy-induced hypertension, HELLP (hemolysis, elevated liver enzymes, and low-platelet count in association with preeclampsia) syndrome, preterm labor, anemia, and pulmonary edema (Bruchim and others, 2000; ACOG, 2004). The patient has an increased risk for persistent GTN as well.

GESTATIONAL TROPHOBLASTIC NEOPLASIA

GTN is persistent trophoblastic proliferation. It may develop after a hydatidiform mole, an abortion, or an ectopic or normal pregnancy. GTN is divided into non-metastatic, metastatic low risk, and metastatic high risk disorders (Hernandez, 2008). Common metastasis sites are lungs (80%), vagina (30%), pelvis (20%), liver (10%), and brain (10%) (Cohn and Herzog, 2000).

Etiology

Approximately 50% to 60% of these tumors follow a hydatidiform mole. The risk for occurrence after an ectopic pregnancy or a spontaneous abortion is approximately 25%. A GTN can occur after an apparently normal term pregnancy (Smith, Kohorn, and Cole, 2005).

Signs and Symptoms

After any type of delivery, the following signs may indicate a GTN:

- Irregular bleeding—continuous or intermittent irregular bleeding related to uterine subinvolution caused by the presence of trophoblastic tissue
- Metastatic vaginal or vulvar tumors
- Bloody sputum related to pulmonary metastasis

- Intraperitoneal hemorrhage caused by perforation of the uterus as the result of continuous trophoblastic growth throughout the uterus

Maternal Effects

There is virtually a 100% cure rate after nonmetastatic and low risk metastatic GTN if treated early and appropriately. The risk for maternal mortality is 10% to 15% after high risk metastatic GTN (ACOG, 2004), usually the result of hemorrhage or pulmonary insufficiency. When metastasis occurs to the brain or liver, the prognosis is poorer (Ngan, 2003).

Diagnostic Testing

During the intense follow-up program after a hydatidiform mole or anytime abnormal postdelivery bleeding occurs, persistent or rising hCG levels in the absence of another pregnancy indicates GTN. Once a diagnosis is made, the stage of the tumor must be established to determine the tumor severity and the appropriate initial therapy. The International Federation of Gynecologists and Obstetricians (FIGO) along with the Committee of the International Society for the Study of Trophoblastic Diseases (ISSTD), the International Society for Gynecological Cancer (ISGC), and the World Health Organization (WHO) have provided a universal standardized scoring system that considers the stage and risk factors for GTN (Table 18-1). First any patient diagnosed with GTD is allocated a stage from I to IV. Second a risk factor score is determined from the sum of the risk factors, as outlined in Table 18-1. This is written by first indicating the stage as a roman numeral, followed by a colon, and then the risk factor number (example II:4). A risk score of 0 to 6 is classified as the low risk category. A score of 7 or higher is classified as the high risk group (Kohorn, 2001).

To employ the scoring system, the following workup is essential:
- Complete blood count (CBC), platelet determination, clotting function studies, blood type, and antibody screen
- Renal and liver function tests
- Pretreatment hCG titer
- Pelvic ultrasonography
- Chest radiograph
- Computed tomographic scan or magnetic resonance imaging of brain, lungs, liver, and pelvis to determine presence or level of metastasis

Usual Medical Management

Refer to an oncologic specialist for treatment for GTN with chemotherapy whenever the serum level of hCG rises or plateaus for more than 3 consecutive weeks or when signs of metastasis are detected during examinations. The initial treatment plan is dependent on tumor staging and risk factors as described in the preceding section and in Table 18-1 or the less complicated clinical classification of gestational trophoblastic neoplasia (Table 18-2).

Nonmetastatic Gestational Trophoblastic Neoplasia (GTN)

Single-agent chemotherapy such as methotrexate or actinomycin D is usually effective (Hernandez, 2008).

Table 18-1   Revised FIGO Stage and Risk Factor Scoring System for GTN

Stage	Description
Stage I	Disease confined to the uterus
Stage II	GTN metastasis outside of the uterus to the genital structures
Stage III	GTN metastasis to the lungs, with or without metastasis to the genital structures
Stage IV	Metastasis to the brain, liver, spleen, kidney

Risk Factor Score	0	1	2	4
Age	<40 years	40 years or more	—	—
Antecedent pregnancy	Hydatidiform mole	Abortion	Term pregnancy	—
Interval from index pregnancy (months)	<4	4-6	7-12	>12
Pretreatment hCG level (mIU/ml)	<1000	1000-10,000	>10,000-100,000	>100,000
Largest tumor size including uterus (cm)	—	3-4 cm	5 cm or larger	—
Site of metastases	Lung, vagina	Spleen, kidney	Gastrointestinal tract	Brain, liver
Number of metastases identified	0	1-4	5-8	>8
Previous failed chemotherapy	—	—	Single drug	Two or more drugs
Total				

Modified from Kohorn E: Negotiating a staging and risk factor scoring system for gestational trophoblastic neoplasia: a progress report, *J Reprod Med* 47(6):445-450, 2002; Kohorn E: The new FIGO 2000 staging and risk factor scoring system for gestational trophoblastic disease: description and clinical assessment, *Int J Gynecol Cancer* 1(1):73-77, 2001.
GTN, Gestational trophoblastic neoplasia.

Table 18-2   Clinical Classification of Gestational Trophoblastic Neoplasia

Type	Description
Nonmetastatic	Neoplasm confined to uterus
	Cure rate virtually 100%
Metastatic	Neoplasm has spread outside uterus
Low risk; good prognosis	Neoplasm present <4 months
	No liver, brain, or peritoneal metastases
	Metastases limited to lungs or vagina
	No prior chemotherapy
	Cure rate virtually 100%
High risk; poor prognosis	Serum hCG level <40,000 mIU/L
	Liver, brain, or peritoneal metastases
	Failed prior chemotherapy
	Neoplasm after term pregnancy
	Cure rate 75% depending on type
	of chemotherapy used

Modified from Cohn D, Herzog T: Gestational trophoblastic diseases: new standards for therapy, *Curr Opin Oncol* 12(5):492–496, 2000.

Low Risk Metastatic Gestational Trophoblastic Neoplasia

Treatment for low risk metastatic GTN usually starts with methotrexate, single-agent chemotherapy (Hernandez, 2008). However, according to the Cochrane Review, dactinomycin is more effective with fewer side effects then methotrexate (Alazzam and others, 2009).

High Risk Gestational Trophoblastic Neoplasia (GTN)

Treatment for a high risk GTN with a risk factor score of less than 7 has been effective with single-agent chemotherapy such as methotrexate or actinomycin D (Ngan and others, 2006). The MAC regimen (methotrexate, actinomycin D, and cyclophosphamide) is frequently used as well (Lurain, 2002; Soper, 2006). With a risk factor score of 7 or greater, multiagent chemotherapy such as the EMA-CO regimen of etoposide, methotrexate, actinomycin D, cyclophosphamide, and vincristine is frequently used (Lurain, Singh, and Schink, 2006). Multiagent chemotherapy is tolerated well and does not appear to affect future fertility (Dobson and others, 2000; Schorge and others, 2000; Ngan, 2003).

Follow-Up

After the initial treatment, serum hCG levels are evaluated every 1 to 2 weeks. As long as the hCG level is regressing, further chemotherapy is withheld. A plateau or rise in the level indicates a need for additional chemotherapy. When hCG is undetectable for 3 consecutive weeks, remission has occurred. Serial hCG levels are usually checked monthly for 1 year. To check the serial hCG levels accurately, the patient should avoid becoming pregnant during the follow-up period.

NURSING MANAGEMENT

Prevention

Because the cause of a hydatidiform mole is unknown, there is no known prevention. However, malnutrition and stress might play parts in influencing its development; therefore instructions should be given to all patients who are planning a pregnancy regarding the importance of stress management and a balanced diet high in protein and vitamin A.

Assessment

Hydatidiform Mole

Transvaginal ultrasound is used on any pregnancy not progressing normally to detect a hydatidiform mole early. Signs such as uterine bleeding, small or large uterine size for gestational dates, hyperemesis gravidarum, preeclampsia before 24 weeks of gestation, passage of grapelike vesicles, or inability to detect FHR using Doppler FHR device after 10 to 12 weeks of gestation should be evaluated immediately.

Gestational Trophoblastic Neoplasia

Because a GTN may develop after a normal delivery, an ectopic pregnancy, or an abortion, all patients should be taught the importance of reporting any unusual bleeding after any reproductive event. In these cases hCG levels should be determined to detect a GTN early.

Nursing Interventions for Evacuation of Mole

- Monitor for evidence of hemorrhage such as abnormal vital signs, abdominal pain, uterine status, and vaginal bleeding.
- Start intravenous infusion with an 18-gauge intracatheter.
- Prepare for surgery according to preoperative protocol, and type and cross-match 2 to 4 units of packed red blood cells as ordered.
- Avoid using oxytocin or prostaglandins before beginning surgery because of the risk for trophoblastic embolization with uterine contractions in the presence of a molar.

Postevacuation Nursing Interventions

- Monitor for postoperative complications such as the following: hemorrhage; respiratory compromise; congestive heart failure precipitated by anemia, hyperthyroidism, or iatrogenic fluid overload; and altered urinary elimination related to the antidiuretic effect of oxytocin.
- Initially continue any added postoperative intravenous infusions of oxytocin to facilitate uterine contractions and decrease uterine bleeding.
- Do not massage a boggy uterus if ovaries are enlarged, because the massage can cause ovarian rupture related to the theca lutein cysts stimulated by the high hCG levels.
- Do not use methylergonovine maleate (Methergine) postoperatively, because it can precipitate a hypertensive crisis.

- If the patient is RhD negative and unsensitized, be prepared to administer Rh_o (D) immune globulin (RhoGAM; HypRho-D). The usual dose is one vial, which equals approximately 300 mcg.

Nursing Interventions to Allay Fear

- Provide time for the patient and her family to express their concerns regarding the possible outcome and inconvenience to the mother and family during the treatment and long-term follow-up assessment period. Encourage them to vent any feelings, fears, and anger they may be experiencing.
- Assess family's support system and coping mechanisms.
- Provide information to the family regarding the disease process, plan of treatment, and risk for the patient.
- Explain all treatment modalities and reasons.
- Keep patient informed of health status and results of tests.
- Discuss risk for a GTN based on whether the patient had a partial or complete mole.
- Reassure patient that she can anticipate normal future reproduction even if she was treated for persistent GTN (Hurteau, 2003).
- Refer to social services for financial concerns if the family is without health benefits.

Nursing Interventions for Anticipatory Grieving

- Assess significance of the loss to all family members and level of guilt or blame.
- Assess family's communication pattern and support systems.
- Reaffirm their losses with the family, and let them know you are aware that these are real.
- Provide physical care such as a back rub or nourishment as needed.
- Consider any significant cultural beliefs or values.
- Spiritual assistance might help the family work through their grief. Refer to the chaplain or family's own clergy.
- Refer to psychiatric services when deemed necessary.

Follow-up Nursing Interventions for Early Detection of Gestational Trophoblastic Neoplasia

- Assess the patient's and family's understandings of the disease and the risks of an ongoing GTN.
- Explain the disease and plan of treatment.
- Educate the patient about the importance of the follow-up assessment for early detection of a GTN because it is almost 100% curable.
- Educate the patient during the follow-up assessment about the importance of avoiding pregnancy to prevent masking the hCG rise of a GTN to obtain better future pregnancy outcome.
- Teach the patient that any effective contraceptive method may be used except an IUD because of bleeding irregularities associated with the IUD. Oral contraceptives are the preferred method because they are highly effective (ACOG, 2004).
- Explain the treatment program if a GTN develops.

- Facilitate future family planning by reassuring the couple that even after chemotherapy they can anticipate a normal reproductive outcome in the future with no increased risk for congenital fetal malformations. The risk for a repeat molar pregnancy is 1% to 2%. After two molar pregnancies, the risk is about 20% (Hurteau, 2003).

CONCLUSION

The goals of the nurse in treating patients who have had a hydatidiform mole are twofold. First the nurse must emphasize the importance of the follow-up assessment. To determine whether a GTN is going to occur, serum hCG levels should be checked closely. The hCG levels should progressively decline and by 10 to 12 weeks be nondetectable. Second the nurse must help the patient work through the loss of an expected baby, a defective pregnancy, the fear of the development of proliferative trophoblastic disease, and the fear of recurrence in subsequent pregnancies.

The goal of GTN management is early detection because there is an almost 100% cure rate with appropriate treatment. To detect all GTNs early, keep in mind that they may occur after any reproductive event; therefore any abnormal bleeding should be evaluated as a possible indication of this disorder.

BIBLIOGRAPHY

Alazzam M, Tidy J, Hancock BW, Osborne R: First line chemotherapy in low risk gestational trophoblastic neoplasia, *Cochrane Database Syst Rev* (Issue 1), 2009.

American College of Obstetricians and Gynecologists (ACOG): *Diagnosis and treatment of gestational trophoblastic disease*, Practice Bulletin No. 53, 2004. Author.

Bentley R: Pathology of gestational trophoblastic disease, *Clin Obstet Gynecol* 46(3):513–522, 2003.

Berkowitz R, Goldstein D: Gestational trophoblastic diseases. In Hoskins W, and others, editors: *Principles and practice of gynecologic oncology*, Philadelphia, 2005, Lippincott Williams & Wilkins.

Berkowitz R, Goldstein D: Molar pregnancy, *N Engl J Med* 36(16):1639–1645, 2009.

Bruchim I, and others: Complete hydatidiform mole and a coexistent viable fetus: report of two cases and review of the literature, *Gynecol Oncol* 77(1):197–202, 2000.

Cohn D, Herzog T: Gestational trophoblastic diseases: new standards for therapy, *Curr Opin Oncol* 12(5):492–496, 2000.

Cunningham F, Leveno K, Bloom S, Hauth J, Rouse D, Spong C: *Williams obstetrics*, ed 23, New York, 2010, McGraw-Hill, Medical.

Dobson L, and others: Persistent gestational trophoblastic disease, *Br J Cancer* 8(9):1547–1552, 2000.

Fallahian M: Familial gestational trophoblastic disease, *Placenta* 24(7):797–799, 2003.

Hernandez E: Gestational trophoblastic neoplasia, *eMedicine Obstetrics and Gynecology* September 24, 2008. Retrieved from http://emedicine.medscape.com/article/279116.

Hurteau J: Gestational trophoblastic disease: management of hydatidiform mole, *Clin Obstet Gynecol* 46(3):557–569, 2003.

Kohorn E: The new FIGO 2000 staging and risk factor scoring system for gestational trophoblastic disease: description and clinical assessment, *Int J Gynecol Cancer* 1(1):73–77, 2001.

Lurain J: Advances in management of high-risk gestational trophoblastic tumors, *J Reprod Med* 47(6):451–459, 2002.

Lurain J, Singh D, Schink J: Primary treatment of metastatic high-risk gestational trophoblatic neoplasia with EMA-CO chemotherapy, *J Reprod Med* 51(10):767–772, 2006.

Ngan H: Gestational trophoblastic disease, *Curr Obstet Gynaecol* 13:95, 2003.

Ngan H, Odicino F, Maisonneuve P, and others: Gestational trophoblastic neoplasia: FIGO 6th annual report on the results of treatment in gynecological cancer, *Int J Gynaecol Obstet* 95(Suppl 1): S193–S203, 2006.

Royal College of Obstetricians and Gynaecologists (RCOG): *The management of gestational trophoblastic neoplasia*. London (UK): Royal College of Obstetricians and Gynaecologists (RCOG): 2004 Feb. 7 (Guideline 38). Retrieved from http://www.guideline.gov.

Schorge J, and others: Recent advances in gestational trophoblastic disease, *J Reprod Med* 45(9):692–700, 2000.

Smith J, Kohorn E, Cole L: Choriocarcinoma and gestational trophoblastic disease, *Obstet Gynecol Clin North Am* 32(4):661–684, 2005.

Soper J: Staging and evaluation of gestational trophoblastic disease, *Clin Obstet Gynecol* 46(3):570–578, 2003.

Soper J: Gestational trophoblastic disease, *Obstet Gynecol* 108(1):176–187, 2006.

19

Placental Abnormalities

pproximately 5% of all pregnant women experience some type of vaginal bleeding during their third trimester of pregnancy (Morgan and Arulkumaran, 2003). The major causes of this bleeding are abruptio placentae and placenta previa (MacMullen, Dulski, and Meagher, 2005). This chapter focuses on these two main causes and contrasts the treatments of both. Other causes of third trimester bleeding are heavy bloody show, cervical carcinoma, polyps, cervical or vaginal infection, cervical trauma, varicosities, invasive placenta, and vasa previa. Invasive placenta and vasa previa are briefly covered in this chapter as well.

ABRUPTIO PLACENTAE

An *abruptio placentae* is the premature separation, either partial or total, of a normally implanted placenta from the decidual lining of the uterus after 20 weeks of gestation. It is normally classified into one of three categories: mild, moderate, or severe (Table 19-1). Some medical personnel refer to grades 1, 2, or 3 instead. Mild abruptio placentae is a grade 1; moderate, a grade 2; and severe, a grade 3. Maternal bleeding in any class can be marginal, concealed, or both (Fig. 19-1), depending on whether it is trapped in the uterus.

Maternal bleeding is classified as one of the following:
- *Marginal or apparent.* The separation is near the edge of the placenta, and the blood is able to escape.
- *Central or concealed.* The separation is somewhere in the center of the placenta, and the blood is trapped.
- *Mixed or combined.* Part of the separation is near the edge, and part is concealed in the center area.

Incidence

Abruptio placentae is clinically recognized in approximately 1% of pregnancies (Salihu and others, 2005). However, the incidence may be as high as 4% based on postdelivery placental examination (Ananth, Smulian, and Vintzileos, 2003). There is a ten to twenty times greater risk in a subsequent pregnancy (Rasmussen, Irgens, and Dalaker, 2000; Morgan and Arulkumaran, 2003).

Table 19-1 Comparison of Three Classifications of Abruptio Placentae

	Mild: Grade 1	Moderate: Grade 2	Severe: Grade 3
Definition	Less than ⅙ of placenta separates prematurely	From ⅙ to ½ of placenta separates prematurely	More than ½ of placenta separates prematurely
Incidence	48%	27%	24%
Signs and symptoms	Total blood loss less than 500 ml	Total blood loss 1000-1500 ml	Total blood loss more than 1500 ml
		15%-30% of total blood volume	More than 30% of total blood volume
	Dark vaginal bleeding (mild to moderate)	Dark vaginal bleeding (mild to severe)	Dark vaginal bleeding (moderate to excessive)
	Vague lower abdominal or back discomfort	Gradual or abrupt onset of abdominal pain	Usually abrupt onset of uterine pain described as tearing, knifelike, and continuous
	No uterine tenderness	Uterine tenderness present	Uterus boardlike and highly reactive to stimuli
	No uterine irritability	Uterine tone increased	
Hypovolemia	Vital signs normal	Mild shock	Moderate-to-profound shock common
		Normal maternal blood pressure	Decreased maternal blood pressure
		Maternal tachycardia	Maternal tachycardia significant
		Narrowed pulse pressure	Narrowed pulse pressure
		Orthostatic hypotension	Orthostatic hypotension severe
		Tachypnea	Significant tachypnea
DIC	Normal fibrinogen of 450 mg/dl	Early signs of DIC common	DIC usually develops unless condition is treated immediately
		Fibrinogen 150-300 mg/dl	Fibrinogen less than 150 mg/dl
Fetal effects	Normal FHR pattern	FHR shows nonreassuring signs of possible fetal distress	FHR shows signs of fetal distress and death can occur

DIC, Disseminated intravascular coagulation; FHR, fetal heart rate.

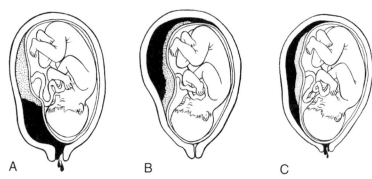

Figure 19-1 Classification of abruptio placentae, **A,** Marginal or apparent. **B,** Central or concealed. **C,** Missed or combined.

Etiology

The actual cause of an abruptio placentae is unknown. Conditions frequently associated with abruptio placentae are listed below:

- *Pregnancy-induced or chronic hypertension.* This is the most common cause of an abruption and is more likely than the other causes to result in a severe abruption (Oyelese and Ananth, 2006).
- *Previous abruption.* There is a 10% increased risk for recurrence after one abruption and a 25% increased risk for recurrence after two abruptions (Cunningham and others, 2010).
- *Trauma.* A placental abruption may result from a direct blow to the abdomen, most commonly as the result of a motor vehicle collision or maternal battering.
- *Cigarette smoking.* Smoking causes approximately 40% of abruptions by vasoconstriction of the spiral arteriole, which can lead to decidual necrosis (Morgan and Arulkumaran, 2003).
- *Cocaine abuse.* Cocaine causes vasoconstriction and hypertension, which can interfere with placental adherence to the uterine wall (Addis and others, 2001; Morgan and Arulkumaran, 2003).
- *Preterm premature rupture of membranes.* A 5% risk for developing an abruptio placentae after premature rupture of membranes exists (Morgan and Arulkumaran, 2003).
- *Thrombophilia.* Inherited thrombophilic disorders such as Factor V Leiden mutation, prothrombin gene mutation, and thermolabile variant of methylene tetrahydrofolate reductase (MTHFR) deficiency causing hyperhomocystein-uria increase the risk of abruptio placentae (Weintraub, Press, Wiznitzer, and Sheiner, 2007).

Normal Physiology

The blastocyst normally implants into the endometrium, now called the *decidua*, by sending out threadlike projections called *chorionic villi* from the trophoblast cells. These villi open up intervillous spaces, which fill with maternal blood. These spaces are supplied by the spiral arteries. At the same time, the trophoblast cells send out anchoring cords to attach themselves to the uterus.

Pathophysiology

An abruptio placentae is commonly caused by degeneration of the spiral arterioles that nourish the decidua (endometrium) and supply blood to the placenta, causing decidua basalis necrosis in the presence of arterial bleeding. When this process takes place, rupture of that spiral arteriole occurs and bleeding quickly results because the uterus is still distended and cannot contract sufficiently to close off the opened blood vessels.

Separation of the placenta takes place in the area of the hemorrhage. If the tear is at the margin of the placenta or if it separates the membranes from the decidua, vaginal bleeding is evident. Otherwise, the blood is concealed between the placenta and the decidua. If it is concealed, enough pressure can build up for blood to be forced through the fetal membranes into the amniotic sac or into the myometrial muscle fibers. This increases uterine tone and irritability. Clotting occurs simultaneously with the hemorrhage because the decidual tissue is rich in thromboplastin. This leads to the formation of a retroplacental or a subchorionic hematoma, causing the release of large quantities of thromboplastin into the maternal circulation. This can lead to disseminated intravascular coagulation (DIC).

In approximately 20% of the cases, the origin of rupture is venous rather than arterial (Elliott, Gilpin, Strong, and Finberg, 1998), separating the membrane from the decidua. Initially, visible bleeding is rare but can occur weeks later. This is the most common cause of a chronic abruption.

Signs and Symptoms

Classic Manifestations

The classic manifestations of an abruptio placentae follow:
- Dark vaginal, nonclotting bleeding (80%)
- Abdominal or low back pain (50%)
- Uterine hypertonus (17%)
- Uterine contractions (17%)
- Uterine tenderness
- Fetal distress signs or fetal death
- Signs of hypovolemia beyond those expected on the basis of observed external blood loss

The presence and degree of each sign are related to the amount of concealed blood trapped between the placenta and the decidua and the degree of separation. If the separation occurs at the margin of the placenta, the blood usually tears the membranes away from the decidua and escapes externally. The blood appears dark because it has had time to begin clotting. If the separation is in the center of the placenta, blood is trapped between the placenta and the decidua.

Concealed blood causes pressure and myometrial contractions, and this results in abdominal pain and uterine tenderness. With no way to escape, pressure builds up and can force blood into the myometrial tissue of the uterus, causing increased uterine irritability. Increasing uterine size and decreasing serial hematocrits are other signs of concealed bleeding. If some of this trapped blood is forced through the fetal membranes into the amniotic cavity, the amniotic fluid is bloody.

An abruption that does not result in delivery within seven days is termed a chronic abruption. In a chronic abruption, there is a 60% risk of oligohydramnios developing without membrane rupture. This condition is termed chronic abruption-oligohydramnios sequence (CAOS) (Elliott, Gilpin, Strong, and Finberg, 1998). Preterm premature rupture eventually occurs in a large percentage of these pregnancies.

Mild Abruptio Placentae: Grade 1

Mild forms of abruptio placentae usually develop gradually and produce mild to moderate dark vaginal bleeding without uterine tenderness. Signs of fetal distress are absent, and the mother's vital signs remain stable. There are no signs of DIC. This type of abruption can be self-limiting or can progress into a more advanced form.

Moderate Abruptio Placentae: Grade 2

A moderate abruptio placentae can develop gradually or abruptly and produce persistent abdominal pain accompanied by visible dark vaginal bleeding. The uterus may be tender on palpation and may remain firm between contractions if the mother is in labor. This can make auditory appraisal of the fetal heart rate (FHR) difficult. Fetal distress may be present, depending on the extent of placental separation and the amount of maternal blood loss. Signs of shock may be present.

Severe Abruptio Placentae: Grade 3

A severe abruptio placentae usually develops suddenly, causing excruciating, unremitting abdominal pain often referred to as *knifelike* or *tearing*. The uterus is often board-like and tender and fails to relax. Profuse bleeding results, although it may not be evident vaginally if the blood is trapped behind the placenta. In situations in which the blood is trapped, the uterus shows signs of enlarging. Shock can ensue, although the signs of shock may not be in proportion to the amount of visible blood loss. Signs of fetal distress are usually evident, and fetal death may result.

Posteriorly Implanted Abruptio Placentae

In a few instances, when an abruptio placentae occurs in a posteriorly implanted placenta, no signs of uterine tenderness or pain are manifested. In these cases, the classic signs are only vaginal bleeding and backache.

Complications

Shock

Shock results as the body attempts to protect the vital organs, especially the brain and heart, from a reduction of effective circulating blood volume. When blood is lost from the vascular system, venous return is diminished and cardiac output is consequently reduced. Physiologic compensatory mechanisms are then activated. The decrease in arterial pressure initiates powerful sympathetic reflexes that stimulate vasoconstriction of the arterioles and venules in the kidneys, liver, lungs, gastrointestinal tract, muscles, skin, and uterus. Blood is then redistributed to the heart and brain from these areas.

The heart and respiratory rates increase in an attempt to compensate by delivering increased volume and better oxygenated blood to the vital organs. A slower compensatory mechanism is activated that stimulates the absorption of fluid from the intestinal tract and stimulates the kidneys to increase reabsorption of sodium and water. Therefore the results are classic signs of hypovolemic shock, which include hypotension; oliguria; rapid, thready pulse; shallow, irregular respirations; cold and clammy skin; pallor; syncope; and thirst. Should severe bleeding continue, the compensatory mechanisms cannot keep up with tissue needs, and cardiac deterioration, loss of vasomotor tone, and release of toxins by ischemic tissue result; cellular death ensues.

Because of the normally increased maternal blood volume during pregnancy, the classic signs of shock are not always present until after the fetal circulation is affected. During pregnancy, signs of shock usually do not present until after 25% to 30% of maternal blood volume is lost. Shunting of blood away from the placenta occurs before this 25% to 30% blood loss. Table 19-2 lists the manifested symptoms of blood loss.

Disseminated Intravascular Coagulation

An abruptio placentae is the most common cause of DIC. This coagulation defect results because of placental tissue fragments (thromboplastin) being forced into the circulatory system. These substances activate widespread intravascular clotting. Soon, the coagulation factors are consumed. Therefore the platelet count is usually decreased, fibrinogen is low, and circulating fibrin degradation products (FDPs) are increased (see Chapter 20).

Other Complications

Renal failure can develop as a result of hypoxia if shock, vascular spasms, or DIC have occurred. Pituitary necrosis (Sheehan syndrome) occasionally results from the same conditions that cause renal failure. In the presence of pituitary necrosis, lactation does not occur because pituitary hormones regulate lactation.

Maternal Effects

In less than 1% of cases, maternal death occurs from hemorrhagic shock. This low maternal mortality is mainly due to the availability of blood replacement therapy. However, maternal morbidity is significant. Because of the potential for massive bleeding, the patient is at high risk for developing shock and DIC at any time before delivery. In rare cases, a fetal-to-maternal hemorrhage may occur, which can cause the RhD-negative mother to become sensitized.

During the postpartum period, mothers who had experienced an abruptio placentae are at an increased risk for anemia, development of an infection related to prolonged separation of the placenta, postpartum hemorrhage related to a poorly contracted uterus caused by blood infiltrating the uterus, and DIC. Other complications that can develop as a result of ischemia are renal failure and anterior pituitary necrosis (Sheehan syndrome). Because of increased blood flow to the pituitary gland during pregnancy, it is more sensitive to hypoxia during pregnancy.

Table 19-2   Manifested Symptoms of Blood Loss

Percentage of Blood Loss	Manifested Symptoms	Treatment
15% = 900 ml	Minimal tachycardia Normal blood pressure Normal pulse pressure Normal respiratory rate Normal capillary refill	Stabilize with crystalloid solution
20%-25% = 1200-1500 ml	Tachycardia Tachypnea (rate doubles) Increased blood pressure, especially diastolic Narrowing pulse pressure Delayed hypothenar refilling Orthostatic blood pressure changes	Usually successful when stabilized with crystalloid solution
30%-35% = 1800-2100 ml	Significant tachycardia (30–50 bpm) Decreased blood pressure especially systolic Decreased pulse pressure Significant tachypnea (30–50 breaths/min) Classic shock signs of cold, clammy extremities	Infuse 1–2 L of a crystalloid solution Infuse blood component therapy, such as packed RBCs
40% or greater 2400 ml or greater	Marked tachycardia Significant depression of blood pressure Narrow pulse pressure Significant tachypnea Oliguria Syncope, shortness of breath, headaches, chest pain Skin cold and pale	Infuse 1–2 L of crystalloid solution Then infuse blood component therapy Whole blood Infuse platelets and fresh frozen plasma after several units of whole blood

Data from Benedetti T: Obstetric hemorrhage. In Gabbe S, Niebyl J, and Simpson J, editors: *Obstetrics: normal and problem pregnancies,* ed 4, New York, 2002, Churchill Livingstone.

Fetal and Neonatal Effects

Perinatal mortality is approximately 14 in 1000, depending on the degree of abruption, causing 12% of all third trimester stillbirths (Salihu and others, 2005). In surviving infants, the most common causes of morbidity are fetal hypoxia, neonatal prematurity, and intrauterine growth restriction neurologic defects. These conditions result when approximately 50% of the placental surface has separated or maternal blood loss is 2000 ml or greater.

Fetal Hypoxia

Fetal hypoxia is caused by uteroplacental insufficiency resulting from placental separation or decreased uterine perfusion resulting from maternal hypovolemia, uterine hypertonus, or less often, fetal hemorrhage. Total anoxia may develop.

Neonatal Prematurity

The neonate is frequently premature because of early delivery necessitated by fetal distress or preterm labor.

Intrauterine Growth Restriction

Even if the bleeding and separation stop, the decreased placental surface area that remains intact may not be adequate to meet the increased needs of the growing fetus.

Neurologic Defects

The infant who survives is at increased risk for a neurologic defect such as cerebral palsy (Cunningham and others, 2010).

Diagnostic Testing

Diagnosis usually is made on the basis of presenting symptoms and a physical assessment. Severe abruptio placentae and moderate abruptio placentae are easier to diagnose; a patient presents with one or more of the classic symptoms. A mild abruptio placentae is more difficult to diagnose; it is easily confused with a placenta previa because vaginal bleeding may be the only presenting symptom. Therefore ultrasound is usually used to rule out a placenta previa and is accompanied by a clinical examination to rule out other less common causes of third trimester bleeding. However, at present, no diagnostic method is available to determine the degree of placental separation.

Usual Medical Management and Protocols for Nurse Practitioners

Treatment of an abruptio placentae depends on the severity of blood loss, fetal maturity, and fetal well-being.

Expectant Management

If the abruptio placentae is mild and there are no signs of hypovolemia or anemia, gestational age of the fetus is determined first. With an immature fetus of less than 36 weeks of gestation without signs of fetal distress, expectant management is usually the treatment. The components of expectant management follow:

- Hospitalize in a facility that can immediately intervene by cesarean delivery because the placenta may further separate at any time and, very quickly, seriously compromise the fetus unless cesarean delivery can be performed immediately. Corticosteroids to accelerate fetal lung maturity may be part of the plan.
- Closely observe for signs of concealed or external bleeding.
- Do continuous FHR monitoring until 72 hours have passed without bleeding, hypertension, or abnormal FHR pattern.

- Monitor for preterm uterine contractions, which can be stimulated by prostaglandin release from placental separation. Tocolytic therapy is usually contraindicated. If a tocolytic agent is used, magnesium sulfate is the drug of choice (Cunningham and others, 2010). Beta-sympathomimetics can cause maternal tachycardia and thereby falsely indicate hemorrhage. Calcium channel blockers can cause hypotension and thereby adversely affect maternal perfusion of the uterus.
- Obtain baseline laboratory data such as complete blood cell count, coagulation studies, abnormal bleeding panel, serum electrolytes panel, and renal function studies such as serum blood urea nitrogen.

Emergency Management

If the abruptio placentae is moderate to severe, the following are the objectives of treatment:
- Monitor maternal volume status continuously.
- Restore blood loss quickly.
- Continuously monitor the fetus.
- Correct coagulation defect if present.
- Expedite delivery.

Maternal volume status must be monitored continually with (1) an indwelling Foley catheter to determine urine output and (2) serial hematocrits every 2 to 3 hours. If urine output drops below 30 ml/hr despite vigorous volume replacement, Swan-Ganz monitoring is needed to determine intravascular volume status.

Fluid replacement is usually accomplished with a crystalloid solution, such as lactated Ringer's, and blood component therapy as soon as it is available. Intravenous (IV) lactated Ringer's solution and blood are usually administered at a rate adequate to maintain the hematocrit at 30% or greater and urinary output at 30 ml/hr or greater. In rare instances, the patient's blood loss is rapid and massive, leading to severe shock. In these cases, volume expanders or immediate transfusions with type O, RhD-negative blood may be given until matched blood is available. Oxygen should be administered with a face mask because it increases oxygen tension and increases oxygen delivery to end-organs.

The fetus must be monitored continuously until delivery takes place. Keep in mind that a maternal heartbeat may be picked up through the fetal scalp electrode in the event of fetal death. Therefore the FHR should be compared with the maternal pulse.

If a coagulation defect develops (fibrinogen level, 150 mg/dl), replacement of the clotting factors is the usual treatment. This can be accomplished by administering cryoprecipitate or fresh frozen plasma to replace fibrinogen and a platelet transfusion if the platelet count is below 50,000/mm³. Heparin was once used to treat DIC in the presence of an abruptio placentae, but it is no longer an acceptable treatment. Within 24 hours after delivery, the coagulation defect normally corrects itself. The platelet count may not return to a normal level for 2 to 4 days. Table 19-3 lists guidelines for blood component replacement.

Delivery

Delivery should be started if the abruption is moderate to severe, if the fetus is older than 36 weeks, or at any time fetal distress is noted. If the fetus is mature and in a cephalic presentation, a vaginal delivery may be attempted with

Table 19-3   Guidelines for Blood Component Replacement

Conditions	Blood Component	Volume per Unit	Dose	Effect	Administration
Acute blood loss	Volume expansion with crystalloid solutions (lactated Ringer's and NS) Fresh whole blood transfusions rarely used. Blood component therapy is preferred. Other volume expanders: albumin, hydroxyethyl starch, dextran, purified protein fractions	1000 ml 500 ml/unit	Depends on amount of blood lost Depends on amount of blood lost	1 unit increases Hct 3%	If bleeding stops and BP rises after 1-2 L, blood components may not be necessary. Immediate transfusion with type O, Rh-negative blood until matched blood is available
Hgb 7 g/dl or less Hct 21% or less • Syncope • Shortness of breath • Chest pain • Oliguria • Tachycardia	Packed RBCs to restore oxygen-carrying capacity	300 ml	Depends on Hgb/Hct levels and amount of continued bleeding	1 unit will increase Hgb 1 g/dl and Hct 3%.	Packed RBCs have an Hct of 70% and therefore increased viscosity; if need to infuse rapidly, mix with 200 ml of NS per unit
Deficiency in clotting factors (II, V, VII, IX, XI) indicated by PT or PTT 1.5 × normal or greater • PT >18 sec • PTT >55sec	Fresh frozen plasma	250 ml	Normal dose: 2 bags	1 unit will increase each clotting factor by 2%-3%.	

Continued

Table 19-3 Guidelines for Blood Component Replacement—cont'd

Conditions	Blood Component	Volume per Unit	Dose	Effect	Administration
Platelet count less than 50,000/mm^3 with active bleeding or surgery Abnormal function as indicated by normal platelet count with bleeding time more than 9 min	Platelet transfusions	50 ml	1 unit × 10 kg of body weight	1 unit will increase platelet count 5000/mm^3.	Approximately 0.5 ml of RBCs are present in platelet transfusions; if ABO and CBE (Rh) type-specific platelets are not available, a D-negative woman can be sensitized with D-positive platelets; administer RhoGAM (one vial needed for every 15 ml of RBCs)

Deficiency in one or more of the following clotting factors: • Fibrinogen (less than 200 mg/dl) • Factor VIII or XIII • von Willebrand factor	Cryoprecipitate contains factors VIII and XIII, fibrinogen, fibronectin, von Willebrand factor	40 ml frozen	For hypofibrino-genemia: 1 bag × 5 kg of body weight	1 unit will increase fibrinogen 10 mg/dl	All blood products should be administered through a Y-type blood administration set with a filter designed to remove debris; only NS should be infused through the same line
Total blood loss exceeds 25% of total blood volume	Packed RBCs and FFP or whole blood	200 ml 500 ml			

Data from Cunningham F, Leveno, K, Bloom S, Hauth J, Rouse D, Spong C: *Williams' obstetrics*, ed 23, New York, 2005, McGraw-Hill Medical; Hull A, Resnik R: Placenta previa, placenta accreta, abruptio placentae, and vasa previa. In Creasy R, Resnik R, Iams J, and others, editors: Creasy & Resnik's *Maternal-Fetal medicine: principles and practice*, ed 6, Philadelphia, 2009, Saunders.
BP, Blood pressure; *FFP*, fresh frozen plasma; *Hct*, hematocrit; *Hgb*, hemoglobin; *NS*, normal saline; *PT*, prothrombin time; *PTT*, partial thromboplastin time; *RBCs*, red blood cells.

continuous fetal monitoring in an environment where a cesarean delivery can be performed immediately. If the woman is not in labor and fetal heart rate pattern is normal, vaginal delivery can be initiated by an amniotomy or a labor stimulant such as oxytocin, provided that the patient is in a tertiary care center in which rapid emergency measures can be initiated if further abruption occurs with contractions. If the fetus is not in a cephalic presentation or if, during the induction of labor, bleeding increases, the uterus fails to relax between contractions, fetal distress occurs, or labor fails to progress actively, a cesarean delivery is performed.

In the presence of a severe abruptio placentae, if the fetus is alive, a cesarean delivery should be performed as soon as possible. If the fetus is dead, a vaginal delivery is preferred unless bleeding cannot be controlled.

PLACENTA PREVIA

Placenta previa occurs when the placenta attaches to the lower segment of the uterus, near (within 2 cm) or over the internal os, instead of in the body or fundal segment of the uterus. It is normally classified into one of three categories, depending on the degree of coverage of the cervix (Fig. 19-2):
1. *Marginal.* The placenta lies within 2 to 3 cm of the internal os.
2. *Partial.* The placenta implants near and partially covers the internal os.
3. *Total.* The placenta completely covers the internal os.
If the placenta is more than 3 cm from the os, there is no risk of bleeding.

Incidence

The incidence of placenta previa is 0.33% with a 4% to 8% recurrence risk (Martin and others, 2002).

Etiology

The actual cause of placenta previa is unknown. However, damage to the endometrium or myometrium or any process that interferes with placental migration increases the risk for a placenta previa. Women of Asian descent who are living in

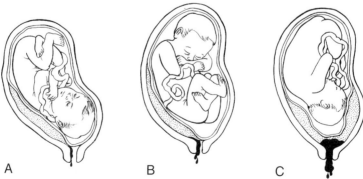

Figure 19-2 Classifications of placenta previa. **A,** Marginal. **B,** Partial. **C,** Total.

the United States have an increased risk as well. Therefore it is frequently associated with endometrial scarring, impeded endometrial vascularization, and increased placental mass.

Endometrial Scarring

Endometrial scarring can result from a previous placenta previa, an abortion, a cesarean delivery, an increased parity 4 or greater, or closely spaced pregnancies (Gesteland and others, 2004). Subsequent pregnancies, after a cesarean delivery, have a 1.5% greater likelihood of a placenta previa complication (Morgan and Arulkumaran, 2003).

Impeded Endometrial Vascularization

Factors that interfere with adequate blood supply to the endometrium, such as hypertension or diabetes, uterine tumor, drug usage (e.g., cocaine), cigarette smoking, or advancing maternal age can cause placenta previa (Hull and Resnik, 2009).

Increased Placental Mass

A multiple pregnancy leads to more than one placenta and therefore increases the risk for placenta previa.

Normal Physiology

The blastocyst normally implants into the upper anterior portion of the uterus, where the vascular blood supply is rich. After implantation of the blastocyst, the trophoblastic tissue sends out threadlike projections, chorionic villi, which grow into the decidua (endometrium). At first, these chorionic villi surround the blastocyst; however, soon after, the portion of the chorionic villi in contact with the decidua basalis proliferates to form the placenta, and the villi, in contact with the decidua capsularis, atrophies.

The chorionic villi are of two types. One type opens up intervillous spaces, which fill with maternal blood to form an area of exchange between the embryonic and maternal circulatory systems. Another type of villi forms anchoring cords to stabilize the placenta and embryo in the uterus. The chorionic villi growth is normally confined to the endometrium because of the fibrinoid layer of Nitabuch, which separates the decidua from the myometrium and stops chorionic villi growth.

Pathophysiology

With placenta previa, the blastocyst implants itself in the lower uterine segment, over or very near the internal os. A large percentage, approximately 90%, of placentas that initially implant low migrate upward. This results because the chorionic villi grow in the direction of improved blood supply and remain dormant in another (Bhide and Thilaganthan, 2004). In the presence of more than a 2-cm placental cervical overlap, migration is rare (Oppenheimer and others, 2001).

The decidua basalis is less developed in the lower segment of the uterus. The fibrinoid layer of Nitabuch, which stops chorionic villi growth, may be absent. Therefore placental tissue may come into direct contact with the myometrium and a placenta accreta, increta, or percreta may develop.

Signs and Symptoms

The two classical presentations of placenta previa are antepartum hemorrhage and fetal malpresentation in later pregnancy.

Painless, Bright Red, Vaginal Bleeding

Normally, during the latter half of pregnancy, the lower uterine segment elongates as the fundal segment of the uterus hypertrophies. Toward the end of the pregnancy, the cervix begins to efface and dilate. When the placenta is implanted in the lower uterine segment over or around the internal cervical os, separation or tearing of portions of the placenta can occur with subsequent bleeding. Usually, the greater the percentage of placenta covering the os, the earlier the first episode of bleeding occurs. Because the normal uterine changes occur gradually until labor begins, the initial bleeding episode is usually slight, presents commonly in the third trimester, and ceases spontaneously as clot formation occurs. This is not always the case, however. The bleeding is usually painless and bright red in color without associated uterine tenderness because the blood is not trapped behind the placenta. In about 20% of the cases, uterine contractions accompany the bleeding (Carter, 1999). Recurrence is unpredictable and can take place at any time.

Fetal Malpresentation

The presenting part of the fetus usually remains high even in late pregnancy because the placenta occupies the lower uterine segment. For this same reason, the risk for malpresentations, such as transverse, oblique, or breech, increases.

Maternal Effects

The incidence of maternal mortality is less than 1%. The most common morbidity factors follow:

- *Hemorrhage and hypovolemic shock.* Placenta previa can cause maternal hemorrhage and hypovolemic shock in the antepartum, intrapartum, and postpartum periods. Puerperal hemorrhage can occur even in the presence of a firmly contracted uterus. This is because the lower uterine segment does not have the contractility of the upper uterine segment, and as a consequence, there is less compression of the open vessels, resulting from the removal of the placenta. This risk for hemorrhage is further increased by the larger than normal surface area denuded by the removal of the placenta.
- *Invasive placenta (includes accreta, increta, and percreta).* The risk for invasive placenta is 5% to 10% with any placenta previa, and if the woman had a previous cesarean delivery, the risk is 10% to 25% (Hull and Resnik, 2009). The risk for invasive placenta can be more than 50% in a pregnancy after multiple cesarean deliveries and a history of placenta previa (Hull and Resnik, 2009).
- *Septicemia.* The opened blood vessels are near the cervical os and can become infected easily.
- *Thrombosis*
- *Renal failure*
- *Rh incompatibility.* An RhD-negative woman can become sensitized during any antepartum bleeding episode (ACOG, 2006).
- *Postpartum anemia.* Puerperal anemia is the result of increased blood loss.

Fetal and Neonatal Effects

- Risk for perinatal mortality is less than 10% with a placenta previa (Ananth, Smulian, and Vintzileos, 2003). However, there is an increased risk for stillbirth. There is also a greater risk for neonatal morbidity. Such effects include the following:
  - *Prematurity.* Prematurity is the greatest cause of mortality (Morgan and Arulkumaran, 2003).
  - *Malpresentation.* The risk for malpresentation is increased with placenta previa.
  - *Intrauterine growth restriction.* Intrauterine growth restriction occurs if the placental exchange is chronically compromised (Morgan and Arulkumaran, 2003).
  - *Fetal anemia.* Anemia is in proportion to maternal blood loss and, if the anemia is severe, it may predispose to fetal hypoxia and death (Crane and others, 1999).

Diagnostic Testing

Determining Placental Location

When any pregnant woman complains of vaginal bleeding after 20 weeks of gestation, placenta previa is considered. To diagnose placenta previa, the location of the placenta must be determined. Both transabdominal and transvaginal ultrasonography facilitate diagnosis; however, transvaginal is more accurate and just as safe (RCOG, 2005).

Ruling Out Other Causes of Bleeding

A speculum examination is usually done to rule out other causes of bright red vaginal bleeding such as cervicitis, cervical polyps, heavy show, or cervical carcinoma.

Determining Gestational Age

An amniocentesis may be included in the diagnostic workup to determine fetal lung maturity. If the lecithin/sphingomyelin (L/S) ratio is 2:1 or phosphatidylglycerol is present, indicating fetal pulmonary lung maturity, delivery is probably the treatment of choice.

Early Diagnosis of Placenta Previa

An asymptomatic placenta previa, which is identified before the latter half of the third trimester, has a 90% chance of changing to a normal placenta (Oppenheimer and others, 2001).

Usual Medical Management and Protocols for Nurse Practitioners

Expectant Management

Treatment of placenta previa depends on the gestational age and the extent of bleeding. If the gestational age is less than 36 weeks, the fetus has a reassuring FHR tracing, the bleeding is mild (less than 250 ml) and stops, the patient is not in labor, and a cesarean delivery can be performed immediately when indicated, the treatment of choice is expectant management. The purpose is to allow the fetus time to mature to lessen the chance of perinatal mortality from prematurity and perhaps allow time for placental migration. When expectant management is chosen, it usually includes the following:

- Hospitalize initially, and use clinical judgment to consider outpatient management once a bleeding episode has occurred (RCOG, 2005).
- Initiate bedrest with bathroom privileges with the intent of improving blood flow to the uterus and increasing fetal growth. Complete bedrest is almost never necessary. To decrease bedrest complications while improving uterine blood flow, bathroom privileges can be interpreted as allowing the woman to be up to use the bathroom and shower and move around the room for 15 to 30 minutes at a time, four times a day.
- Closely observe for signs of bleeding.
- Start IV infusions with a 14- to 16-gauge needle, unless bleeding is minimal; then a heparin lock may be left in place and changed as needed.
- Have a maternal blood sample available at all times in the blood bank for immediate type and cross-match for blood component therapy. If there are no antibodies on the antibody screen, blood does not need to be held. Periodic blood component therapy may be given to maintain hemoglobin at 8 or above. See Table 19-3 for a list of guidelines for blood component replacement.
- Establish continuous fetal monitoring to facilitate early detection of fetal distress during bleeding episodes; otherwise, assess every 4 hours with a Doppler FHR device.
- Perform a nonstress test (NST) with amniotic fluid index, a modified biophysical profile, twice weekly to determine fetal well-being because of the increased risk for stillbirth. Contraction stress tests are contraindicated.
- Use antepartum corticosteroids such as betamethasone (Celestone) or dexamethasone to enhance fetal pulmonary maturity between 24 and 34 weeks of gestation.
- Monitor for signs of preterm uterine contractions stimulated by prostaglandin release from placental separation. Tocolytic therapy can be useful to slow cervical change (Sharma, Suri, and Gupta, 2004).
- Initiate antenatal iron supplementation to facilitate tolerance to mild and moderate blood loss (Morgan and Arulkumaran, 2003).
- Perform amniocentesis between 34 and 36 weeks of gestation to determine fetal lung maturity because risk for bleeding increases with increasing gestational age.

After stabilization and 48 hours without vaginal bleeding, home management is appropriate for some patients (Oppenheimer, 2007). The family should be instructed to comply with the activity level of bedrest with bathroom privileges and pelvic rest. The patient must remain within 15 minutes of the hospital, have a telephone, have 24-hour access to transportation, and have close supervision by family in the home. Fetal activity charts should be kept daily, and a modified biophysical profile should be done weekly or more often as indicated with weekly clinic visits.

Delivery

Expectant management is terminated as soon as the fetus is mature, excessive bleeding occurs, active labor begins, or any other obstetric reason to terminate the pregnancy develops, such as an intraamniotic infection.

If the bleeding is profuse, the gestational age is 36 or more weeks, the L/S ratio is 2:1, or phosphatidylglycerol is present, immediate delivery is usually the treatment of choice. Cesarean delivery is the accepted method of delivery in all women when the placenta lies within 2 cm of the cervical os documented by late trimester TVU (Hull and Resnik, 2009). They are at risk for an invasive placenta. Table 19-4 compares placenta previa and abruptio placentae.

INVASIVE PLACENTA (PLACENTA CRETAS)

There are three types of invasive placenta: accreta, increta, and percreta. *Placenta accreta* is an uncommon condition in which the chorionic villi adhere to the myometrium. Its more advanced forms are placenta increta and placenta percreta. *Placenta increta* is invasion of the chorionic villi into the myometrium, and *placenta percreta* is growth of the chorionic villi through the myometrium. This causes the placenta to adhere abnormally to the uterus. The abnormal placental adherence may involve a single cotyledon (focal), a few cotyledons (partial adherence), or all the cotyledons (total adherence).

Incidence

In the presence of a placenta previa, there is a 5% to 10% risk for invasive placenta. The risk is 10% to 25% with a history of one cesarean delivery, increasing to 50% with a history of two or more cesarean deliveries (Hull and Resnik, 2009).

Etiology

Placenta accreta can occur if there is an inadequate or absent decidua basalis and fibrinoid layer of Nitabuch. Predisposing factors are those that contribute to an abnormal decidua (endometrium). These factors include prior uterine surgery such as cesarean delivery and women who have a current placenta previa (Usta and others, 2005; Silver and others, 2006). Other risk factors are advanced maternal age, increased parity, and smoking.

Diagnosis

Antepartum

Usually, there is no clinical evidence until after delivery. Because of the increased risk in the presence of a placenta previa, ultrasonographic evaluation of all placentae previae for invasive placenta should be done. Ultrasound imaging or magnetic resonance imaging can confirm or exclude the presence of an invasive placenta (Hull and Resnik, 2009).

Postpartum

Placenta accreta is usually diagnosed soon after delivery when the placenta fails to normally separate from the uterine wall and spontaneously deliver. In a focal or partial adherence, the placenta may separate only partially, opening blood vessels while leaving part of the placenta attached. Profuse hemorrhage results because the uterus cannot contract. In a totally adhering placenta, there is no bleeding until attempts are

Table 19-4   Comparison of Placenta Previa and Abruptio Placentae

Parameter	Placenta Previa	Abruptio Placentae
Description Classification	Implantation of placenta in lower segment of uterus near or over internal os Marginal: placenta implanted near but does not cover any part of internal os Partial: placenta implants near and partially covers internal os Total: placenta completely covers internal os	Premature separation of normally implanted placenta after 20 weeks of gestation Mild: less than 1/6 of placenta is separated, mild-to-moderate bleeding, and no uterine tenderness; maternal vital signs of FHR normal Moderate: 1/6 to 1/2 of placenta is separated; abdominal pain; increased uterine tone; maternal vital signs may show mild hypovolemia; FHR may indicate distress Severe: more than 1/2 of placenta is separated; profuse bleeding; persistent and severe abdominal pain and increased tenderness; signs of shock or coagulopathy frequently present with fetal distress or death resulting
Etiology	Unknown: theoretic considerations include a defective vascularization of decidua resulting from uterine scarring or interference with adequate blood supply to endometrium; increased placental mass; early or late ovulation *Associated conditions* • Multiparity of more than five children • Previous placenta previa • Prior uterine scar related to history of suction curettage or previous cesarean birth • Smoking or drug addiction • Uterine tumor • Multiple pregnancy	Unknown: theoretic considerations include degeneration of spiral arteriole, which causes rupture of involved blood vessels and bleeding; bleeding under placenta separates placenta from decidua *Associated conditions* • Gestational hypertensive disorder • Previous abruption • Trauma from motor vehicle collision or maternal battering • Cigarette smoking • Cocaine use • PROM

Signs and symptoms	Painless, bright red bleeding; onset of bleeding usually slight-to-moderate and ceases spontaneously Presenting part high or displaced Uterus soft and nontender During labor, uterus relaxes between contractions Blood usually clots normally	Painful, dark red bleeding unless only marginal; onset of bleeding is slight to profuse and usually continues Presenting part engaged Uterus tender or rigid (moderate-to-severe abruption) During labor, uterus usually has increased resting tone Clotting defects may be present According to signs and symptoms
Diagnosis	Ultrasound No vaginal examination except under double setup	Serial hematocrits to assess concealed bleeding
Treatment	If initial bleeding episode is slight and gestational age is less than 37 weeks, expectant management is usual choice of treatment Close observation of fetal well-being and amount of bleeding Limited physical activity No douches, enemas, or sexual intercourse Delivery when fetus is mature or hemorrhage dictates When bleeding is profuse, gestational age greater than 36 weeks, or L/S ratio 2:1 or greater, delivery is choice of treatment; if placenta previa is: • Marginal, a vaginal delivery may be attempted • Partial or complete, a cesarean delivery is performed	In presence of mild abruptio placentae and gestational age is less than 36 weeks, expectant management is usual choice of treatment; close observation of fetal well-being and amount of bleeding Delivery when fetus is mature or hemorrhage dictates; in presence of mild abruptio placentae, with gestational age of 36 weeks or more, delivery is usual choice of treatment In presence of moderate-to-severe abruptio placentae: • Restore blood loss • Correct coagulation defect if present • Facilitate delivery • Vaginal delivery is attempted if there is no evidence of fetal or maternal distress with fluid and blood replacement, fetus is in cephalic presentation, labor progresses actively, or fetus is dead. • Cesarean delivery is indicated for severe abruption if fetus is alive, fetal or maternal distress develops with fluid and blood replacement, labor fails to progress actively, or fetal presentation is not cephalic.

Continued

Table 19-4 Comparison of Placenta Previa and Abruptio Placentae—cont'd

Parameter	Placenta Previa	Abruptio Placentae
Maternal outcome	Less than 1% maternal mortality	Less than 1% maternal mortality
Maternal complications	Hemorrhage and hypovolemic shock	Hemorrhage and hypovolemic shock
	Placenta accreta/increta/percreta	DIC
	Premature rupture of membranes	D-sensitization
	D-sensitization	Couvelaire uterus
	Puerperal infection	Puerperal infection
	Puerperal anemia	Puerperal anemia
	Puerperal hemorrhage	Puerperal hemorrhage
		Puerperal DIC
		Renal failure
		Pituitary necrosis
Fetal outcome	Perinatal mortality 10.7 in 1000	Perinatal mortality 14.3 in 1000
Neonatal complications	Prematurity	Prematurity
	Intrauterine hypoxia	Intrauterine hypoxia
	Malpresentation	Small for gestational age
	Small for gestational age	Central nervous system malformations
	Congenital abnormalities	
	Velamentous inserted umbilical cord	
	Vasa previa	
	Neonatal anemia	

DIC, Disseminated intravascular coagulation; FHR, fetal heart rate; L/S, lecithin/sphingomyelin; PROM, premature rupture of membranes.

made to manually remove it. Resulting tears in the placenta or partial removal then causes profuse hemorrhage.

Maternal and Fetal Effects

The fetus is rarely affected by this condition unless uterine rupture or extensive bleeding occurs during the pregnancy related to a placenta previa. The mother is at extreme risk for hemorrhage, infection, and pelvic organ damage. Shock and even death can occur. Maternal mortality is approximately 7% (ACOG, 2002).

Usual Medical Management

If there is any evidence of increased risk for invasive placenta, consideration of a cesarean hysterectomy should be discussed before delivery with the family. This surgery should take place at a facility with excellent blood banking capabilities. A team of physicians, including a surgeon who is skilled in pelvic surgery, should assist. Hypotensive anesthesia can reduce blood loss.

Unexpected invasive placenta treatment depends on the number of cotyledons involved and the depth of penetration. In a focal accreta, the one cotyledon can usually be gently removed from the myometrium. The increased bleeding that results is treated with massage and oxytocin. With more extensive involvement, treatment begins with immediate blood replacement therapy and, nearly always, prompt hysterectomy. Conservative treatment may be attempted in some cases if preservation of fertility is desired.

VASA PREVIA

Vasa previa is a rare developmental disorder of the umbilical cord that may occur with a *velamentous inserted umbilical cord.* Velamentous inserted umbilical cord is a condition in which the umbilical blood vessels are separated when they leave the placenta and are not protected with Wharton jelly as they course between the amnion and chorion before uniting to form the umbilical cord (Fig. 19-3). Vasa previa occurs when velamentous vessels cross the region of the internal os and occupy a position ahead of the presenting part. These vessels are easily compressed or ruptured, which causes immediate fetal distress or death.

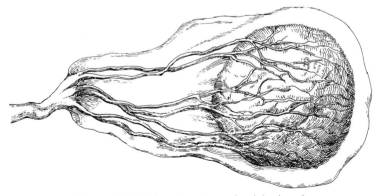

Figure 19-3 Velamentous inserted umbilical cord.

Etiology

One postulated cause of vasa previa is that it is the result of the blastocyst failing to implant with the area of the embryonic disk first into the endometrium. This causes the umbilical cord and the placenta to lie opposite each other. Another possible cause may be the result of one side of the placenta growing toward the vascularized uterine fundus and the other side remaining dormant (Oyelese and Smulian, 2006).

Maternal Effects

Vasa previa presents no danger to the mother because her circulatory system is not involved.

Fetal Effects

Death

The unprotected umbilical vessels are vulnerable to tearing. If one of the umbilical vessels ruptures, death is virtually certain. When the fetal membranes rupture, 60% of the time velamentous umbilical vessels will rupture as well (Hull and Resnik, 2009). Therefore if not identified prior to labor, there is an approximately 60% risk of fetal loss. However, if diagnosed prior to labor, neonatal survival rate has been shown to be as high as 97% (Oyelese, Catanzarite, Prefumo, and others 2004).

Diagnosis

Vasa previa may be diagnosed prenatally using ultrasound. Therefore routine ultrasound should include assessment of the placenta cord insertion site (Hull and Resnik, 2009).

Management

Once vasa previa is confirmed by TVU, a cesarean delivery is usually planned between 34 and 35 weeks of gestation without confirmation of fetal lung maturity testing. Antepartum corticosteroids are routinely used to increase fetal lung maturity (Oyelese and Smulian, 2006). According to Hull and Resnik (2009), the patient can be followed as an outpatient as long as cervical length is 2.5 cm or greater. Provide the patient and her family with educational materials about the condition. A valuable resource is The International Vasa Previa Foundation (*http://www.vasaprevia.com*).

NURSING MANAGEMENT

Prevention

Because inadequate blood supply to the decidua (endometrium) before implantation may be the underlying cause of a placenta previa and because inadequate blood supply to the decidua during pregnancy may be the underlying cause of an abruptio placentae, any condition that would decrease the uterine blood supply should be avoided if possible. Because cigarette smoking decreases uterine blood supply, the mother should not smoke.

Adequate contraceptive instructions should be given so that couples can plan the time and number of their children, preventing therapeutic abortions and closely spaced pregnancies. Hypertensive disorders of pregnancy are the most common causes of abruptio placentae. Use of cocaine is known to cause transient acute hypertensive episodes, which can initiate abruption of the placenta. For this reason and others, illicit drugs should be avoided altogether during pregnancy (see Chapter 27).

Assessment of Blood Loss

- Obtain a history of onset, duration, amount, color, and consistency of bleeding; obtain a history regarding associated symptoms, prior bleeding episodes, and activity at onset of bleeding.
- Visually record blood loss in cubic centimeters or by weighing saturated pads, linen protectors, or linen (1 g = 1 ml).
- Estimate blood loss related to manifested symptoms. Record blood pressure, pulse, and respiratory rate, determining pulse pressure (difference between systolic and diastolic pressures), orthostatic blood pressure changes, hypothenar refilling (by blanching the fleshy elevation of the ulnar side of the palm of the hand; normal refill is 1 to 2 seconds), skin temperature, and color of skin and mucous membranes. Vital signs may be misleadingly normal even in the presence of severe blood loss. This is related to the normal increase of 40% to 50% in the circulatory blood volume during pregnancy. In fact, after week 32 of gestation, the pregnant patient can lose 25% to 30% of her blood volume without exhibiting signs of shock. The blood supply to the placenta is affected before a 25% to 30% decrease in the maternal blood volume. See Table 19-2 for an interpretation of these symptoms.
- Monitor urinary output as indicated by severity. Because of increased peripheral resistance, cerebral and cardiac perfusion may be preserved, but renal blood flow is often jeopardized because it is sensitive to lack of perfusion. Therefore urinary output during pregnancy is the best noninvasive indicator of circulatory volume. Less than 30 ml/hr indicates decreased circulatory volume to the uterus.
- Monitor laboratory data such as complete blood count, electrolyte panel, renal function with blood urea nitrogen, and coagulation factors such as bleeding time, fibrinogen, platelet count, FDPs, prothrombin time, and partial thromboplastin time. Serial hematocrits can facilitate early detection of concealed blood loss.
- Do a clot observation test for DIC if the bleeding is moderate to severe.
- Check for abdominal pain, uterine tenderness, or rigidity.
- Observe fundal height changes.
- Assess for fetal well-being and gestational age.
- Assess fetal presentation. Transverse or oblique position is common with a placenta previa because the placenta usually interferes with engagement.
- Assess level of consciousness.
- Obtain baseline breath sounds before starting fluid replacement.
- If the patient is hemodynamically unstable despite apparently adequate fluid replacement or has an underlying renal, cardiac, or pulmonary disease, a triple-lumen Swan-Ganz catheter may be placed for a more accurate assessment of central venous pressure, pulmonary capillary wedge pressure, and cardiac output.

Nursing Interventions for Mild Bleeding (Less Than 15% Blood Loss)

- Continue the assessment as indicated.
- Do not perform vaginal or rectal examinations and do not give enemas or douches in the presence of vaginal bleeding. If there is a placenta previa, enemas and douches can initiate further separation, and profuse bleeding would result. In the presence of an abruptio placentae, when delivery is not to be initiated immediately, no vaginal or rectal examinations should be carried out to avoid disturbing the injured placenta any further.
- Implement bedrest with bathroom privileges. To decrease bedrest complications while improving uterine blood flow, bathroom privileges can be interpreted as up to bathroom and shower, around the room for 15 to 30 minutes at a time, four times a day.
- Establish an IV access with a 14- or 16-gauge IV catheter to allow for fluid and blood component therapy if necessary. Once bleeding has stopped and the hematocrit level is within normal limits, a heparin lock may be placed.
- Have a maternal blood sample in the blood bank at all times for immediate type and cross-match for blood component therapy, and be prepared to transfuse to maintain hemodynamic stability.
- Prevent constipation and excessive stool straining by educating as to the importance of a high-fiber diet. Administer a stool softener as ordered.
- Decrease risk for anemia by teaching the importance of foods high in iron (e.g., whole grains, green leafy vegetables, legumes), vitamin C (e.g., citrus, strawberries, potatoes, broccoli), and protein. Administer ferrous gluconate as ordered between meals to facilitate the absorption of supplemental iron.
- Monitor for signs of preterm uterine contractions and administer tocolytic therapy, preferably magnesium sulfate, for treatment of uterine activity. Terbutaline is contraindicated if hemodynamically unstable because it relaxes vascular beds, decreasing the body's natural compensatory mechanism.

Nursing Interventions for Moderate (20% to 25% Blood Loss) to Severe Bleeding (30% to 35% Blood Loss)

- Complete bedrest in a quiet environment optimizes the outcome. Activity and sensory stimulation can increase the bleeding and elevate the basal metabolic rate, which increases oxygen consumption. Encourage the mother to lie on either side to prevent pressure on the vena cava and further compromise of the fetal circulation.
- Tilt the uterus to the left by placing a folded sheet under the patient's right hip to keep the gravid uterus off the vena cava, if for any reason the patient must be positioned on her back.
- Start an IV line immediately with a 14- or 16-gauge intracatheter to allow for blood administration; two lines if the patient is hemodynamically unstable.
- Aim fluid therapy at maintaining an adequate circulating blood volume and a hematocrit of 30% or greater.
- Have blood available for type and cross-matching. Administer 2 units of packed red blood cells at the time of each bleeding episode. A lactated Ringer's solution can be administered until blood component therapy is available; it is a better

volume expander than dextrose in water. Volume expanders can also be ordered while waiting for properly matched blood components. Prepare for blood component therapy as ordered by having 250 ml of normal saline available. Administer blood component therapy or volume expanders as ordered. See Table 19-3 for a list of guidelines for blood component replacement.

- Allow nothing by mouth unless otherwise ordered.
- Assess for fetal well-being. FHR is usually normal unless excessive blood loss, maternal shock, or major placental detachment compromises the placental exchange.
- Continue to assess for signs of bleeding as severity of condition indicates.
- Keep an accurate intake and output record, and assess urine specific gravity intermittently to determine kidney perfusion.
- Monitor oxygen saturation with pulse oximeter and blood gases as indicated. A maternal oxygen saturation of at least 95% and a Po_2 of at least 65 mm Hg are necessary for adequate fetal oxygenation.
- Observe for signs of hypovolemic shock.
- After stabilization of the patient with adequate blood component replacement, be prepared to facilitate delivery. Be prepared to assist with an amniotomy and administer a labor stimulant as ordered. Prepare patient for possible cesarean delivery.
- Treat postpartum hemorrhage with uterine massage, with direct compression, by ensuring there are no retained placental fragments, and by using pharmacologic agents for uterine atony such as 10 to 40 units of oxytocin in 1000 ml of Ringer's lactate or normal saline at an infusion rate to control bleeding; methylergonovine maleate (Methergine) 0.2 mg intramuscularly in the deltoid every 2 to 4 hours for a maximum of five times (Weiner and Buhimschi, 2009). If oxytocin and Methergine are ineffective, Carboprost (Hemabate) 250 mcg intramuscular may be ordered (Weiner and Buhimschi, 2009). Rule out vaginal and cervical lacerations. Oxytocin can cause hypotension and has a marked antidiuretic effect when a large dose is given. Methylergonovine maleate is contraindicated in hypertensive, increased intraocular pressure, hepatic dysfunction, or renal dysfunction patients. Gastrointestinal side effects are common with the use of carboprost.
- Report to the primary care provider any change in the patient's bleeding pattern, signs of shock, or failure to respond to treatment.

Critical Care Interventions for Hypovolemic Shock (40% Blood Loss or Greater)

- Restore the blood volume and oxygen-carrying capacity. Begin with lactated Ringer's solution while blood is being typed and cross-matched. It has a 3:1 replacement ratio, 3 ml of solution per 1 ml of estimated blood loss. O-negative packed red bloods cells follow as soon as possible until type-specific cross-matched blood is available. See Table 19-3 for guidelines for blood component replacement.
- Assess for risks caused by using blood and blood components such as hypothermia, dysrhythmias, acidosis, or electrolyte imbalance.

- Administer oxygen at 8 to 10 L/min by face mask to increase oxygen tension and increase oxygen delivery to end-organs.
- Improve autotransfusion by placing patient in modified Trendelenburg position (only elevate legs) to increase blood perfusion to vital organs until blood volume replacement is achieved without contributing to respiratory impairment.
- Always keep the uterus off the vena cava by using a wedge under the hip.
- Continuously monitor blood pressure to evaluate fluid replacement therapy.
- In the presence of a live fetus, continuously monitor FHR until delivery. Keep in mind that a maternal heart beat may be picked up through the fetal scalp electrode in the event of fetal death.
- Monitor input and output with a Foley catheter hourly. *Note*: 30 ml/hr or greater of urine indicates adequate organ perfusion and oxygenation.
- Treat the underlying cause of hemorrhage.
- Use invasive hemodynamic monitoring with a pulmonary artery catheter to evaluate fluid replacement therapy if the hypovolemic shock is unresponsive to initial volume resuscitation and to prevent fluid overload.
- Use the pulmonary artery catheter to obtain direct measurement of the heart rate, central venous pressure, pulmonary artery systolic and diastolic pressures, pulmonary capillary wedge pressure (PCWP), and cardiac output.
- Continuously monitor electrocardiograph as indicated.
- Assess for fluid overload with signs of pulmonary congestion, such as dyspnea, cough, or crackles, by auscultating lung fields every shift.
- Continue to monitor laboratory data as indicated.
- If fluid replacement is inadequate in restoring optimal cardiovascular function, vasopressor agents are indicated as the last resort. Administer dopamine hydrochloride as a continuous infusion starting at 2 to 5 mg/kg/min and titrate according to hemodynamic response. Remember that these agents decrease blood flow to the uterus while increasing maternal myocardial contractility, cardiac output, and systemic vascular resistance without affecting myocardial oxygen consumption. Norepinephrine and ephedrine are two other vasopressor drugs that are used.
- If hypovolemic shock occurred, assess for the possible development of pituitary necrosis (Sheehan syndrome) during the postpartum period by assessing for the onset of lactation. Instruct patient to notify physician if onset of lactation does not occur by the fifth postpartum day.
- Evaluate for urinary output greater than 30 ml/hr with clear breath sounds. If a Swan-Ganz catheter is in place, pulmonary capillary wedge pressure should be maintained between 10 and 15 mm Hg and central venous pressure between 12 and 15 cm.

Critical Care Interventions for Disseminated Intravascular Coagulation

- Observe for signs of DIC such as oozing of blood from the IV site, easy bruising, or petechiae.
- Monitor the DIC profile, which includes fibrinogen, platelet count, prothrombin time, partial thromboplastin time, fibrin split products, and fibrin degradation products (FDPs) with a D-dimer test. A sensitive test for diagnosis of abruptio-related DIC is the determination of FDP with a D-dimer test. Prothrombin

time and partial thromboplastin time are late indicators because 50% or more of the clotting factors must be consumed before these tests are abnormal. It should be noted that normal measurements during pregnancy are bleeding time less than 4 minutes, fibrinogen levels of 400 to 650 mg/dl, platelets between 100,000 and 350,000/mm³, prothrombin time 12 to 14 seconds, and partial prothrombin time between 14 and 36 seconds.

- Serial clot observation tests may be done at the bedside to assess for severe DIC. To carry this out, the nurse places 5 ml of venous blood in a test tube, hangs it in the room, and observes the time it takes to clot. If it does not form a clot within 6 to 8 minutes, a significant coagulation defect is usually present.
- Treat the underlying disease process and bleeding. Administer procoagulants such as platelets, clotting factors with fresh frozen plasma, and factor VIII and fibrinogen with cryoprecipitate. Heparin is rarely needed. See Chapter 20 for management. *Note*: Minimal clotting factor levels for surgery are fibrinogen above 100 mg/dl and platelets greater than 50,000/mm³.
- DIC usually resolves spontaneously after delivery.

Nursing Interventions for Antepartum Fetal Surveillance

- Assess FHR. It is usually normal unless excessive blood loss, maternal shock, or major placental detachment compromises the placental exchange.
- Determine gestational age.
- Monitor FHR as indicated (depending on severity).
- Evaluate FHR for tachycardia, bradycardia, late or variable decelerations, and loss of long- or short-term variability.
- During labor, check uterine contractions for duration, frequency, and uterine resting tone. Observe amniotic fluid for meconium staining.
- Prevent vena caval syndrome by keeping the patient positioned on her left or right side; if she must be on her back, tilt uterus to the left by placing folded sheet under the right hip.
- Administer oxygen as indicated with face mask at 8 to 10 L/min.
- Prepare the patient for fetal well-being and maturity studies as ordered. Modified biophysical profiles, ultrasound, and amniocentesis are usually ordered on a frequent basis in an attempt to determine the optimal time for delivery.
- Antepartum corticosteroids such as betamethasone or dexamethasone are indicated to enhance fetal pulmonary maturity between 24 and 34 weeks of gestation.
- Be prepared to intermittently assess blood to determine whether it is of fetal origin by a Kleihauer-Betke analysis or APT (alum-precipitated toxoid) test because of the increased risk for vasa previa associated with a placenta previa.
- If vaginal bleeding occurs immediately after rupture of membranes, vasa previa is suggested.
- Notify physician if a baseline or periodic FHR change is noted or if there is a nonreactive NST or amniotic fluid index less than 8.
- During a trial of labor, notify the physician of a hypertonic uterus, increased signs of bleeding, a labor that progresses abnormally slowly, or any signs of fetal stress.
- Once delivery is imminent, notify the intensive care nursery of a possible high risk infant.

Nursing Interventions to Manage Fear Related to Effect on Health Status and Threat of Fetal or Neonatal Death

- Assess level of maternal anxiety. Parents are usually very concerned about the health and well-being of the baby and the mother's safety. They may also be experiencing some common fears or worries such as wondering what they might have done to cause this to happen. Therefore the expectant parents should be encouraged to express their feelings and concerns. In this way, the nurse knows how to better individualize emotional support.
- Assess other family members' feelings of guilt, such as wondering what they might have done to cause this to happen.
- Assess the family's coping strategies and resources.
- Encourage expression of feelings, concerns, and labor experience.
- Clarify any misconceptions. Explain that the cause of the condition is unknown but it is not related to patient's activity at time of occurrence.
- Provide information to the patient and her family regarding the pregnancy complication, plan of treatment, and implications for mother and fetus in understandable terms. Discuss with the expectant parents the possibility of a cesarean delivery. The parents are then more prepared if the event arises.
- Explain all treatment modalities and reasons for each.
- Keep parents informed of health status, test results, and fetal well-being. Focus on the positive signs of fetal well-being such as a normal FHR, fetal activity, and reactive NSTs.
- Compliment the patient for her cooperation in adhering to medical therapy.
- Refer to the social worker if inadequate coping is noted.
- Refer to pastor, priest, or chaplain per parents' request.
- Evaluate. The patient and her family will be able to communicate their fears and concerns openly.

Nursing Interventions for Altered Role Performance Related to Prolonged Hospitalization and Treatment with Bedrest

- Assess the patient's responsibilities to determine difficulties she will have in implementing prescribed bedrest.
- Teach patient importance of bedrest in the lateral position with bathroom privileges.
- Help the family problem solve if difficulties arise in implementing bedrest.
- Refer to Sidelines high risk support group (*http://www.sidelines.org/*).
- Make needed referrals, such as to social worker, if problems are identified.
- Encourage participation in her care and decision making as much as possible.
- Evaluate the patient's plan that will take care of all her work- and family-related responsibilities during her absence.

Diversional Activity for Therapeutic Management of Bedrest

- Assess patient's interest in various diversional activities within the activity limit.
- Provide activities such as crafts, reading, and puzzles that can be done in bed, or encourage patient to have these items brought in.
- Provide classes in preparation for childbirth by way of video, hospital television, or group classes that can be attended while reclining.

- Refer to a diversional therapist or volunteer to provide reading materials, handicrafts, or other interesting materials.
- Evaluate. Ask the patient to verbalize various appropriate activities she would like to do while maintaining bedrest.

Nursing Interventions to Prevent RhD Alloimmunization in an RhD-Negative Mother Carrying an RhD-Positive Fetus

- Monitor the RhD antibody titer with an antibody screen, indirect Coombs test at 28 weeks of gestation, and then again at the time of admission. An antibody titer may be repeated after any bleeding episode if a fetal-maternal bleed is suggested.
- Administer Rh_o (D) immune globulin (RhoGAM; HypRho-D) 300 mcg intramuscularly in the deltoid as ordered at 28 weeks, after any suspected fetal-maternal bleed, and within 72 hours postpartum.
- After any antepartum bleed, evaluate for fetal cells in the maternal circulation. If fetal cells are found, be prepared to order a Kleihauer-Betke stain to assess the amount of fetal blood in the maternal circulation. If the bleed is greater than 30 ml of fetal whole blood (15 ml packed RBCs), administer additional Rh_o (D) immune globulin based on this formula: PRBCs divided by 2; then divided by 15 = number of vials (Weiner and Buhimschi, 2009).

CONCLUSION

The ultimate goal of treatment for both an abruptio placenta and a placenta previa is early recognition and appropriate intervention to prevent hemorrhage and its resulting complications of shock, DIC, multisystem failure, and ultimately death of mother or fetus. At the same time, premature delivery must be avoided as long as intrauterine hypoxia is not present.

BIBLIOGRAPHY

Addis A, and others: Fetal effects of cocaine: an updated meta-analysis, *Reprod Toxicol* 15:341, 2001.

American College of Obstetricians and Gynecologists (ACOG): *Placenta accreta*. Committee Opinion, No. 266, Washington, DC, 2002, Author.

American College of Obstetricians and Gynecologists (ACOG): *Management of alloimmunization during pregnancy*, Clinical Management Guidelines for Obstetricians-Gynecologists, No. 75, Washington, DC, 2006, Author.

Ananth C, Smulian J, Vintzileos A: The effect of placenta previa on neonatal mortality: a population-based study in the United States, 1989 through 1997, *Am J Obstet Gynecol* 188(5):1299–1304, 2003.

Benedetti T: Obstetric hemorrhage. In Gabbe S, Niebyl J, and Simpson J, editors: *Obstetrics: normal and problem pregnancies*, ed 4, New York, 2002, Churchill Livingstone.

Bhide A, Thilaganthan B: Recent advances in the management of placenta previa, *Curr Opin Obstet Gynecol* 16(6):447–451, 2004.

Carter S: Overview of common obstetric bleeding disorders, *Nurse Pract* 24(3):50–58, 1999.

Crane J, and others: Neonatal outcomes with placenta previa, *Am Coll Obstet Gynecol* 93:541, 1999.

Cunningham F, Leveno K, Bloom S, Hauth J, Rouse D, Spong C: *Williams obstetrics*, ed 23, New York, 2010, McGraw-Hill Medical.

Elliott J, Gilpin B, Strong T, Finberg H: Chronic abruption-oligohydramnios sequence, *J Reprod Med* 43(5):418–422, 1998.

Gesteland K, and others: Rates of placenta previa and placental abruption in women delivered only vaginally or only by cesarean section, Abstract No. 403, *J Soc Gynecol Investig* 11:208A, 2004.

Hull A, Resnik R: Placenta previa, placenta accrete, abruptio placentae, and vasa previa. In Creasy R, Resnik R, Iams J, and others, editors: *Creasy & Resnik's maternal-fetal medicine: principles and practice,* ed 6, Philadelphia, 2009, Saunders.

MacMullen N, Dulski L, Meagher B: Red alert: perinatal hemorrhage, *MCN Am J Matern Child Nurs* 30(1):46–51, 2005.

Martin J, and others: Births: final data for 2001, *National Vital Statistics Reports,* vol 51, No 2, Hyattsville, MD, National Center for Health Statistics, 2002.

Morgan K, Arulkumaran S: Antepartum heamorrhage, *Curr Obstet Gynaecol* 13(2):81, 2003.

Neilson JP. Interventions for suspected placenta praevia, *Cochrane Database Syst Rev* (Issue 2), Art. No.: CD001998, 2003.

Oppenheimer L: Society of Obstetricians and Gynaecologists of Canada: Diagnosis and management of placenta previa, *J Obstet Gynaecol Can* 29(3):261–266, 2007. Retrieved from http://www.guideline. gov.

Oppenheimer L, and others: Diagnosis of low-lying placenta: can migration in the third trimester predict outcome?, *Ultrasound Obstet Gynecol* 18(2):100–102, 2001.

Oyelese Y, Ananth C: Placental abruption, *Obstet Gynecol* 108:1005–1016, 2006.

Oyelese Y, Catanzarite V, Prefumo F, and others: Vasa previa: the impact of prenatal diagnosis on outcomes, *Obstet Gynecol* 103:937–942, 2004.

Oyelese Y, Smulian J: Placenta previa, placenta accrete, and vasa previa, *Obstet Gynecol* 107:927–941, 2006.

Rasmussen S, Irgens L, Dalaker K: Outcome of pregnancies subsequent to placental abruption: a risk assessment, *Acta Obstet Gynecol Scand* 79:496–501, 2000.

Royal College of Obstetricians and Gynaecologists (RCOG). *Placenta praevia and placenta praevia accreta: diagnosis and management,* Guideline No. 21, London, 2005, RCOG Press. Retrieved from http://www.rcog.org.uk/index.

Salihu H, and others: Perinatal mortality associated with abruptio placenta in singletons and multiples, *Am J Obstet Gynecol* 193(1):198–203, 2005.

Sharma A, Suri V, Gupta I: Tocolytic therapy in conservative management of symptomatic placenta previa, *Int J Gynaecol Obstet* 84:109–113, 2004.

Silver R, Landon M, Rouse D, and others: Maternal morbidity associated with multiple repeat cesarean deliveries, *Obstet Gynecol* 107:1226–1232, 2006.

Usta I, Hobeika E, Musa A, and others: Placenta previa-accreta: risk factors and complications, *Am J Obstet Gynecol* 193:1045–1049, 2005.

Weiner C, Buhimschi C: *Drugs for pregnant and lactating women,* ed 2, Philadelphia, 2009, Saunders.

Weintraub A, Press F, Wiznitzer A, Sheiner E: Maternal thrombophilia and adverse pregnancy outcomes, *Expert Rev Obstet Gynecol* 2(2):203–216, 2007.

20

Disseminated Intravascular Coagulation

D isseminated intravascular coagulation (DIC) is not a primary disease but rather a secondary event activated by a number of severe illnesses. It occurs when a severe illness causes a generalized activation of the coagulation process (Samuels, 2004). If coagulation factors are consumed faster than the liver can replace them, depletion occurs. At that point, the process of fibrinolysis is activated in response to coagulation. The result is rampant coagulation and simultaneous massive bleeding (Becker and Wira, 2009).

INCIDENCE

The incidence of DIC is rare and has not been reported (Francois and Foley, 2007).

ETIOLOGY

The following stimuli are known to activate the coagulation syndrome during pregnancy (Samuels, 2004; Anthony, 2006; Becker and Wira, 2009):
- Tissue damage and inflammation
- Severe injury to endothelial cells
- Red cell or platelet injury seen in hemolytic processes
- Bacterial debris or endotoxins
- Immune reactions
- Thrombocytopenia
- Chemical and physical agents

Some of the conditions that commonly activate this process are listed (Samuels, 2004; Becker and Wira, 2009):
- Greater than expected blood loss with inadequate crystalloid or colloid replacement
- Placental abruption
- Severe preeclampsia, eclampsia or the HELLP (*h*emolysis, *e*levated *l*iver enzymes, and *l*ow-*p*latelet count in association with preeclampsia) syndrome
- Sepsis
- Acute fatty liver of pregnancy

- Retained dead fetus
- Major trauma
- Anaphylactoid syndrome of pregnancy (see Chapter 15)

NORMAL PHYSIOLOGY

The processes of clot formation and clot breakdown (*fibrinolysis*) must be understood to comprehend DIC. Clot formation and fibrinolysis are intertwined with the activation of factors maintaining a homeostasis under normal circumstances.

Whenever blood vessels or tissues become damaged and bleeding occurs, several factors attempt hemostasis. First, central nervous system reflexes cause vascular spasms, reducing blood flow to the area. Second, platelets attempt to plug the break. Finally, clot formation occurs. Clot formation can be activated by intrinsic and extrinsic factors. The intrinsic factors exist within the vascular system and are activated with blood vessel damage. The extrinsic factors are within the tissue and are activated in response to tissue trauma. When either process is activated, prothrombin activator is formed. Prothrombin activator, along with calcium and phospholipids, acts as a catalyst to convert inactive plasma prothrombin into thrombin. The enzyme *thrombin* converts inactive plasma fibrinogen into fibrin. Fibrin, along with platelets, causes the red blood cells (RBCs) and plasma to mesh, and a clot is then formed (Fig. 20-1).

Fibrinolysis normally occurs simultaneously with clot formation as long as activators are present. Plasminogen, a plasma euglobulin, is activated into plasmin. Plasmin then breaks fibrin down into fibrin split products and fibrinogen into fibrinogen split products. This process consumes factors V, VIII, and XII (intrinsic

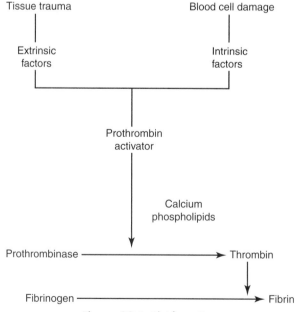

Figure 20-1 Clot formation.

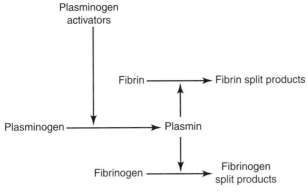

Figure 20-2 Fibrinolysis.

factors) and prothrombin. Anticoagulants, antithrombin III, and heparin also facilitate fibrinolysis. Antithrombin III neutralizes thrombin, plasmin, and factors VII, X, and XII, which are intrinsic and extrinsic factors (Fig. 20-2) (Samuels, 2004; Becker and Wira, 2009).

In pregnancy, fibrinogen, platelet adhesiveness, and factor VIII are increased. Antithrombin III and the activators for plasminogen are decreased. Plasminogen itself is increased. Therefore the equilibrium of coagulation and fibrinolysis is skewed toward procoagulation. Factors in pregnancy that can promote this include feto-placental hormones, pregnancy-specific hormones, immunologic complexes, and entry of placental thrombin into maternal circulation through the vascular interfaces (Samuels, 2004; Auerbach and Lockwood, 2006).

The listed clotting factors are the important ones for DIC. See Chapter 19 for placental abnormalities and Chapter 22 for hypertensive disorders and their relationships to DIC.

PATHOPHYSIOLOGY

DIC occurs when factor consumption of the coagulation-fibrinolysis processes exceed the liver's capacity to produce factors. The coagulation process is stimulated by endothelial or tissue injury. When coagulation factors are depleted, equilibrium is disrupted and bleeding occurs because of deficient coagulation factors. The body continues to attempt clot formation in the presence of bleeding, which further depletes coagulation factors. Small clots can plug the small blood vessels and lead to organ ischemia (Samuels, 2004).

Anaphylactoid syndrome of pregnancy is currently thought to occur when the entry of amniotic fluid and fetal cells into the maternal circulation in certain patients triggers an anaphylactic reaction. This anaphylactic response initiates a cascade of activation of both the coagulation and the fibrinolysis processes, as well as simultaneous respiratory and cardiac arrest (Martin and Foley, 2009) (see Chapter 15).

When the products of conception are retained after intrauterine fetal demise, thromboplastic material can seep into the maternal circulation. This infusion of tissue extract activates the overwhelming depletion of coagulation factors.

In preeclampsia and eclampsia, damage to vessel walls occurs secondary to oxidative stress and ischemic endotoxin substance released by the placenta. The vessel wall damage causes products of cellular breakdown to come in contact with the surface of the platelets, and the coagulation-fibrinolysis process occurs simultaneously. The process then consumes massive amounts of coagulation-fibrinolysis factors, and the liver is unable to replace factors as rapidly as is necessary (Anthony, 2006).

Hemorrhage and shock can also precipitate disequilibrium of coagulation-fibrinolysis. Hypovolemia causes decreased cardiac output, decreased arterial pressure, and decreased systemic blood flow. This results in decreased nutrition to the brain and vascular system. The hypoxic vascular endothelium triggers intravascular coagulation. Intravascular coagulation releases toxins that increase capillary permeability, further diminishing circulating volume. Brain anoxia results in cardiac depression and further compromises cardiac output.

SIGNS AND SYMPTOMS

Early symptoms of DIC include epistaxis, gingival bleeding, ecchymoses, and bleeding into the urine or at the site of an intravenous (IV) line. As DIC develops, these early signs may rapidly progress to the following severe signs of shock:
- Respirations progress from rapid and deep to rapid, shallow, and irregular and finally to barely perceptible.
- Pulse rate becomes rapid, weaker, irregular, and thready.
- Blood pressure may initially be normal but then begins falling until the systolic pressure is below 60 mm Hg or is not palpable.
- Skin color may then begin to pale and cool, progressing rapidly to being cold, clammy, and cyanotic.
- Urinary output initially remains stable and then quickly begins to decrease to less than 30 ml/hr.
- Level of consciousness changes from apprehension to increasing restlessness, lethargy, and finally coma.
- Central venous pressure and pulmonary artery wedge pressure drop.

Laboratory signs of DIC include decreased platelet count, fibrinogen, and antithrombin III levels, as well as increased fibrin split products, abnormal prothrombin fragment 1 and 2, abnormal fibrinopeptide A, and the presence of FDP/D-dimer.

MATERNAL EFFECTS

DIC can and often does result in maternal death. If it does not result in maternal death, few mothers survive neurologically intact. Damage ranges from relatively minor to very profound.

FETAL AND NEONATAL EFFECTS

DIC can result in fetal death or severe hypoxia. Possible neonatal sequelae to severe hypoxia are intracranial bleeding and brain death.

DIAGNOSTIC TESTING

The medical diagnosis is made based on a history of predisposing conditions, the early signs of ecchymosis formation, and bleeding from the IV site or urinary tract. Definitive diagnosis is made based on the laboratory data previously listed.

USUAL MEDICAL MANAGEMENT AND PROTOCOLS FOR NURSE PRACTITIONERS

When DIC occurs in the antepartum period, the initial treatment is to correct the underlying cause, which usually means emptying the uterus by the most expeditious means. To improve the circulatory volume, fluid replacement is essential. Blood replacement with packed cells, fresh frozen plasma (FFP), cryoprecipitate, and platelets may be necessary to replace volume and depleted coagulation factors. Simultaneously, the primary disease must be stabilized and corrected.

Blood Replacement

Red Blood Cell Transfusions

The main blood replacement is red blood cells (RBCs). These may come as packed RBCs, which contain RBCs and plasma—usually 250 ml of RBCs and 50 ml of plasma—and have a hematocrit level of approximately 80%. This replacement thus reduces the risk for fluid overload.

Platelet Concentrates

Platelets are separated from whole blood and suspended in small amounts of plasma and a small amount of serum-bound RBCs. Caution should be exercised in an Rh-negative woman.

Fresh Frozen Plasma (FFP)

FFP is extracted from whole blood within 6 hours of collection and then frozen. It contains 700 mg of fibrinogen. It is indicated to correct deficiencies of multiple clotting factors, including factors V, VIII, X, and XIII. It also increases fibrinogen level.

Cryoprecipitate

Cryoprecipitate is extracted from frozen whole blood, which has then thawed at a controlled, refrigerated temperature. FFP precipitates under these conditions and is then rich in Factor VIII and fibrinogen.

Recombinant Human Activated Protein C

This protein inhibits coagulation by blocking factors Va and VIIIa in the clotting cascade.

Antithrombin III

Antithrombin III may be used in severe DIC to suppress coagulation by suppressing thrombin, plasmin, and other coagulation factors such as VIIa, IXa, Xa, XIa, and XIIa.

Supportive Measures

Supportive measures for monitoring fluid replacement and cardiac output are necessary. These include cardiac monitoring, hemodynamic monitoring, and blood pressure recordings every 5 to 15 minutes depending on clinical presentation of the patient. Because clinical signs of DIC may be rapid in onset, the emergency initially threatens the mother's life and fetal considerations are excluded. Once factor replacement is instituted for the mother, the fetus is often delivered before continuous monitoring of the fetal heart rate (FHR) can be initiated. Fetal delivery may be accomplished simultaneously with resuscitation of the pregnant woman. Two teams, one for trauma response and one for perinatal response, are usually required for this type of approach.

Anticoagulants

Heparin and antithrombolytic therapy is rarely used unless clotting continues 4 to 6 hours after initiation of blood replacement therapy to decrease the risk for progressive renal failure and gangrene (Becker and Wira, 2009).

NURSING MANAGEMENT

Secondary Prevention

When the mother has a condition that might predispose her to development of DIC, the nurse must be alert for early signs of ecchymosis: blood in the urine or bleeding from the gums, the IV insertion site, or other venous puncture sites. A simple test to confirm early signs of possible DIC is the clot retraction test, in which 5 ml of blood is drawn into a test tube, capped, and taped to the bedside wall. If a clot does not form and the serum does not separate from the cells within 8 to 10 minutes, DIC is possible and the physician should be notified. Late signs of disequilibrium are watched for as well. These signs include progressive changes in respiration, pulse, blood pressure, skin color, and urinary output, as well as indications of mild to moderate shock and acute renal failure (see Chapter 12).

Tertiary Prevention

During the recovery phase, care should include early detection and treatment of infection and transfusion hepatitis. Grief management is an important component of the recovery phase if maternal or fetal loss occurred. Maternal death occurs in approximately 75% to 85% of cases, and fetal loss occurs at a rate that is equally as high or higher. See Chapter 7 for information about perinatal loss and grief.

Critical Care Nursing Interventions for Disseminated Intravascular Coagulation

- Observe patients with complications precipitating DIC for early signs of shock.
- Evaluate vital signs for evidence of shock; that is, increased pulse rate preceding a drop in blood pressure (in fact, early signs may include a slight rise in blood pressure), restlessness, and loss of sensorium.
- Evaluate bedside clot retraction test by placing 5 ml of blood in test tube and observing after 8 to 10 minutes to see whether a clot has formed.

- Start an IV line with at least a 14-gauge angiocatheter and infuse physiologic saline solution.
- Notify laboratory trauma support personnel for possible need for uncrossed-matched blood and blood products.
- Prepare to transfuse rapidly with cryoprecipitate, packed cells, and FFP.
- Administer oxygen, 8 to 10 L/min by face mask.
- Position patient off her back, using a rolled towel under her right hip.
- Involve the intensive care or trauma team so that they can assist with fluid replacement and monitoring or refer.
- Assist with insertion of invasive hemodynamic lines.
- Monitor vital signs and hemodynamic data as indicated.
- Report vital signs, hemodynamic monitoring data, amount of continued bleeding, and laboratory data immediately to the physician in charge of fluid replacement therapy.
- Assess for the potential complication of acute renal failure.
- Institute fetal monitoring as soon as the intensive care team or trauma team begins managing the maternal emergency. The labor nurse's responsibility shifts to the fetus.
- Prepare for an emergent (agonal) cesarean birth if the mother is not immediately stabilized before delivery and the fetus is viable.
- Notify the neonatal team.
- During postpartum recovery phase, monitor for signs of infection such as pneumonia, septic shock, or transfusion hepatitis.

CONCLUSION

The primary goal of care of the pregnant woman with DIC is to prevent shock and its sequelae. Early recognition of conditions that predispose a woman to DIC can help prevent maternal death or unexpected long-term sequelae as well as promote a healthy newborn outcome. When a pregnant woman presents with a severe medical condition and has developed DIC, it is important to attempt rapid stabilization of the mother before attempting an emergency or agonal cesarean delivery.

BIBLIOGRAPHY

Anthony J: Major obstetric hemorrhage: disseminated intravascular coagulation. In James D, and others, editor: *High risk pregnancy: management options*, ed 3, Philadelphia, 2006, Saunders.

Auerbach R, Lockwood C: Clotting disorders. In James D, and others, editors: *High risk pregnancy: management options*, ed 3, Philadelphia, 2006, Saunders.

Becker J, Wira C: Disseminated intravascular coagulation, *eMedicine*, 2009. Retrieved from http://emedicine.medscape.com/article/779097-overview.

Francois K, Foley M: Antepartum and postpartum hemorrhage. In Gabbe S, Niebyl J, Simpson J, editors: *Obstetrics: normal and problem pregnancies*, ed 5, Philadelphia, 2007, Churchill Livingstone.

Martin S, Foley M: Intensive care monitoring of the critically ill pregnant patient. In Creasy R, Resnik R, Iams J, Lockwood C, Moore T, editors: *Creasy & Resnik's maternal-fetal medicine: principles and practice*, ed 6, Philadelphia, 2009, Saunders.

Samuels P: Disseminated intravascular coagulopathy and thrombocytopenia complicating pregnancy: an acute approach. In Foley M, Strong T, Garite T, editors: *Obstetric intensive care*, ed 2, New York, 2004, McGraw-Hill.

21

Hemolytic Incompatibility

Hemolytic incompatibility occurs when a pregnant woman is sensitized to produce immunoglobulin G antibodies against fetal red blood cells, usually from the CDE (Rh) or ABO blood group. The antibodies, returning to the fetal circulation, can cause erythrocyte destruction in the fetus and subsequent fetal anemia with liver failure and congestive heart failure (hydrops).

INCIDENCE

With the routine use of Rh_o (D) immune globulin, alloimmunization occurs in less than 1% of all live births (Moise, 2008). Although RhD incompatibility is the most common and usually the most serious, other hemolytic incompatibilities do occur. Hemolytic disease is seen in 10% of the ABO blood group incompatibilities. ABO and RhD incompatibilities account for 98% of all hemolytic disease in the fetus. Of the remaining 2%, rare antibodies, such as C, c, E, e, Kell, or Duffy antibodies, are implicated. The pathophysiologic processes for all incompatibilities are similar (Weiner, 2006).

ETIOLOGY

ABO incompatibility occurs when the mother's blood type is O and the fetal blood type is A, B, or AB. Compared with the CDE (Rh) system, the ABO system is weakly antigenic to its own factors for two reasons. First, A and B antibodies do not cross the placenta. Second, fewer A and B antigenic sites exist on fetal red cells. Therefore there is only a 5% risk for an ABO incompatibility, and it seldom causes hydrops fetalis.

Rh incompatibility occurs primarily when the mother is RhD-negative and the fetus is RhD-positive. However, it can also occur if the fetus has any antigen C, c, E, or e and the mother does not (Weiner, 2006).

NORMAL PHYSIOLOGY

Blood Type Genetics
Each father and mother, having received half of their blood type from each parent, can be said to be homozygous or heterozygous. Thus in the ABO system, combinations occur. All people with type O blood are homozygous. When the mother is

type O, she is homozygous, having received an O from both parents. If the father is type O also, there are no antigenic possibilities for the fetal ABO system; the fetus must be type O. If the father is type A, he could be AO heterozygous or AA homozygous. If the father is type B, he could be BB homozygous or BO heterozygous. If the father is type AB, he is heterozygous. To understand the possible fetal blood types from heterozygous fathers with type A, B, or AB and homozygous O mothers or from homozygous type A or B fathers and homozygous O mothers, the following examples may be helpful:

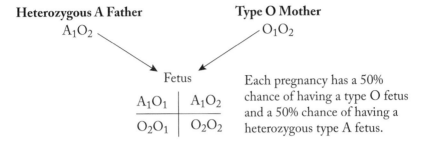

Heterozygous A Father
A_1O_2

Type O Mother
O_1O_2

Fetus

A_1O_1	A_1O_2
O_2O_1	O_2O_2

Each pregnancy has a 50% chance of having a type O fetus and a 50% chance of having a heterozygous type A fetus.

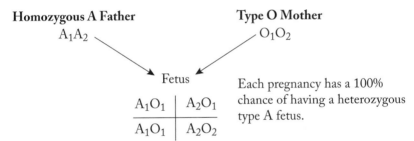

Homozygous A Father
A_1A_2

Type O Mother
O_1O_2

Fetus

A_1O_1	A_2O_1
A_1O_1	A_2O_2

Each pregnancy has a 100% chance of having a heterozygous type A fetus.

- The heterozygous type A fetus carried by a type O mother has antigen A that can evoke antibody formation in the type O mother. Type B works the same way.

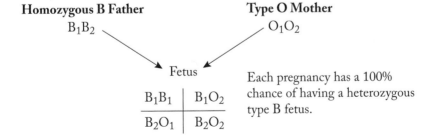

Homozygous B Father
B_1B_2

Type O Mother
O_1O_2

Fetus

B_1B_1	B_1O_2
B_2O_1	B_2O_2

Each pregnancy has a 100% chance of having a heterozygous type B fetus.

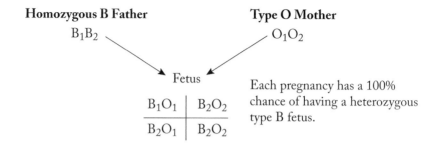

Homozygous B Father   **Type O Mother**

<table>
<tr><td>B_1O_1</td><td>B_2O_2</td></tr>
<tr><td>B_2O_1</td><td>B_2O_2</td></tr>
</table>

Each pregnancy has a 100% chance of having a heterozygous type B fetus.

- The heterozygous type B fetus has the B antigen, which can evoke antibody formation in the type O mother.
- Type AB fathers are always heterozygous. Their children from a type O mother have the following chances:

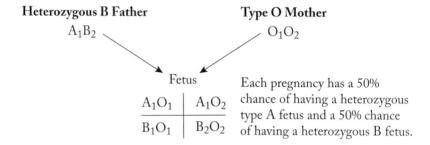

Heterozygous B Father   **Type O Mother**

Each pregnancy has a 50% chance of having a heterozygous type A fetus and a 50% chance of having a heterozygous B fetus.

- Because type AB fathers having children with type O mothers always produce heterozygous A or heterozygous B children, each fetus has the potential of antigenic factors evoking antibody formation by the type O mother. All have antigenic factors that are relatively weak compared with the CDE blood system.
- If a mother is RhD-negative, she is always homozygous, having received the RhD-negative gene from both parents. The RhD-positive father may be RhD-positive heterozygous or RhD-positive homozygous. The following examples demonstrate this.

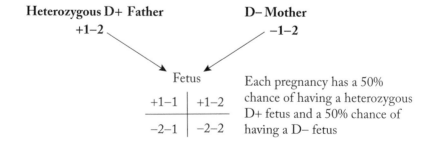

Heterozygous D+ Father   **D− Mother**

Each pregnancy has a 50% chance of having a heterozygous D+ fetus and a 50% chance of having a D− fetus

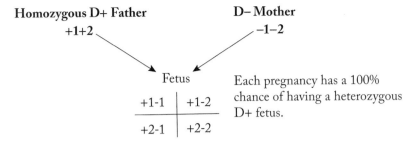

Homozygous D+ Father   D− Mother

+1+2   −1−2

Fetus

+1-1	+1-2
+2-1	+2-2

Each pregnancy has a 100% chance of having a heterozygous D+ fetus.

- The RhD fetus has a strong RhD antigen on the surface of each red blood cell. These antigens evoke antibody formation in the RhD mother. The degree of sensitivity to the fetal D antigen varies but is assumed to be related to the total number of RhD fetal red blood cells entering the maternal circulation (Weiner, 2006; Moise, 2009).

ABO Blood Group System

The ABO blood group system has the following antigens:
- A has antigen A.
- B has antigen B.
- AB has both antigens A and B.
- O has none.

The person who does not have the AB antigen probably has the antibody against the respective antigen.

CDE (Rh) Blood Group System

More than 400 red cell antigens have been identified. The person who lacks a specific red cell antigen and is exposed to that antigen can potentially produce an antibody against the antigen. It is fortunate that many of these red cell antigens are rare and many have low immunogenicity capability. The greatest immunogenicity capability is seen with the RhD (rhesus factor) antigen. If the mother is Rh-positive, she probably has the RhD antigen. If the mother is Rh-negative, she does not have the antigen and is extremely vulnerable to the formation of anti-D antibodies if she is exposed to the D antigen. However, recognition is growing of immunogenicity in the Rh system if factor E, c, C, or e (listed in order of frequency) is present (Weiner, 2006).

Placental Transport

The placenta provides a large area in which exchange of nutrients and waste can take place across the placental membrane. This membrane consists of fetal tissues that separate maternal and fetal blood. As the pregnancy advances, the placental membrane, which also serves as a barrier, becomes progressively thinner. Because of the thinning of this membrane, some fetal blood cells may pass into the maternal blood in the intervillous space. It has been established that small numbers of fetal erythrocytes pass into the maternal circulation normally throughout pregnancy. Typically, a greater amount enters at the time of delivery when the separation of the placenta traumatically forces entry of cells through the ciliated, open maternal vessels.

However, small separations of the placenta can occur during pregnancy or with any potentially traumatic procedure such as amniocentesis. In most instances, the fetal-maternal transfusion is small enough to evoke no sensitivity or involves no incompatibilities from the CDE or ABO system.

PATHOPHYSIOLOGY

The pathophysiology for all the hemolytic incompatibilities is similar. D incompatibility, the most common type, is used here to describe the process of Rhesus alloimmunization. Alloimmunization occurs when the mother is sensitive to the fetal cells; thus it is also called *sensitization* (Weiner, 2006).

Fetal erythrocytes, with the paternal D antigen, gain entry across the placental membrane into the intervillous blood, which is made up entirely of maternal blood. The fetal erythrocytes mix with the maternal blood and are then carried into the mother's circulation.

The breakthrough of fetal erythrocytes carrying the RhD antigen into the maternal circulation requires certain conditions favorable to sensitization of the mother and antibody formation. The widely dilated uteroplacental vessels encouraging blood flow also facilitate this process. Maximum maternal blood volume increasing between 28 and 32 weeks of gestation further facilitates dilation of these vessels. Changes in fetal blood pressure are responsive to changes in blood flow in the maternal circulation and presumably could increase the chance of a few fetal erythrocytes, under increased pressure, breaking into the intervillous space. For this reason, the second most likely time for Rhesus alloimmunization to occur in the mother is at approximately 28 weeks of gestation.

The most likely time for fetal erythrocytes to escape into maternal circulation is at the time of delivery. The wide open vessels at the site of placental separation allow rapid back pressure as the uterus relaxes, and large numbers of fetal erythrocytes can escape into the maternal circulation.

The formation of antibodies is gradual in the mother. Conditions favoring small areas of placental separation such as placenta previa, marginal abruption, or trauma to the placenta during amniocentesis can also favor the entry of increased numbers of fetal erythrocytes carrying the D antigen into the maternal circulation.

SIGNS AND SYMPTOMS

Evidence of antibody formation in the RhD-negative woman can be detected with an indirect Coombs test and positive identification of the specific antibody on a screen. A titer of 1:4 or greater is significant and indicates maternal sensitization.

In the fetus, signs of anemia and impending hydrops include the following:
- A baseline heart rate of 180 beats per minute (bpm) or greater
- Late decelerations or loss of short-term variability with presence of regular sine-wave long-term variability (sinusoidal pattern) (Fig. 21-1)
- Decreased fetal activity
- Fetal ascites or congestive heart failure on ultrasound examination

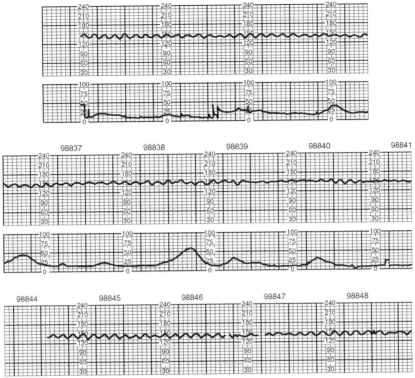

Figure 21-1 *Top:* D-isoimmunized woman at 30 weeks of gestation. Nonstress test after fourth amniocentesis. *Middle and bottom:* The following-day strip shows sinusoidal pattern. (Courtesy John P. Elliott, MD, Phoenix, Ariz.)

MATERNAL EFFECTS

There are no negative physiologic effects on the well-being of the mother other than discomfort if polyhydramnios occurs with fetal hydrops. If the mother is sensitized and desires future pregnancies, she may experience significant psychologic difficulties. The various feelings evoked depend on the circumstances leading to the Rhesus alloimmunization.

FETAL AND NEONATAL EFFECTS

Harmful effects of rhesus alloimmunization of the mother are seen as hemolysis of fetal erythrocytes. If the sensitization process begins in one pregnancy, the effects will be seen in future pregnancies.

The current pregnancy may be in jeopardy if the process of sensitization is undetected. This can occur if minute placental tissue fragments enter maternal circulation during an amniocentesis, at 28 weeks of gestation, or as a result of placenta previa or abruptio placentae. The current pregnancy may also be jeopardized because sensitization occurred inadvertently with a previous pregnancy.

Hemolysis of fetal erythrocytes can lead to various degrees of fetal anemia. When anemia becomes severe, large amounts of bilirubin, resulting from hemolysis of the erythrocytes, place an overwhelming burden on the fetal liver. As a result, swelling occurs in the liver and portal pressure increases, causing abdominal ascites and congestive heart failure. This phenomenon is called hydrops fetalis and can be fatal to the fetus if not corrected by intrauterine transfusion or by delivery so that exchange transfusion of the neonate can occur (Moise, 2009).

Because of excessive bilirubin breakdown from rapid, increased hemolysis of fetal erythrocytes, the fetus attempts to excrete as much bilirubin as possible. It is excreted in abnormally large amounts into the amniotic fluid and gives it a characteristic yellow-brown appearance.

A fetal sign of hypoxia unique to hemolytic anemia or anemia from fetal-maternal hemorrhage is loss of variability in the fetal heart rate (FHR). The pattern is that of regular smooth oscillations resembling a sine wave and is called a *sinusoidal pattern*. There are no accelerations or variations from the regular smooth oscillations around the baseline. A sinusoidal pattern (see Fig. 21-1), if left untreated, is terminal or may have serious consequences for neonatal outcome (Nageotte and Gillstrap III, 2009).

DIAGNOSTIC TESTING

Antibody Screen

Diagnosis of a hemolytic incompatibility is made by routine prenatal screening, which should be done in all patients, regardless of Rh factor, on the initial prenatal visit. The test that is used is an antibody screen or indirect Coombs test. The RhD-negative mother who is not sensitized at the beginning of the pregnancy is rescreened at 28 weeks because by this time, the placental membrane becomes thin enough for fetal red cells to cross (transplacental transfusion), making it the second most common time for sensitization to occur.

Severity of Fetal Bleed

In the event that a large fetal-maternal hemorrhage is suspected in the RhD-negative woman, a Kleihauer-Betke blood test is done on the mother. This test detects the number of fetal cells that have entered the maternal circulation. If more than 15 ml of fetal cells have entered the maternal circulation, the usual Rh_o (D) immune globulin dose of 300 mcg is not sufficient to prevent sensitization.

Severity of Disease

If the mother has been RhD-alloimmunized from a previous pregnancy, fetal erythroblastosis must be detected early to promote optimal fetal outcome by either early delivery or intrauterine transfusions (IUT). Unless previous obstetric history indicates earlier involvement, the fetal erythroblastosis is followed by serial maternal antibody titers beginning at 16 to 18 weeks of gestation. When a critical antibody titer of 32 is reached, serial ultrasounds for peak middle cerebral artery (MCA) Doppler velocity or serial amniocenteses are begun.

Ultrasound for Peak Middle Cerebral Artery (MCA) Doppler Velocity

MCA Doppler velocity measures the fetal hemoglobin in order to detect fetal anemia. The cerebral artery can be easily visualized with color-flow Doppler. Pulsed Doppler is then used to measure the peak systolic velocity of the middle cerebral artery. In the presence of anemia the increased fetal output and a drop in blood viscosity causes an increased blood flow velocity in the cerebral artery (ACOG, 2006; Moise, 2008).

Amniocentesis

Bilirubin, a breakdown product of red blood cells, can be measured in the amniotic fluid. The breakdown product is identified as delta-OD 450. Liley, of Auckland, New Zealand, developed a graph for measuring the optical density of delta-OD in the amniotic fluid. He divided the levels of bilirubin optical density into "zones" of safety, based on gestation. Levels of delta-OD should decrease with increasing gestation. If the level of bilirubin optical density for delta-OD is increased, it indicates abnormal erythrocyte destruction (Moise, 2008). The current trend is to use MCA Doppler velocity measures versus bilirubin when available (ACOG, 2006).

Cordocentesis

In cordocentesis, a direct fetal blood sample is obtained from the umbilical cord vessels to evaluate the fetal hemoglobin and hematocrit. An anemic fetus is indicative of abnormal erythrocyte destruction (Moise, 2008). Currently cordocentesis is performed when the MCA is greater than 1.5 MoM to determine if a transfusion is indicated.

USUAL MEDICAL MANAGEMENT AND PROTOCOLS FOR NURSE PRACTITIONERS

Prevention

To prevent rhesus alloimmunization in unsensitized RhD-negative women, Rh_o (D) immune globulin is used. Rh_o (D) immune globulin is a specially prepared gamma globulin that contains a specific concentration of D antibodies. These antibodies neutralize the RhD-positive fetal antigens that have entered the maternal circulation. For this reason, Rh_o (D) immune globulin cannot correct sensitization but can prevent it from occurring if given within 72 hours of the potential fetal-maternal red blood cell infusion (Crowther and Middleton, 1997; Weiner and Buhimschi, 2009).

Because the antibody formation in the mother is gradual, it is also apparently effective in preventing sensitization during pregnancy. When Rh_o (D) immune globulin is given at 28 weeks of gestation to unsensitized women, the incidence of Rhesus alloimmunization has been further reduced (Crowther and Middleton, 1999; Weiner and Buhimschi, 2009). Rh_o (D) immune globulin is also given any time a traumatic fetal-maternal bleed is likely to occur, such as after a genetic amniocentesis, a chorionic villi sampling, maternal abdominal trauma from MVC, abuse or fall, termination of an ectopic pregnancy or hydatidiform mole, spontaneous or induced abortion, placenta previa with bleeding, suspected abruption, or external cephalic version (U.S. Preventive Services Task Force, 2004).

The usual dose of Rh_o (D) immune globulin is 300 mcg at 28 weeks of gestation, at the time of any amniocentesis and within 72 hours after delivery. Woelfer and others (2004) studied serum Rh_o (D) immune globulin levels in relationship to maternal weight. If the expectant mother's BMI is more than 27 kg per m^2, serum anti-D levels were significantly lower, indicating a possible need of a larger dosage of anti-D.

If a test such as the Kleihauer-Betke indicates that more than 30 ml of fetal blood or 15 ml of fetal red blood cells has entered the maternal circulation, a higher dose may be required to prevent sensitization. A first-trimester spontaneous or induced abortion, an ectopic pregnancy, or a chorionic villi sampling requires a minidose of 50 mcg within 72 hours (U.S. Preventive Services Task Force, 2004). There are no immunoglobulins for prevention of other blood group sensitization incompatibilities.

Treatment for Hemolytic Incompatibility

Follow-Up

If a hemolytic incompatibility is present, the usual medical management depends on the severity of fetal anemia. Two tests are currently being used to monitor for fetal anemia. The less invasive procedure measures by direct evaluation; the fetal hemoglobin and hematocrit method, by way of middle cerebral artery (MCA) Doppler velocity. An older alternative method measures bilirubin levels by optical density (Delta OD) in the amniotic fluid, which are obtained by serial amniocenteses. Testing is usually started around 19 weeks of gestation. When the level of bilirubin is low for a particular gestational age or the hemoglobin and hematocrit are normal, the test is repeated in 3 weeks. If the bilirubin level rises or the hemoglobin and hematocrit levels decrease, evaluation may be repeated in 1 to 2 weeks. Extremely abnormal levels for a particular gestation indicate a need for intrauterine transfusion in the very immature fetus. Cesarean delivery may be necessary when this occurs after 34 to 35 weeks of gestation (Moise, 2008).

Fetal Surveillance

By 26 weeks of gestation, FHR monitoring should be started. A nonstress test may be done biweekly, a contraction stress test may be done weekly, or some combination of testing methods may be used. Between FHR monitorings, the mother should keep daily fetal activity charts.

Intrauterine Transfusion

If the fetus becomes anemic any time after 18 weeks of gestation, an intrauterine transfusion is indicated to allow more time for the immature or nonviable fetus to remain in utero (Moise, 2008). The transfusion must be done by a skilled physician, usually a perinatologist, who has learned the procedure during postgraduate training in maternal-fetal medicine (see Chapter 4). The intrauterine transfusion can be performed intravascularly or intraperitoneally (although the later is rarely used with the current skills of perinatologists).

Intravascular Transfusion (IVT)

When an intravascular transfusion is performed, the fetal umbilical vein is used. The mother is medicated with a uterine relaxant and an antianxiety or tranquilizer agent. The procedure is done under ultrasound direction. A 22-gauge spinal needle is guided through the mother's abdomen and the uterine wall into the umbilical vein at the site of placental insertion. Either washed, packed, leuko-reduced O RhD-negative blood or negative blood matched to the mother's blood type may be used (Moise, 2008). Prophylactic antibiotics are given to the mother following the procedure.

Intraperitoneal Transfusion

Originally fetal alloimmune-induced hemolytic anemia was treated by intraperitoneal transfusion. This practice has been replaced with the intravascular transfusion because a hemolytic anemic fetus absorbs transfused red cells poorly. If done, the procedure for intraperitoneal transfusion is performed under ultrasound direction. Approximately 50 to 150 ml of negative blood, cross-matched to the mother, is used. It is spun down to increase the hematocrit to 70% to 80%. Rh-negative blood from a donor must be used because it contains no antibodies to the fetal Rh-positive blood.

The mother is given a narcotic or tranquilizer to quiet the baby for the procedure. After an abdominal scrub of the amniocentesis site and with the direction of ultrasound, a large-gauge intracatheter is inserted through the maternal abdomen, into the uterus, and into the fetal abdomen, just under the fetal diaphragm. The intracatheter tubing, the attached intravenous tubing, and the syringe for the blood are all preflushed with normal saline. A small amount of normal saline can be injected to confirm placement on ultrasonic view. The syringe with the specially prepared blood is connected to an infusion pump designed for constant speed infusion via syringe. Depending on fetal gestation, 50 to 150 ml of blood is infused over a 1-to 2-hour period. The fetus is monitored before and during the procedure if greater than 26 weeks of gestation. If the fetus is less than 26 weeks, frequent auscultation of the FHR is usually done. During the next 3 to 4 days, the fetal diaphragmatic lymph system absorbs the blood, and improvement in fetal anemia can be expected.

Amniocentesis for Fetal Lung Maturity

Amniocentesis for fetal lung maturity is usually initiated at 35 weeks of gestation. If fetal lungs are mature, induction is the standard of care at 38 weeks of gestation. If fetal lungs are immature and fetal bilirubin is high, the mother is treated with 30 mg of oral phenobarbital 3 times a day for 1 week to accelerate fetal hepatic maturity and therefore enhance neonatal conjugation of bilirubin. If the fetal lungs are immature but fetal bilirubin is low, amniocentesis is usually repeated in 2 weeks.

Outcome

With intrauterine transfusions to prevent fetal alloimmune-induced hemolytic anemia, fetal survival rate is high (Moise, 2008). Success of intrauterine transfusion generally depends on a number of factors. If the fetus is extremely immature or if there are significant liver and congestive heart failure, the potential for improved fetal well-being is less likely and death in utero can ensue in a few days. The earlier the transfusions must be started, the greater the number required for the fetus to gain maturity while maintaining well-being. This puts the fetus at higher risk for intra-uterine infection or premature rupture of membranes and therefore interferes with the potentially successful outcome for the fetus.

NURSING MANAGEMENT

Prevention

The prenatal nurse caring for the pregnant woman must recognize the importance of antibody screening in all pregnant patients not only for D incompatibility but also for any blood system incompatibility. Education of the patient regarding necessary prenatal laboratory work should include the need for antibody screening. Patients can be given this information in early prenatal classes, as well as during early office visits.

To prevent rhesus alloimmunization, all RhD-negative women should receive Rh₀ (D) immune globulin (Rhophylac, RhoGAM, HyperRho, WinRho SDF) at the following times:

- At 28 weeks of gestation
- Postnatally, within 72 hours, to unsensitized women who have given birth at any gestation to an RhD-positive or untyped fetus (Crowther and Middleton, 1997; Weiner and Buhimschi, 2009)
- In the event of a third-trimester bleed
- Following any procedure during pregnancy that may breach the integrity of the choriodecidual space and lead to a potential fetomaternal bleed (e.g., chorionic villus sampling, amniocentesis, cordocentesis, percutaneous fetal procedures, or external cephalic version)
- Even in situations in which the woman intends to undergo tubal ligation, the woman should be instructed regarding potential future problems should steril-ization fail or should she ever choose to have a surgical reversal of the steriliza-tion after becoming sensitized with this pregnancy. She also risks no longer being safe to receive uncrossed-matched universal donor blood should she expe-rience a future emergent need for this blood.

Nursing Interventions for Administering Rh₀ (D) Immune Globulin

Assess the RhD-negative woman's understanding of when sensitization can take place. Educate the patient in a reassuring manner regarding the use of Rh₀ (D) immune globulin at all recommended times.

- At the initial prenatal visit, determine the mother's blood type and screen for the presence of antibodies by an indirect Coombs test (antibody screen). The RhD-negative unsensitized pregnant woman should be screened again at 26 to 28 weeks of gestation.
- Administer Rh₀ (D) immune globulin by appropriate route, either intramuscu-larly or intravenously.
- Prepare patient for such potential side effects as temporary soreness at the site of injection and a low-grade fever. In rare instances, an anaphylactic reaction occurs. For this reason, the patient should remain in the health care setting for 15 to 30 minutes following the injection.

- Fill out an identification card confirming the injection, and give it to the patient to keep. Instruct her to keep it with her identification papers. Of women who receive Rh_o (D) immune globulin antepartum prophylaxis, 15% to 20% will subsequently have passive acquired D antibodies at the time of delivery. This could lead to misinterpretation and withholding of eligible Rh_o (D) immune globulin. In the event of confusion, the mother should be instructed to present her identification card (PDR Drug Information, 2006).
- Fill out the blood bank form. Return the form and empty ampule or syringe to the blood bank. In the event of an allergic reaction, the blood bank needs the information these provide.
- Be prepared to discuss the issue of risk for transmission of HIV through Rh_o (D) immune globulin. According to PDR Drug Information (2006), the risk is eliminated because the preparing process is effective in removing any enveloped viruses such as HBV, HCV, and HIV.

Antepartum Nursing Interventions for Alloimmunization

- Obtain the patient's history to ascertain first day of last menstrual period, regularity of menstrual cycles, type of birth control used, date of a positive pregnancy test, and ultrasound to determine the estimated date of delivery. This will be invaluable in determining when necessary interventions should be instituted.
- Assess fetal growth with fundal height measurement. Concern for fetal growth should occur if fundal growth stops or decreases. If the fetus becomes anemic, the decreased oxygenation can lead to decreased growth rate. If the fetus becomes hydropic, fundal height can be abnormally large because of associated polyhydramnios.
- Assess FHR for tachycardia at each prenatal visit after 10 weeks.
- Monitor FHR during and after treatment for alloimmunization for evidence of sinusoidal FHR pattern or for nonreassuring features such as persistent late decelerations or loss of variability. Because of maternal sedation during intrauterine transfusion, baseline variability can be depressed (but without tachycardia, late decelerations, or a sinusoidal pattern) and should be compared with the strip before premedication and with the strip 1 hour after medication.
- Understand the importance of ultrasound examinations at least every 3 weeks after 20 weeks of gestation when alloimmunization has already occurred.
- Teach the mother to keep a daily fetal movement chart after 26 weeks of gestation. An active fetus is assumed to be adequately oxygenated.
- Explain special evaluation procedures and treatment.
- Assist with monitoring FHR during fetal evaluation by amniocentesis or ultrasound-directed fetal blood sampling. A baseline FHR should be determined before the procedure, and a 20-to 30-minute fetal monitoring strip should be run to assess FHR for signs of fetal compromise. Such signs include tachycardia, late decelerations, or absent long-term variability with the presence of short-term variability (sinusoidal pattern) (see Fig. 21-1).
- Assist with intrauterine fetal transfusion. During the initiation of the catheter insertion into the fetus, assist with ultrasound guidance and evaluation of the fetal well-being.

- Refer to a nurse specialist for patient education specific to tertiary level care and referral.
- Make appropriate referrals based on expressed psychosocial and financial needs.

Intrapartum Nursing Interventions for Alloimmunization

- Monitor FHR continuously with an electronic fetal monitor during labor for nonreassuring or preterminal patterns or events. If fetal anemia has developed, labor can further stress the fetus.
- Prepare the patient and her family for the possible necessity of a cesarean delivery if the fetus shows signs of hypoxia.
- Refer signs of fetal stress to the physician immediately because these fetuses are very sensitive.
- Assess the mother and her family for level of anxiety related to fear for the fetus or infant and potential outcome.
- Determine the family's support system. Assess the couple's support of each other.
- Keep the parents informed of the status of their fetus or neonate.
- If the neonate is sick or premature, assess the level of parental attachment behaviors such as frequent visitation, early touching and stroking, calling the infant by name, and attempting to establish eye contact.
- Encourage and facilitate early and close contact with the nursery personnel.

CONCLUSION

For the unsensitized RhD-negative woman, prevention is the primary goal. This can be accomplished (1) through antibody screening at the first prenatal visit; (2) through antibody screening at 26 to 28 weeks of gestation and by giving Rh_o (D) immune globulin by 28 weeks of gestation, after delivery, with potential placental accidents, and after an abortion. Education regarding indications for Rh_o (D) immune globulin and times of greatest risk can improve the future protection of RhD-negative women from unintentional Rhesus alloimmunization. As yet, there is no protective therapy for other hemolytic incompatibilities.

For the sensitized woman, the primary goal is to promote an optimal neonatal outcome through close monitoring of fetal well-being and through institution of therapy at the earliest safe time. High risk perinatal nurses should encourage the RhD-negative woman to seek information about new, proven methods of evaluation and treatment, such as those described in Chapter 4.

BIBLIOGRAPHY

American College of Obstetricians and Gynecologists (ACOG): *Management of alloimmunization during pregnancy,* Clinical Management Guidelines for Obstetricians-Gynecologists, No. 75, Washington, DC, 2006, ACOG.

Crowther C, Middleton P: Anti-D administration after childbirth for preventing Rhesus alloimmunisation, *Cochrane Database Syst Rev* (Issue 2), Art. No.: CD000021. Last assessed as up-to-date: June 26, 2007, 1997.

Crowther CA, Middleton P: Anti-D administration in pregnancy for preventing Rhesus alloimmunization, *Cochrane Database Syst Rev* 1999, (Issue 2), Art. No.: CD000020. Last assessed as up-to-date: June 26, 2007.

Moise K: Management of rhesus alloimmunization in pregnancy, *Obstet Gynecol* 112(1):164–176, 2008.

Moise K: Hemolytic disease of the fetus newborn. In Creasy R, Resnik R, Iams J, and others, editors: *Creasy & Resnik's maternal-fetal medicine: principles and practice*, ed 6, Philadelphia, 2009, Saunders.

Nageotte M: Gilstrap III l: Intrapartum fetal surveillance. In Creasy R, Resnik R, Iams J, and others, editors: *Creasy & Resnik's maternal-fetal medicine: principles and practice*, ed 6, Philadelphia, 2009, Saunders.

PDR Drug Information: *Rho (D) immune globulin (Human), Drugs.com, 2006.* Retrieved from http://www.drugs.com/pdr/rho__d__immune_globulin_human_.html.

U.S. Preventive Services Task Force: *Screening for Rh(D) Incompatibility: Recommendation Statement,* Rockville, Md, 2004, Agency for Healthcare Research and Quality. Retrieved from http://ahrq.gov/clinic/3rduspstf/rh/rhrs.htm.

Weiner C: Fetal hemolytic disease. In James D, and others, editors: *High risk pregnancy: management options,* ed 3, Philadelphia, 2006, Saunders.

Weiner C, Buhimschi C: *Drugs for pregnant and lactating women,* ed 2, Philadelphia, 2009, Saunders.

Woelfer B, and others: Postdelivery levels of anti-D IgG prophylaxis in D-mothers depend on maternal body weight, *Transfusion* 44(4):512–517, 2004.

22

Hypertensive Disorders

The specific terminology for hypertensive disorders of pregnancy is inconsistent. According to the National High Blood Pressure Education Program Working Group (2000), hypertensive disorders of pregnancy are classified into one of four disorders. Table 22-1 summarizes these classifications. Hypertensive disorders of pregnancy, and preeclampsia in particular, are a leading cause of maternal and neonatal morbidity and mortality. Preeclampsia is associated with the release of antiangiogenic factors, plasma volume is contracted, and widespread effects on vascular endothelium lead to the maternal syndrome of preeclampsia (Khalil and others, 2009). Two of these disorders, gestational hypertension and preeclampsia/eclampsia, develop during pregnancy, labor, or the early postpartum period in a previously normotensive, nonproteinuric woman. The other two disorders, chronic hypertension and preeclampsia superimposed on hypertension, are related to a preexisting condition. This chapter first covers chronic hypertension and then focuses on preeclampsia. The primary pathophysiology of chronic hypertension is elevated blood pressure. Preeclampsia is a multisystemic, pregnancy-induced syndrome resulting from an endothelial cell dysfunction. Hypertension is a primary sign of the underlying disorder, most often developing after 20 weeks of gestation.

Both chronic hypertension and preeclampsia can be subclassified as either mild or severe. For chronic hypertension, subclassification is dependent on systolic and diastolic values. For preeclampsia, subclassification is dependent on the severity of end organ involvement. Severe forms of hypertension are HELLP syndrome and eclampsia. HELLP syndrome (Hemolysis of red blood cells [RBCs], Elevated Liver enzymes, and Low Platelets) is a multisystem disease. Eclampsia is the development of seizures in the preeclamptic patient. Approximately 15% of patients with HELLP syndrome and 20% of patients who develop eclampsia are normotensive (Sibai, 2005).

Gestational hypertension is divided into mild and severe development of an elevated blood pressure during pregnancy or early postpartum without other preeclampsia symptoms or previous hypertension. Mild gestation hypertension that develops after 35 weeks of gestation is usually benign and treated like mild preeclampsia (National High Blood Pressure Education Program Working Group, 2000). Severe gestational hypertension should be treated like severe preeclampsia because of the increase morbidity risks of abruption, preterm birth, and small-for-gestational-age fetus (Sibai, 2009).

416

Table 22-1   Classification of Hypertensive States of Pregnancy

Type	Description
Gestational hypertension	Development of mild hypertension during pregnancy in previously normotensive patient without proteinuria and with normal laboratory test
	Blood pressure returns to normal by 6 weeks postpartum.
Preeclampsia	Development of hypertension and proteinuria in previously normotensive patient after 20 weeks of gestation or in early postpartum period; in presence of trophoblastic disease, it can develop before 20 weeks of gestation
Eclampsia	Development of seizures in the preeclamptic patient
Chronic hypertension	Hypertension occurring before pregnancy or a blood pressure of 140/90 or higher before 20 weeks of gestation on two occasions, 6 hours apart
Preeclampsia super-imposed on chronic hypertension	Development of preeclampsia or eclampsia in patient with chronic hypertension

INCIDENCE

Hypertension occurs in approximately 5% of all pregnancies (Erogul, 2008). Preeclampsia accounts for about 80% of these cases and chronic hypertension for about 20% (von Dadelszen and Magee, 2005). The strongest risk factors for preeclampsia are a primigravida younger than 19 years or older than 40 years, a first pregnancy with a new father (Dekker and Sibai, 1999), or a history of severe preeclampsia (Al-Mulhim and others, 2003; Gudnasson, Dubiel, and Gudmundsson, 2004). Other factors associated with a higher-than-normal incidence of preeclampsia are as follows:

- Familial history
- Connective tissue disease such as lupus or rheumatoid arthritis (Barton and Sibai, 2008)
- Acquired or congenital thrombophilia (Barton and Sibai, 2008)
- Limited sperm exposure such as donor insemination or oocyte donation (Barton and Sibai, 2008)
- Partner who fathered preeclamptic pregnancy in another woman (Barton and Sibai, 2008)
- Woman born as small-for-gestational-age (Barton and Sibai, 2008)
- Adverse outcome in a previous pregnancy such as fetal growth restriction, abruptio placentae, or fetal death (Barton and Sibai, 2008)
- Preexisting vascular disease such as diabetes, renal disease, chronic hypertension, or collagen disease
- Exposure to a superabundance of trophoblastic tissue, such as in multiple gestation and hydatidiform mole

- Thrombophilia disorder such as in acquired antiphospholipid syndrome or inherited Factor V Leiden mutation (Lin and August, 2005)
- Obesity (increases the risk three-fold)
- Periodontal disease (Boggess and others, 2003)
- African-American descent (Flack and others, 2002)

CHRONIC HYPERTENSION

Chronic hypertension occurs in approximately 4% to 5% of all pregnancies, with 21% of these women developing superimposed preeclampsia (Walfisch and Hallak, 2006). Chronic hypertension in pregnancy is usually classified as mild or severe (depending on the hypertensive stage) according to the staging system by the Joint National Committee (JNC VII, 2003). Table 22-2 lists stages of hypertension.

Preconception screening is ideal. During this visit, lifestyle changes are discussed, such as the DASH (Dietary Approaches to Stop Hypertension) diet with adequate potassium, calcium, and magnesium, and sodium limited to 2.4 g; aerobic exercise until pregnant and then no exercise; no smoking or alcohol use; if overweight, loss of weight before but not during pregnancy (Paruk and Moodley, 2005). The patient should be trained in home blood pressure monitoring. Baseline laboratory studies such as renal function and urinary protein excretion may be helpful for later comparison. Counseling should include review of pregnancy risk associated with hypertension. With mild chronic hypertension, 10% of pregnant women went on to develop superimposed hypertension (Egerman and Sibai, 2001). The other 90% had favorable pregnancy outcomes. In the presence of severe chronic hypertension, there is an increased risk for perinatal mortality starting in the first trimester and continuing throughout pregnancy, related to superimposed preeclampsia, abruptio placentae, or preterm delivery.

Current management should be evaluated and needed changes made for pregnancy. For stage 1 hypertension without complications such as left ventricular hypertrophy, peripheral arterial disease, renal disease, or retinopathy, the best therapy is periodic bedrest of 45 minutes in the middle of the day and 1 hour before the evening meal to promote uterine blood flow. A regimen of tapering and stopping hypertensive medication is usually tried (National High Blood Pressure Education Program Working Group, 2000).

When the diastolic blood pressure exceeds 100 mm Hg, systolic exceeds 160 mm Hg, or left ventricular hypertrophy is present, drug therapy is usually initiated. The

Table 22-2   Stages of Hypertension

Blood Pressure Stages—JNC VII	Blood Pressure Reading
Prehypertension	Systolic 120–139 or diastolic 80–89
Stage 1 Hypertension	Systolic 140–159 or diastolic 90–99
Stage 2 Hypertension	Systolic >160 or diastolic >100

Reference: Joint National Committee (JNC VII): *Prevention, detection, evaluation, and treatment of high blood pressure,* NIH Publication No. 035233, Bethesda, MD, 2003, U.S. Department of Health and Human Services. Retrieved from http://www.nhlbi.nih.gov/guidelines/hypertension/jncintro.htm.

Table 22-3 Antihypertensive Medications for Chronic Hypertension During Pregnancy

Medication	Drug Classification	Usual Dosage	Maximum Dosage
Methyldopa (Drug of choice: Aldomet)	Central-acting antiadrenergic agent	250 mg orally bid or tid	2000 mg
Labetalol (Trandate)	Beta-blocker	Start at 100 mg orally bid Increase 100 mg bid q 2 to 3 weeks	1200 mg
Pindolol (Visken)	Beta-blocker	5 mg orally bid Increase by 10 mg/day q 3 to 4 weeks	60 mg
Nifedipine (Procardia)	Calcium channel blocker	10 mg orally tid	180 mg

Reference: Weiner C, Buhimschi C: *Drugs for pregnant and lactating women*, ed 2, Philadelphia, 2009, Saunders.
bid, Twice daily; *q*, every; *tid*, three times daily.

drug of choice continues to be methyldopa (Aldomet) (National High Blood Pressure Education Program Working Group, 2000). The usual dose of methyldopa is 750 to 2000 mg/day. The alternative drugs used to treat chronic hypertension during pregnancy are beta-blockers, such as atenolol (Tenormin), labetalol (Trandate, Normodyne), or pindolol (Visken), and calcium channel blockers, such as nifedipine. Table 22-3 lists common dosages of these antihypertensive medications. The new angiotensin-converting enzyme inhibitors or angiotensin II receptor antagonists are contraindicated during pregnancy because they decrease uterine blood flow and may increase the chance of intrauterine growth restriction (IUGR) or fetal death (National High Blood Pressure Education Program Working Group, 2000). Diuretics are not used as the first-line drug therapy because of their effect on plasma volume. If a diuretic is indicated, thiazide has the safest record. Furosemide is contraindicated because of its added risk for embryotoxicity. All pregnant patients with chronic hypertension should be monitored carefully for an abruption, as well as superimposed preeclampsia, renal failure, and disseminated intravascular coagulation (DIC). They have a 0.7% to 1.5% increased risk for an abruption. The preeclampsia rate is 15% in those who have mild hypertension before conception or early in pregnancy, whereas it approaches 50% in those with severe prepregnancy hypertension (Barton and Sibai, 2008). Antepartum fetal assessment should begin at 28 to 30 weeks of gestation because the fetus is at greater risk for IUGR and fetal mortality increases 10-fold.

If renal failure occurs during pregnancy, volume overload may result, requiring sodium restriction, diuretic use, or dialysis. Magnesium sulfate is hazardous in the presence of renal failure and, if needed, dose is based on every 1- to 2-hour magnesium levels. Phenytoin may be a better alternative drug (National High Blood Pressure Education Program Working Group, 2000).

During postpartum recovery, monitor for such complications as pulmonary edema, renal failure, heart failure, and encephalopathy. If the mother is breastfeeding and in stage 1 or 2 hypertension, consider withholding any antihypertensive agent until cessation of breastfeeding. For women in stage 3 hypertension, give the lowest dose and monitor mother and infant. Methyldopa is the preferred drug. If a beta-blocker is indicated, labetalol or propranolol is preferred. There is no available evidence-based data about calcium-channel blockers. Angiotensin-converting enzyme inhibitors and angiotensin II receptor antagonists are contraindicated for the same reasons as during pregnancy. Diuretics may have a negative effect on milk production.

PREECLAMPSIA

Normal Physiology

Although the triggering factor of preeclampsia is unknown, much of the pathophysiology of the disease is understood. To understand the pathophysiology of preeclampsia, the nurse should be familiar with the normal physiologic changes of pregnancy, which are summarized in the following sections.

Cardiovascular System

Plasma blood volume is increased 30% to 50%; stroke volume and heart rates are increased as well. Increased plasma blood volume accounts for the 40% increased in cardiac output. There appear to be increased oxidative stress and an increased maternal antioxidant related to increased lipid peroxidation capacity (Spinnato and Livingston, 2005).

Renal Function

The normal glomerular filtration rate is increased by approximately 50% related to increased renal plasma flow. Serum creatinine normally decreases with an increase in creatinine clearance.

Fluid Balance

Renin, angiotensin II, and aldosterone levels are increased. These substrates, along with increasing estrogen, facilitate the normal expansion of the blood volume by 40% to 50% above nonpregnant levels (Baylis and others, 1998).

Placentation

Early in pregnancy, the muscular components of the uterine spiral arteries begin to be replaced by cytotrophoblast. To further increase fetoplacental blood flow, the trophoblast erodes the myometrial portions of the uterine spiral arteries so that they widen and lose their vasoconstrictive properties, increasing the diameter four to six times from their nonpregnant size.

Vasodilatory State

Angiotensin II is a potent pressor substance that stimulates a rise in blood pressure. In normal pregnancy, although the levels of angiotensin II are elevated, blood pressure does not rise. This is because healthy pregnant women have an increased resistance to the presser effects of angiotensin II (Baylis and others, 1998; Vedernikov, Saade, and Garfield, 1999; Walfisch and Hallack, 2006) related to increased levels of endothelial-derived vasodilator prostacyclin (PGI_2) and nitric oxide (Myatt and

Miodovnik, 1999). The diastolic blood pressure normally drops 7 to 10 mm Hg during the first and second trimesters and returns to nonpregnant levels during the third trimester (National High Blood Pressure Education Program Working Group, 2000).

A delicate balance between vasodilator and vasopressor activity must be maintained during pregnancy to maintain a normotensive state. The placenta and intact endothelium that line the blood vessel walls produce prostacyclin. Prostacyclin stimulates the renin-angiotensin-aldosterone cycle, which is important for fluid balance. Prostacyclin is a potent vasodilator because of its resistance to the presser effects of angiotensin II. It prevents platelet clumping and promotes increased uteroplacental blood flow as well. Nitric oxide is another vasodilator substance that is important to maintaining low basal blood vessel tone but at the same time weakening the action of vasoconstrictors (Ghabour and others, 1995) and inhibiting platelet aggregation (Lowenstein, Dinerman, and Snyder, 1994). Nitric oxide is derived from the endothelial blood vessel cells.

Active vasopressors are thromboxane, endothelins (endothelin-1), and increased lipid peroxides. Thromboxane is a vasoconstrictor, a stimulant of platelet aggregation, and a uterine-stimulating prostaglandin (Wang and others, 1991a, b). Thromboxane is produced by the placenta and, in lesser amounts, by the platelets. Endothelin-1 production normally increases during pregnancy (Branch, Dudley, and Michell, 1991; Nova and others, 1991; Clark and others, 1992). In the event of endothelial damage, endothelin-1 is produced in abnormally increasing amounts, which causes inactivation of nitric oxide (Wang and others, 2004).

Fluid Shifts

Fluid moves from the intravascular space to the extracellular space in the dependent limbs. The fluid shift is related to plasma colloid osmotic pressure that decreases below 23 mm Hg secondary to the normal hemodilution of the blood. Fluid shift is also related to the increased venous capillary hydrostatic pressure in the dependent limbs secondary to the gravid uterus pressing on the inferior vena cava, interfering with the blood returning to the heart. The net result is physiologic edema in the dependent limbs during the last trimester of pregnancy. Physiologic edema should disappear after 8 to 12 hours of bedrest.

Pathophysiology

In preeclampsia it appears that the cytotrophoblastic tissue of the placenta fails to adequately migrate down the maternal spiral arteries and displace the musculoelastic structures of these arteries, *decreasing spiral artery remodeling* (Levine and Karumanchi, 2005). Therefore these arteries do not widen as they normally do, which means that the perfusion to the placenta is suboptimal. This suboptimal perfusion is referred to as a *defective placentation* (Myatt and Miodovnik, 1999). Multiorgan system involvement results because of the ensuing *endothelial cell dysfunction* (van Beck and Peeters, 1998; Myatt and Miodovnik, 1999; Roberts and Funai, 2009). Endothelial cells line all blood vessels, providing blood vessel wall integrity, preventing intravascular coagulation, modulating smooth muscle contractility, and mediating immune and inflammatory responses. Figure 22-1 presents a summary of the manifestations of damaged endothelial cells in preeclampsia.

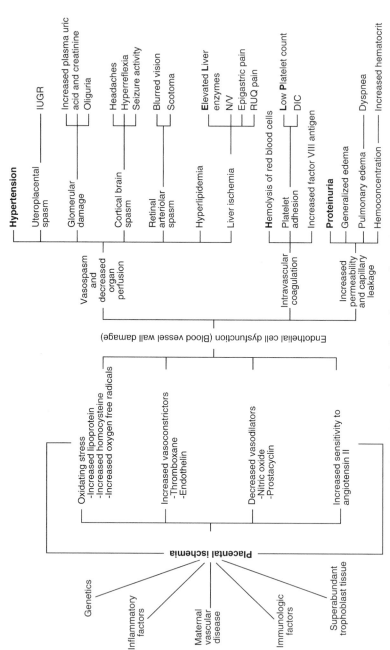

Figure 22-1 Pathophysiologic changes of preeclampsia.

It is currently postulated that endothelial cell dysfunction is caused by placental ischemia stimulating the release of a substance that is toxic to endothelial cells, and antiendothelial factors such as sFlt-1 (van Beck and Peeters, 1998; Var and others, 2003; Levine and others, 2004; Levine and Karumanchi, 2005), increasing oxidative stress response (Myatt and Miodovnik, 1999), and inflammatory released cytokines (tumor necrosis factor-alpha) (Taylor, 1997). Oxidative stress is the imbalance of prooxidants (homocysteine, low-density lipoprotein, hypertriglyceridemia, increased iron) and antioxidants (high-density lipoprotein and transferrin, a blood protein that binds with iron), leading to the formation of oxygen free radicals and lipid peroxides. Lipid peroxides and oxygen free radicals are directly toxic to the endothelial cells and increase the release of cytokines, which cause damage to the endothelial lining of blood vessel walls (Dekker, 2001; Cotter and others, 2003; Var and others, 2003; Mignini and others, 2005; Roberts and Funai, 2009).

With endothelial damage, there is significantly less production of vasodilators such as prostacyclin and nitric oxide (Myatt and Miodovnik, 1999; Var and others, 2003; Spinnato and Livingston, 2005), upsetting the delicate balance between prostacyclin and thromboxane (Mills and others, 1999). Decreased production of nitric oxide and increased production of thromboxane cause platelet adhesion to the surface of the trophoblast, resulting in intervillous thrombi (Ghabour and others, 1995), which further alters blood flow to the fetus. Damaged endothelial cells cause increased release of endothelin-1, which inactivates nitric oxide (Wang and others, 2004). Increased production of oxygen free radicals and lipid peroxides results, which further inactivates the vasodilator effect of nitric oxide (Myatt and Miodovnik, 1999) and further damages endothelium.

Multiple-organ endothelial cell injury ensues (Hayman, 2004). Generalized vasospasm results, leading to poor tissue perfusion to all organ systems, increased total peripheral resistance with subsequent elevation of blood pressure, and increased endothelial cell permeability, which allows intravascular protein and fluid loss that leads to decreased plasma osmotic pressure and plasma volume (Patrick and Roberts, 1999). Vascular endothelial cell injury may initiate coagulation pathways as well (Myatt and Miodovnik, 1999).

Resulting Pathophysiologic Changes

Other specific pathophysiologic changes result from preeclampsia; a discussion of these follows.

Uteroplacental Insufficiency

Uteroplacental perfusion is compromised, even before preeclamptic symptoms, related to pathologic spiral arteriole lesions and a deficiency of prostacyclin. The uteroplacental perfusion is further reduced as the disease progresses. The fetal blood flow is decreased related to constriction of umbilical vessels.

Renal Damage

In 70% of preeclamptic patients, glomerular endothelial damage, fibrin deposition, and resulting ischemia reduce renal plasma flow and glomerular filtration rate (National High Blood Pressure Education Program Working Group, 2000). Protein, mainly in the form of albumin, is lost into the urine. Uric acid, creatinine, and calcium clearance are decreased, and oliguria develops as the condition worsens. Therefore proteinuria and increased plasma uric acid levels are signs of preeclampsia, and oliguria is a sign of severe preeclampsia and kidney damage.

Fluid and Electrolyte Imbalance

Serum albumin is decreased as the result of serum protein lost into extracellular spaces and into the urine by way of damaged capillary walls. Decreased serum albumin causes a decrease in the plasma colloid osmotic pressure, an increase in intracellular edema, and failure of the normal expansion of the intravascular plasma volume (ACOG, 2002). Although there is intravascular hemoconcentration, the production of renin, angiotensin, and aldosterone decreases, resulting in an increased hematocrit.

Worsening Pathophysiologic Changes

As preeclampsia progresses, the following systemic changes, which are signs that the condition is worsening, may occur.

Pulmonary Involvement

Pulmonary edema may develop and is related to one of three factors. The most common factor is volume overload as a result of left ventricular failure caused by extremely high vascular resistance, excessive fluid infusion during treatment of the disease, or postpartum diuresis. The other two factors are related to a further decreased colloid osmotic pressure or an endothelial injury that increases pulmonary capillary permeability, resulting in a fluid leak or a noncardiogenic pulmonary edema.

Central Nervous System Involvement

Endothelial damage to the cortical region of the brain, resulting in fibrin deposition, edema, and cerebral hemorrhage, may lead to hyperreflexia and severe headaches and can progress to seizure activity (eclampsia) (National High Blood Pressure Education Program Working Group, 2000).

Ophthalmic Involvement

Visual changes, such as scotoma, photophobia, blurring, or double vision, can occur related to retinal arteriolar spasms caused by arteriolar narrowing (Walfisch and Hallak, 2006).

Hemodynamic Changes

Severe preeclampsia or eclampsia manifests with varying hemodynamic patterns related to the disease process. For example, elevated blood pressure may be related to increased vascular resistance or increased cardiac output. Pulmonary edema may result from volume overload and is the result of left ventricular failure from extremely high vascular resistance or excessive fluid infusion during treatment of the disease. Volume overload can also occur during the postpartum period when normal mobilization of the third-space fluid occurs.

The two other factors that can cause pulmonary edema are: (1) further reduced colloid osmotic pressure and (2) increased pulmonary capillary permeability related to capillary wall damage. Oliguria is related to decreased renal blood flow as the result of intravascular volume depletion or severe vascular resistance, either of which can cause left ventricular failure. Occasionally, specific renal arteriospasms disproportionate to the systemic vasospasms can cause oliguria.

Coagulation Involvement

Endothelial damage causes activation of the clotting cascade. Fewer platelets are created. When platelets drop below 100,000 cells/mm^3, preeclampsia is severe. Abnormalities of blood coagulation sufficient to cause DIC are present in only about 10% of patients with preeclampsia.

Hepatic Involvement

Hepatic ischemia and fibrin deposition can cause anywhere from mild hepatocellular necrosis indicated by a mild increase in aminotransferase and lactate dehydrogenase to the ominous HELLP syndrome. In approximately 10% of these patients, hepatic involvement can lead to periportal hemorrhagic necrosis in the liver, which can cause a subcapsular hematoma (Williamson and Girling, 2006). Warning signs of hepatic involvement, such as right upper quadrant pain or epigastric pain, can indicate impending eclampsia.

HELLP Syndrome Development

In 5% of patients with preeclampsia, the HELLP syndrome, a severe form of preeclampsia characterized by hemolysis of RBCs, elevated liver enzymes, and low platelets, may develop (Weinstein, 1985; Martin and others, 1991; Sibai and others, 1993; Roberts and Funai, 2009). This cascade of events is the result of systemic capillary endothelial cell damage exposing the basement membrane, which activates platelet adherence and fibrin deposition. Platelets are then decreased, and RBCs, which are torn while trying to pass through the narrowed vessels, are deposited along with the fibrin. Activation of platelets results in release of more thromboxane, and endothelial damage leads to further reduction in prostacyclin production, thus setting up a vicious cycle (Walsh, 1990; Barton and Sibai, 2008). Hyperbilirubinemia *(jaundice)* may develop as a result of hemolysis of the RBCs. At the same time, endothelial damage and fibrin deposition in the liver may lead to impaired liver function and can result in hemorrhagic necrosis, indicated by right upper quadrant tenderness or epigastric pain, nausea, and vomiting (Phelan and Easter, 1990). Liver enzymes are elevated when liver tissue is necrotic. In rare cases, a subcapsular hematoma develops in the liver. Normal blood pressure is found in approximately 15% of the patients with HELLP syndrome and 13% do not have proteinuria (Sibai, 2007).

Eclampsia

Eclampsia is the occurrence of seizure activity in the presence of preeclampsia. Eclampsia is normally thought to be trigged by severe cerebral vasospasm, hemorrhage, ischemia, or edema. Occasionally, encephalopathy may trigger the seizure activity. Severe, persistent headache, visual disturbances, epigastric pain, and restlessness can be warning signs of impending eclampsia. Normal blood pressure is found in approximately 20% of patients with eclampsia (Anumba and Robson, 1999; Mattar and Sibai, 2000; Sibai, 2007).

Etiology

The cause of preeclampsia remains unknown. Because of characteristic changes in the placental vessels, it is currently thought to be a placentation defect mediated by the interplay of three or more factors (Williamson, 2005).

Immunologic Maladaptation and Activation of Inflammatory Factors

The immunologic influence is supported by epidemiologic studies to be an impaired maternal immune response directed against the trophoblastic invasion and subsequently causing a defective placentation. This impaired immune response is postulated to be the result of decreased human leukocyte antigen (HLA) G protein normally produced to facilitate the mother's tolerance to the immunologically foreign placenta components (Moreau and others, 2008) or decreased formation of blocking antibodies to immunoprotect the immunologically partly foreign placenta (Cunningham and others, 2010). Repeated sperm exposure may prevent this impaired immunologic response, thus explaining the increased risk in primipaternity, use of barrier contraceptives, and donor insemination (Hayman, 2004; Sibai, Dekker, and Kupfermine, 2005).

This immune response or other variable may activate an inflammatory response. Oxidative stress caused by increased cytokines and interleukins damages the endothelial cells of the placenta, resulting in decreased nitric oxide and interference with the thromboxane-to-prostacyclin balance (Var and others, 2003; Freeman and others, 2004; Wang and others, 2004).

Genetic Predisposition

There appears to be a familial tendency toward preeclampsia related to a single recessive gene (Chesley and Cooper, 1986), a dominant gene with incomplete penetrance (Dekker, 2001), or multifactorial inheritance (Hayman, 2004) that increases one's susceptibility to preeclampsia if other variables are present. Other research indicates that it might be the result of a growth-restricting effect on the daughter born to a woman with severe preeclampsia. A patient with a history of having a child who was IUGR is at considerable risk for hypertension, insulin resistance, and dyslipidemia later in life. Therefore the woman experiencing preeclampsia might have undiagnosed cardiovascular complications that increase her susceptibility to preeclampsia (Dekker and Sibai, 1999; Manten and others, 2005).

Vascular-Mediated Factors

The presence of a vascular defect caused by a disease such as diabetes, chronic hypertension, or collagen vascular disease or hidden abnormal metabolic factors such as the presence of anticardiolipin antibodies, hyperhomocystinemia, insulin resistance, metabolic syndrome, or obesity may interact with reduced placental perfusion to increase susceptibility to preeclampsia. It is postulated to influence the development of preeclampsia in one of three ways:

- Defective placentation
- Placental ischemia
- Endothelial cell dysfunction

Other Factors

Obesity (O'Brien, Ray, and Chan, 2003) and thrombophilia are two other risk factors of preeclampsia (Mello, Parretti, Marozio, 2005).

Maternal Effects

Preeclampsia is a very serious disease and is the second leading cause of maternal mortality (National High Blood Pressure Education Program Working Group, 2000; USDHHS, 2000), accounting for 16% to 18% of all maternal deaths (ACOG, 2002; Cox, Kilpatrick, and Geller, 2004). If preeclampsia is treated early and effectively, maternal mortality is low. If the disease is allowed to progress to the HELLP syndrome or eclampsia, maternal mortality increases to as high as 24%, and morbidity levels are even higher. The most common causes of maternal mortality or morbidity are related to abruptio placentae, pulmonary edema, adult respiratory distress syndrome (ARDS), stroke, renal or hepatic failure, cardiopulmonary arrest, DIC, and cerebral hemorrhage (Barton and Sibai, 2008). Women who receive no prenatal care are 12 times as likely to die from preeclamptic complications as women who do receive prenatal care (MacKay, Berg, and Atrash, 2001).

Fetal and Neonatal Effects

Perinatal mortality related to mild preeclampsia ranges from 1% to 8%, increasing to an overall average of 12% in severe preeclampsia, with a higher incidence found with early onset and lower incidence if the onset develops after 37 weeks of gestation (Sibai, 2005). If the disease progresses into the HELLP syndrome or eclampsia, or exists in the presence of preexisting chronic hypertension, perinatal mortality can be as high as 60% (Barton and Sibai, 2008). The majority of perinatal losses are related to placental insufficiency, which causes fetal growth restriction, prematurity associated with preterm delivery, hypoxia/acidosis, or abruptio placentae (Barton and Sibai, 2008).

Signs and Symptoms

Cardinal Signs

The cardinal signs of preeclampsia are hypertension and proteinuria (National High Blood Pressure Education Program Working Group, 2000). Except in the presence of a hydatidiform mole, these signs develop after 20 weeks of gestation. An elevated blood pressure is usually the first symptom in the early stages of this disease; therefore the disease may be diagnosed without the presence of proteinuria.

Hypertension

Hypertension is diagnosed if one of the following is present:
- Systolic blood pressure is 140 mm Hg or greater.
- Diastolic blood pressure is 90 mm Hg or greater.

Proteinuria

Proteinuria is diagnosed if one of the following is present:
- More than 0.3 g (300 mg/dl) of protein per liter of urine is found in a 24-hour urine collection.

- More than 0.1 g of protein per liter is found in at least two random urine specimens collected on two or more occasions at least 6 hours apart when the specific gravity is 1.030 or less and the pH is less than 8. (This is indicated as 1 or greater on a dipstick.)
- The following guidelines should be kept in mind when evaluating the urine for protein:
  - Vaginal discharge, blood, amniotic fluid, and bacteria can contaminate the specimen and give a false-positive reading.
  - The specimen should be obtained by either a voided midstream collection or catheterization to avoid contamination with vaginal discharge. One study suggests that a midstream clean catch collection may be as effective as catheterization (Chen and others, 2008a).
  - Alkaline urine or very concentrated urine (specific gravity greater than 1.030) may give a false-positive reading (Davey and MacGillivray, 1988).
  - Dilute urine (specific gravity less than 1.010) may give a false-negative reading.

Subjective Signs

Subjective signs of preeclampsia suggesting end-organ involvement include the following:

- Headaches
- Visual changes, such as blurred vision
- Rapid-onset edema of the face or abdomen or pitting edema in the feet or legs after 12 hours of bedrest
- Oliguria less than 500 ml/24 hours
- Hyperreflexia
- Nausea or vomiting
- Epigastric or right upper quadrant pain

HELLP Syndrome Signs

Signs of the HELLP syndrome follow:

- Vague symptoms before the onset of HELLP syndrome and increase in blood pressure and proteinuria develop
- Right upper quadrant tenderness or epigastric pain, which occurs in patients with HELLP syndrome and is related to obstructed hepatic blood flow because of fibrin deposition (O'Brien and Barton, 2005)
- Nausea or vomiting related to hepatic stretching occurs in 50% of patients.
- Headache
- Influenza-like symptoms, such as malaise, occur 90% of the time.
- Jaundice
- Hematuria
- One third of the time, HELLP syndrome develops in the postpartum period within 48 hours after delivery but may not be evident until the sixth day.

Comparison of Mild and Severe Preeclamptic Signs

Preeclampsia is usually categorized in grades of mild or severe for the purpose of treatment (Table 22-4).

Table 22-4   Comparison of Mild and Severe Preeclampsia

	Mild	Severe
Blood pressure		
Systolic	140–160 mm Hg	>160 mm Hg
Diastolic	90–110 mm Hg	≥110 mm Hg
Proteinuria (24 hr)	0.3–4.0 g	≥5g
Dipstick	+2/+3	+4
Urinary output	>30 ml/hr	<20 ml/hr
	>650 ml/24 hr	<500 ml/24 hr
Pulmonary edema	Not present	Can be present
Subjective signs	Not present	Can be present
HELLP syndrome signs	Not present	Can be present

HELLP, Hemolysis, Elevated Liver enzymes, and Low Platelet count in association with preeclampsia.

Eclampsia

If coma or convulsions occur, preeclampsia is then classified as eclampsia. Severe persistent headaches, epigastric pain, hyperreflexia with clonus, and restlessness are warning signs of impending eclampsia. However, in the presence of only edema, some normal women have hyperreflexia.

In an eclamptic seizure, the convulsive activity begins with facial twitching followed by generalized muscle rigidity. During the convulsion, respiration ceases because of muscle spasms. Coma usually follows the seizure-like activity, and respiration naturally resumes.

Diagnostic Testing

Diagnostic Signs

The most easily diagnosed symptom of preeclampsia is a rise in blood pressure. To detect blood pressure diagnostic of early preeclampsia, one must consider two elements. First, the blood pressure, mainly the diastolic pressure, normally drops slightly during the second trimester of pregnancy and then gradually returns to its original baseline level during the third trimester. Second, the systolic blood pressure is more affected by cardiac output changes, whereas the diastolic blood pressure is more affected by peripheral vascular resistance changes (Foley, 2001). Therefore the diastolic blood pressure is the more diagnostic of the two.

Obtaining Accurate Blood Pressure Readings

To obtain an accurate blood pressure reading, the blood pressure cuff must cover approximately 80% of the upper arm. Because position can lead to variability in the blood pressure reading, blood pressure should be measured in the same arm and with the patient in a sitting position with the arm at heart level (National High Blood Pressure Education Program Working Group, 2000). The blood pressure should be taken after a 10-minute rest period without caffeine or tobacco use for at least 30 minutes.

During pregnancy, Korotkoff phase V most accurately reflects intraarterial pressure (Brown and others, 1998). Therefore the National High Blood Pressure Education Program Working Group (2000) currently recommends that the Korotkoff phase V sound be used.

A second controversy exists as to the device used to take blood pressure. The question is whether blood pressure readings obtained by the standard mercury sphygmomanometer (manual) and the automated blood pressure device (electronic) can be used interchangeably. Brown and others (1998) found the auscultatory (manual) systolic pressures were 7 to 10 mm Hg lower than the oscillatory (electronic) values. Auscultatory diastolic pressures were 5 to 7 mm Hg higher than oscillatory values. Therefore use caution when interpreting blood pressure values taken with different devices (Green and Froman, 1996).

Diagnostic Tests

Tests of biochemical markers that assist in the diagnosis of preeclampsia are found in Table 22-5. Diagnostic tests that can be helpful in diagnosing HELLP syndrome are summarized in Table 22-6.

Predictive Tests

Because the hypertensive disease process begins long before signs and symptoms appear, various researchers have attempted to develop a predictive test. More than 100 clinical biophysical and biochemical tests have been evaluated for predicting patients at risk for preeclampsia. Inconsistent and contradictory predictive abilities have limited their usefulness. According to the World Health Organization systematic review (Conde-Agudelo, Villar, and Lindheimer, 2004), there is currently no ideal predictive test. However, Doppler ultrasonography is a useful method to assess the velocity of uterine artery blood flow in pregnancy. An abnormal uterine artery Doppler velocimetry in the first or second trimesters has been proposed as a good screening test to predict preeclampsia. Pregnancies complicated by abnormal uterine

Table 22-5   Summary of Diagnostic Tests Used in the Diagnosis of Preeclampsia

Condition Evaluated	Diagnostic Test	Significant Finding
Hemoconcentration	Hematocrit	>35 and rising
Kidney involvement	Uric acid test	>6.1 mg
	BUN test	>10 mg/dl
	Serum creatinine test	>2 mg/dl
Coagulopathy	FSP test	>40 mg/ml
	Platelet count	<100,000/mm^3
Bleeding time prolonged	Fibrinogen levels	<300 mg/dl
Endothelial damage	Albumin levels	<2.5
	Fibronectin levels	Increased 2 to 3 times
Hepatic involvement	AST	>41 units/L
	ALT	>30 units/L

ALT, Alanine transaminase; *AST*, aspartate transaminase; *BUN*, blood urea nitrogen; *FSP*, fibrin split products.

Table 22-6 Summary of Diagnostic Tests Used in the Diagnosis of HELLP

Condition Evaluated	Diagnostic Test	Significant Finding
Hemolysis	Peripheral smear	Abnormal
		Schistocytes or burr cells present
	Bilirubin	>1.2 mg/dl
	LDH	>600 units/L
Hepatic involvement	Liver enzymes	
	AST (SGOT)	>72 units/L
	ALT (SGPT)	>50 units/L
	LDH	>600 international units/L
Thrombocytopenia	Platelet count	<100,000/mm^3

ALT, Alanine transaminase; *AST*, aspartate transaminase; *HELLP*, hemolysis, elevated liver enzymes, and low platelet in association with preeclampsia; *LDH*, lactate dehydrogenase; *SGOT*, serum glutamic oxaloacetic transaminase; *SGPT*, serum glutamic pyruvate transaminase.

artery Doppler findings in the second trimester are associated with a more than six-fold increase in the rate of preeclampsia (Barton and Sibai, 2008). Previous studies that evaluated the predictiveness of placental growth factor (PIGF) in urine have been inconclusive. However, one study has shown that the tyrosine kinase (sFLt) and serum placental growth factor (PIGF) ratio at 22 to 26 weeks was highly predictive of early-onset preeclampsia (Barton and Sibai, 2008).

USUAL MEDICAL MANAGEMENT AND PROTOCOLS FOR NURSE PRACTITIONERS

The only cure for preeclampsia is termination of the pregnancy. The goal of management is to prevent eclampsia and other severe complications while allowing the fetus to mature. Because fetuses are usually immature when the disease develops, the severity of the disease and the maturity of the fetus must be considered in determining when delivery should take place.

If the pregnancy has progressed 36 weeks or more or fetal maturity is confirmed by a lecithin/sphingomyelin (L/S) ratio of 2:1, delivery is the treatment of choice after the condition is stabilized. If the pregnancy is fewer than 36 weeks of gestation or the fetus is immature, interventions are instituted to attempt to arrest or improve preeclampsia and allow time for the fetus to mature. However, if the HELLP syndrome develops, signs of impending eclampsia are present, or symptoms manifest indicating the condition is worsening, immediate delivery is necessary at any gestational age.

Expectant Management

Medical interventions depend on the severity of the disease and gestational age. In mild preeclampsia when the gestational age is 36 weeks or greater, the patient is usually treated with intravenous (IV) magnesium sulfate and oxytocin to induce labor. In mild preeclampsia when the fetus is immature, the patient is usually hospitalized with decreased activity to attempt to arrest the disease or at least stabilize the disease to allow the fetus time to mature without jeopardizing the mother's health. If the patient becomes normotensive with no significant proteinuria (less than 500 mg/24 hours), research has indicated similar outcomes with home management (either in a day care unit or with home health care) as with in-patient hospital care (Crowther, Bouwmeester, and Ashurst, 1992; Tuffnell and others, 1992; Barton and others, 1994, 1995, 1997). Refer to home care guidelines for treatment of mild preeclampsia under the Nursing Management section of this chapter.

If the disease is severe—as indicated by worsening maternal symptoms, diagnostic tests showing evidence of end-organ dysfunction, or deterioration of the fetus—or if HELLP syndrome develops, the current treatment is to prevent convulsions with an anticonvulsant, control the blood pressure within a safe range with an antihypertensive agent, and evaluate maternal and fetal well-being frequently. Then expeditious delivery is initiated as the woman's condition indicates. If the patient manifests a bleeding tendency, fresh frozen plasma (FFP) and packed RBCs are usually transfused.

Activity Restriction

Resting in bed in the lateral recumbent position takes the pressure of the gravid uterus off the inferior vena cava. This facilitates venous return, thereby increasing the circulatory volume, which increases renal blood flow and promotes diuresis (Dekker, 2001). Blood pressure normally drops as a result, enhancing blood flow to the placenta and fetus. How much of the day should be spent in bed is currently controversial. According to the National High Blood Pressure Education Program Working Group (2000), there is lack of scientific support for the effectiveness of continuous bedrest when compared with maternal risks associated with bedrest (see Chapter 1).

Diet

A diet adequate in protein is therapeutic in promoting cellular growth, replacing the protein lost in the urine, and lowering the risk for hypertension. During pregnancy, the RDA for protein increases by 10 grams (IFIC, 2008; Wardlaw and Smith, 2008). Protein also increases the plasma colloid osmotic pressure. As the plasma colloid osmotic pressure increases, it pulls fluid from the intracellular spaces back into the circulatory system. Adequate calcium (Atallah, Duley, and Hofmeyr, 2007) and folic acid (Chen, Perkins, Rennicks-White, and others, 2008) have both been shown to reduce the risk of preeclampsia and hypertensive disorders. Vitamins C and E, because of their antioxidant effect, were thought to decrease the risk of preeclampsia (Perkins, 2006). However, current research evidence has refuted this and actually found them to influence the risk of low birth weight (Barton and Sibai, 2008). Therefore Vitamins C and E supplementation is not currently recommended.

Sodium intake should not exceed 6 g daily. According to the Cochrane Review (Duley, Henderson-Smart, and Meher, 2005), the patient should be instructed to salt foods to taste. An excessive salt intake can increase angiotensin II sensitivity and cause increased vasoconstriction. On the other hand, an inappropriate dietary sodium restriction below 1.5 g can further reduce the blood volume and decrease placental perfusion (IFIC, 2008; Roberts and Funai, 2009). However, if the patient has salt-sensitive chronic hypertension or renal disease and was on a sodium-restricted diet before pregnancy, she should continue this diet during her pregnancy.

Fetal Surveillance

The most commonly used methods of fetal surveillance are serial ultrasounds to estimate fetal growth, amniotic fluid index (AFI) studies, biophysical profile (BPP) with nonstress test, and daily fetal movement counts to assess uteroplacental perfusion.

Pharmacologic Therapy

The following medications are commonly used in the treatment of preeclampsia.

Anticonvulsive Therapy

Magnesium sulfate is still the anticonvulsant drug of choice to prevent seizure activity with severe preeclampsia and to treat eclampsia (National High Blood Pressure Education Program Working Group, 2000; Duley, Gülmezoglu, and Henderson-Smart, 2003). However, there is no evidence-based data concerning the use of prophylactic magnesium in mild preeclampsia. Phenytoin may be used as an alternative therapy when magnesium is contraindicated such as in renal failure and myasthenia gravis. It is not as effective as magnesium for prophylaxis or treatment of eclampsia seizures. For anticonvulsant therapy, refer to the section on critical case interventions for anticonvulsant therapy later in this chapter.

Antihypertensive Therapy

A recent Cochrane analysis of antihypertensive drug therapy for mild to moderate hypertension during pregnancy reviewed 40 studies; 24 studies compared antihypertensive drug with placebo or no antihypertensive drug. The authors reported a halving the risk of developing severe hypertension; however, there was no difference in the risk of developing preeclampsia or proteinuria (Barton and Sibai, 2008). Antihypertensive therapy in preeclampsia does not appear to improve perinatal outcomes (Abalos and others, 2006). However, in situations in which the diastolic blood pressure goes above 110 or the systolic goes above 160 to 180, there are significant renal, hepatic, and neurologic risks, such as cerebrovascular accident, to the mother. Antihypertensive therapy is indicated. Treatment should be implemented to reduce the blood pressure to a level that provides a margin of maternal safety without compromising adequate uterine perfusion.

Hydralazine (Apresoline) has been the antihypertensive drug of choice in the United States because it is more effective in lowering MAP to safe levels than other drugs (National High Blood Pressure Education Program Working Group, 2000). However, it has been shown to be associated with more maternal side effects and low Apgar scores at 1 minute (von Dadelszen and Magee, 2005). Labetalol has extensively been used during pregnancy. Another antihypertensive agent being tried is oral nifedipine (Procardia). However, it is not approved by the Food and Drug Administration for treating hypertensive emergencies (National High Blood Pressure Education Program Working Group, 2000). For antihypertensive therapy, refer to the section on critical case interventions for acute antihypertensive therapy later in this chapter.

Corticosteroid Therapy

The use of a single course of corticosteroids to facilitate fetal lung maturity is recommended if delivery is imminent between 24 and 34 weeks of gestation (NIH, 2000). In the presence of severe preeclampsia or HELLP syndrome, glucocorticoids have been shown to significantly decrease the rate of respiratory distress syndrome, as well as decrease neonatal intraventricular hemorrhage and infection (Amorium, Santas, and Faundes, 1999; Anumba and Robson, 1999).

Blood Component Replacement

In the presence of severe persistent thrombocytopenia, FFP or packed RBCs are usually infused. Platelet transfusions are ineffective because platelet consumption occurs soon after administration (Mabie, 2001).

Intensive Hemodynamic Monitoring

Intensive hemodynamic monitoring is not considered a standard of practice for severe preeclampsia or eclampsia according to the National High Blood Pressure Education Program Working Group (2000). However, many clinicians find it helpful in determining appropriate therapy in the presence of pulmonary edema or oliguria or in situations in which blood pressure is unresponsive to therapy results.

Delivery

Vaginal delivery is preferred unless caesarean delivery is indicated for other obstetric reasons. Cervical ripening agents or oxytocin for induction or augmentation can be used to expedite labor within 24 hours. Regional anesthesia such as epidural, spinal, or combination spinal and epidural are safe. Laryngoscopy and tracheal intubation with a general anesthesia can increase hypertension. Pretreatment with an antihypertensive agent may decrease this risk.

NURSING MANAGEMENT

Prevention

Because the etiology of the disease is unknown, it is difficult to outline a protocol for prevention. Based on scientific studies, some general principles, however, appear to decrease the incidence of this disease.

Adequate Nutrition

All pregnant patients should receive instructions regarding the benefits of eating a nutritious, balanced diet containing at least 70 to 80 g of protein, 1200 mg of calcium, and an adequate amount of zinc, magnesium, sodium (salt), and folic acid every day (Atallah, Duley, and Hofmeyr, 2007; Chen, Perkins, Rennicks-White, and others 2008b; Roberts and Funai, 2009; Gundersson, 2003). According to the Cochrane Trials, supplementation of magnesium or zinc has not been shown to be beneficial (Makrides and Crowther, 2001; Mahomed, Bhutta, and Middleton, 2007). With evidence that oxidative stress influences the disease process, a diet with adequate antioxidants such as lycopene, selenium, and melatonin may decrease the incidence (Scholl and others, 2005; Spinnato and Livingston, 2005). Drinking six to eight glasses of water or fluid per day should be included in the instructions. According to the Cochrane Database of Systematic Review, a calcium supplement reduces the risk for preeclampsia especially in patients that have diets deficient in calcium (Hofmeyr, Atallah, and Duley, 2006).

Adequate Rest

Bedrest facilitates venous return, increasing the circulatory volume, enhancing renal and placental perfusion, and lowering blood pressure. Therefore high risk patients may benefit from 8 to 12 hours of sleep each night with a rest period in the middle of the day. Bedrest also mobilizes edematous fluid back into the intravascular space. However, according to the Cochrane Review, complete bedrest should not be considered unless the disease is severe (Meher, Abalos, and Carroli, 2007).

Water Therapy

In the presence of severe edema, research has demonstrated that shoulder-deep immersion in water can mobilize extravascular fluid, initiate diuresis, and decrease the renin, angiotensin, aldosterone, and vasopressin levels (Katz and others, 1990, 1992; Kent and others, 1999; DiPasquale and Lynett, 2003). Therefore water therapy may help prevent or slow the progression of preeclampsia. It has also been shown to help reverse oligohydramnios resulting from uteroplacental insufficiency (Strong, 1993).

Heparin Therapy

Heparin therapy may reduce the risk of severe preeclampsia in the presence of thrombophilia caused by protein S deficiency, Factor V Leiden mutation, or anticardiolipin antibodies (Kupferminc, Fair, Mary, and others, 2001; Stella, Ghulmiyyah, and Sibai, 2006).

Early and Appropriate Prenatal Care

Early, appropriate treatment is effective in preventing the severe form of preeclampsia or eclampsia. Therefore early detection of its development is effective in lowering the high maternal and fetal mortality associated with the disease (MacKay, Berg, and Atrash, 2001).

Detection begins on the first prenatal visit early in pregnancy. The nurse practitioner or nurse obtains an in-depth patient history that includes age and parity, a medical history of such things as diabetes and persistent hypertensive disorders, and a familial history of preeclampsia or eclampsia. On each prenatal visit, the patient is weighed, an accurate blood pressure reading is obtained, and an early-morning urine specimen is checked for protein. If protein is noted in the urine, it should be checked for bacteria and another specimen obtained by clean-catch midstream collection because bacteria, vaginal discharge, blood, and amniotic fluid can give a false-positive result. If urine protein is 11 or greater, follow up with a 24-hour urine test for protein and creatinine clearance.

Low-Dose Aspirin

A recent Perinatal Antiplatelet Review of International Studies (PARIS) Collaborate Group performed a meta-analysis of the effectiveness and safety of antiplatelet agents (predominantly aspirin) for the prevention of preeclampsia. The reviewers concluded that there is a small to moderate benefit when used for prevention of preeclampsia, and it was also found to be safe. However, more information clearly is required to assess which women are most likely to benefit from this therapy as well as when treatment is optimally started and what dose to use (Barton and Sibai, 2008). Aspirin selectively inhibits thromboxane production with minimal effect on prostacyclin synthesis. Therefore it restores the prostacyclin/thromboxane balance. This low dose appears to have no harmful effects on the fetus or neonate and is safe for the mother, and epidural anesthesia is safe with the use of low-dose aspirin (CLASP Collaborative Group, 1995). Further studies are needed to assess which women would benefit and when treatment should be initiated (Duley and others, 2007).

Home Health Care for Mild Preeclampsia[*]

Criteria Selection

- Blood pressure lower than 150/100 mm Hg sitting and lower than 140/90 mm Hg in the left lateral position
- Proteinuria lower than 500 mg/day
- Platelet count more than 125,000/µl
- Normal liver enzymes: aspartate transaminase (AST) less than 50 units/L, alanine transaminase (ALT) less than 50 units/L, lactate dehydrogenase (LDH) less than 200 units/L
- Serum creatinine less than 1.32 mg/dl
- Reassuring fetal status with no intrauterine fetal growth restriction
- No worsening signs present
- A compliant, reliable patient

Home Care Protocols

- Limited home activity with 12 hours sleep each night and rest periods during the day to facilitate renal and placental perfusion by mobilizing the movement of extracellular fluid back into the intravascular space
- Bed exercises to keep the muscles toned and increase blood flow; leg exercises, such as foot circles at least twice each day; the super Kegel and abdominal tightening exercises to keep the perineal and abdominal muscles in tone. If the patient complains of back pain, the pelvic rock can help relieve this discomfort (see Box 1-1).
- Balanced diet containing at least 60 to 70 g of protein, 400 mcg of folic acid, 1200 mg of calcium; adequate zinc and sodium (2 to 6 g); and six to eight glasses of water per day
- Blood pressure monitored every 4 to 6 hours daily (while awake)
- Daily weighing at the same time
- Urine tested for protein using first-voided specimen of the day
- Understanding of the signs and symptoms that indicate the condition is worsening with instructions to report them immediately:
  - Headaches, severe and not relieved by acetaminophen
  - Vision changes, such as blurry vision or seeing spots
  - Epigastric pain or right upper quadrant (RUQ) pain

---

[*]Friedman and others, 2001.

- Increased edema indicated by a weight gain of more than 2 pounds in 1 day or 5 pounds in 1 week
- Vaginal bleeding or changes in vaginal discharge
- Severe abdominal pain
- Watery fluid leading from the vagina
- Uterine tightening
- Decreased fetal movements or fetal movements of fewer than four in 1 hour
- Instruct patient to expect home health nurse visits two times per week with daily telephone contact.
- Schedule weekly prenatal visits.
- Perform initial and frequent diagnostic laboratory assessments as follows:
  - 24-hour urine sample for protein and creatinine clearance
  - Serum creatinine and uric acid levels
  - Hematocrit
  - Serum albumin
  - Platelet count
  - Liver enzymes, such as AST, ALT, and LDH, if platelet count is low
- Instruct patient in fetal surveillance:
  - Daily fetal movement counts
  - Frequent evaluations with BPP, nonstress test (NST), and Amniotic Fluid Volume (AFV)
  - Fetal growth by ultrasound every 3 weeks
- Admit patient to hospital for worsening status

Nursing Assessment for Severe Preeclampsia

General Criteria

The goal is *early* detection of indicators that the condition is deteriorating.

Instruct the patient to check her blood pressure every 4 hours while she is awake or more often if indicated. The blood pressure should be taken on the same arm with the patient in the same position each time. Preferably, the patient is lying on her left side with the cuff on the right arm.

Cardiovascular Alterations

- Measure pulse rate; assess quality and rhythm.
- Evaluate degree of edema every 8 hours and score as shown in Table 22-7.
- Obtain daily weight before breakfast.

Table 22-7   Degree of Edema

Physical Findings	Score
Minimal edema of lower extremities	1
Marked edema of lower extremities	2
Edema of lower extremities, face, hands	3
Generalized massive edema including abdomen and sacrum	4

- Check capillary refill and neck vein distention.
- Evaluate serum albumin to check for endothelial leakage.

Renal Alterations

- Evaluate urine for protein, specific gravity, pH, and glucose daily or every 8 hours with dipstick. The gram equivalent of protein, as indicated on the dipstick, is outlined in Table 22-8. A 24-hour urine collection for protein and creatinine clearance may be ordered if the dipstick protein is +1 or greater. The loss of 5 g or more of protein in 24 hours indicates severe preeclampsia.
- Measure intake and output every 1 to 4 hours, and keep a record. If the urinary output is less than 30 ml/hour or 120 ml/4 hours, oliguria is present. This indicates that the condition is deteriorating. If output is increased, monitor electrolytes for indications of high output renal failure such as serum creatinine greater than 1.
- Measure serum creatinine and uric acid levels.

Central Nervous System Alterations

- Check deep tendon reflexes (DTRs) daily or more often if indicated. The easiest DTR to check is the patellar reflex (knee jerk). The response elicited should be graded as shown in Table 22-9.
- Determine whether clonus is present. In clonus, dorsiflexion of the foot causes spasms of the muscle. This is seen as a convulsive movement of the foot and indicates neuromuscular irritability.

Table 22-8   Proteinuria

Dipstick Reading	Protein
Trace	5–20 mg/L
1	30 mg/L
2	100 mg/L
3	300 mg/L
4	>1000 mg/L

Reference: Chernecky C, Berger B: *Laboratory tests and diagnostic procedures*, ed 5, Philadelphia, 2007, Saunders.

Table 22-9   Deep Tendon Reflex Grading

Physical Result	Grade
None elicited	0
Sluggish or dull	1
Active, normal	2
Brisk	3
Brisk with transient (few beats) or sustained (continuous) clonus	4

Reference: Hallett M: National Institute of Neurological Disorders and Stroke (NINDS) myotatic reflex scale, *Neurology* 43(12):2723, 1993.

- Assess for severe headaches not relieved by acetaminophen or visual changes that are indicative that the condition is worsening. Additionally, note changes in level of consciousness or changes in behavior.

Pulmonary Alterations

- Check respiration rate every 4 hours while the patient is awake or more often if indicated.
- Auscultate lung fields for wheezing or crackles, which can indicate pulmonary edema. Signs of dyspnea, tightness of the chest, shallow respirations, or a cough should be noted.
- Assess skin color and mucous membranes for cyanosis.
- Monitor oxygenation with pulse oximetry as indicated.

Hepatic Alterations

- Assess for epigastric pain, right upper quadrant pain, nausea, vomiting, and jaundice; these are all possible signs of liver injury.
- If platelet count is low, assess liver enzymes such as AST, ALT, and LDH to monitor for HELLP.
- Assess for hypoglycemia and coagulation defects in the presence of severe hepatic involvement.

Hematology Alterations

- Hematocrit for hemoconcentration
- Peripheral smear for hemolysis of RBCs
- Platelet counts to monitor for HELLP (If patient has been on low-dose aspirin therapy, platelet function may be below normal even if platelet count is adequate.)
- Follow-up coagulation studies, such as fibrinogen, D-dimers, prothrombin, and partial thromboplastin time, if platelet count is lower than 100,000 mm^3
- Indications of possible DIC development include signs of bleeding, such as oozing from IV sites, nosebleeds, and petechiae.

Reproductive System Status

- Assess for the presence of uterine contractions because decreased uteroplacental blood flow can initiate labor.
- Assess for signs of an abruptio placentae, including dark red vaginal bleeding, sustained abdominal pain, uterine tenderness, tetanic contractions, and increasing fundal height.

Fetal Surveillance Status

- Check fetal heart rate every 4 to 6 hours with a Doppler FHR device or a continuous electronic fetal monitor, if the condition indicates.
- Record fetal movements daily. Fetal movements have been shown to correlate with fetal well-being. Fewer fetal movements from the patient's previous pattern may indicate fetal hypoxia. Instruct the patient to report decreased fetal movements compared with the movements of the previous day or when there are fewer than 10 fetal movements in any 2-hour period (ACOG, 1999).

- Monitor for IUGR. Use serial ultrasounds and AFV for oligohydramnios.
- Severe uteroplacental insufficiency: Appropriate fetal surveillance tests, such as NST, or BPP with frequent AFV, are carried out at appropriate intervals after 28 to 30 weeks of gestation.

Nursing Interventions for Severe Preeclampsia

- *Manage the patient in a tertiary care center* on a high risk obstetric unit that has a neonatal intensive care unit.
- *Follow systematic assessments* (as outlined under Nursing Assessment for Severe Preeclampsia) if critical to the ongoing management.
- *Limit activity to bathroom privileges.* Help the patient and her family problem-solve difficulties that implement limited activity.
- *Make appropriate referrals,* for example, to Sidelines or a social worker.
- *Encourage family participation* in the patient's care and decision making as much as possible.
- *Encourage bed exercises* because they are important in keeping the muscles in tone and in increasing blood flow to decrease a thromboembolism. The patient should be instructed to do leg exercises such as foot circles at least twice each day. She should also be instructed to do the super Kegel and abdominal tightening exercises to keep the perineal and abdominal muscles in tone. If the patient complains of back pain, the pelvic rock can help relieve this discomfort (see Box 1-1).
- *If IV fluids are indicated to promote plasma volume expansion, administer isotonic crystalloid fluids or colloid-containing fluids* to increase colloid osmotic pressure, or albumin. Avoid the use of hypotonic fluids in fluid replacement therapy because they may further decrease the serum osmolarity.
- *Base initial intake of fluid* on the need to combat dehydration. (The usual amount for the first 24 hours is 1500 to 3000 ml of fluid. Therefore if the patient is not dehydrated, fluid intake equals amount of urinary output of the previous 24 hours plus 1000 ml, except in acute renal failure, in which case intake should not exceed 500 ml.) If oliguria develops, fluid administration is best guided by pulmonary capillary wedge pressure.
- *Monitor maternal and fetal status* and for signs the condition is worsening (as outlined under Nursing Assessment for Severe Preeclampsia).
- *Monitor baseline and frequent diagnostic laboratory assessments* (as outlined under Nursing Assessment for Severe Preeclampsia).
- *Monitor for HELLP* (see Table 22-6).
- *Prevent eclampsia* with anticonvulsant therapy (refer to Critical Care Intervention for Anticonvulsant Therapy, later in this chapter).
- *Administer antithrombotic agents* such as low-dose aspirin as ordered.
- *Treat hypertension* if blood pressure is higher than 160 to 180/110 mm Hg (refer to Critical Care Intervention for Antihypertensive Therapy, later in this chapter).
- *Initiate corticosteroid therapy* to improve premature fetal lung maturity and to decrease HELLP syndrome severity (Box 22-1).
- *Allay anxiety* by providing time for the patient and her family to express their concerns regarding the possible outcomes for the baby and the inconvenience to the mother and family during the treatment. Encourage them to vent any feelings,

Box 22-1   Corticosteroid Therapy

Betamethasone

Action

Corticosteroid therapy stimulates the production of a more mature surfactant in the fetal lung between 24 and 34 weeks of gestation. It has no effect in enhancing fetal lung maturity after 34 weeks of gestation (Odendaal, 2001). Optimal benefit begins 24 hours after initiation of therapy and lasts 7 days. This period of time is called the steroid window.

Dosage

Betamethasone, two doses of 12.5 mg are given intramuscularly 24 hours apart or Dexamethasone 6 mg is administered intramuscularly every 12 hours for 4 doses (NIH, 2000; Weiner and Buhimschi, 2009).

---

fears, and anger they may experience. Provide understandable information to the patient and her family regarding the disease process, plan of treatment, and implications for mother and fetus. Explain all treatment modalities and reasons for each. Keep patient informed of health status, results of tests, and fetal well-being.

- *Refer to a community support group* such as Sidelines (*http://www.sidelines.org*).
- *Refer to a spiritual counselor or chaplain* on request.
- *Suggest diversional activities.* Assess the patient's interest in various diversional activities within her activity limit. Provide crafts, reading, and puzzles that can be done in bed, or encourage patient to have these things brought in. Provide classes in preparation for childbirth by way of video, the hospital television, or group classes that can be attended while reclining. Refer to a diversional therapist or volunteer to provide reading materials, handicrafts, or other activities of interest.
- *Prepare for delivery when indicated as outlined by Odendaal (2001)*:
  - Fetal lung maturity
  - Fetal stress
  - Abruptio placenta
  - Uncontrolled blood pressure
  - Oliguria
  - Pulmonary edema
  - Persistent symptoms of HELLP
  - Imminent eclampsia
- *Postpartum considerations.* There is an increased risk for recurrence of preeclampsia of approximately 10% to 25% (Hayman, 2004). There is an increased risk for cardiovascular disease later in life. Van Pampus and Aarnoudse (2005) consider preeclampsia as a first manifestation of atherosclerosis. Lifestyle changes should be advised as indicated, as well as ongoing screening such as hyperlipidemia, hyperhomocystinemia, and thrombophilia. Overall, 35% of patients develop chronic hypertension later in life (Witlin, 1999). This risk can be affected by or be related to lifestyle health habits, stress level, and current partner (Egerman and Sibai, 2001). Long-term follow-up is important because of possible underlying medical problems such as coagulation disturbances, protein S and C deficiencies, hyperhomocystinemia, and anticardiolipin antibodies (Odendaal, 2001).

Critical Care Interventions for Anticonvulsant Therapy: Magnesium Sulfate

- *Administer magnesium sulfate.* Normal dosing guidelines are provided in Box 22-2.
- *Set the goal of therapy* to be decreased but not absent DTRs.
- *Assess for magnesium toxicity* in any patient receiving magnesium sulfate in the following manner:
  - DTRs should be checked every hour if the patient is on continuous IV drip and before administering each dose if the patient is on intermittent therapy (Table 22-10).

Box 22-2   Anticonvulsive Therapy in Preeclampsia

Magnesium Sulfate
The drug of choice to treat eclampsia.
Action
Decreases central nervous system irritability and blocks neuromuscular conduction by blocking the release of acetylcholine at neuromuscular junctions. Acetylcholine is the excitatory substance that transmits nerve messages across the synapse.
Other Beneficial Actions
Magnesium sulfate has been shown to cause peripheral vasodilation, increase uterine and renal blood flow, increase prostacyclin production by endothelial cells, reduce platelet aggregation, and decrease the action of plasma renin and angiotensin (Eclampsia Trial Collaborative Group, 1995). It is superior to phenytoin or diazepam (Duley, Gülmezoglu, and Henderson-Smart, 2003; Duley and Henderson-Smart, 2003a, 2003b).
Intravenous Dosage
Therapeutic administration of magnesium sulfate usually consists of an initial loading dose of 4 to 6 g by IV in 100 ml of fluid administered over 15 to 20 minutes, followed by a maintenance dose of 1–2 g/hr diluted in 5% dextrose and lactated Ringer's solution administered by an infusion pump to maintain serum magnesium levels with a therapeutic range of 4 to 7 mEq/L.
Intramuscular Dosage
The maintenance dose can also be administered intramuscularly. The normal dosage is 5 g every 4 hours in alternate buttocks. Intramuscular injections of magnesium sulfate are seldom used because the rate of absorption cannot be controlled, tissue necrosis can develop, and the injections are painful. If magnesium sulfate is administered intramuscularly, Z-track technique should be used with a 3-inch, 20-gauge dry needle to ensure that the medication is injected deep into the gluteal muscle, and the site should be gently massaged to facilitate absorption. A local anesthetic agent can be added to the magnesium sulfate solution to minimize the discomfort.
Side Effects
Frequently experienced side effects are lethargy, sensations of heat or burning, headache, nausea and vomiting, blurry vision, and constipation. The patient should be prepared for these normal side effects. Because magnesium sulfate decreases smooth muscle contractility by moving calcium out of the smooth

Box 22-2   Anticonvulsive Therapy in Preeclampsia—cont'd

muscle, it decreases uterine activity and can prolong labor. However, it is ineffective in suppressing uterine activity once labor becomes active. Because magnesium blocks neuromuscular and cardiac transmission of nerve impulses and depresses the central nervous system, respiratory paralysis and cardiac arrest can result if serum magnesium levels rise too high. Plasma levels of 4 to 7 mEq/L are very effective in preventing convulsions, demonstrated by depressed deep tendon reflexes (DTRs). Plasma levels between 8 and 10 mEq/L cause a loss of DTRs, which is the first sign of toxicity. Other early signs are nausea, a feeling of warmth, flushing, somnolence, double vision, slurred speech, and weakness.

Plasma levels greater than 13 to 15 mEq/L can cause respiratory paralysis, and levels greater than 20 to 25 mEq/L can cause cardiac arrest (see Table 22-10). Therefore, serum magnesium levels should be assessed daily. Neonatal neuromuscular and respiratory depression has been seen with hypermagnesemia delivery.

Fetal Effect

Magnesium crosses the placenta, but there is no clear evidence of adverse effects from short-term therapy (Weiner and Buhimschi, 2009).

Contraindications

Myasthenia gravis and myocardial ischemia or infarct (Aagaard-Tillery and Belfort, 2005)

Phenytoin

Can be used in situations when magnesium is associated with increased risk.

Action

Suppresses the influx of sodium ions across cell membranes during potential repetitive neuronal activity and blocks the changes in the concentrations of potassium and calcium ions that occur before seizure activity, thus lowering the neuronal excitation threshold.

Dosage

The therapeutic loading dose is usually 10 mg/kg of current weight, diluted in 250 ml of normal saline or lactated Ringer's solution. A dextrose solution should not be used, because a precipitation will occur (Lucas and Jordan, 1997). The rate of infusion should be between 25 and 40 mg/min. An additional dose of 5 mg/kg is given 2 hours later. Because the half-life of this drug is 12 hours, which is relatively long compared with that of magnesium sulfate, a maintenance dose may not be needed. It is given based on the serum phenytoin levels. The therapeutic range for phenytoin is 10 to 20 mg/ml.

Side Effects

Hypotension, the most common side effect, occurs if the IV infusion is given too rapidly (Lucas and Jordan, 1997). Other side effects seen are cardiac dysrhythmias, bradycardia, hypotension, and heart block; ataxia, slurred speech, mental confusion, and decreased coordination; nausea and vomiting; and double or blurred vision (Weiner and Buhimschi, 2009). Phenytoin has no effect on suppression of labor. Mothers are more alert, awake, and able to breastfeed compared with mothers who received magnesium sulfate (Lucas and Jordan, 1997).

Table 22-10   Serum Magnesium Levels

Magnesium Levels (mEq/L)	Magnesium Levels (mg/dl)	Interpretation
1.5–2.5	1.7–2.4	Normal
4–7	5–8.4	Therapeutic
7–8	8.5–10	Depression of deep tendon reflexes
8–10	10–12	Loss of deep tendon reflexes
10–12	12–15	Respiration depression
12–15	15–18	Respiratory paralysis
15–20	18–25	Heart block
Above 20	Above 25	Cardiac arrest

Data from Nick J: Deep tendon reflexes, magnesium, and calcium: assessments and implications, *J Obstet Gynecol Neonatal Nurs* 33(2):221-230, 2004; Roberts J, Funai F: Pregnancy-related hypertension. In Creasy R, Resnik R, Iams J, Lockwood C, Moore T, editors: *Creasy & Resnik's maternal-fetal medicine: principles and practice*, ed 6, Philadelphia, 2009, Saunders; Sibai, B: Hypertension. In Gabbe S, Niebyl J, Simpson J, editors: *Obstetrics: normal and problem pregnancies*, ed 5, New York, 2009, Churchill Livingstone.

- Check the respiratory pattern and rate, pulse, blood pressure, oxygen saturation, and level of consciousness frequently if the patient is receiving a continuous IV drip or before administering each dose if the patient is receiving intermittent therapy.
- Monitor the patient's intake and output closely and insert a Foley catheter because magnesium is excreted largely in the urine; the patient with kidney involvement can develop toxicity rapidly. If the patient is receiving a continuous IV drip, the urinary output should be at least 30 ml/hour. If the patient is receiving intermittent doses of magnesium, the urinary output should be obtained every 4 hours and should be at least 120 ml/4 hours.
- To decrease the risk for pulmonary edema, limit the total fluid intake for 24 hours, not to exceed 2000 ml.
- Use serum magnesium levels to assess magnesium toxicity. Therapeutic levels are between 4 and 7 mEq/L and are effective in preventing convulsions, demonstrated by depressed DTRs. Plasma levels between 8 and 10 mEq/L cause a loss of DTRs, which is the first sign of toxicity. Other early signs are nausea, a feeling of warmth, flushing, somnolence, double vision, slurred speech, and weakness. Plasma levels above 13 to 15 mEq/L can cause respiratory paralysis, and levels greater than 20 to 25 mEq/L can cause cardiac arrest (see Table 22-10). Therefore assess serum magnesium levels daily. Magnesium can have some detrimental effects on the fetus as well. Relatively less FHR variability at therapeutic levels and neonatal neuromuscular and respiratory depression have been seen.
- *Signs of magnesium toxicity.* Discontinue or withhold magnesium sulfate and notify the attending physician if any of the following signs of magnesium toxicity develop:
  - No DTR or a sudden change in the DTR
  - Respirations fewer than 14/min or change in breath sounds
  - Oxygen saturation below 95%
  - Urinary output less than 30 ml/hour or 120 ml/4 hours

- Significant drop in pulse or blood pressure
- Double or blurred vision
- Signs of fetal distress
- Serum magnesium levels 8 mEq/L or greater
- *Use calcium chloride as the antidote* for magnesium toxicity because calcium stimulates the release of acetylcholine at the nerve synapse. The normal dose is 500 mg IV by slow infusion over 30 minutes (Weiner and Buhimschi, 2009).
- *Prevent pulmonary edema* by closely monitoring the IV and oral fluids to avoid exceeding 125 ml/hour.
- *If magnesium sulfate* is contraindicated, use phenytoin. (Refer to Box 22-1 for dosage administration.)
- *Postpartum considerations:*
  - Continue magnesium sulfate or another anticonvulsant for 24 to 48 hours following delivery or longer if the HELLP syndrome coexists (Friedman and others, 2001).
  - Monitor closely for pulmonary edema related to fluid replacement and mobilization of accumulated fluid back into the intravascular spaces.

Critical Care Interventions for Acute Antihypertensive Therapy

- *Initiate antihypertensive therapy* if the diastolic blood pressure is greater than 105 to 110 mm Hg or the systolic blood pressure is greater than 160 to 180 mm Hg.
- *Goal of therapy.* Maintain blood pressure below 160/100 mm Hg but above 140/90 mm Hg to reduce blood pressure for mother's benefit while maintaining uteroplacental perfusion for fetal oxygenation.
- *Two of the most commonly used drugs* are hydralazine and labetalol. Nifedipine is used occasionally. Box 22-3 provides a listing of antihypertensive medications to use for acute hypertensive crisis during pregnancy.
- *Stabilization for transport* may be accomplished with hydralazine 5 mg intramuscularly or nifedipine 10 to 20 mg orally (Odendaal, 2001).
- *Check the blood pressure* every minute for the first 5 minutes following administration of antihypertensive medication and then every 5 minutes for the next 30 minutes, preferably with an automatic blood pressure cuff.
- *To prevent treatment-induced severe hypotension*, consider the need for 200 to 300 ml of IV fluid before drug administration unless contraindicated.

Critical Care Interventions for HELLP Syndrome

- Transfer the patient to a tertiary care center, if possible.
- Assess and stabilize maternal condition.
- Implement the same monitoring protocol as for the severe preeclamptic patient.
- Provide oxygen, 8 to 10 L/min via face mask to improve oxygen flow to vital organs and the placenta.
- Prevent eclampsia with anticonvulsant therapy. The infusion dose of magnesium sulfate is adjusted based on serum magnesium levels, patellar reflexes, and urinary output. The risk for magnesium toxicity is increased because of the possibility of renal dysfunction and hematoma in the presence of thrombocytopenia. Refer to Critical Care Interventions for Anticonvulsant Therapy.

| **Box 22-3** | Antihypertensive Medications for Acute Hypertensive Crisis during Pregnancy |

Hydralazine

Action

Directs peripheral vasodilation by relaxing smooth muscle; increases cardiac output and heart rate.

Dosage

Administer 5 to 10 mg by intravenous (IV) push over 1 to 2 minutes. The dose can be repeated every 20 minutes until the diastolic blood pressure is between 90 and 100 mm Hg or a maximum of 30 mg is reached. The diastolic blood pressure should not be allowed to fall below 90 mm Hg to prevent further reduction in blood flow to the placenta, cerebrum, and kidneys. Hydralazine is administered whenever the diastolic blood pressure again reaches 110 mm Hg.

Side Effects

Possible side effects are tachycardia, dizziness, faintness, headache, palpitations, numbness, tingling of the extremities, and disorientation. Fetal effects, such as adverse fetal heart rate and low Apgar score at *1 minute,* may occur.

Contraindication

Do not use in patients with hypertension and tachycardia because hydralazine is ineffective in treating hypertension caused by elevated cardiac output.

Labetalol

Action

Labetalol is a combined alpha- and beta-blocker that decreases peripheral vascular resistance without changing cardiac output or causing tachycardia. Therefore it is the drug of choice for hypertensive patients with tachycardia (Weiner and Buhimschi, 2009). It is less effective in black Americans.

Dosage

Administer 20 mg by a bolus IV injection. If effect is suboptimal, give 40 mg 10 minutes later and 80 mg 10 minutes after that, up to a maximum of 300 mg.

Side Effects

The patient may experience nausea, vomiting, orthostatic hypotension, sweating, dizziness, headaches, bronchospasm, and dyspnea (Weiner and Buhimschi, 2009). Fetal effects such as respiratory depression and bradycardia can occur.

Contraindication

Labetalol is contraindicated in patients with asthma, congestive heart failure, hypoglycemia, or with hepatotoxicity.

- Treat severe acute hypertension. Refer to Critical Care Interventions for Antihypertensive Therapy.
- When DIC is present, correct coagulopathy.
- Be aware that the patient is at increased risk for abruptio placentae, pulmonary edema, acute renal failure, eclampsia, and subcapsular hematoma of the liver.
- Consider the differential diagnosis of acute fatty liver of pregnancy (AFLP). AFLP is a rare but potentially fatal third trimester complication that can manifest with symptoms similar to HELLP syndrome. A diagnostic laboratory

finding that differs between AFLP and HELLP is that AFLP has prolonged prothrombin and partial thromboplastin, hypoglycemia, and increased ammonia.
- Observe more closely for a subcapsular hematoma, which is rare but life-threatening. Possible signs are a sudden exacerbation of severe epigastric or RUQ pain or unexplained hypotension (Williamson and Girling, 2006). If subcapsular hematoma is suspected, abdominal ultrasound is indicated for diagnosis. If subcapsular hematoma of the liver develops, perform the following:
  - Follow with serial abdominal ultrasounds.
  - Type and cross-match packed RBCs (30 units), FFP (20 units), and platelet concentration (30 to 50 units).
  - Monitor the hemodynamic state closely by assessing signs of shoulder pain, ascites, respiratory difficulty, and shock.
  - Be prepared for emergency surgery and aggressive management of coagulopathy if rupture occurs.
- *Provide continuous electronic monitoring of FHR*, and carry out ordered fetal surveillance studies such as an NST or BPP.
- *Be prepared to assist with fetal lung maturity studies* if less than 35 weeks of gestation.
- *Initiate corticosteroid therapy* if indicated to improve fetal lung maturity and effect a more rapid improvement of the condition (see Box 22-1).
- In the presence of significant hemorrhage when the platelet count is less than 20,000 mm^3, be prepared to administer a platelet transfusion either before or after delivery (Sibai, 2007).
- *Prepare for delivery.* If the fetus is immature, attempts may be made to stabilize the patient, undelivered, until corticosteroids can be administered. If the fetus is mature, vaginal delivery is preferred. Induction with oxytocin and or prostaglandins may be attempted if the patient's condition is stable. If a cesarean delivery is indicated and the platelet count is below 40,000 mm^3, 10 units of platelets should be administered before the surgery.
- *Postpartum considerations*:
  - Continue intensive monitoring for 48 hours postpartum.
  - Consider corticosteroid therapy to shorten the disease process and improve recovery time (see Box 22-1).
  - Be aware that the onset of the HELLP syndrome develops 30% of the time during the postpartum period. Clinical manifestations of the syndrome usually occur within the first 48 hours postpartum.
  - There is a 19% to 27% risk for recurrence in subsequent pregnancies with the highest risk correlating with the severity of abnormal laboratory findings and a 15% risk for developing a non-HELLP preeclampsia (Witlin, 1999).

Critical Care Nursing Interventions for Eclampsia

Seizure Precautions
- *Assess for signs of impending eclampsia*, such as epigastric or right upper quadrant pain, nausea and vomiting, headache, jaundice, and hematuria.
- *Implement seizure precautions* by having oxygen, suction, a padded tongue blade, and supplies to pad side rails at bedside.

- *Provide a quiet, pleasant environment* with limited lighting so as not to further activate the already overstimulated central nervous system.
- *Limit visitors* except the patient's family.
- *Administer magnesium sulfate* or other anticonvulsant therapy as ordered. Refer to Critical Care Interventions for Anticonvulsant Therapy.
- *Assess for signs of magnesium toxicity,* such as absence of DTRs, respirations fewer than 12/min, or a significant drop in pulse or blood pressure. Monitor urinary output, because magnesium sulfate is excreted by way of the kidneys. Note serum magnesium levels.
- *Have the antidote of calcium gluconate* at the bedside.
- *Notify the attending physician of any worsening signs,* including signs of magnesium sulfate toxicity.

During the Seizure

- Remain with the patient.
- Reduce the risk for aspiration and establish airway patency by lowering and turning the head to one side to keep the airway open. Suction any secretions from the mouth.
- Observe seizure activity for time of occurrence, length of seizure, and type of seizure activity.
- Call for help by turning on the patient's call light.
- Maintain adequate oxygenation by administering supplemental oxygen via face mask at 8-10 L/min (Sibai, 2005).
- Notify the attending physician at the first sign of convulsive activity.
- Prevent maternal injury. If possible, a padded tongue blade should be inserted with care between the teeth to prevent tongue injury and to facilitate the insertion of an airway if needed. Make sure the side rails are up and padded if possible.

After the Seizure

- *Assess airway and suction* if needed. Maintain adequate oxygenation by administering oxygen via face mask at 10 L/min.
- *Start an IV line* as soon as possible. Monitor IV fluid closely with infusion pump.
- *Ensure maternal oxygenation after seizure.* Monitor oxygenation with pulse oximetry, assess breathing pattern, and administer oxygen at 10 L/min by tight face mask as needed to increase the maternal oxygen concentration and improve the oxygen supply to the fetus, which is lessened during a convulsion. Assess blood pressure, pulse, and respirations every 5 minutes until stable. Auscultate lung sounds to rule out aspiration.
- *Ensure fetal oxygenation after seizure.* Assess the FHR continuously with a fetal monitor because the hypoxic and acidotic state of a seizure may cause fetal distress. Change the patient's position from left lateral to right lateral every 30 minutes to increase uterine and renal blood flow.
- *Provide a quiet environment.*
- *Establish seizure control with magnesium sulfate.* Magnesium sulfate therapy is usually initiated as soon as the seizure stops. Start an IV line with an 18-gauge

intracatheter if it has not already been inserted. The normal dosage is a 4-g IV loading dose followed by a continuous infusion of 1-2 g/hour. Closely monitor delivery of IV fluid, and avoid exceeding 125 ml/hour to decrease risk for pulmonary edema. Insert a Foley catheter to measure hourly output, proteinuria, and specific gravity. Refer to Critical Care Interventions for Anticonvulsant Therapy.

- *Assess frequently for uterine contractions*, since a seizure frequently stimulates labor. During the coma phase, restlessness may indicate uterine contractions.
- *Assess for abruptio placentae*, which occurs in 7% to 10% of eclamptic patients (Sibai, 2005), by checking for fundal height changes, uterine hyperactivity, vaginal bleeding, or fetal bradycardia.
- *Assess for signs of the HELLP syndrome and DIC.* There is a high frequency of HELLP syndrome (8%) and DIC (7% to 11%) in eclamptic patients (Sibai, 2005).
- *The environment should be kept as quiet as possible* throughout the delivery of care, and bright lights should be avoided to decrease central nervous system stimulation.
- *Assess and treat severe hypertension if present.* Blood pressure is checked according to previously stated protocol as soon as possible to determine whether a hypertensive agent will be needed. Be prepared to administer an antihypertensive agent, such as hydralazine, if the diastolic blood pressure is higher than 110 mm Hg. Refer to Critical Care Interventions for Antihypertensive Therapy.
- *Assess urine for protein.*
- *Keep hourly input and output measures.*
- *Correct maternal acidemia.* Obtain blood gas levels following a seizure, and administer sodium bicarbonate only if pH is lower than 7.10.
- *Initiate delivery.* Once the mother and fetus have been stabilized, delivery is usually initiated. If labor is not already underway, induction by a labor stimulant is usually attempted if there is no fetal malpresentation or distress and if the fetus is at least 33 weeks of gestation. If the fetus is less than 33 weeks of gestation but the cervix is ripe, labor induction may be attempted. Cesarean birth is the choice of delivery for all others.

Postpartum Considerations

- Remember that approximately 30% of eclampsia cases develop during the postpartum period (Sibai, 2005).
- *Monitor closely for 48 hours* vital signs, fluid intake and output, laboratory values and pulse oximetry.
- *Monitor closely for pulmonary edema* related to fluid replacement and mobilization of accumulated fluid back into the intravascular spaces as well as *compromised renal function.*
- Remember that although the risk for recurrence of eclampsia in the next pregnancy is 2%, 22% to 35% do experience some form of preeclampsia; however, most is of the mild form (Sibai, 2005). According to Witlin (1999), the risk for developing chronic hypertension later in life is 24%. Therefore the postpartum nurse should discuss lifestyle modifications for the prevention of hypertension after pregnancy as presented by the National Institutes of Health (JNC VII, 2003).

Critical Care Interventions for Invasive Hemodynamic Monitoring

- Recommended indications for use of invasive hemodynamic monitoring: Because it is impossible to differentiate clinically among the varying causative factors of severe preeclampsia or eclampsia, invasive hemodynamic monitoring is being recommended for severe preeclampsia or eclampsia complicated with pulmonary edema, oliguria unresponsive to fluid challenge, or severe hypertension unresponsive to hydralazine treatment (ACOG, 2002).
- A pulmonary artery catheter (Swan-Ganz catheter) that continuously evaluates central vein and pulmonary artery pressures and intermittent measurement of central venous pressure and pulmonary capillary wedge pressure should be used for hemodynamic monitoring. This allows precise assessment of the underlying pathophysiology, thus allowing the medical team to specifically tailor and evaluate the therapy.
- Table 22-11 lists manifestations of preeclampsia that should be evaluated with invasive hemodynamic monitoring and treatment protocols.
- *Oliguria*, defined as less than 25 ml of urine over 2 consecutive hours, requires fluid challenge of 500 to 1000 ml of normal saline or Ringer's lactate over 30 minutes. An unresponsive urine output in a patient not ready to deliver indicates the need for invasive hemodynamic monitoring.
- *Acute pulmonary edema* usually responds to the following treatment plan:
  - Have the patient sit upright.
  - Administer oxygen by face mask at 8 to 10 L/min to increase arterial oxygen saturation.
  - Reduce anxiety and dilate the pulmonary and systemic veins by administering morphine sulfate at 2 to 5 mg IV every 10 minutes unless near the time of delivery.
  - Improve diuresis with furosemide 40 mg IV. Although furosemide is one of the medications of choice for treatment of CHF and pulmonary edema in pregnancy, the therapeutic value for the maternal patient must be weighed against the potential risks to the fetus.
  - The goal is 1800 to 2000 ml diuresis to improve pulmonary edema.
  - Use invasive hemodynamic monitoring.

Intrapartum Interventions for Preeclampsia

- *Delivery* is indicated in the preeclamptic patient for the following reasons: deterioration of fetal well-being, treatment ineffective in improving the disease as evidenced by worsening maternal symptoms or laboratory evidence of end-organ dysfunction, or eclampsia or warning signs of eclampsia.
- *Vaginal delivery* is usually attempted and achieved after induction with oxytocin.
- *Cesarean birth* is the method of delivery if the following conditions are present: labor does not begin promptly after attempted induction, vaginal delivery is contraindicated for other obstetric reasons, or the fetus weighs less than 1500 g.
- *Continue to assess and implement precise care* that was outlined for the antepartum period.
- *Continuous IV* of 5% D_5W and lactated Ringer's solution at 100 to 150 ml an hour or as assessment indicates is needed.

Table 22-11   Manifestations of Preeclampsia That Should Be Evaluated with Invasive Hemodynamic Monitoring

Disease Manifestation	Causes	Hemodynamic Values	Possible Treatment
Hypertensive crisis	Increased cardiac output related to increased heart rate and stroke volume Increased systemic vascular resistance	Normal preload High cardiac output Increased PCWP (≥18 mm Hg)	Reduce cardiac preload with beta-blocker agents and vasodilators Reduce systemic vascular resistance Bedrest in left lateral position Antihypertensive therapy such as hydralazine hydrochloride
Pulmonary edema	Noncardiogenic • Decreased colloid osmotic pressure • Increased pulmonary capillary permeability	Normal PCWP (<18 mm Hg) Normal PCWP	Administer colloid fluids Maintain filling pressures in lower-normal range
	Cardiogenic • Volume overload related to left ventricular failure resulting from high vascular resistance	Increased PCWP (>18 mm Hg)	Decrease afterload with bedrest and antihypertensive therapy
	• Volume overload related to iatrogenic fluid overload	Increased CVP	Attempt diuresis with diuretic such as furosemide, O_2, morphine
	• Volume overload related to normal postpartum mobilization of third-space fluid (diuresis)	Normal or increased PCWP	

Continued

Table 22-11   Manifestations of Preeclampsia That Should Be Evaluated with Invasive Hemodynamic Monitoring—cont'd

Disease Manifestation	Causes	Hemodynamic Values	Possible Treatment
Oliguria	*Hypovolemic:* Decreased renal blood flow related to intravascular volume depletion	Decreased PCWP Decreased cardiac output Increased SVR	Administer colloid or crystalloid fluid boluses
	Hypervolemic: Decreased renal blood flow related to severe vascular resistance causing left ventricular failure	Increased PCWP (>18 mm Hg) Increased SVR Decreased cardiac output Decreased vascular resistance	Decrease vascular resistance Bedrest in the left lateral position Aggressive afterload reduction and diuresis Antihypertensive drugs such as hydralazine hydrochloride
	Renal arteriospasms: Specific renal arteriospasms disproportionate to systemic vasospasms	Normal PCWP Normal cardiac output Normal SVR	Treat with low-dose dopamine infusion (1–5 mcg 1 kg/min)

CVP, Central venous pressure; PCWP, pulmonary capillary wedge pressure; SVR, systemic vascular resistance.

- *Hourly input and output* is evaluated.
- *Monitor labor progress* closely because the patient may not be aware of the strength and frequency of her contractions.
- *Continuous electronic fetal monitoring* is required because the uteroplacental blood flow is already compromised, and the added stress of labor may be too much for the fetus. Magnesium sulfate crosses the placenta readily. It can cause decreased beat-to-beat variability as seen on the fetal monitor strip. However, there is no indication that it adversely affects the fetus as long as the mother's serum magnesium level does not reach toxic levels.
- *Allay anxiety.* The patient is usually very anxious about the well-being of the fetus and her own condition. Most women with preeclampsia or eclampsia are transferred to a high risk center. This can mean that they are a long way from home without any family members available. This adds to the anxiety and stress of the condition. Therefore it is important for nurses who are providing skilled care to attempt to allay anxiety.
- *Analgesia during labor* is limited to small doses and is withheld during the 2 hours before delivery. If the fetus is premature, analgesics should be avoided;

they further depress an already compromised fetus. Administering anesthesia to a patient with preeclampsia has added risks. Regional anesthesia such as intrathecal or epidural block is the preferred method except in the presence of coagulopathy. Because of the hemorrhagic risk, regional anesthesia should not be used in the presence of severe thrombocytopenia (platelet count less than 75,000/mm^3) (ACOG, 2002). A general anesthesia may further elevate the blood pressure, especially during induction and awakening.

Postpartum Interventions for Preeclampsia

Nursing Interventions

If the patient has been receiving magnesium sulfate or another anticonvulsant, it is usually continued for 24 to 48 hours following delivery or longer if the HELLP syndrome coexists (Sibai, 2007). During this time, the patient's condition is monitored as closely as before; her condition can still deteriorate. This risk may be enhanced by normal postpartum diuresis. As diuresis takes place, an increased loss of magnesium leads to a drop in serum magnesium below therapeutic levels, and a convulsion could result. Blood loss is not tolerated as well as in the healthy postpartum patient because of the reduced blood volume caused by the disease process. Therefore the nurse should monitor the blood loss closely. Because of the increased risk of pulmonary edema, assess intake and output, pulse oximetry, and auscultate breath sounds. These patients are also at increased risk of stroke and thromboembolism.

If the HELLP syndrome coexists, platelets, AST, ALT, and LDH levels are appropriate indicators of severity and progress toward recovery. There is a direct correlation between severity of the disease and the length of time for recovery.

Psychologic needs are great during the postpartum period. If the mother was not fully alert for all or part of the labor and delivery, it is important to fill in the gaps of the event for her. Most parents are also very concerned about their neonate's well-being. If the neonate was born prematurely or has IUGR and is in the intensive care nursery (ICN), the mother should be shown pictures of the infant and kept informed about the infant's condition. The father should be encouraged to visit the ICN. Then, when the mother's condition becomes stable, arrangements should be made for her to visit the ICN. Even if the neonate is healthy, the mother will need extra support because she will be separated from her infant for a large portion of the first day or two following delivery. The mother needs limited neuromuscular stimulation and therefore is kept in a dark, quiet environment with limited visitors.

The parents might be concerned about the effects of magnesium on their neonate. It is a relatively safe drug in relationship to the disease process (Weiner and Buhimschi, 2009). The neonate may appear hypotonic at first. The parents should be informed that this is a temporary condition and it does not indicate neurologic damage. The mother may also be concerned about breastfeeding and the effects of magnesium. She should be reassured that no negative effect has been implicated and that the levels of magnesium in breast milk are usually even less than in some formulas (Weiner and Buhimschi, 2009).

On the other hand, the patient who has chronic hypertension and must continue on hypertensive therapy should understand that antihypertensives are excreted in breast milk. The effect on the infant is unknown. If the patient has mild hypertension, the health care provider may withhold the medication during breastfeeding and closely observe the patient's blood pressure. For the patient with severe hypertension, the same antihypertensive drugs that are recommended during pregnancy seem to be the safest during breastfeeding, as long as they are taken at the lowest dose possible for hypertensive management (National High Blood Pressure Education Program Working Group, 2000).

Long-term effects are listed under the respective nursing intervention sections. However, the increased risk for preeclampsia and hypertension and cardiovascular disease later in life direct the nurse to encourage lifestyle modifications for the prevention of hypertension as outlined by the National Institutes of Health (Irgens and others, 2001; JNC VII, 2003; Kestenbaum and others, 2003; Freeman and others, 2004; Van Pampus and Aarnoudse, 2005).

All types of contraception are available to hypertensive women, provided that compliance and close follow-up can be guaranteed, according to Repke (2001). However, the risks of oral contraceptives must be discussed completely if that method is considered. Estrogen has a negative effect on various clotting factors, total cholesterol, triglycerides, and angiotensinogen. Progesterone has a negative effect on high-density lipoprotein, low-density lipoprotein, and insulin resistance. In contrast, the benefits of these methods should also be presented.

CONCLUSION

The ultimate goal of the nurse is to prevent hypertensive disorders of pregnancy or to assist in early diagnosis and appropriate treatment of these disorders to maximize outcome. Preeclampsia is a much studied disease of pregnancy, but the triggering factor remains unknown. This makes prevention difficult; however, because research indicates that several factors, such as early appropriate prenatal care, adequate fluid intake, and optimal nutrition, play important roles, the nurse should include these in the prenatal instructions. When a patient develops preeclampsia during pregnancy, the goal becomes the prevention of eclampsia and uteroplacental insufficiency while attempting to facilitate fetal maturity. Therefore, preeclampsia is treated in hopes of stabilizing the condition until fetal maturity is reached. If treatment is effective, diuresis should occur within 18 to 36 hours. Positive signs of stabilization are increased output and a decrease in weight, blood pressure, edema, and proteinuria. If preeclampsia does not respond to treatment, delivery is the treatment of choice to prevent eclampsia and uteroplacental insufficiency.

Other hypertensive disorders of pregnancy are treated to keep the diastolic blood pressure below 100 mm Hg to prevent maternal cardiovascular complications and uterine insufficiency.

BIBLIOGRAPHY

Aagaard-Tillery K, Belfort M: Eclampsia: morbidity, mortality, and management, *Clin Obstet Gynecol* 48(1):12–23, 2005.

Abalos E, Duley L, Steyn DW, Henderson-Smart DJ: Antihypertensive drug therapy for mild to moderate hypertension during pregnancy, *Cochrane Database Syst Rev* (Issue 4), Art. No.: CD002252, 2006.

Al-Mulhim A, and others: Pre-eclampsia: maternal risk factors and perinatal outcome, *Fetal Diagn Ther* 18(4):275–280, 2003.

American College of Obstetricians and Gynecologists (ACOG): *Antepartum fetal surveillance,* ACOG Tech Bull, No. 9, Washington DC, 1999, ACOG.

American College of Obstetricians and Gynecologists (ACOG): *Diagnosis and management of preeclampsia and eclampsia,* ACOG Pract Bull, No. 33, Washington DC, 2002, ACOG.

Amorium M, Santas L, Faundes A: Corticosteroid therapy for prevention of respiratory distress syndrome in severe preeclampsia, *Am J Obstet Gynecol* 180:1283, 1999.

Anumba D, Robson S: Management of pre-eclampsia and haemolysis, elevated liver enzymes, and low platelets syndrome, *Curr Opin Obstet Gynecol* 11(2):149–156, 1999.

Atallah A, Duley L, Hofmeyr G: Dietary calcium supplementation for prevention of preeclampsia and related problems: a systematic review and commentary, *Intl J Obstet Gynaecol* 114:933–943, 2007.

Barton J, and others: Does advanced maternal age affect pregnancy outcomes in women with mild hypertension remote from term? *Am J Obstet Gynecol* 176(6):1236–1240, 1997.

Barton J, and others: Monitored outpatient management of mild gestational hypertension remote from term in teenage pregnancies, *Am J Obstet Gynecol* 173(6):1865–1868, 1995.

Barton J, Sibai B: Prediction and prevention of recurrent preeclampsia, *Obstet Gynecol* 112(2):359–372, 2008.

Barton J, Stanziano G, Sibai B: Monitored outpatient management of mild gestational hypertension remote from term, *Am J Obstet Gynecol* 170(3):765–769, 1994.

Baylis C, and others: Recent insights into the roles of nitric oxide and renin-angiotensin in the pathophysiology of preeclamptic pregnancy, *Semin Nephrol* 18(2):208–230, 1998.

Boggess K, and others: Maternal periodontal disease is associated with an increased risk for preeclampsia, *Obstet Gynecol* 101(2):227–231, 2003.

Branch D, Dudley D, Michell M: Preliminary evidence for homeostatic mechanism regulating endothelin production in preeclampsia, *Lancet* 337(8747):943–945, 1991.

Brown M, and others: Randomised trial of management of hypertensive pregnancies by Korotkoff phase IV or phase V, *Lancet* 352(9130):777–781, 1998.

Chen B, and others: Correlation of catheterized and clean catch urine protein/creatinine ratios in preeclampsia evaluation, *Obstet Gynecol* 112(3):606–610, 2008.

Chen X, Perkins S, Rennicks-White R, and others: Folic acid supplementation in early second trimester and the risk of preeclampsia, *Am J Obstet Gynecol* 198:45–47, 2008.

Chesley L, Cooper D: Genetics of hypertension in pregnancy: possible single gene control of pre-eclampsia and eclampsia in the descendants of eclamptic women, *Br J Obstet Gynaecol* 93(9): 898–908, 1986.

Clark B, and others: Plasma endothelin levels in preeclampsia: elevation and correlation with uric acid levels and renal impairment, *Am J Obstet Gynecol* 166(3):962–968, 1992.

CLASP Collaborative Group: Low dose aspirin in pregnancy and early childhood development: follow up of collaborative low dose aspirin study in pregnancy, *Br J Obstet Gynaecol* 102(11):861–868, 1995.

Conde-Agudelo A, Villar J, Lindheimer M: World Health Organization systematic review of screening tests for preeclampsia, *Obstet Gynecol* 104(6):1367–1391, 2004.

Cotter A, and others: Elevated plasma homocysteine in early pregnancy: a risk factor for the development of nonsevere preeclampsia, *Am J Obstet Gynecol* 189(2):391–394, 2003.

Cox S, Kilpatrick S, Geller S: Preventing maternal deaths, *Contemp Ob Gyn,* 49(9):78-80, 2004.

Crowther C, Bouwmeester A, Ashurst H: Does admission to hospital for bedrest prevent disease progression or improve fetal outcome in pregnancy complicated by nonproteinuric hypertension? *Br J Obstet Gynaecol* 99(1):13–17, 1992.

Cunningham F, Leveno K, Bloom S, Hauth J, Rouse D, Spong C: *Williams' obstetrics,* ed 23, New York, 2010, McGraw-Hill Medical.

Davey D, MacGillivray I: The classification and definition of the hypertensive disorders of pregnancy, *Am J Obstet Gynecol* 158(4):892–898, 1988.

Dekker G: Prevention of preeclampsia. In Sibai B, editor: *Hypertensive disorders in women,* Philadelphia, 2001, Saunders.

Dekker G, Sibai B: The immunology of preeclampsia, *Semin Perinatol* 23(1):24–33, 1999.

DiPasquale L, Lynett K: The use of water immersion for treatment of massive labial edema during pregnancy, *MCN Am J Matern Child Nurs* 28(4):242–245, 2003.

Duley L, Gülmezoglu AM, Henderson-Smart DJ: Magnesium sulphate and other anticonvulsants for women with pre-eclampsia, *Cochrane Database Syst Rev* (Issue 1), 2003, Art. No.: CD000025.

Duley L, Henderson-Smart DJ: Magnesium sulphate versus diazepam for eclampsia, *Cochrane Database Syst Rev* (Issue 3), Art. No.: CD000127, 2003a.

Duley L, Henderson-Smart DJ: Magnesium sulphate versus phenytoin for eclampsia, *Cochrane Database Syst Rev* (Issue 3), Art. No.: CD000128, 2003b.

Duley L, Henderson-Smart DJ, Meher S: Altered dietary salt for preventing pre-eclampsia, and its complications, *Cochrane Database Syst Rev* (Issue 4), Art. No.: CD005548, 2005.

Duley L, Henderson-Smart DJ, Meher S, King JF: Antiplatelet agents for preventing pre-eclampsia and its complications, *Cochrane Database Syst Rev* (Issue 1), Art. No.: CD004659, 2007.

Eclampsia Trial Collaborative Group: Which anticonvulsant for women with eclampsia? Evidence from the collaborative eclampsia trial, *Lancet* 345(8963):1455–1463, 1995.

Egerman R, Sibai B: Preconception counseling for women with a history of hypertensive disorders. In Sibai B, editor: *Hypertensive disorders in women*, Philadelphia, 2001, Saunders.

Erogul M: Pregnancy, preeclampsia, *EMedicine specialties*, 2008. Retrieved from http://www.emedicine.com/emerg/topic480.htm.

Flack J, and others: Hypertension in special populations, *Cardiol Clin* 20(2):303–319, 2002.

Foley M: *Hypertensive emergencies during pregnancy: a general overview*, Phoenix, AZ, April 7, 2001, Presented at Obstetrical Challenges of the New Millennium.

Freeman D, and others: Short- and long-term changes in plasma inflammatory markers associated with preeclampsia, *Hypertension* 44(5):708–714, 2004.

Friedman S, and others: Mild gestational hypertension and preeclampsia. In Sibai B, editor: *Hypertensive disorders in women*, Philadelphia, 2001, Saunders.

Ghabour M, and others: Immunohistochemical characterization of placental nitric oxide synthase expression in preeclampsia, *Am J Obstet Gynecol* 173(3 Pt 1):687–694, 1995.

Green L, Froman R: Blood pressure measurement during pregnancy: auscultatory versus oscillatory methods, *J Obstet Gynecol Neonatal Nurs* 25(2):155–159, 1996.

Gudnasson H, Dubiel M, Gudmundsson S: Preeclampsia: abnormal uterine artery Doppler is related to recurrence of symptoms during the next pregnancy, *J Perinat Med* 32(5):400–403, 2004.

Gundersson E: Nutrition during pregnancy for the physically active woman, *Clin Obstet Gynecol* 46(2):390–402, 2003.

Haddad B, Sibai S: Expectant management of severe preeclampsia: proper candidates and pregnancy outcome, *Clin Obstet Gynecol* 48(2):430–440, 2005.

Hayman R: Hypertension in pregnancy, *Curr Opin Obstet Gynecol* 14(1):1–10, 2004.

Hofmeyr GJ, Atallah ÁN, Duley L: Calcium supplementation during pregnancy for preventing hypertensive disorders and related problems, *Cochrane Database Syst Rev* (Issue 1), Art. No.: CD001059, 2006.

International Food Information Council Foundation (IFIC): *Healthy eating during pregnancy*, Washington, DC, 2008, Author. Retrieved from http://www.ific.org/publications/brochures/upload/2008HealthyEatingPregnancy.pdf.

Irgens H, and others: Long term mortality of mothers and fathers after pre-eclampsia: population based cohort study, *BMJ* 323(7323):1213–1217, 2001.

Joint National Committee (JNC VII): *Prevention, detection, evaluation, treatment of high blood pressure*, NIH Publication No. 03–5233, Bethesda, Md, 2003, U.S. Dept. of Health and Human Services. Retrieved from http://www.nhlbi.nih.gov/guidelines/hypertension/jncintro.htm

Katz V, and others: A comparison of bed rest and immersion for treating the edema of pregnancy, *Obstet Gynecol* 75(2):147–151, 1990.

Katz V, and others: Effect of daily immersion on the edema of pregnancy, *Am J Perinatol* 9(4):225–227, 1992.

Kent T, and others: Edema of pregnancy: a comparison of water aerobics and static immersion, *Obstet Gynecol* 94(5 Pt 1):726–729, 1999.

Kestenbaum B, and others: Cardiovascular and thromboembolic events following hypertensive pregnancy, *Am J Kidney Dis* 42(5):982–989, 2003.

Khalil A, Jauniaux E, Harrington K: Antihypertensive therapy and central hemodynamics in women with hypertensive disorders in pregnancy, *Obstet Gynecol* 113(3):646–654, 2009.

Kupferminc M, Fair G, Mary A, and others: Low molecular weight heparin for the prevention of obstetric complications in women with thrombophilia, *Hypertens Pregnancy* 20:35, 2001.

Levine R, and others: Two-stage elevation of cell-free fetal DNA in maternal sera before onset of preeclampsia, *Am J Obstet Gynecol* 190(3):707–713, 2004.

Levine R, Karumanchi S: Circulating angiogenic factors in preeclampsia, *Clin Obstet Gynecol* 48(2): 372–386, 2005.

Lin J, August P: Genetic thrombophilias and preeclampsia: a meta-analysis, *Obstet Gynecol* 105(1): 182–192, 2005.

Lowenstein C, Dinerman J, Snyder S: Nitric oxide: a physiologic messenger, *Ann Intern Med* 120(3):227–237, 1994.

Lucas L, Jordan E: Phenytoin as an alternative treatment for preeclampsia, *J Obstet Gynecol Neonatal Nurs* 26(3):263–269, 1997.

Mabie W: Life-threatening complications of hypertension in pregnancy. In Sibai B, editor: *Hypertensive disorders in women*, Philadelphia, 2001, Saunders.

MacKay A, Berg C, Atrash H: Pregnancy-related mortality from preeclampsia and eclampsia, *Obstet Gynecol* 9(4):533–538, 2001.

Mahomed K, Bhutta ZA, Middleton P: Zinc supplementation for improving pregnancy and infant outcome, *Cochrane Database Syst Rev* (Issue 1), Art. No.: CD000230, 2007.

Makrides M, Crowther CA: Magnesium supplementation in pregnancy, *Cochrane Database Syst Rev* (Issue 3), Art. No.: CD000937, 2001.

Manten G, and others: The role of lipoprotein (a) in pregnancies complicated by pre-eclampsia, *Med Hypotheses* 64(1):162–169, 2005.

Martin J, and others: The natural history of HELLP syndrome: patterns of disease progression and regression, *Am J Obstet Gynecol* 164(6 Pt 1):1500–1509, 1991.

Mattar F, Sibai B: Eclampsia VIII risk factor for maternal morbidity, *Am J Obstet Gynecol* 182:307, 2000.

Meher S, Abalos E, Carroli G: Bed rest with or without hospitalisation for hypertension during pregnancy, *Cochrane Database Syst Rev* (Issue 4), Art. No.: CD003514, 2007.

Mello G, Parretti E, Marozio L: Thrombophilia is significantly associated with severe preeclampsia: results of a large scale case-controlled study, *Hypertension* 46:1270, 2005.

Mignini L, and others: Mapping the theories of preeclampsia: the role of homocysteine, *Obstet Gynecol* 105(2):411–425, 2005.

Mills J, and others: Prostacyclin and thromboxane changes predating clinical onset of preeclampsia: a multicenter prospective study, *JAMA* 282(4):356–362, 1999.

Moreau P, Contu L, Alba F, and others: HLA-G gene polymorphism in human placentas: possible association of G*0106 allele with preeclampsia and miscarriage, *Biol Reprod* 79:459–467, 2008.

Myatt L, Miodovnik M: Prediction of preeclampsia, *Semin Perinatol* 23(1):45–57, 1999.

National High Blood Pressure Education Program Working Group: Report on high blood pressure in pregnancy, *Am J Obstet Gynecol* 183(1):S1–S22, 2000.

National Institutes of Health (NIH): *Antenatal corticosteroids revisited.* Consensus development conference statement, Maryland, 2000, NIH. Retrieved from http://consensus.nih.gov.

Nick J: Deep tendon reflexes: the what, why, where, and how of tapping, *J Obstet Gynecol Neonatal Nurs* 32(3):297–306, 2003.

Nick J: Deep tendon reflexes, magnesium, and calcium: assessments and implications, *J Obstet Gynecol Neonatal Nurs* 33(2):221–230, 2004.

Nova A, and others: Maternal plasma level of endothelin is increased in preeclampsia, *Am J Obstet Gynecol* 165(3):724–727, 1991.

O'Brien J, Barton J: Controversies with the diagnosis and management of HELLP syndrome, *Clin Obstet Gynecol* 48(2):460–477, 2005.

O'Brien J, Milligan D, Barton J: Impact of high-dose corticosteroid therapy for patients with HELLP (hemolysis, elevated liver enzymes, and low platelet count) syndrome, *Am J Obstet Gynecol* 183(4):921–924, 2000.

O'Brien T, Ray J, Chan W: Maternal body mass index and the risk of preeclampsia: a systematic overview, *Epidemiology* 14:368, 2003.

Odendaal H: Severe preeclampsia eclampsia. In Sibai B, editor: *Hypertensive disorders in women*, Philadelphia, 2001, Saunders.

Paruk F, Moodley J: Antihypertensive therapy for the management of mild-to moderate hypertension? In Studd J, editor: *Progress in obstetrics and gynaecology*, Edinburgh, 2005, Churchill Livingstone.

Patrick T, Roberts J: Current concepts in preeclampsia, *MCN Am J Matern Child Nurs* 24(4):193–200, 1999.

Perkins A: Endogenous antioxidants in pregnancy and preeclampsia, *Aust N Z J Obstet Gynaecol* 46:77–83, 2006.

Phelan J, Easter T: HELLP syndrome: the great masquerader, *Female Patient* 15(2):79, 1990.

Repke J: Contraception in the woman with hypertension. In Sibai B, editor: *Hypertensive disorders in women*, Philadelphia, 2001, Saunders.

Roberts J, and others: Summary of the NHLBI Working Group on research on hypertension during pregnancy, *Hypertension* 41(3):437–445, 2003.

Roberts J, Funai F: Pregnancy-related hypertension. In Creasy R, Resnik R, Iams J, and others, editors: *Creasy & Resnik's maternal-fetal medicine: principles and practice*, ed 6, Philadelphia, 2009, Saunders.

Scholl T, and others: Oxidative stress, diet, and the etiology of preeclampsia, *Am J Clin Nutr* 81(6): 1390–1396, 2005.

Sibai B: Diagnosis, prevention, and management of eclampsia, *Obstet Gynecol* 105(2):402–410, 2005.

Sibai B: Hypertension. In Gabbe S, Niebyl J, Simpson J, editors: *Obstetrics: normal and problem pregnancies*, ed 5, New York, 2007, Churchill Livingstone.

Sibai B, and others: Maternal morbidity and mortality in 442 pregnancies with hemolysis, elevated liver enzymes, and low platelets (HELLP syndrome), *Am J Obstet Gynecol* 169(4):1000–1006, 1993.

Sibai B, Dekker G, Kupfermine M: Pre-eclampsia, *Lancet* 365:785, 2005.

Spinnato J, Livingston J: Prevention of preeclampsia with antioxidants: evidence from randomized trials, *Clin Obstet Gynecol* 48(2):416–429, 2005.

Stella C, Ghulmiyyah L, Sibai B: Thrombophilia and adverse maternal-perinatal outcomes, *Female Patient* 31:42–48, 2006.

Strong T: Reversal of oligohydramnios with subtotal immersion: a report of five cases, *Am J Obstet Gynecol* 169(6):1595–1597, 1993.

Taylor R: Review: immunobiology of preeclampsia, *Am J Reprod Immunol* 37(1):79–86, 1997.

Tuffnell D, and others: Randomised controlled trial of day care for hypertension in pregnancy, *Lancet* 339(8787):224–227, 1992.

U.S. Department of Health and Human Services (USDHHS): *Healthy People 2010: understanding and improving health*, Washington, DC, 2000, USDHHS.

van Beck E, Peeters L: Pathogenesis of preeclampsia: a comprehensive model, *Obstet Gynecol Surv* 53(4):233–239, 1998.

Van Pampus M, Aarnoudse J: Long-term outcomes after preeclampsia, *Clin Obstet Gynecol* 48(2): 489–494, 2005.

Var A, and others: Endothelial dysfunction in preeclampsia: increased homocysteine and decreased nitric oxide levels, *Gynecol Obstet Invest* 56(4):221–224, 2003.

Vedernikov Y, Saade G, Garfield R: Vascular reactivity in preeclampsia, *Semin Perinatol* 23(1):34–44, 1999.

von Dadelszen P, Magee L: Antihypertensive medications in management of gestational hypertension-preeclampsia, *Clin Obstet Gynecol* 48(2):441–459, 2005.

Walfisch A, Hallak M: Hypertension. In James D, and others, editors: *High risk pregnancy: management options*, ed 3, Philadelphia, 2006, Saunders.

Walsh S: Physiology of low dose aspirin therapy for the prevention of preeclampsia, *Semin Perinatol* 14(2):152–170, 1990.

Wang Y, and others: Maternal levels of prostacyclin, thromboxane, vitamin E, and lipid peroxides throughout normal pregnancy, *Am J Obstet Gynecol* 165(6 Pt 1):1690–1694, 1991a.

Wang Y, and others: The imbalance between thromboxane and prostacyclin in preeclampsia is associated with an imbalance between lipid peroxides and vitamin E in maternal blood, *Am J Obstet Gynecol* 165(6 Pt 1):1695–1700, 1991b.

Wang Y, and others: Evidence of endothelial dysfunction in preeclampsia: decreased endothelial nitric oxide synthase expression is associated with increased cell permeability in endothelial cells from preeclampsia, *Am J Obstet Gynecol* 190(3):817–824, 2004.

Wardlaw G, Smith A: *Contemporary nutrition*, ed 7, Boston, 2008, McGraw-Hill.

Weiner C, Buhimschi C: *Drugs for pregnant and lactating women*, ed 2, Philadelphia, 2009, Saunders.

Weinstein L: Preeclampsia/eclampsia with hemolysis, elevated liver enzymes, and thrombocytopenia, *Obstet Gynecol* 66(5):657–660, 1985.

Williamson C: Molecular biology related to pre-eclampsia, *Institute Reprod Dev Biol* 1279:282, 2005.

Williamson C, Girling J: Hepatic gastrointestinal disease. In James D, and others, editors: *High risk pregnancy: management options*, ed 3, Philadelphia, 2006, Saunders.

Witlin A: Counseling for women with preeclampsia and eclampsia, *Semin Perinatol* 23(1):91–98, 1999.

23

Preterm Labor and Multiple Gestation

PRETERM LABOR

Preterm labor (PTL) can be defined as regular uterine contractions that cause progressive dilation of the cervix after 20 weeks of gestation and before 36 completed weeks. Late preterm birth is a recent term used for preterm birth between 34 0/7 and 36 6/7 completed weeks of gestation.

MULTIPLE GESTATION

A multiple gestation can result from fertilization of one egg by one sperm that splits, which is called *monozygotic multiple fetus*. Multiple gestations can also result from fertilization of two or more eggs called *dizygotic*. Or multiple gestations can result from a combination of these two processes.

Because of the increased likelihood for infertile couples who become pregnant with any fertility method to have twins or more, we now see many more successful pregnancy outcomes. However, with this success comes an increased incidence of preterm births of the multiples. Currently, some perinatal programs are reporting equally successful outcomes with quadruplet and triplet births as with twin births (Elliott, 2000). Although quadruplets and triplets are more likely to deliver by 32 to 34 weeks than are twins, ultimately their outcome successes rival twins (Elliott, 2000). Multiple gestations with more than four fetuses have an extremely high loss rate of all fetuses and probably fall more in the "miraculous" survival rather than a statistical prediction model (Elliott, 2000).

PTL with multiple gestation is more difficult for the pregnant woman to identify. It can be confused with the extra aches and pains from rapid stretching and pressure, and it can be confused with kicks and movements of multiple babies. In addition, the overdistention of the uterus contributes to increased irritability of the uterus.

INCIDENCE

Approximately 13% of all pregnancies end in PTL (Hamilton, Martin, Ventura, and others, 2007). Approximately 76% of all PTL occurs in the late preterm period (McIntire and Leveno, 2008). Prematurity in the newborn continues to account for

75% to 80% of neonatal morbidity and mortality (Hamilton and others, 2007). The rate of multiple gestations is rapidly rising (19% increase), secondary to new technologies in infertility treatment. Twins have a 50% preterm birth rate, and triplets and higher-order multiples have a 90% preterm birth rate (Russell and others, 2002). In addition, there are significant racial differences in preterm birth rates: whites, 10.4%; blacks, 18.2%; Native Americans, 13.3%; Hispanics, 10.5%; and Asians, 11% (Behrman and Stith, 2007). Sociodemographics affect preterm birth as well, with rates of preterm birth being highest among the lower educated (Behrman and Stith, 2007).

ETIOLOGY

PTL is currently thought to be a chronic, long-term, multifactorial process with a genetic component (Ward and others, 2005; Crider, Whitehead, and Buus, 2006). Four intertwined pathways are being proposed to influence the risk of spontaneous preterm uterine contractions and cervical changes: altered uterine and cervical factors, placental ischemia; inflammation, and stress. Bacterial infections account for 25% to 40% of all preterm births because endotoxins have a preinflammatory effect and stimulate prostaglandin production. In multiparas, the strongest risk factor is a history of previous preterm delivery frequently related to a short cervix, bacterial infection, or short-interval between pregnancies. Box 23-1 provides a summary of the predisposing factors of each PTL pathway.

Late preterm labor accounts for most of the increased rate of singleton prematurity in the United States in recent years. Recent research indicates that elective (without medical indication) inductions and cesarean births before 39 weeks account for this increase (Davidoff, Dias, Damus, and others, 2006; Bettegowda and others, 2008; MOD, 2009b).

NORMAL ANATOMY OF THE CERVIX

The cervix is composed mainly of connective tissue (collagen) that normally keeps the cervix strong and resists cervical effacement and dilation during the pregnancy. Normal cervical lengths, according to gestation, are as follows:
- 14 to 22 weeks of gestation: 35 to 40 mm cervical length
- 24 to 28 weeks of gestation: 35 mm cervical length
- 32 weeks or more of gestation: 30 mm cervical length

NORMAL PHYSIOLOGY OF LABOR CONTRACTIONS

Muscle contraction and relaxation occur in response to the movement of the thick (myosin) and the thin (actin) filaments. The flow of calcium regulates the movement of the filaments. Multiple mechanisms regulate the flow of calcium affecting the balance between muscle relaxation and contraction. Hormones are one important regulator of myometrial contraction.

To have a physiologic understanding of possible causes and current medical treatments for preterm labor, one must understand the physiology of labor contractions. A fetal signal (surfactant protein A [SP-A]) from the maturing lungs probably

Box 23-1   Predisposing Factors of Each PTL Pathway

Altered Uterine and Cervical Factors
- Multiple gestation
- Polyhydramnios
- Uterine anomalies (Zlopasa, Skrablin, and Kalafatic, 2007)
- Trauma, motor vehicle collision (Ananth and others, 2001)
- Assisted reproductive technology (ART)
- Cervical injury from an elective abortion or prior cervical surgery related to treatment of HPV or diethylstilbestrol (DES) exposure (Jorgensen, 2008)
- Short interconception interval (DeFranco, O'Brien, Adair, and others, 2007)
- Smoking: decreases serum vitamin C levels, which is important for collagen formation and strength of the cervix (Galan and others, 2005) and increases sensitivity of the myometrium to oxytocin (Nakamoto and others, 2006)

Placental Ischemia
- Abruptio placentae
- Gestational and chronic health conditions such as:
  - Diabetes
  - Hypertensive disorders
  - Hereditary thromboembolic disorders
  - Obesity (Rosenberg, Garber, Lipkind, and others, 2005)
  - Anemia
  - Cardiovascular disease
  - Renal disease
  - Hepatitis
  - Cholestasis
- Smoking (Cnattingius, 2004; Tikkanen, Nuutila, Hiilesmaa, and others 2006; Nabet, Lelong, Ancel, and others, 2007)
- Alcohol or illicit drug use (Behrman and Stith, 2007)
- Altered nutrition that leads to low body mass index (Hendler, Goldenberg, Mercer, and others, 2005)

Inflammation
- Bacterial infections including *Mycoplasma* of the genital tract, pyelonephritis, asymptomatic bacteriuria, and pneumonia (Goldenberg, Culhane, and Johnson, 2005)
- Gonorrhea or Chlamydia
- Symptomatic BV or trichomoniasis

Stress
- High stress level in general (Rich-Edwards and Grizzard, 2005; Giurgescu, 2009)
- Domestic violence (Jasinski, 2004)
- Single marital status (Zhong-Cheng, Wilkins, and Kramer, 2004)
- Socially disadvantaged or low education status (Thompson, Irgens, Rasmussen, and others, 2006; Reedy, 2007; Smith, Draper, Manktelow, and others, 2007)
- African American Ethnicity (Behrman and Stith, 2007)
- Long working hours, night shift, or strenuous work (Hobel, 2004; Lawsen, Whelan, Hibert, and others, 2009)

initiates normal labor (Condon and others, 2004). Following initiation, there is strong scientific evidence that various hormones interplay to influence uterine activity.

PROSTAGLANDINS

The fetal adrenal glands' production of dehydroepiandrosterone (DHEA), related to certain fetal maturational milestones, may interrupt the support of systems that serve to promote uterine quiescence and maintain pregnancy (Lockwood, 1999). This unknown fetal signal appears to stimulate macrophage-like decidua, the endometrium of pregnancy, to release interleukin-1-beta (IL-1β). IL-1β, an immune hormone, causes hydrolysis of glycerophospholipids found in the decidua, fetal membranes, and myometrium. Esterified arachidonic acid, which is stored in the glycerophospholipids, is released to free arachidonic acid (Norwitz and Lye, 2009). The release of arachidonic acid is accomplished either directly by phospholipase A2 or indirectly by phospholipase C. Both of these agents hydrolyze the membrane to release arachidonic acid.

Free arachidonic acid is then converted into prostaglandins (PGs) and thus stimulates the platelet-activating factor. Each tissue synthesizes a type of PG. For example, the decidua produces primarily $PGF_{2\alpha}$ and a small amount of PGE_2. The amniotic and chorionic fetal membranes produce PGE2, and the myometrium produces prostacyclin (PGI_2) and a small amount of $PGF_{2\alpha}$.

During labor, prostaglandins PGF_{2a} and PGE_2 and platelet-activating factor accumulate in the amniotic fluid. Along with arachidonic acid and IL-1β, $PGF_{2\alpha}$, PGE_2, and platelet-activating factor remain active for 4 to 6 hours.

Thromboxane, $PGF_{2\alpha}$, and PGE_2 prepare the myometrial muscle for labor by promoting the development of gap junctions, which are cell-to-cell contact areas, and coordinate smooth muscle contractions. These three substances stimulate myometrial contractions by facilitating the movement of calcium into the smooth muscle so that the muscle can contract and promote cervical ripening.

During pregnancy, PGI_2 quiets the uterus by inhibiting the function of gap junctions, by inhibiting release of phospholipases A2 and C, and by blocking movement of calcium into cells. Production of PGI_2 is suppressed during labor secondary to high levels of maternal and fetal cortisol (Lockwood, 2000).

Estrogen

Estrogen is produced by the corpus luteum for the first 2 to 4 weeks of gestation. Then the placenta takes over the production. Low-density lipoprotein (LDL) cholesterol is used by the fetal and maternal adrenal glands to secrete a precursor for placental estrogen. Near term, the adrenal gland, the largest fetal organ, is the primary source for placental estrogen precursor. Estriol, one form of placental estrogen, stimulates the fetal membranes and decidua to deposit glycerophospholipids.

Estrogen influences the increased number of cells and size of the myometrium, stimulates Braxton-Hicks contractions, facilitates the development of gap junctions (Castracane, 2000), and promotes oxytocin receptors. It is for this reason that oxytocin is an ineffective stimulator of myometrial contractions until late in pregnancy when estrogen levels are high. Estrogen also stimulates prostaglandin biosynthesis and inhibits progesterone synthesis in fetal membranes, thus effecting a local change in the progesterone-estrogen ratio in amniotic fluid at term.

Progesterone

Progesterone is produced by the corpus luteum for the first 4 to 6 weeks of gestation. Then it is produced by the fetal syncytiotrophoblasts at an increasing rate until 32 to 34 weeks of gestation by converting maternal plasma LDL cholesterol into progesterone. Then progesterone is maintained at a constant level, approximately 250 mg/day, until birth. During pregnancy progesterone promotes myometrial quiescence, down regulates gap junction formation, regulates cervical remodeling, and decreases production of chemokines decreasing the inflammatory response (Romero and Lockwood, 2009).

Oxytocin

It was once thought that oxytocin initiated normal labor, but it is now known to maximize uterine contraction of second-stage labor and, after delivery, to stimulate decidual prostaglandin release. Oxytocin is ineffective at stimulating uterine contractions during early pregnancy because high estrogen levels are necessary first for the formation of oxytocin receptors in the uterus. Oxytocin is also ineffective at promoting gap junctions and cervical ripening.

NORMAL PHYSIOLOGIC ADAPTATION OF MULTIPLE GESTATION

In a multiple gestation, cardiac output is increased 20% to 40% more than in a singleton pregnancy. Renal plasma flow increases and the systemic vascular resistance decreases more than in a singleton pregnancy. Placentation may differ as well. In monozygotic multiples, the fetal membranes may surround one or more fetuses and their placentas may be separate or fused. When splitting of the zygotic occurs, dichorionic diamniotic placentation results. When the splitting occurs during the morula phase, the placentation is usually monochorionic and diamniotic. If the splitting occurs after the eighth day, the placentation is monochorionic and monoamniotic.

PATHOPHYSIOLOGY

PTL is usually influenced by a breakdown in the multifactorial process that maintains the hormonal balance that preserves uterine quiescence in patients with a genetic predisposition (Crider, Whitehead, and Buus, 2006).

Infection

Inflammatory cytokines or bacterial endotoxins can stimulate prostaglandin release directly or indirectly by stimulating the release of corticotropin-releasing hormone (CRH) or interleukin (IL). In this manner, a urinary tract, vaginal, uterine, or fetal infection may stimulate PTL. Infection may be predictive as a marker in preterm birth at least 40% of the time (Goldenberg, Culhane, and Johnson, 2005; Klebanoff and Searle, 2006).

Altered Uterine Factors

Uterine factors such as myometrial stretch, hyperosmolarity, rupture of fetal membrane, or uterine trauma cause lysosomes to release phospholipase A2. Prostaglandins are then produced, stimulating the myometrium to contract. In this way, preterm premature rupture of membranes (PROM), abdominal trauma, multiple gestations, uterine anomalies causing overdistention of the uterus, and polyhydramnios can stimulate PTL.

Stress

Emotional stress can increase pro-inflammatory cytokines (interleukin-1β and tumor necrosis factor [TNF-α]) and lower levels of anti-inflammatory cytokines interleukin-4 and interleukin 10 (Giurgescu, 2009). Both elevated levels of pro-inflammatory cytokines and low levels of anti-inflammatory cytokines can activate the hypothalamus to secrete corticotrophin-releasing hormone (CRH). This hormone increases the production of prostaglandins from the fetal membranes and uterine decidua and stimulates the fetal pituitary gland to release adrenocorticotropin (ACTH) and the fetal adrenal gland to release DHEAS, enhancing oxytocin and prostaglandin receptors.

Placental Ischemia

Factors that decrease blood flow to the uterus may also cause the release of CRH. Therefore conditions during pregnancy that interfere with uterine or placental blood flow can trigger PTL. Some of these conditions are preeclampsia, poorly controlled diabetes, heart disease, renal disease, abruptio placentae, or placenta previa. Altered nutrition, smoking, or illicit drug use may stimulate PTL in this manner as well.

Table 23-1 summarizes the interrelationships among the different endocrine factors that contribute to the control of labor or the development of PTL.

MATERNAL EFFECTS

Preterm Labor

The most common direct effect on the mother is psychologic stress from the threat of a preterm delivery on the health and well-being of the expected baby. Other maternal consequences are related to the side effects of the medical treatment, such as prolonged bedrest and the use of labor suppressant drugs, on the mother's health.

Multiple Gestation

Complications such as pregnancy-induced hypertension, abruptio placentae, and anemia are more likely in the multiple gestation pregnancy. Labor suppressant drugs place the multifetal gestation at higher risk than a singleton pregnancy, especially to pulmonary edema. When one fetus dies, disseminated intravascular coagulation results.

FETAL AND NEONATAL EFFECTS

Preterm Labor

PTL leads to the birth of an infant whose body processes are immature. These infants have an increased risk for birth trauma and an increased difficulty adjusting to extrauterine life. Special problems seen in the preterm infant are as follows:
- Respiratory distress syndrome
- Intraventricular or pulmonary hemorrhage
- Patent ductus arteriosus

Table 23-1 Factors Influencing Uterine Activity

Factor	Role	Maintain Pregnancy	Promote Labor
Cervix	Collagen and fibrous connective tissue (ground substance) resist gravity force.	Closure of cervix maintained by progesterone	Cervix ripened by: • Breakdown of collagen by collagenase • Breakdown of connective tissue • Addition of more water Estrogen increases collagenase activity. Prostaglandin E_2 increases cervical extensibility. Cervical trauma can cause early cervical dilation.
Gap junctions	Cell-to-cell contact areas that coordinate smooth muscle contraction	Kept inactive by prostacyclin	Formed by: • Estrogen • Thromboxane
Calcium	Free calcium in the cytoplasm of the cell essential for smooth muscle contractions	Decreases in intracellular calcium favor myometrial relaxation: • Prostacyclin Calcium channel blockers: • Nifedipine • Magnesium calcium substitution	Increases intracellular calcium: • Oxytocin • Prostaglandin F_{2a} • Thromboxane
Autonomic nervous system	Innervates uterus • Beta receptors—inhibit uterine contractility • Alpha receptors—stimulate uterine contractility	Medications that stimulate beta receptors: • Terbutaline	Hormone that stimulates alpha receptors: • Norepinephrine Stress stimulates norepinephrine release.
Progesterone	Placenta hormone of pregnancy	Normally promotes uterine relaxation. Keeps cervical collagen together.	As estrogen-to-progesterone ratio increases, collagenase is released, breaking down cervical collagen; cervical softening results. When combined with oxytocin and prostaglandins, relaxation effect may be lost.
Relaxin	Protein hormone produced by the corpus luteum	Suppresses myometrial contraction with progesterone	Promotes cervical ripening Increased levels increase preterm labor

Oxytocin	Promotes uterine contractility if oxytocin receptors are present. Oxytocin receptors are myometrial cell components that allow oxytocin to attach.	Normally held in check by: • Progesterone. Oxytocin antagonist may be beneficial in stopping preterm labor. Oxytocin sensitivity decreased in postterm patients	Estrogen promotes formation of oxytocin receptors in the myometrial muscle. Levels normally do not rise before labor but during active labor enhance contraction strength. Uterine oxytocin release is stimulated by: • DHEA • Fetal hormone • Estrogen • Stress such as immobility or bedrest
Prostaglandins	Prostaglandins E_2, F_{2a}, thromboxane cause uterine contractions and cervical ripening	Production suppressed by: • Progesterone • Prostaglandin synthetase inhibitors help arrest: • PTL • Indomethacin	Production stimulated by: • Estrogen • Uterine hypoxia caused by maternal smoking, drug use (e.g., cocaine), or hypertension
Vasopressin	Antidiuretic hormone related structurally to oxytocin. Primary action is to conserve body water	Hydration can reduce secretion of and decrease uterine contractile activity.	Dehydration can cause increased release and uterine contractile activity.
Endothelin and cytokines	Potent uterine contractility substances that are released during an infectious process	Early diagnosis and treatment of bacterial infections including gonorrhea and chlamydia of the genital tract, pyelonephritis, asymptomatic bacteriuria, and pneumonia	Infection releases endothelin and cytokines, which stimulate increased release of oxytocin and prostaglandins.

DHEA, Dehydroepiandrosterone sulfate; *PTL*, preterm labor; *UTIs*, Urinary tract infections.

Reference: Castracane V: Endocrinology of preterm labor, *Clin Obstet Gynecol* 43(4):717–726, 2000; Ruiz R: Mechanism of full-term and preterm labor: factors influencing uterine activity, *J Obstet Gynecol Neonatal Nurs* 27(6):652–660, 1998.

- Necrotizing enterocolitis
- Retinopathy
- Hyperbilirubinemia
- Increased susceptibility to infections
- Anemia
- Ineffective temperature regulatory mechanism
- Developmental delay
- Chronic lung disease
- Later in life, increased risk for type 2 diabetes mellitus (Hofman and others, 2004)

The severity of each of these problems depends greatly on the gestational age of the infant. The greatest potential problem the preterm infant has is respiratory distress. If it is severe, hypoxia can ensue and cerebral hemorrhage, seizure disorders, and neonatal death can result. In fact, PTL accounts for 75% to 85% of all neonatal mortality and morbidity (Bernhardt and Dorman, 2004).

Emerging evidence suggests that late preterm infants are premature and have an increased mortality and morbidity risk. They experience an initial increased incidence of respiratory distress, hypoglycemia, hypothermia, hyperbilirubinemia, and feeding problems (Shaw, 2008; Clark, Miller, Belfort, and others, 2009; Tita, Landon, Spong, and others, 2009). The baby's brain is about $\frac{1}{3}$ less developed as at term (Shaw, 2008). These infants have an increased risk of SIDs (Fuchs and Wapner, 2006) and long-term neurologic deficits that can lead to hyperactivity disorders as well as learning and behavioral problems (Adams-Chapman, 2006; Engle and others, 2007).

Multiple Gestation

Prematurity is the greatest risk that occurs in multiple gestations. Diamniotic (two amniotic sacs) and monochorionic placentation is associated with high fetal uncertainty because of the risk for twin-to-twin transfusion syndrome (Jackson and Mele, 2009). This type of placentation usually results in vascular communication between placentas. One fetus tends to receive a volume overload, leading to polyuria and polyhydramnios at the expense of another fetus who becomes hypovolemic, resulting in oligohydramnios. Both fetuses are at extreme risk if untreated.

NATIONAL EFFECTS

Despite technologic and pharmacologic advances in the treatment of PTL, the preterm birth rate is higher in the United States than in 18 other industrialized nations. At the same time, the economic importance of preterm births has direct and indirect effects on us as a nation. Neonatal intensive care, primarily because of premature births, is the most expensive care service in our health care system, with estimated costs of $26 billion annually or $51,600 per preterm infant (Behrman and Butler, 2007; Galson, 2008).

DIAGNOSTIC TESTING

Risk Assessment

No routine screening tool has been effective in predicting those at high risk for PTL. Current biochemical markers being used to assist in the diagnosis of PTL in symptomatic high risk patients are listed next.

Fetal Fibronectin

Fibronectins are a family of proteins found in extracellular matrix. Fetal fibronectins (fFns) are found in fetal membranes and decidua throughout pregnancy. As the gestational sac implants and attaches to the interior of the uterus in the first half of pregnancy, fFns are normally found in cervicovaginal fluid. After 22 weeks, the presence of fFns normally is no longer detected in normal vaginal secretions until approximately 2 weeks prior to the onset of delivery, term or preterm. It is suggested that fFns be released into the cervix and the vagina when mechanical- or inflammatory-mediated damage occurs to the membranes (McParland, Jones, and Taylor, 2004).

This test is done during a speculum examination by taking a sterile Dacron polyester swab and collecting vaginal and cervical secretions near the external os of the cervix. The swab should remain in place approximately 10 seconds and then be transferred to a tube of sample buffer for transport. This test is for women who have PTL signs and symptoms and who are at 24 to 35 weeks of gestation to assist in avoiding unnecessary interventions (ACOG, 2001). A positive fFn (50 ng/ml or greater) in a singleton pregnancy is a moderate predictor that more significant preterm cervical changes are likely within 1 to 2 weeks (Andersen, 2000; Iams, 2003; Ruiz, Fullerton, and Brown, 2004). A negative fFn is a strong predictor that preterm delivery in the next 2 weeks is unlikely (Lockwood, 2003). False positives may result from recent sexual intercourse, vaginal bleeding, amniotic fluid, or recent cervical examination.

Cervical Length

Transvaginal ultrasound to measure cervical length is also being used to assess risk for PTL. Women with short cervical length have an increased risk for PTL. According to Farine, Dodd, Basso, and others (2008), cervical length less than 15 mm between 22 and 24 weeks of gestation indicates an increased risk for PTL. The role of cervical length in assessing risk for PTL in multiple gestations is less defined (Welsh and Nicolaides, 2002).

Clinical Markers

Clinical markers are being investigated that identify at risk patients earlier than fFN and cervical changes. Such markers are increased salivary cortisol or corticotropin-releasing hormone that indicates maternal stress (Giurgescu, 2009), or placental abnormality by elevated levels of thrombin-antithrombin III complex (Baker, 2008). If an infection is the precipitating cause, inflammation can be detected by a systemic infection such as pyelonephritis, asymptomatic bacteriuria, or pneumonia. Inflammation also can be detected by an ascending genital tract infection such as gonorrhea, Chlamydia, or bacterial vaginitis because their presence correlates with an increased risk of preterm birth, but treatment and eradication does not decrease its risk (Iams, Romero, Creasy, and others, 2009); periodontal disease may be another marker (Klebanoff and Searle, 2006).

Criteria for Diagnosis of Preterm Labor

When a patient comes in experiencing regular, rhythmic uterine contractions, the medical team must first determine whether the patient is in true labor. The diagnosis is usually made in the presence of (1) four contractions in a 20-minute period, (2) a cervix that is beginning to dilate more than 2 cm, and (3) 80% or greater cervical effacement (ICSI, 2009). Therefore the diagnosis of PTL requires both uterine contractions and cervical change. Cervical length and fetal fibronectin are used to facilitate diagnosis. A fibronectin swab must be obtained at the initial speculum exam to prevent a false positive. If the patient is experiencing uterine contractions but the cervix is less than 80% effaced and 3 cm dilated, cervical length is usually determined with transvaginal ultrasound. A cervical length of more than 25 mm indicates that preterm labor is unlikely (ICSI, 2009).

USUAL MEDICAL MANAGEMENT AND PROTOCOLS FOR NURSE PRACTITIONERS:

PRIMARY PREVENTION

Preconception

The current thinking regarding preterm labor prevention and treatment is prompted by the recent theory that spontaneous preterm labor is a complex chronic condition. As for all chronic conditions, prevention of complications during pregnancy needs to start preconceptionally by promoting a healthier life style (MOD, 2009). Interventions indicated by research reviews that decrease the risk of preterm labor are:

- Smoking cessation program (Lumley and others, 2004)
- Routine screening and treatment for asymptomatic bacteriuria (Smaill and Vazquez, 2007)
- Screening high-risk patients for bacterial vaginosis and treating symptomatic women with metronidazole; it has not proved beneficial to screen or treat asymptomatic low-risk pregnant women (ICSI, 2009)
- Use of a laminaria for women undergoing second trimester dilation and evacuation (Kalish, Chasen, Rosenzweig, and others, 2002)
- Preconception medical management of medical conditions such as diabetes, seizures, asthma, or hypertension (Haas, Fuentes-Afflick, Stewart, and others, 2005)

Prenatal

During pregnancy, primary prevention is focusing on patient education about significance and symptoms of PTL and clinical management of women who are at risk for PTL.

Patient education

Research indicates that approximately 50% of pregnant women knew the symptoms of PTL and 70% do not view PTL as any major health concern (Green, Ryan, Shusterman, and others, 2003). Therefore prenatal education is important for early identification of signs of PTL when treatable causes can be effectively managed.

Clinical evaluation for "at risk" patients

Assess patients prenatally for predisposing factors in the four pathways: altered uterine and cervical factors, placental ischemia, inflammation, and stress (as outlined in Box 23-1). Examples of areas of assessment for "*at risk*" patients include:

- Smoking habits using the 5 As and intervention
- Substance use, if substance abuse is determined (see Chapter 27 for interventions)
- Medical risks

- Symptomatic and asymptomatic bacteriuria and other clinical markers of inflammation
- Domestic violence: Provide appropriate intervention and referrals if identified (see Chapter 25).
- Stress level: Discuss with the patient and her family the link between increased stress, increased cortisol levels and the correlation to preterm birth (Giurgescu, 2009). Problem-solve with the patient and her family ways to lower stress and make appropriate referrals as indicated.
- Anxiety, as well as economic or family stressors: Teach relaxation techniques to decrease the effects of stress (Hobel, 2004). Encourage problem solving to reduce stress by avoiding or altering stressful situations. Make appropriate referrals as needed.

Close surveillance of patients with a positive history

Research indicates close surveillance of cervical length and fetal fibronectin for patients with a positive history of PTL or previous preterm PROM without a medical indication.

Progesterone

In patients with a prior history of preterm labor and with a short cervix, clinical trials suggest that progesterone given by injection or vaginally may be helpful in preventing recurrent PTL. Various randomized control trials and research reviews indicate significant reduction of PTL, especially in a singleton pregnancy with a history of preterm labor and a short cervical length (Da Fonseca, Bittar, Carvalho, and others, 2003; Meis, Klebanoff, Thom, and others, 2003; Fonseca, Celik, Parra, and others, 2007; O'Brien, Adair, Lewis, and others, 2007; Dodd and others, 2008; Farine, Dodd, Basso, and others, 2008; Weiner and Buhimschi, 2009). Progesterone (17P) injections, administered weekly between 16 and 20 weeks of gestation, have been shown to decrease the chance of preterm labor in the current pregnancy by 33% (Petrini and others, 2005). The same results have not been shown to be effective for a multiple gestation (Thorp, Mercer, Sorokin, and others, 2009).

SECONDARY PREVENTION

Once preterm labor symptoms have manifested, secondary prevention focuses on determination of any treatable cause and whether further continuation of the pregnancy will be beneficial or harmful to the fetus or harmful to the mother. The choice of treatment depends on the following diagnostic results and the age and maturity of the fetus.

Clinical Evaluation of Patients Who Present with PTL Symptoms

Diagnostic data include the following:

- Blood studies: a complete blood cell count with differential and platelets; WBC count is normally elevated in pregnancy and in labor, but a WBC count above 18,000 is considered significant for infection
- Urinalysis: note presence of WBCs, RBCs, bacteria, nitrites, or leukocytes
- Urine culture and sensitivity to rule out a urinary tract infection

- Sterile speculum exam to visualize the cervix for bleeding, pooling of amniotic fluid, and effacement
- Collect specimens such as:
  - Fetal fibronectin (fFN)
  - Cervical cultures for group B streptococcus, Chlamydia, and gonorrhea
  - Wet mount for bacterial vaginosis and trichomonas vaginalis
  - Samples for assessing amniotic fluid with either ferning, nitrazine paper, or Amnisure.
- Drug screen if indicated
- Fetal surveillance studies to determine signs of fetal compromise
- Fetal lung maturity
- Transvaginal ultrasound to determine cervical length

Contraindications to Halting Preterm Labor

In 25% of the cases that present in PTL, delivery is indicated because of a medical or obstetric reason (Ananth and Vintzileos, 2006), such as the following:
- Mature fetus as demonstrated by a lecithin/sphingomyelin (L/S) ratio of 2:1 or greater or the presence of phosphatidylglycerol in the amniotic fluid
- Fetal death
- Fetal anomaly incompatible with life
- Intrauterine growth restriction related to an unfavorable intrauterine environment
- Fetal compromise
- Active hemorrhage
- Intraamniotic infection
- Severe preeclampsia, heart disease, or significant bleeding from placenta previa or abruptio placentae

Nontreatable Cause Preterm Labor Management

No treatment has been shown to effectively stop nontreatable cause preterm labor. There is some clinical evidence that some tocolytic agents used to initially suppress uterine contractions for an acute episode of PTL may have limited benefit by delaying delivery for a few days, thus allowing time for steroid administration and maternal transport to a tertiary care center (Hollier, 2005; Anotayanonth and others, 2006). According to the Cochrane Database of Systematic Review, data are too inadequate to identify one specific tocolytic agent over another (Anotayanonth and others, 2006) and all these drugs have risks. Tocolytic drugs assigned for "off-label" use for acute tocolysis per U.S. Food and Drug Administration (FDA) include magnesium sulfate; terbutaline, a beta-mimetic agonist; nifedipine, a calcium channel blocker; and indomethacin, a prostaglandin synthetase inhibitor. According to the Cochrane Database of Systematic Reviews, there is little evidence that Atosiban, an oxytocin antagonist, should be used as a tocolytic agent. It is not superior to other tocolytics and is associated with more infant deaths (Papatsonis, Flenady, Cole, and others, 2005).

According to several systematic reviews of relevant published random-control clinical trials by Gyetvai and others (1999); Nanda, Cook, Gallo, and others (2007); Sanchez-Ramos and Huddleston (2003); and Caritis, 2005, maintenance tocolytic therapy with the subcutaneous infusion pump or oral tocolytic therapy, after acute tocolytic therapy, does not significantly reduce the rates of recurrent PTL. Therefore because of the risk, consequences, and substantial expense of the medication, routine use of maintenance tocolytic therapy is not currently recommended (Svigos, Robinson, and Vigneswaran, 2006; Nanda, Cook, Gallo, and others, 2007).

Current management options to treat PTL include the following:

- Evaluate the symptomatic patient by assessing her contraction pattern, obtaining a vaginal swab for fibronectin, ruling out rupture of membranes and vaginal bleeding, and assessing the cervical status of effacement and dilation. If the cervix is less than 80% effaced, perform a transvaginal ultrasound, assessing length of the cervix.
- Determine whether possible contributing causes, such as infection or PROM, are present.
- Antibiotics may be indicated if a bacterial infection such as pyelonephritis, asymptomatic bacteriuria, and pneumonia is diagnosed or in the case of premature rupture of membranes (Klein and Gibbs, 2004; Smaill and Vasquez, 2007). Prophylactic antibiotic therapy for GBS is appropriate (as outlined in Chapter 26).
- Prophylactic antibiotic therapy is ineffective in treating preterm labor (King, Flenady, and Murray, 2002; Simcox, Sin, Seed, and others, 2007).
- Monitor intake and output (I&O).
- Hydrate with 500 ml of isotonic crystalloid solution if the patient is dehydrated (Stan and others, 2002); if the patient is not dehydrated, this may lead to pulmonary edema if tocolytic drugs are used.
- Initially monitor fetal heart rate (FHR) and uterine activity continuously, then periodically.
- Transfer to a tertiary care center if possible.
- Initially use tocolytic agents to suppress uterine contractions for an acute episode of PTL until the patient can be transported to tertiary care or complete corticosteroid therapy are initiated (Anotayanonth and others, 2006).
- Use a single course of corticosteroids to facilitate fetal lung maturity if delivery is imminent before 34 weeks of gestation (NIH, 2000; Dalziel, 2006; Roberts and Dalziel, 2006).

Abdominal Surgery Management

If a surgical emergency presents itself before 36 weeks of gestation, regardless of previous risk, the pregnant patient is at high risk for PTL and delivery. It is postulated that the higher production of prostaglandins for the healing process increases the likelihood of preterm contractions. The pregnant woman may find it difficult or impossible to distinguish preterm contractions from abdominal pain at the surgical site. Add pain medication, which masks contraction discomfort as well, and it becomes even more unlikely that contractions will be the identified complaint. After abdominal surgery, it is a good idea to monitor with an electronic monitor the contraction pattern of the uterus. Some providers treat with subcutaneous terbutaline every 2 to 4 hours or with IV magnesium sulfate as a preventative for 24 to 48 hours after abdominal surgery, if the woman is more than 20 weeks pregnant.

Late Preterm Labor Prevention

Prevention of late preterm labor starts with accurate pregnancy dating, with a reliable last normal menstrual period (LNMP) or early ultrasound dating (Gardosi, Reynir, and Geirsson, 2005). The next step is to discuss the importance of spontaneous labor for all normal uncomplicated pregnancies. Then the American College of Obstetrics and Gynecology (ACOG, 2008) recommends no elective induction or cesarean birth before 39 weeks without medical indication or documentation of fetal lung maturity because of the increased risk of prematurity related to inadequate gestational dating.

Multiple Gestation Management

The most common components of multiple gestation management are increased nutritional requirements (see Chapter 1), increased rest, PTL prevention, and antepartum testing every 3 to 4 weeks after 25 weeks.

Bedrest, except for being allowed up to the bathroom and for meals, is still the preferred treatment once signs of preterm cervical changes are identified. Usually, larger doses of magnesium sulfate or other tocolytics are needed than with a singleton preterm pregnancy. Tocolytic home therapy with the terbutaline pump is more successful than any of the other home tocolytic therapies. Ultimately, the most effective tocolytic is IV magnesium sulfate. There is no evidence to support hospitalization for bedrest in the absence of significant cervical changes. Prolonged hospitalized bedrest does not reduce the risk for preterm birth or perinatal death. There is some suggestion that hospitalization may increase fetal growth in the higher order multiples (e.g., more than twins) (Crowther, 2000).

Other complications also are more likely with a multiple gestation pregnancy, including pregnancy-induced hypertension, which may be modified by hydrotherapy beginning at 24 to 26 weeks, thus allowing the fetuses more time in utero. Hydrotherapy has a number of beneficial effects:
- Forces fluid from tissue back into the circulating volume
- Improves blood flow to the uterus and thus to the babies, thereby improving growth potential in multiple gestation
- Buoyancy with water relieves weight from the skeletal structures and muscles and therefore improves comfort.

There is no doubt that multiple gestation presents management problems to the provider, as well as self-management challenges for the patient and her family. Bedrest is the ultimate treatment of choice. This places an additional strain on the family unit. It requires additional support financially, physically, and emotionally. The emotional strain can be a prenatal precursor to postpartum depression even when the infant outcomes are optimal. The deconditioning from prolonged inactivity makes recovery more difficult and the fatigue factor more pronounced. Counseling prenatally and postpartum can help to shorten the term of depression or avoid most or all of the more serious sequelae.

NURSING MANAGEMENT

Prevention

Preventive measures must center on counteracting or improving the modifiable risk factors for PTL while keeping in mind that 33% or more of patients who experience PTL have no identifiable risk factors. Thus any prevention program must consider the inclusion of all pregnant women (ICSI, 2009; MOD, 2009). It is the single most important aspect of obstetric management of multiple gestation (Elliott, 2007).

Prevention consists of first screening all pregnancies for risk. If a patient is found to be at moderate to high risk, extra evaluation and more frequent evaluation can help identify signs and symptoms before advanced changes occur. If the patient is not at risk, she should be made aware of early signs of PTL and be made to feel comfortable reporting these for evaluation by her health care provider. PTL cannot be diagnosed over the phone and must be evaluated by seeing the patient, talking with her, and physically examining her for early signs of cervical change.

The antepartum preterm prevention program should include the following general education components to be taught to all pregnant women to facilitate lifestyle modification and risk reduction:

- Plan pregnancies with at least an interval of 16 months between births.
- Encourage smoking cessation using the 5 As (refer to Chapter 27).
- Encourage preconception of medical management of medical conditions.
- Screen for substance abuse, depression, and domestic violence and refer to services for appropriate treatment
- Encourage early and regular prenatal care.
- Provide nutritional counseling to achieve appropriate weight for height and avoid fasting, which can cause accelerated ketosis and release stress hormones (Hobel, 2004).
- Provide oral health education to decrease periodontal disease; however, random control trails do not support the correlation of periodontal disease and increased risk of preterm labor but rather may serve as a clinical marker for PTL (Michalowicz, Hodges, DiAngelis, and others, 2006).
- Encourage patients to drink 8 ounces of water or fruit juice every waking hour except for the last couple of hours before sleep to decrease release of ADH and oxytocin from the posterior pituitary gland and increase uterine blood flow, thereby stabilizing decidual lysosomes. Drinks containing caffeine should be avoided.
- Instruct the patient to empty her bladder every 2 hours while awake. A full bladder can stimulate the uterus to contract and increase the risk for urinary tract infections.
- Help the patient avoid infection. Because of the stimulating effect of cytokines and bacterial endotoxins in prostaglandin production, infection prevention should be taught. Prevention of urinary tract and vaginal infections is most important. Adequate fluid, perineal hygiene, wearing cotton-lined underwear, the avoidance of scented bath salts, and limiting sexual contacts to only one person are beneficial in lowering the risk for these infections. The patient should understand the signs of an infection and the need to report any signs immediately.
- Encourage rest periods during the day to prevent fatigue, to decrease pressure of the fetus on the cervix, and to increase blood flow to the uterus. However, remember that bedrest, hydration, and pelvic rest are not effective in decreasing the risk for preterm birth (ACOG, 2003).
- Emphasize that appropriate exercise such as walking or swimming can be beneficial in decreasing fatigue and stress.

The antepartum preterm prevention program includes the following specific education components. It is to be taught to all pregnant women and their significant others between 20 and 36 weeks of gestation to enhance early recognition:

- PTL is subtle.
- Contractions may feel like a tightening sensation; they are not necessarily painful. (Avoid use of the term *Braxton-Hicks contractions.*)
- Uterine contractions should be felt for twice a day for 1 hour.
- Symptoms of PTL that should be reported to the health care provider include menstrual-like cramps, low dull backache, pelvic pressure, changes in vaginal discharge, and intestinal cramping with or without diarrhea.
- If any PTL symptoms occur, the patient should empty her bladder, lie down on her side, drink two to three glasses of fluid, and palpate for uterine contractions. She should come in for a vaginal examination if the symptoms continue or if she experiences four or more contractions in 1 hour. If symptoms stop, she may resume light activity. If the symptoms resume, she should call the health care provider or go directly to the hospital.
- The nurse should provide sensitive care when women report symptoms of PTL, making a through evaluation and reinforcing the importance to continue to report any symptoms experienced.

Hospitalization Management of Preterm Labor

- Determine estimated age of delivery through history and an ultrasound for fetal growth and gestational age assessment.
- Place the electronic fetal monitor to continually assess FHR, fetal well-being, and uterine contraction pattern.
- Obtain urinalysis.
- Assess for bacterial infections such as pyelonephritis, asymptomatic bacteriuria, and pneumonia.
- Initiate orders for treatment of PTL contractions within 30 minutes of initial hospital evaluation if the patient reports symptoms.
- Treat preterm contractions by having the patient void and placing her in a lateral recumbent position.
- Use IV hydration only if patient manifests signs of dehydration (Freda and Patterson, 2001; Stan and others, 2002).
- If tocolytic drugs are to be used, administer as outlined in this chapter under the respective tocolytic drug therapy (Box 23-2). Tocolytic agents are currently divided into four classes: (1) beta-sympathomimetics, (2) magnesium sulfate, (3) calcium antagonists, and (4) prostaglandin inhibitors.
- Assess for signs of infection by palpating for abdominal tenderness unassociated with contractions; assess for changes in vaginal discharge (either watery, bloody, with increased mucus, or foul-smelling); assess laboratory data for rapid rise in white blood cells; evaluate FHR for tachycardia, late decelerations, and absence of variability; assess maternal vital signs for temperature rise or drop in blood pressure.
- Educate patient as to the importance of promotion of fetal lung maturity with corticosteroids between gestational weeks 24 and 34 to decrease respiratory distress syndrome, intraventricular hemorrhage, and necrotizing enterocolitis (ACOG, 2003).

Box 23-2   Tocolytic Therapy for Preterm Labor

Terbutaline Sulfate

Action

Terbutaline sulfate is a beta-adrenergic agonist. A Cochrane Review concludes that beta-mimetic drugs can delay delivery by 48 hours but have greater maternal side effects than other tocolytic agents. Its long term use is not supported (Anotayanonth and others, 2006).

Contraindications

Contraindications for beta sympathomimetics are cardiovascular disease, cardiac dysrhythmias, hypertension, uncontrolled maternal hyperthyroidism, chorioamnionitis, and migraine headaches. Because beta sympathomimetics antagonize the body's normal compensatory mechanism for blood loss by their effects on heart rate and systolic and diastolic blood pressure, these drugs should not be used if there are any indications that bleeding is present.

Acute Dosage for Intravenous Terbutaline

Subcutaneous injections of 0.25 mg every 30 to 60 minutes up to 3 doses or 2.5 to 10 mcg/minute IV up to 30 mcg/minute are used to treat acute preterm labor (Weiner and Buhimschi, 2009). A dose should be held if the maternal pulse is greater than 120 beats a minute. Continuous use is not recommended (ICSI, 2009). Baseline electrocardiogram (ECG) is recommended. Electrolyte monitoring and strict fluid status are important.

Maternal Side Effects

Side effects that frequently occur with terbutaline include the following:
- Slight hypotension or a widening of maternal pulse pressure related to a slight increase in systolic and a slight decrease in diastolic pressure, thereby decreasing coronary perfusion
- Lightheadedness, tremors, and a flushed feeling related to relaxation of vascular smooth muscle
- Restlessness, emotional upset, and anxiety related to epinephrine release
- Maternal and fetal tachycardia, heart palpitations, and frequent skipping of a heartbeat related to cardiac stimulation
- Transient maternal hyperglycemia related to drug stimulation of the liver and muscle, causing glycogenolysis, gluconeogenesis, and decreased uptake of glucose by peripheral tissue
- Elevated lactate and free fatty acids, related to hyperglycemia, cause drug stimulation of the pancreas
- Decreased serum potassium caused by intracellular shift from the extracellular space
- Decreased hematocrit by 20% to 25% related to plasma volume expansion
- Nausea and vomiting
- Increased insulin and glucagon secretion related to decreased intestinal motility
- Bronchial relaxation

    Intolerable side effects are maternal tachycardia greater than 120 beats/minute, drop in blood pressure to less than 90/60, chest pain or tightness, and cardiac dysrhythmias.

Continued

Box 23-2   Tocolytic Therapy for Preterm Labor—cont'd

Life-threatening complications are pulmonary edema, which may result from myocardial failure and fluid overload; subendocardial myocardial ischemia; cardiac dysrhythmias, such as premature ventricular contractions, premature nodal contractions, and atrial fibrillation; or cerebral vasospasm in patients who have a history of migraine headaches.

Long-Term Fetal Effects of Terbutaline

The major side effect to the fetus is tachycardia, but other side effects are hyperinsulinemia, hyperglycemia, hypocalcemia, myocardial hypertrophy, and ischemia (Hearne and Nagey, 2000).

Magnesium Sulfate

Action

Relaxes smooth muscle by competing with calcium at the motor end plate (reducing the release of acetylcholine) or at the cell membrane decreasing calcium influx into the cell. Cochrane Review concludes that magnesium sulfate has limited effect as a tocolytic agent, with severe risk factors such as pulmonary edema and cardiovascular problems (Crowther, Hiller, and Doyle, 2002).

Contraindications

A contraindication for magnesium sulfate is myasthenia gravis (ACOG, 2003).

IV Dosage

A loading IV piggyback dose of 4 to 6 g, given over 20 to 30 minutes, is usually recommended in the treatment of preterm labor, followed by a maintenance dose of 2 to 4 g/hour for 48 hours (Weiner and Buhimschi, 2009). The patient being treated for preterm labor can tolerate a much higher dose of magnesium than the preeclamptic patient. Kidney function usually is not compromised in the preterm labor patient as it can be in the preeclamptic patient.

Signs of Toxicity

Signs of toxicity are fewer than 12 respirations/minute, absence of deep tendon reflexes, severe hypotension, or extreme muscle relaxation.

Side Effects

During the loading dose, the patient frequently complains of hot flashes, nausea, vomiting, drowsiness, headaches, muscle weakness, and blurred vision. These side effects usually subside when the loading dose is completed. Less common but more problematic side effects are bone demineralization, paralytic ileus, shortness of breath, and pulmonary edema.

Signs of magnesium toxicity include the following:
- Respirations fewer than 12/minute
- Absence of deep tendon reflexes
- Severe hypotension
- Extreme muscle relaxation

Antidote for Magnesium Toxicity

- Calcium chloride 500 mg IV slow infusion (Weiner and Buhimschi, 2009)

Long-Term Effects on Neonate

There is no clear evidence of adverse neonatal effects from short-term use (Weiner and Buhimschi, 2009). However, recent research indicates that magnesium sulfate may have a neuroprotective benefit, protecting the brain of the preterm infant less than 34 weeks or birth weight less than 1500 grams,

Box 23-2 Tocolytic Therapy for Preterm Labor—cont'd

possibly reducing the risk of cerebral palsy (Marret, Marpeau, Zupan-Simunek, and others, 2007; Rouse, Hirtz, Thom, and others, 2008).

Calcium Channel Blockers
Action
Calcium channel blockers, such as nifedipine, do not allow the movement of calcium into the smooth muscle of the uterus. Contraction of smooth muscle depends on the availability of calcium. According to a Cochrane Review (King, Flenady, Papatsonis, and others, 2002) and several meta-analyses (Weiner and Buhimschi, 2009), nifedipine can delay delivery by 2 to 7 days and has a favorable risk to benefit ratio related to decreased adverse side effects. Also, nifedipine is more cost effective then terbutaline or magnesium sulfate (Weiner and Buhimschi, 2009)
Contraindications
Contraindicated in the presence of an intrauterine infection, maternal hypertension, or cardiac disease.
    If nifedipine is given with magnesium sulfate or erythromycin, sudden cardiac arrest can occur (Weiner and Buhimschi, 2009).
Dosage
Initial loading dose: 10 to 40 mg PO; followed by 30 to 60 mg long-acting preparation PO every 8 to 12 hours for a maximum of 48 hours.
Maternal Side Effects
Uncommon side effects related to peripheral vasodilation are flushing, headache, fatigue, mild hypotension, dizziness, and peripheral edema (Weiner and Buhimschi, 2009). Usually mild, less common with long-acting preparations; insignificant decrease in blood pressure (no change in heart rate).
Fetal Side Effects
There are minimal randomized, controlled studies at this time; however, clinical evidence indicates beneficial effects of decreased RDS, intracranial bleeding, and neonatal jaundice.

Prostaglandin Inhibitors
Action
Prostaglandin inhibitors, such as indomethacin, act by inhibiting prostaglandin synthesis. A Cochrane Review concludes that indomethacin significantly reduces contractions for 48 to 72 hours but has greater adverse fetal effects following 1 week of use as compared to nifedipine (King, Flenady, Cole, and Thornton, 2005). Both nifedipine and indomethacin are more cost-effective then terbutaline or magnesium sulfate (Weiner and Buhimschi, 2009).
Contraindications
Prostaglandin inhibitors are contraindicated in patients who have an active peptic ulcer, renal disease, hypertension, nonsteroidal antiinflammatory drug sensitive asthma, or a coagulation disorder.
Dosage
The initial loading dose of indomethacin is 50 mg PO; then 25 mg PO every 6 hours for 2 days maximum (Weiner and Buhimschi, 2009).

Continued

Box 23-2 Tocolytic Therapy for Preterm Labor—cont'd

Maternal Side Effects

Maternal side effects are increased bleeding time; potential to exacerbate hypertensive disorders. They can mask the symptoms of a fever.

Fetal and Neonatal Side Effects

Side effects are premature closure of the ductus arteriosus that can cause oligohydramnios, neonatal pulmonary hypertension, intraventricular hemorrhage, hyperbilirubinemia, and necrotizing enterocolitis. The risk for transient obstruction of the ductus arteriosus increases with increasing gestational age and long duration of treatment. It rarely occurs if the drug is not used after 32 weeks of gestation (Hearne and Nagey, 2000).

- Include supportive family members in all instructions.
- Make needed referrals—for example, to the social worker—if problems are identified.
- Encourage the patient's participation in her own care and decision making as much as possible.
- Provide time for the patient and her family to express their concerns regarding the possible outcome for the baby and inconvenience to the mother and family during treatment. Encourage them to vent any feelings, fears, and anger they may experience.
- Assess the family's support system and coping mechanisms.
- Provide the patient and her family with honest appraisal of the situation and plan of treatment.
- Give adequate information for decisions about alternatives of care.
- Refer to a high risk pregnancy support group such as Sidelines, a national support group for women experiencing a high risk pregnancy (*www.sidelines.org*).
- Refer to a spiritual counselor or chaplain on request or based on your assessment of need and patient acceptance.

Nursing Interventions for Acute Tocolytic Therapy

- Talk with the patient and her family to assess their understanding of the prescribed management plan.
- Obtain a patient history to assess contraindications to the prescribed tocolytic agent or to suppression of labor.
- Obtain such baseline data as FHR, uterine activity, maternal vital signs, weight, electrocardiogram, and laboratory studies that include a complete blood cell count with differential, blood glucose, colloid osmotic pressure, urea nitrogen, and serum electrolytes to determine maternal response to the drug therapy.
- If the IV route is to be used, start an IV infusion of normal saline with an 18-gauge needle to piggyback the IV administration of the drug. Because incremental titration is essential, an infusion pump should be used. (Refer to Box 23-2, Tocolytic Therapy for PTL for normal dosing.)
- Encourage the patient to maintain a left lateral position to minimize the risk for hypotension.

- Provide psychosocial support.
- Use an external monitor to record FHR and uterine activity continuously.
- Monitor blood pressure, pulse rate and rhythm, and temperature closely. Notify health care provider if systolic blood pressure is higher than 140 or lower than 90 mm Hg, diastolic blood pressure is higher than 90 or lower than 50 mm Hg, maternal pulse is higher than 120 beats per minute, or hyperthermia is present.
- Keep total fluid intake below 2500 ml/24 hours to avoid fluid overload and pulmonary edema.
- Accurately measure and record intake and output and a daily weight. Notify the health care provider if output is less than 30 ml per hour.
- Auscultate lung sounds for evidence of pulmonary edema.
- Assess for intolerable side effects and potential life-threatening complications to the drug.
- Have available cardiopulmonary resuscitation equipment and appropriate antidotes such as propranolol (Inderal) or verapamil for beta-sympathomimetics, or calcium chloride 500 mg slow infusion for magnesium sulfate.
- If pulmonary edema develops, be prepared to treat as outlined under Critical Care Interventions for Pulmonary Edema, later in this chapter.
- If beta-sympathomimetics are used, be prepared to obtain diagnostic data, such as serum potassium, hemoglobin, hematocrit, and renal function studies, periodically during the IV treatment. Although hypokalemia can develop as the result of potassium moving from the extracellular space to the intracellular space, there is no change in the total body potassium level. Therefore supplemental potassium is usually not necessary. The potassium level will return to normal within 24 hours after the IV therapy is discontinued.
- If beta-sympathomimetics are used, measure blood glucose twice daily. Patients with diabetes can become hyperglycemic if treated with terbutaline. Therefore they require careful monitoring of plasma glucose and usually require IV insulin administration.
- If magnesium sulfate is being used, check deep tendon reflex every hour and refer to serum magnesium levels daily. Therapeutic serum levels of 4 to 7.5 mEq/L are effective in reducing uterine contractions. Toxicity can develop with levels of 10 mEq/L or greater.
- If prostaglandin inhibitors are being used, be prepared to assist with fetal surveillance studies such as an echocardiogram and amniotic fluid volume. These drugs should not be used after 35 weeks of gestation because of the potential seriousness of the fetal side effects after this gestational age.

Critical Care Interventions for Pulmonary Edema[*]

- Position in upright tilted position.
- Start strict I&O.
- Administer oxygen at a rate indicted by pulse oximetry and arterial blood gases to maintain maternal SaO_2 greater than 95%.

---

*Powrie, 2006.

- Be prepared to use continuous positive airway pressure by face mask if oxygen levels are difficult to maintain.
- Administer diuretics as ordered using the lowest effective dose. Usual dose is furosemide 10 to 80 mg IV. Furosemide is one of the drugs of choice for pulmonary edema during pregnancy (Weiner and Buhimschi, 2009).
- Monitor blood pressure and be prepared to administer IV hydralazine or labetalol as indicated.
- Use invasive hemodynamic monitoring if conservative methods are not effective, if indicated.

Home Management of Preterm Labor
- Instruct regarding the importance of follow up care.
- Encourage no heavy lifting or work.
- Emphasize rest periods but bedrest is ineffective (Simhan and Caritis, 2007).

Nursing Interventions for Preterm Labor in Multiples
- Focus treatment on prevention strategies and early detection of PTL (Elliott, 2007). Start with determining the background uterine activity. The goal is to keep the background uterine activity below 3.5 contractions/hour (Elliott, 2007).
- Lower background uterine activity with increased nutrition, limited activity, hydration, infection prevention, and stress reduction. Progesterone therapy may be of benefit.
- When the background uterine activity exceeds 3.5 contractions/hour, Elliott (2007) recommends prophylactic tocolysis in multiple gestations. He has found that multiple gestations require high dosages of tocolytics as well as multiple drugs such as magnesium sulfate, terbutaline, and indomethacin.

CONCLUSION

The ultimate goal of prevention and treatment of PTL is delivery of a healthy term infant. It is a fact that neonatal outcomes are greatly improved when intrauterine life can be extended until fetal lungs mature. It is therefore suggested that delaying labor for even days can be beneficial. Early and ongoing risk assessment, education of all pregnant women in preterm prevention, and psychosocial intervention regarding smoking, alcohol use, illegal substance use, and domestic violence are important components of primary prevention. Early diagnosis and frequent health care contact can have a positive effect on early treatment of PTL before advanced cervical changes take place. Perinatal nurses can have a positive impact on neonatal morbidity by doing what nurses do so uniquely well. Screening, motivating, providing health care education, and frequent caring and sensitive contact with at-risk pregnant women can make a significant contribution to lowering neonatal morbidity and mortality from preterm delivery.

BIBLIOGRAPHY
Adams-Chapman I: Neurodevelopmental outcome of the late preterm infant, *Clin Perinatol* 33: 947–964, 2006.
American College of Obstetricians and Gynecologists: *Committee on Obstetric Practice: Late-preterm infants*, ACOG Committee Opinion No. 400, Washington, DC, 2008, ACOG.

American College of Obstetricians and Gynecologists: *Committee on Obstetric Practice: Use of pro-gesterone to reduce preterm birth,* ACOG Committee Opinion No. 419, Washington, DC, 2008, ACOG.

American College of Obstetricians and Gynecologists: *Management of preterm labor, ACOG Pract Bull No. 43,* Washington, DC, 2003, ACOG.

American College of Obstetricians Gynecologists: *Clinical management guidelines for obstetrician-gynecologists. Assessment of risk factors for preterm birth,* ACOG Pract Bull No. 31, Washington DC, 2001, Author.

Ananth C, and others: Placental abruption among singleton and twin births in the United States: risk factor profiles, *Am J Epidemiol* 153:773–778, 2001.

Ananth C, Vintzeleos A: Epidemiology of preterm birth and its clinical subtypes, *J Matern Fetal Neonatal Med* 19:773–782, 2006.

Andersen H: Use of fetal fibronectin in women at risk for preterm delivery, *Clin Obstet Gynecol* 43(4):746–758, 2000.

Anotayanonth S, Subhedar NV, Neilson JP, Harigopal S: Betamimetics for inhibiting preterm labour, *Cochrane Database Syst Rev* Issue 2. Art. No.: CD004352, 2006.

Baker V: Prevention of preterm delivery, *Am J Nurse Pract* 33(5):42–46, 2008.

Behrman R, Butler A, editors: *Preterm birth: causes, consequences, and prevention.* Committee on Understanding Premature Birth and Assuring Healthy Outcomes, Washington, DC, 2007, Institute of Medicine.

Behrman R, Stith B, editors: *Institute of Medicine committee on understanding preterm birth and assuring healthy outcomes, preterm birth: causes, consequences, and prevention,* Washington, DC, 2007, National Academies Press.

Bernhardt J, Dorman K: Exploring fetal fibronectin and cervical length for validating risk, *AWHONN Lifelines* 8(1):39–44, 2004.

Bettegowda V, and others: The relationship between cesarean delivery and gestational age among U.S. singleton births, *Clin Perinatol* 35:309–323, 2008.

Caritis S: Adverse effects of tocolytic therapy, *BJOG* 112(s1):74–78, 2005.

Castracane V: Endocrinology of preterm labor, *Clin Obstet Gynecol* 43(4):717–726, 2000.

Chandraharan E, Arulkumaran S: Acute tocolysis, *Curr Opin Obstet Gynecol* 17(2):151–156, 2005.

Clark S, Miller D, Belfort M, and others: Neonatal and maternal outcomes associated with elective term delivery, *Am J Obstet Gynecol* 200(2):156, 2009.

Cnattingius S: The epidemiology of smoking during pregnancy: smoking prevalence, maternal characteristics, and pregnancy outcome, *Nicotine Tob Res* 6(Suppl 2):S125–S140, 2004.

Condon J, and others: Surfactant protein secreted by the maturing mouse fetal lung acts as a hormone that signals the initiation of parturition, *Proc Natl Acad Sci USA* 101(14):4978–4983, 2004.

Crider K, Whitehead N, Buus R: Genetic variation associated with preterm birth: a huge review, *Genet Med* 7:593–604, 2006.

Crowther CA: Hospitalisation and bed rest for multiple pregnancy, *Cochrane Database Syst Rev* Issue 4. Art. No.: CD000110, 2000.

Crowther CA, Hiller JE, Doyle LW: Magnesium sulphate for preventing preterm birth in threatened preterm labour, *Cochrane Database Syst Rev* Issue 4. Art. No.: CD001060, 2002.

Da Fonseca E, Bittar R, Carvalho M, and others: Prophylactic administration of progesterone by vaginal suppository to reduce the incidence of spontaneous preterm birth in women at increased risk: a randomized placebo controlled double-blind study, *Am J Obstet Gynecol* 188:419–424, 2003.

Dalziel R: Antenatal corticosteroids for accelerating fetal lung maturation for women at risk of preterm birth, *Cochrane Database Syst Rev* Issue 3. Art. No.: 2006.

Dames K: Prevention of preterm birth: a renewed national priority, *Curr Opin Obstet Gynecol* 20: 590–596, 2008.

Davidoff M, Dias T, Damus K, and others: Changes in the gestational age distribution among U.S. singleton births: impact on rates of late preterm birth, 1992-2002, *Semin Perinatol* 30:8–15, 2006.

DeFranco E, O'Brien J, Adair C, and others: Vaginal progesterone is associated with a decrease in risk for early preterm birth and improved neonatal outcome in women with a short cervix: a secondary analysis from a randomized, double-blind, placebo-controlled trial, *Utrasound Obstet Gynecol* 30:697–705, 2007.

Dodd JM, Flenady V, Cincotta R, Crowther CA: Prenatal administration of progesterone for preventing preterm birth in women considered to be at risk of preterm birth, *Cochrane Database Syst Rev*, Issue 4. Art. No.: CD004947, 2008.

Dolan S, Gross S, Merkatz I, and others: The contribution of birth defects to preterm birth and low birth weight, *Obstet Gynecol* 110:318–324, 2007.

Elliott J: *Overview of the problem and higher order multiples, what have we learned*, Phoenix, AZ, November, 2000, Presented at Preterm Delivery: A National Disgrace.

Elliott J: Preterm labor in twins and high-order multiples, *Clin Perinatol* 34:599–609, 2007.

Engle W, and others: and the Committee on Fetus and Newborn: "Late-Preterm" infants: a population at risk, *Pediatrics* 120(6):1390–1401, 2007.

Farine D, Dodd J, Basso M, and others: The use of progesterone for prevention of preterm birth, *J Obstet Gynaecol Can* 30(1):67–71, 2008. Retrieved from http://www.guideline.gov

Fonseca E, Celik E, Parra M, and others: Fetal Medicine Foundation Second Trimester Screening Group: Progesterone and the risk of preterm birth among women with a short cervix, *N Engl J Med* 357:462–469, 2007.

Freda M, Patterson E: *Preterm labor: prevention and nursing management*, ed 2, White Plains, NY, 2001, March of Dimes.

Fuchs K, Wapner R: Elective cesarean section and induction and their impact on late preterm births, *Clin Perinatol* 33:793–801, 2006.

Galan P, and others: Serum concentrations of beta-carotene, vitamins C and E, zinc and selenium are influenced by sex, age, diet, smoking status, alcohol consumption and corpulence in a general French adult population, *Eur J Clin Nutr* 59(10):1181–1190, 2005.

Galson S: Preterm birth as a public health initiative: surgeon general's perspectives, *Public Health Rep* 123:548–550, 2008.

Gardosi J, Reynir T, Geirsson R: Routine ultrasound is the method of choice for dating pregnancy, *BJOG* 105:933–936, 2005.

Giurgescu C: Are maternal cortisol levels related to preterm birth? *J Obstet Gynecol Neonatal Nurs* 38(4):377–390, 2009.

Goldenberg R, Culhane J, Johnson D: Maternal infection and adverse fetal and neonatal outcomes, *Clin Perinatol* 32:523–559, 2005.

Goldenberg R, Iams J, Mercer B, and others: What we have learned about the predictors of preterm birth, *Semin Perinatol* 27(3):185–193, 2003.

Green N, Ryan C, Shusterman H, and others: Understanding pregnant women's perspectives on preterm birth, *Contemp Ob Gyn* 1:70–87, 2003.

Gyetvai K, and others: Tocolytics for preterm labor: a systematic review, *Obstet Gynecol* 94(5 Pt 2): 869–877, 1999.

Haas J, Fuentes-Afflick E, Stewart A, and others: Pre-pregnancy health status and the risk of preterm delivery, *Arch Pediatr Adolesc Med* 159:58–63, 2005.

Hamilton B, Martin J, Ventura S, and others for the Division of Vital Statistics: *Preliminary data for 2006: Infant and maternal health, National Vital Statistics Reports*, Hyattsville, MD, 2007, National Center for Health Statistics.

Hearne A, Nagey D: Therapeutic agents in preterm labor: tocolytic agents, *Clin Obstet Gynecol* 43(4):787–801, 2000.

Hendler I, Goldenberg R, Mercer B, and others: The preterm prediction study: association between maternal body mass index and spontaneous and indicated preterm birth, *Am J Obstet Gynecol* 192(3):882–886, 2005.

Hobel C: Stress and preterm birth, *Clin Obstet Gynecol* 47(4):856–880, 2004.

Hofman P, and others: Premature birth and later insulin resistance, *N Engl J Med* 351(21):2179–2186, 2004.

Hollier L: Preventing preterm birth: what works, what doesn't, *Obstet Gynecol Surv* 60(2):124–131, 2005.

Iams J: Prediction and early detection of pre-term labor, *Obstet Gynecol* 101(2):402–412, 2003.

Iams J, Romero R, Creasy R: Preterm labor and birth. In Creasy R, Resnik R, Iams J, and others, editors: *Creasy & Resnick's maternal-fetal medicine: principles and practice*, ed 6, Philadelphia, 2009, Saunders.

Institute for Clinical Systems Improvement (ICSI): *Management of Labor Guideline*, Bloomington, MN, 2009, Institute for Clinical Systems Improvement.

Jackson K, Mele N: Twin-to-twin transfusion syndrome: what nurses need to know, *Nurs Womens Health* 13(3):225–233, 2009.

Jasinski J: Pregnancy and domestic violence: a review of the literature, *Trauma Violence Abuse* 5(1):47–64, 2004.

Jeavons W: Sterile speculum exams and fFN collection, *AWHONN Lifelines* 9(3):237–240, 2005.

Jorgensen A: Late preterm birth: a rising trend, *Nurs Womens Health* 12(4):308–314, 2008.

Kalish R, Chasen S, Rosenzweig L, and others: Impact of midtrimester dilation and evacuation on subsequent pregnancy outcome, *Am J Obstet Gynecol* 187:882–885, 2002.

Kenyon S, Boulvain M, Neilson J: Antibiotics for preterm rupture of membranes, *Cochrane Database Syst Rev*, Issue 2. Art. No.: CD001058, 2003.

King J, Flenady V, Cole S, Thornton S: Cyclo-oxygenase (COX) inhibitors for treating preterm labour, *Cochrane Database Syst Rev*, Issue 2. Art. No.: CD001992, 2005.

King JF, Flenady V, Murray L: Prophylactic antibiotics for inhibiting preterm labour with intact membranes, *Cochrane Database Syst Rev*, Issue 3. Art. No.: CD000246, 2002.

King JF, Flenady V, Papatsonis D, and others: Calcium channel blockers for inhibiting preterm labour, *Cochrane Database Syst Rev*, Issue 3. Art. No.: CD002255, 2002.

Klebanoff M, Searle K: The role of inflammation in preterm birth: focus on periodontitis, *BJOG* 113(Suppl 3):43–45, 2006.

Klein L, Gibbs R: Use of microbial cultures and antibiotics in the prevention of infection-associated preterm birth, *Am J Obstet Gynecol* 190:493–502, 2004.

Lawsen C, Whelan E, Hibert B, and others: Occupational factors and risk of preterm birth in nurses, *Am J Obstet Gynecol* 200(1):51.e1–51.e8, 2009.

Lockwood C: Stress-associated preterm delivery: the role of corticotropin releasing hormone, *Am J Obstet Gynecol* 180(1 Pt 3):S264–S266, 1999.

Lockwood C: *Biochemical predictors of preterm delivery*, Phoenix, AZ, November 2000, Presented at Preterm Delivery: a national disgrace.

Lockwood C: Testing for risk of preterm delivery, *Clin Lab Med* 23:345–360, 2003.

Lumley J, Oliver SS, Chamberlain C, Oakley L: Interventions for promoting smoking cessation during pregnancy, *Cochrane Database Syst Rev*, Issue 4. Art. No.: CD001055, 2004.

Malone F, D'Alton M: Anomalies peculiar to multiple gestations, *Clin Perinatol* 27(4):1033–1046, 2000.

March of Dimes Foundation (MOD) (2009a): Effectiveness of progesterone in reducing preterm births may be altered by genetic predisposition. *Science Daily* February, 2009. Retrieved July 31, 2009, from http://www.sciencedaily.com/releases/2009/01/090130084153.htm.

March of Dimes (MOD) (2009b): Premature birth, 2009. Retrieved from http://www.marchofdimes.com/printableArticle/21326_1157.asp.

March of Dimes (MOD) (2009c): Resource library: preterm labor assessment toolkit, 2009. Retrieved from: http://www.marchofdimes.com/pretermlabor.

Marret S, Marpeau L, Zupan-Simunek V, and others for the PREMAG Trial Group: Magnesium sulphate given before very-preterm birth to protect infant brain: the randomized controlled PREMAG trial, *BJOG* 114:310–318, 2007.

Maxwell C, Amankwah K: Alternative approaches to preterm labor, *Semin Perinatol* 25(5):310–315, 2001.

McIntire D, Leveno K: Neonatal mortality and morbidity rates in late preterm births compared with births at term, *Obstet Gynecol* 111(1):35–41, 2008.

McParland P, Jones G, Taylor D: Preterm labour and prematurity, *Curr Obstet Gynaecol* 14:309–319, 2004.

Meis P, Klebanoff M, Thom E, and others: Prevention of recurrent preterm delivery by 17 alpha-hydroxyprogesterone caproate, *N Engl J Med* 348:2379–2385, 2003.

Mercer B, and others: The preterm prediction study: effect of gestational age and cause of preterm birth on subsequent obstetric outcome, *Am J Obstet Gynecol* 181(5 Pt 1):1216–1221, 1999.

Michalowicz B, Hodges J, DiAngelis A, and others: Treatment of periodontal disease and the risk of preterm birth, *N Engl J Med* 355(18):1885–1894, 2006.

Nabet C, Lelong N, Ancel P, and others: Smoking during pregnancy according to obstetric complications and parity: results of the EUROPOP study, *Eur J Epidemiol* 22:715–721, 2007.

Nakamoto T, and others: Cigarette smoke extract enhances oxytocin-induced rhythmic contractions of rat and human preterm myometrium, *Reproduction* 132(2):343–353, 2006.

Nanda K, Cook LA, Gallo MF, Grimes DA: Terbutaline pump maintenance therapy after threatened preterm labor for preventing preterm birth, *Cochrane Database Syst Rev* Issue 2. Art. No.: CD003933, 2007.

National Institute of Child Health and Human Development: *Perinatology research branch annual report excerpt on pathophysiology of premature labor and complications of prematurity*, Washington, DC, 2001, NICHHD, Retrieved from http://dir2.nichd.nih.gov.

National Institutes of Health (NIH): *Antenatal corticosteroids revisited, Consensus development conference statement*, Maryland, 2000, NIH. Retrieved from http://consensus.nih.gov.

Nohr B, Tabor A, Frederiksen K, Kjaer S: Loop electrosurgical excision of the cervix and the subsequent risk of preterm delivery, *Acta Obstet Gynecol Scand* 85:596–603, 2007.

Norwitz E, Lye S: Biology of parturition. In Creasy R, Resnik R, Iams J, and others, editors: *Creasy & Resnik's maternal-fetal medicine: principles and practice*, ed 6, Philadelphia, 2009, Saunders.

O'Brien J, Adair C, Lewis D, and others: Progesterone vaginal gel for the reduction of recurrent preterm birth: primary results from a randomized, double-blind, placebo-controlled trial, *Ultrasound Obstet Gynecol* 30(5):687–696, 2007.

Olsen S: Is supplementation with marine omega-3 fatty acids during pregnancy a useful tool in the prevention of preterm birth? *Clin Obstet Gynecol* 47(4):768–774, 2004.

Papatsonis D, Flenady V, Cole S, Liley H: Oxytocin receptor antagonists for inhibiting preterm labour, *Cochrane Database Syst Rev* Issue 3. Art. No.: CD004452, 2005.

Petrini J, and others: Estimated effect of 17 alpha-hydroxyprogesterone caproate on preterm birth in the United States, *Am College Obstet Gynecol* 105(2):267–272, 2005.

Powrie R: Respiratory disease. In James D, and others, editors: *High risk pregnancy: management options*, ed 3, Philadelphia, 2006, Saunders.

Reedy N: Born too soon: the continuing challenge of preterm labor and birth in the United States, *J Midwifery Womens Health* 52:281–290, 2007.

Rich-Edwards J, Grizzard R: Psychosocial stress and neuroendocrine mechanisms in preterm delivery, *Am J Obstet Gynecol* 192:530–535, 2005.

Roberts D, Dalziel SR: Antenatal corticosteroids for accelerating fetal lung maturation for women at risk of preterm birth, *Cochrane Database Syst Rev* 2006, Issue 3. Art. No.: CD004454.

Romero R: Prevention of spontaneous preterm birth: the role of sonographic cervical length in identifying patients who may benefit from progesterone treatment, *Ultrasound Obstet Gynecol* 30(5):675–686, 2007.

Romero R, and others: The preterm parturition syndrome, *BJOG* 113(Suppl 3):17–24, 2006.

Romero R, Lockwood C: Pathogenesis of spontaneous preterm labor. In Creasy R, Resnik R, Iams J, and others, editors: *Creasy & Resnik's maternal-fetal medicine: principles and practice*, ed 6, Philadelphia, 2009, Saunders.

Rosenberg T, Garber S, Lipkind H, Chiasson A: Maternal obesity and diabetes as risk factors for adverse pregnancy outcomes: differences among 4 racial groups, *Am J Public Health* 95:1545–1551, 2005.

Ross M, Cousins L, Baxter-Jones R, and others: Objective cervical length measurements: consistency and efficacy of screening for a short cervix, *J Reprod Med* 52(5):385–389, 2007.

Rouse D, Cartiitis S, Peaceman A, and others: A trail of 17 alpha-hydroxyprogesterone caproate to prevent prematurity in twins. National Institute of child health and Human Development Maternal-Fetal Medicine units network, *N Engl J Med* 357:454–461, 2007.

Rouse D, Hirtz D, Thom E, and others: A randomized, controlled trial of magnesium sulfate for the prevention of cerebral palsy, *N Eng J Med* 359(9):895–905, 2008.

Ruiz R: Mechanism of full-term and preterm labor: factors influencing uterine activity, *J Obstet Gynecol Neonatal Nurs* 27(6):652–660, 1998.

Ruiz R, Fullerton J, Brown C: The utility of fFN for the prediction of preterm birth in twin gestations, *J Obstet Gynecol Neonatal Nurs* 33(4):446–454, 2004.

Russell R, and others: The changing epidemiology of multiple births in the United States, *Obstet Gynecol* 101(1):129–135, 2002.

Sanchez-Ramos L, and others: Efficacy of maintenance therapy after acute tocolysis: a meta-analysis, *Am J Obstet Gynecol* 181(2):484–490, 1999.

Sanchez-Ramos L, Huddleston J: The therapeutic value of maintenance tocolysis: an overview of the evidence, *Clin Perinatol* 30:841–854, 2003.

Sfakianaki A, Norwitz E: Mechanisms of progesterone action in inhibiting prematurity, *J Matern Fetal Neonatal Med* 19:763–772, 2006.

Shaw R: Late preterm birth: a new nursing issue, *MCN* 33(5):287–293, 2008.

Simcox R, Sin W, Seed P, and others: Prophylactic antibiotics for the prevention of preterm birth in women: a meta-analysis, *Aust N Z J Obstet Gynecol* 47:368–377, 2007.

Simhan H, Caritis S: Prevention of preterm delivery, *N Engl J Med* 357:477–487, 2007.

Sjoborg K, Vistad I, Myhr S, and others: Pregnancy outcome after cervical cone excision: a case-control study, *Acta Obstet Gynecol Scand* 86:423–428, 2007.

Smaill FM, Vazquez JC: Antibiotics for asymptomatic bacteriuria in pregnancy, *Cochrane Database Syst Rev* Issue 1. Art. No.: CD000490, 2007.

Smith L, Draper E, Manktelow B, and others: Socioeconomic inequalities in very preterm birth rates, *Arch Dis Child Fetal Neonatal Educ* 92:F11–F14, 2007.

Stan C, and others: Hydration for treatment of preterm labour, *Cochrane Database Syst Rev* Issue 2. Art. No.: CD003096, 2002.

Svigos J, Robinson J, Vigneswaran R: Threatened and actual preterm labor including mode of delivery. In James D, and others, editors: *High risk pregnancy: management options*, ed 3, Philadelphia, 2006, Saunders.

Thompson J, Irgens L, Rasmussen S, Daltveit A: Secular trends in socio-economic status, and the implications for preterm birth, *Paediatr Perinat Epidemiol* 20:182–187, 2006.

Thorp J, Mercer B, Sorokin Y, and others: Prevention of preterm birth in triplets using 17 hydroxprogesterone caproate: a randomized controlled trial, *Obstet Gynecol* 113(2, Part1):285–292, 2009.

Tikkanen M, Nuutila M, Hiilesmaa V, and others: Clinical presentation and risk factors of placental abruption, *Acta Obstet Gynecol Scand* 85:700–705, 2006.

Tita A, Landon M, Spong C, and others: Timing of elective repeat cesarean delivery at term and neonatal outcomes, *N Engl J Med* 360(2):111–120, 2009.

U.S. Department of Health and Human Services: *Healthy People 2010: understanding and improving health*, Washington, DC, 2000, USDHHS.

Ward K, Argyle V, Meade M, Nelson L: The heritability of preterm delivery, *Obstet Gynecol* 106:1235–1239, 2005.

Weiner C, Buhimschi C: *Drugs for pregnant and lactating women*, ed 2, Philadelphia, 2009, Saunders.

Welsh A, Nicolaides K: Cervical screening for preterm delivery, *Curr Opin Obstet Gynecol* 14(2):195–202, 2002.

Zhong-Cheng L, Wilkins R, Kramer M: Disparities in pregnancy outcomes according to marital and cohabitation status, *Obstet Gynecol* 103(6):1301–1307, 2004.

Zlopasa G, Skrablin S, Kalafatic D: Uterine anomalies and pregnancy outcome following resectoscope metroplasty, *Int J Gynecol Obstet* 98:129–133, 2007.

24

Premature Rupture of Membranes

*P*remature or prelabor rupture of membranes (PROM) is defined as rupture of the amniotic sac surrounding the fetus before the onset of labor. *Preterm PROM* is commonly used to refer to the rupture of the membranes when it occurs before 37 weeks of gestation. The period between preterm rupture of membranes and the onset of labor is called the *latency period. Prolonged rupture of membranes* occurs when the latency period extends beyond 24 hours.

INCIDENCE

PROM occurs in less than 1% of pregnancies before 24 weeks of gestation, 2% to 5% of pregnancies between 24 and 34 weeks and 2% to 8% of pregnancies between 34 and 37 weeks. By term, PROM accounts for 8% of pregnancies (ACOG, 2007). Approximately 20% of these cases occur before 36 weeks of gestation (Weitz, 2001; Mercer, 2003).

ETIOLOGY

The cause of PROM is unknown in most cases. Increased intrauterine pressure with multiple gestation and polyhydramnios, inflammatory processes such as cervicitis and amnionitis, placenta previa, abruptio placentae, abnormalities of the internal cervical os, multiple amniocenteses, and therapeutic abortions are factors sometimes associated with PROM.

An inherently weak fetal membrane was once believed to be a cause of PROM. However, when fetal membranes were tested after premature rupture, they were found to be just as strong as membranes from normal term deliveries (Mercer, 2009). Current research reveals bacterial invasions as a precursor for PROM and may possibly cause 30% to 40% of PROM cases. However, the bacterial invasion is usually related to an ascending vaginal infection and does not mean the patient has an intraamniotic infection.

Another etiologic factor for PROM is a positive history in a prior pregnancy (Mercer, 2009). Research indicates that 16% to 32% of patients with preterm PROM experience a prior pregnancy complicated by PROM (Lee, Carpenter, Heber, and others, 2003). The risk for PROM is increased in socioeconomically disadvantaged patients; sexually promiscuous teenagers; patients who have nutritional deficiencies, especially in zinc, vitamins C and E, and copper (Parry and Strauss, 1998; Woods, Plessinger, and Miller, 2001; Bendich and Deckelbaum, 2005; ACOG, 2007); patients who smoke (ACOG, 2007); and patients with decreased immunity.

NORMAL PHYSIOLOGY

The developing fetus is protected from the outside world by two fetal membranes—the amnion, composed of five distinct layers, and the chorion, composed of three layers—which form a sac around the fetus. These membranes are thin but tough. They contain no blood vessels or nerve endings. However, they are rich in collagen, which gives them their strength and elasticity. Regulatory inhibitors control collagenolytic enzymes such as trypsin and collagenase from breaking down the collagen throughout pregnancy (Bryant-Greenwood, 1998).

As the pregnancy nears term, a normal decrease in regulatory inhibitors and an increase in collagenolytic enzyme activity occur. Among these enzymes are relaxin and cytokines. Near term, the phospholipase enzymes activate and assist with converting phospholipids to arachidonic acid, the precursor of prostaglandins. These prostaglandins initiate labor. The decrease in phospholipids creates a rubbing force between the chorion and amnion. During labor, increasing amounts of collagenolytic enzymes and decreasing amounts of phospholipids cause the membranes to rupture.

Amniotic fluid is produced within the amniotic sac, allowing the developing fetus to float freely. The pH of normal vaginal secretions is 4.5 to 5.5. Amniotic fluid is slightly alkaline with a pH 7.0 to 7.5. In early pregnancy, the primary source of the fluid appears to be the amnion, which produces the amniotic fluid by actively transporting solute and passively transporting water from maternal serum to the amniotic fluid space throughout pregnancy. As pregnancy advances, fetal urine and lung fluid significantly contribute to the amount of amniotic fluid. By way of fetal swallowing and breathing, amniotic fluid is reabsorbed. Thus, the amniotic fluid is constantly formed and reabsorbed (Gabbe, Niebyl, and Simpson, 2007). Replacement of amniotic fluids occurs about every 3 hours. At 12 weeks of gestation, the average volume is 50 ml; at 20 weeks, the average volume is 400 ml. The maximum volume of 1000 ml is reached between 36 and 38 weeks.

Amniotic fluid serves many functions. It provides a medium allowing for symmetrical fetal movement, growth, and development without pressure on its delicate tissue. Blood flow is also unrestricted as blood is transported through the umbilical cord. The fluid helps to maintain an even environmental temperature for the fetus.

Normal amniotic fluid contains an antibacterial substance, which gradually increases with gestational age until term and then decreases. The level of this antibacterial substance varies among individuals. A diet deficient in protein, zinc, and antioxidants such as vitamin C may decrease the antibacterial and antiviral activity of the amniotic fluid (Brace, 1997; Connors and Merrill, 2004; Bendich and Deckelbaum, 2005; ACOG, 2007).

PATHOPHYSIOLOGY

Premature rupture of the fetal membranes results from focal weakening, extensive changes in collagen metabolism, or increased intraamniotic pressure (Parry and Strauss, 1998; Woods, Plessinger, and Miller, 2001). In the presence of many bacteria, bacterial proteases and collagenases are produced. These enzymes and the inflammatory response of neutrophils act together, decreasing the collagen content of the membranes; thus, a focal weakening occurs in the membranes' strength and elasticity (Mercer, 2009). Bacterial proteases also activate the prostaglandin cascade.

After prolonged rupture of membranes, an intraamniotic infection often develops as the result of ascending vaginal organisms. The percentage of women with preterm PROM experiencing intraamniotic infections is 13% to 60% (ACOG, 2007). The organisms commonly responsible for intraamniotic infections include *Ureaplasma urealyticum, Mycoplasma hominis, Bacteroides bivius,* group B streptococci, and *Gardnerella vaginalis. Neisseria gonorrhoeae,* herpes simplex virus, cytomegalovirus, and *Candida albicans* have been implicated as well. There are two possible mechanisms contributing to an intraamniotic infection. Some patients have normal inhibitory activity of the amniotic fluid, but when large volumes of bacteria enter the amniotic cavity, they are unable to overpower the inhibitors. In other patients inhibitory activity in the amniotic fluid may be lacking. These patients are susceptible to an intraamniotic infection if any bacteria enter the amniotic fluid.

It is hypothesized that tissue-damaging molecules called *reactive oxygen species* (ROS) damage the integrity of the collagen, causing membrane weakening (Connors and Merrill, 2004). Overproduction of relaxin increases collagenase activity and has been linked with preterm PROM.

MATERNAL EFFECTS

Infection

If an intraamniotic infection develops because of rupture of membranes, it can quickly cause a serious maternal infection leading to septicemia and death if not treated promptly. Maternal sepsis occurs in about 1% of pregnancies complicated by preterm PROM (ACOG, 2007). If maternal infection occurs, it usually develops during the postpartum period (Svigos, Robinson, and Vigneswaran, 2006). Intraamniotic infections in the postpartum period complicate 2% to 13% of deliveries related to preterm PROM (ACOG, 2007).

Abruptio Placentae

Abruptio placentae also occurs more frequently in the woman with preterm PROM.

Postpartum Hemorrhage

Postpartum hemorrhage occurs more frequently related to increased retained placenta and intrauterine infection.

FETAL AND NEONATAL EFFECTS

Prematurity

Preterm PROM causes one third of all preterm births (Weitz, 2001). Before 36 weeks of gestation, respiratory distress syndrome is the main cause of morbidity and mortality of the neonate resulting from a preterm PROM (Svigos, Robinson, and Vigneswaran, 2006; Mercer, 2009).

Fetal and Neonatal Infection

The incidence of fetal/neonatal sepsis is small, 2% to 4%, with the rate correlating directly with the length of time the membranes are ruptured and the gestational age. The earlier the gestation, the greater the risk for an infection (Svigos, Robinson, and Vigneswaran, 2006). If an intraamniotic infection develops, the fetus has a 15% to 20% risk for developing septicemia, pneumonia, or a urinary tract infection (Mercer, 2009).

Fetal Compromise

PROM can cause fetal compromise because of a prolapsed cord or oligohydramnios. The cord can prolapse if the presenting part is not well engaged. If the amniotic fluid volume is affected to a large degree, pressure can be applied on the cord as the fetus moves, thereby causing fetal compromise. Seventy-five percent of patients with PROM will experience variable decelerations related to cord compression (Mercer, 2009). If fetal compromise is allowed to persist for any length of time, fetal hypoxia can result, causing the anal sphincter to relax and release meconium into the amniotic fluid. Deep, gasping respiratory movements are triggered, which moves the meconium-stained amniotic fluid deep into the alveoli increasing the neonate's risk for developing aspiration pneumonia.

Developmental Anomalies

If the membranes rupture before 23 to 26 weeks of gestation and marked oligohydramnios results, the fetus is at an increased risk (20% to 50%) for skeletal compression deformities, amniotic band syndrome, and pulmonary hypoplasia (Mercer, 2009). Pulmonary hypoplasia is more common with PROM because lung development depends more on extrinsic factors such as amniotic fluid than other fetal organs. Amniotic band syndrome occurs when the fetal membranes adhere to and constrict fetal parts causing deformities (Weitz, 2001; ACOG, 2007). Other developmental abnormalities associated with an early rupture are intestinal obstruction, diaphragmatic hernia, clubfoot, scoliosis, and hip dislocation (Weitz, 2001; Mercer, 2003).

DIAGNOSTIC TESTING

Sterile Speculum Examination

When PROM is suspected, a sterile speculum examination is usually done. If amniotic fluid is observed leaking from the cervix and collecting in the posterior fornix of the vagina, a subjective diagnosis of PROM is made. However, semen and other fluids can at times be mistaken for amniotic fluid. A digital vaginal examination should *never* be done if any attempt is to be made in delaying labor. Digital vaginal examinations increase the potential for bacteria to be transported into the cervical canal, thereby increasing the risk for an intraamniotic infection and thus precipitating the need for early delivery (ACOG, 2007; Mercer, 2009).

Nitrazine Test

If there is no visual sign of loss of amniotic fluid from the cervix, the secretions of the posterior fornix of the vagina can be tested with Nitrazine paper for pH determination. Because amniotic fluid is alkaline and vaginal secretions are acidic, the Nitrazine paper turns blue in the presence of amniotic fluid. Blood, cervical mucus, alkaline urine, vaginitis caused by bacterial vaginosis or Trichomonas, and povidone-iodine (Betadine) should not be allowed to contaminate the specimen; they are also alkaline and can cause a false-positive result (Caughey, Robinson, and Norwitz, 2008).

Microscopic Examination

A small amount of the amniotic fluid can be spread on a slide and allowed to dry. Microscopic examination of dried amniotic fluid results in arborization, a fernlike pattern in the presence of amniotic fluid because of the fluid's high concentration of salt. However, this test has a sensitivity (rate at which the test will correctly detect ROM) of 98% for the laboring patient and only 51.4% for the patient not in labor (Caughey and others, 2008).

Immunoassay Test: PAMG-1 Test (AmniSure Assay)

AmniSure detects trace amounts of PAMG-1, a protein expressed by the cells of the decidua and found in the amniotic fluid. Its presence is found in vaginal secretions after the rupture of membranes, with a 99% sensitivity at any gestational age. The test is administered using a sterile polyester swab to obtain vaginal secretions without the need of a speculum. The swab is rinsed in a vial with solvent for one minute and then thrown away. Next the test strip is dipped into the vial for 5 to 10 minutes. After removing the test strip the results are read and interpreted as follows: One line indicates NO membrane rupture, two lines indicate a positive rupture of membranes, and no lines indicate the test is invalid as the quality control line is not present (Lee, Park, Norwitz, and others, 2007; Caughey and others, 2008).

USUAL MEDICAL MANAGEMENT AND PROTOCOLS FOR NURSE PRACTITIONERS

The treatment of PROM is one of the most controversial subjects in obstetrics today because of conflicting scientific research. Management generally depends on variables such as gestational age, presence of fetal stress, presence of maternal or fetal infection, and presence of labor.

Documentation of Fetal Age

Gestational age is usually verified with review of prenatal records and ultrasounds. If this information is unavailable because of late prenatal care, the biparietal diameter may not be accurately determined because the head is low in the pelvis. In this case, femur length, abdominal circumference, or both are used to determine gestational age of the fetus.

Fetal Maturity Assessment

Fetal lung maturity can be determined in one of two ways. First, the amniotic fluid from the vaginal pool can be tested for phosphatidylglycerol (PG); if PG is present, fetal lung maturity is probable (Svigos, Robinson, and Vigneswaran, 2006; Mercer, 2009). Second, fetal lung maturity can be determined by collecting amniotic fluid through amniocentesis and evaluating for lecithin/sphingomyelin (L/S) ratio. An L/S ratio of 1:8 to 2:1 indicates probable lung maturity.

It may be difficult to collect fluid by amniocentesis if the leak is large. Amniocentesis may be facilitated by having the patient drink large amounts of fluids and remain in the Trendelenburg position for a period of time before the procedure. Fluid collected by amniocentesis is less likely to be contaminated by blood than that collected from vaginal pooling, which can create false-positive results. It may then be determined solely by the presence of PG. If lung maturity is positive, delivery is the management decision of choice.

Assessment of Fetal Stressors

Fetal heart rate (FHR) monitoring, fetal movement monitoring, nonstress tests (NSTs), biophysical profiles (BPPs), and amniotic fluid index (AFI) are used to determine fetal compromise in the presence of PROM. Fetal compromise may result from cord compression caused by oligohydramnios. This will manifest itself as variable decelerations of the FHR. An infected fetus is usually lethargic. Therefore, decreased fetal movement may indicate the presence of an infection. A reactive NST is a positive indicator of an uninfected fetus.

In the presence of a nonreactive NST, further testing should be done because of the high false-positive rate of this test (Mercer, 2009). The fetal BPP and AFI have been used to detect early signs of an intraamniotic infection after PROM. Late decelerations accompanying variable decelerations may indicate a coexistent placental abruption.

Assessment of Intraamniotic Infection

Maternal fever, maternal and fetal tachycardia, uterine tenderness, and an elevated maternal white blood cell count are clinical indicators of an intraamniotic infection. Fetal heart rate reactivity can be used as a screening assessment. Nonreactive fetal heart rate is associated with an intraamniotic infection. Laboratory tests such as serial white blood cell differential and C-reactive protein estimates coupled with weekly vaginal cultures can facilitate diagnosis of an intraamniotic infection (James, Mahomed, Stone, and others, 2004). Daily BPPs to assess for a subclinical infection are used. Some obstetricians obtain a culture of the amniotic fluid by way of an amniocentesis. The amniotic fluid is then tested for bacteria by doing a Gram stain and glucose level (Mercer, 2009).

Assessment of Signs of Labor

If the fetal membranes rupture before the onset of labor at term, 70% will begin labor within 24 hours (Parry and Strauss, 1998). The latency period after preterm PROM decreases inversely with gestational age; therefore the earlier the gestation, the longer the latency period.

Expectant Management Before 34 Weeks of Gestation

When the fetus is not mature, no signs of infection are present, and no fetal compromise is identified, expectant management consisting of bedrest with bathroom privileges and observation for signs of infection and fetal compromise is the preferred treatment. This is done in the hope that, by lengthening the pregnancy, fetal lungs may mature and the risk for respiratory distress will decrease in the neonate. It is currently recommended that prophylactic antibiotics and corticosteroids be administered during expectant management of preterm ROM (NIH, 2000; ACOG, 2007). The use of tocolytics is very controversial.

Before 23 weeks of gestation, care must be individualized because of the very early gestation, as well as the risk for maternal infection and fetal developmental abnormalities. Most providers inform and involve parents in the decision-making process (Mercer, 2003, 2009; ICSI, 2007).

Expectant Management After 34 Weeks of Gestation

The preferred treatment of term PROM is delivery. According to *The Cochrane Review* (Dare, Middleton, Crowther, and others, 2006), the woman with gestational rupture of membranes at 34 to 36 weeks should be allowed to choose between labor induction and expectant management after presentation of the risks and benefits of both options. The benefits of induction with oxytocin or prostaglandin have been demonstrated, through research results, to lower the risk for chorioamnionitis and neonatal infection as well as decrease the length of stay in the neonatal intensive care setting without increased risk for cesarean birth or operative vaginal birth. The risks associated with induction were increased use of epidural analgesia at an early stage of labor dilation, use of anesthesia or analgesia, and use of internal FHR monitoring in the presence of prolonged rupture of membranes (Wilkes and Galan, 2004; ACOG, 2007).

Variations in Management

Prophylactic Antibiotic Therapy

According to *The Cochrane Review* (Kenyon, Boulvain, and Neilson, 2004), the use of antibiotic therapy to prevent an ascending infection in patients with preterm PROM has been shown to lengthen the latency period, decrease the incidence of chorioamnionitis, decrease postpartum maternal endometritis, and decrease neonatal morbidity related to sepsis, pneumonia, respiratory distress syndrome (RDS), and necrotizing enterocolitis. One protocol is ampicillin and erythromycin intravenously for 48 hours, followed by amoxicillin (250 mg orally every 8 hours) and erythromycin (333 mg orally every 8 hours) for 5 days (Mercer, 2003; Kenyon, Boulvain, and Neilson, 2004). This regimen does not always treat group B strep. The intrapartum prophylaxis therapy for prevention of neonatal GBS infection should still be followed as outlined by the Centers for Disease Control and Prevention (see below and Chapter 26).

Antenatal Corticosteroids

Antenatal corticosteroids in women with preterm PROM at less than 34 weeks of gestation, in the absence of chorioamnionitis, is recommended according to the National Institutes of Health (NIH, 2000). Antenatal corticosteroids have been shown to significantly reduce RDS and intraventricular hemorrhage in the neonate. According to both the National Institues of Health and *The Cochrane Review* (Roberts and Dalziel,

2006) the corticosteroid treatment consists of a single course of betamethasone or dexamethasone. For betamethasone dosing, give two doses of 12 mg intramuscularly 24 hours apart. For dexamethasone dosing give four doses of 6 mg intramuscularly 12 hours apart (Weiner and Buhimschi, 2009). Although previous scientific data has shown repetitive courses of antenatal corticosteroids to carry potential risks with few or no benefits to the fetus, a recent randomized placebo-controlled trial demonstrated that neonatal outcomes improved significantly with administration of a single "rescue course" of antenatal corticosteroids before 33 weeks, without an evident increase of short-term risks (Garite, Kurtzman, Maurel, and others, 2009).

Tocolysis

The use of tocolysis in the presence of PROM is controversial. Tocolytic agents are less effective when membranes are ruptured, and may increase the risk for or mask the signs of an intrauterine infection (Mercer, 2009). According to the ICSI (2007), if tocolytics are used, they should be used to facilitate transfer; only long enough to allow sufficient time for gestational age and other assessments to be completed; for antibiotics to take effect; or if corticosteroids are used, for there to be sufficient time to have any benefit. (See Chapter 23 for further discussion of drug therapies.)

Intrapartum Prophylaxis for Group B Streptococcus (GBS)

The benefit of narrow-spectrum intrapartum prophylaxis with either intravenous penicillin or ampicillin to prevent transmission of GBS to the neonate is well documented. In the presence of rupture of membranes for 18 hours or more, with unknown GBS status, intrapartum antibiotic prophylaxis is indicated (CDC, 2002; Kenyon, Boulvain, and Neilson, 2004; ACOG, 2007).

NURSING MANAGEMENT

Prevention

Because the actual cause of PROM is unknown, prevention is difficult. However, it may be helpful to look at the risk factors and guard against these during pregnancy. Statistics indicate that socioeconomically disadvantaged patients and teenagers have an increased risk for PROM. The reason for this is unknown, but nutrition probably plays an important role. Therefore, these patients should be instructed early in pregnancy regarding a healthful diet for pregnancy and should be provided with reasons to follow this diet. They may also need referral to sources of financial assistance and food supplement programs, as well as instruction in how to prepare nutritious foods.

Cleanliness can also be a factor in decreasing the risk for PROM. Vaginal bacterial flora should be kept to a minimum. Instructions regarding the importance of daily bathing and wiping the perineum from front to back are important prenatal instructions. Multiple sexual partners increase vaginal bacterial count and should be discouraged.

Any attempt to facilitate increased immunity against infection is beneficial. Therefore maintaining cleanliness; drinking 6 to 8 ounces of fluid per waking hour;

exercising daily; resting adequately to avoid fatigue; and eating an adequate diet that is high in protein, zinc, and antioxidants are all beneficial in guarding against PROM.

A relationship between smoking and PROM has been demonstrated in numerous studies. Patients who smoke while pregnant should be instructed regarding its effect on pregnancy and should be supported in their attempts to stop smoking.

All pregnant women should be instructed regarding the danger signs in pregnancy, and PROM should be pointed out as one of these signs. The signs of membrane rupture and the necessity of prompt notification if these signs occur should be explained early in prenatal care.

Nursing Interventions to Decrease the Risk for Infection After PROM

- Assess and prove membrane rupture with PAMG-1 immunoassay (AmniSure) and/or by a sterile speculum examination (two out of three positive tests proving positive); by positive pooling; by positive ferning on collected slide specimen when viewed under a microscope; or by Nitrazine-positive result (paper turns from yellow to blue).
- Assess temperature every 4 hours or as indicated. (Maternal fever is one of the earlier signs of an intraamniotic infection.)
- Assess maternal pulse and blood pressure as indicated. (Tachycardia is one of the earlier signs of an intraamniotic infection.)
- Assess FHR as indicated. (Fetal tachycardia is one of the earlier signs of an intraamniotic infection.)
- Assess vaginal discharge for odor or color change.
- Assess for uterine tenderness.
- Assess for signs of a urinary tract infection.
- Determine nutritional habits.
- Determine activities since PROM.
- Refer to such diagnostic data as white blood cell count and C-reactive protein. A white blood cell count above 18,000/mm^3 is a significant sign of an infection during pregnancy. A normal C-reactive protein level is a valuable predictor of no intraamniotic infection.
- Assist in obtaining vaginal and urethral cultures for group B streptococci, chlamydia, and gonococcus. If any of these organisms is present, be prepared to start antibiotic therapy to decrease risk of neonatal infection. (Group B streptococcus is the most common cause of neonatal sepsis.)
- Assist with an amniocentesis to measure for gram-positive bacteria.
- Teach the benefits of bedrest with bathroom privileges only.
- Teach the importance of perineal care after each voiding and stool.
- Perform no vaginal examinations until the patient is in active labor.
- Prior to being discharged home for expectant management of PROM, the patient requires educational information about not having sexual intercourse, not performing any vaginal douching, taking temperature twice daily, taking showers only, notifying the physician if temperature is more than 38°C, if amniotic fluid loss increases or becomes foul-smelling, and returning to the clinical laboratory for a white blood cell count twice weekly.

- Notify the provider if temperature is greater than 38°C, fetal or maternal tachycardia develops, foul-smelling amniotic fluid develops, or amniotic fluid changes from straw color.
- If signs of an intraamniotic infection are manifested, be prepared to begin broad-spectrum antibiotic therapy, such as penicillin G and gentamicin, ampicillin and gentamicin, or cephalosporin. If the patient has a cesarean delivery, clindamycin may also be administered.

Nursing Interventions to Decrease Impaired Fetal Gas Exchange

- Continuous FHR monitoring initially and for about 48 to 72 hours after membrane rupture, to rule out fetal stressors.
- Assess maternal temperature, palpable abdominal tenderness unassociated with contractions, and any purulent vaginal discharge.
- During expectant management, periodically monitor FHR for variable decelerations and fetal activity.
- Observe amount of amniotic fluid leakage.
- Reposition the mother, and initiate intrauterine resuscitation measures if variable decelerations occur.
- Instruct the patient to report any decrease in fetal activity.
- Prepare the patient for ordered fetal well-being and maturity studies. BPPs, ultrasound, NSTs, AFI, and amniocentesis are usually ordered on a frequent basis in an attempt to determine the optimal time for delivery.
- Notify the physician if a baseline or periodic FHR change occurs, if an NST is nonreactive, or a BPP of 6 or less is noted.

Nursing Interventions to Decrease Fear and Stress

- Assess the family's anxiety over maternal, fetal, or neonatal well-being.
- Assess the family's coping strategies and resources.
- Encourage expectant parents to communicate openly about their feelings and concerns.
- Clarify any misconceptions.
- Provide information to the patient and her family regarding the pregnancy complication, treatment plan, and implications for mother and fetus in understandable terms.
- Arrange a tour of the intensive care nursery in the event of a possible preterm delivery.
- Refer to the social worker if inadequate coping is noted.
- Refer to a pastor, priest, or chaplain per patient's request.

Nursing Interventions to Promote Prescribed Bedrest

- Assess the patient's responsibilities to determine difficulties she will have in implementing prescribed bedrest.
- Teach the patient and her family about the importance of bedrest in the lateral position.
- Facilitate the family in problem solving if difficulties arise in implementing bedrest.

- Make needed referrals (for example, to the social worker) if problems are identified.
- Encourage the patient's participation in her own care and decision making as much as possible.
- Assess for side effects of prolonged bedrest and implement therapeutic interventions as outlined in Chapter 23.

Nursing Interventions to Decrease Other Antepartum Complications

- Assess for signs of preterm labor.
- Administer tocolytics if ordered.
- Provide routine prenatal education and care, as well as education for special care needs of a premature infant.

Intrapartum Nursing Interventions

- Use continuous fetal monitoring for early detection of nonreassuring FHR changes.
- Be prepared to administer intrapartum prophylaxis for group B streptococcus if vaginal and rectum culture is positive or unknown.
- Assess amniotic fluid for meconium.
- Reposition the patient, decrease uterine activity, begin an intravenous fluid bolus or increase fluid rate of infusion, correct maternal hypotension, begin amnioinfusion, and alter second-stage labor pushing efforts if variable decelerations occur.
- Be prepared to manage a saline amnioinfusion if multiple variable decelerations occur related to decreased amniotic fluid. Refer to Chapter 30 for the nursing interventions.
- Notify the physician at the first signs of a category II or category III FHR pattern.
- Once delivery is imminent, notify the intensive care nursery of a possible high-risk infant.

CONCLUSION

Because infections and lower amniotic fluid immunity play a significant role in PROM, the ultimate goal of the nurse should be to educate the patient. Prenatal education should cover the need for adequate fluids and nutrition, appropriate hygiene, and the significance of reporting any signs of an infection immediately. This decreases the risk for PROM. Once the membranes rupture, the goal of treatment is to allow for fetal maturity by maintaining the pregnancy as long as the uterine environment is healthy. If the uterine environment becomes infected or causes fetal compromise, the fetal outcome may be improved by premature delivery.

BIBLIOGRAPHY

American College of Obstetricians and Gynecologists (ACOG): *Premature rupture of membranes.* ACOG Pract Bull No. 80, 109(4):1007–1019, 2007.
Bendich A, Deckelbaum R: *Preventive nutrition: the comprehensive guide for health professionals,* ed 3, Totowa, NJ, 2005, Humana Press.

Brace R: Physiology of amniotic fluid volume regulation, *Clin Obstet Gynecol* 40(2):280–289, 1997.

Bryant-Greenwood GD: The extracellular matrix of the human fetal membranes: structure and function, *Placenta* 19:1–11, 1998.

Caughey AB, Robinson JN, Norwitz ER: Contemporary diagnosis and management of preterm premature rupture of membranes, *Rev Obstet Gyncol* 1(1):11–22, 2008.

Centers for Disease Control and Prevention (CDC): Prevention of perinatal group B streptococcal disease: revised guidelines from CDC, *MMWR Morb Mortal Wkly Rep* 51:RR-11, 2002.

Connors N, Merrill D: Antioxidants for prevention of preterm delivery, *Clin Obstet Gynecol* 47(4): 822–832, 2004.

Dare MR, Middleton P, Crowther CA, and others: Planned early birth versus expectant management (waiting) for prelabour rupture of membranes at term (37 weeks or more), *Cochrane Database Syst Rev* 2006, Issue 1. Art. No.: CD005302.

Gabbe SG, Niebyl JR, Simpson JL: *Obstetrics: normal and problem pregnancies*, ed 5, Philadelphia, 2007, Churchill Livingstone.

Garite TJ, Kurtzman J, Maurel K, and others: Impact of a 'rescue course' of antenatal corticosteroids: a multicenter randomized placebo-controlled trial, *Am J Obstet Gynecol* 200:248.e1–248.e9, 2009.

Institute for Clinical Systems Improvement (ICSI): *Health care guideline: Management of labor*, Bloomington, Minn, 2007, ICSI. Retrieved from http://www.icsi.org.

James D, Mahomed K, Stone P, and others, editors: *Evidence-based obstetrics: a companion volume to high risk pregnancy*, ed 2, Philadelphia, 2004, Saunders.

Kenyon S, Boulvain M, Neilson JP: Antibiotics for preterm rupture of membranes, *Cochrane Database Syst Rev* Issue 3. Art. No.: CD001058, 2004.

Lee SE, Park JS, Norwitz ER, and others: Measurement of placental alpha-microglobulin-1 in cervicovaginal discharge to diagnose rupture of membranes, *Obstet Gynecol* 109(3):634–640, 2007.

Lee T, Carpenter M, Heber WW, Silver HM: Preterm premature rupture of membranes: risks of recurrent complications in the next pregnancy among a population-based sample of gravid women, *Am J Obstet Gynecol* 188:209–213, 2003.

Mercer B: Premature rupture of membranes. In Creasy R, Resnik R, Iams J, and others, editors: *Creasy & Resnik's maternal-fetal medicine: principles and practice*, ed 6, Philadelphia, 2009, Saunders.

Mercer B: Preterm premature rupture of the membranes, *Obstet Gynecol* 101(1):178–193, 2003.

National Institutes of Health (NIH): *Antenatal corticosteroids revisited*. Consensus development conference statement, Maryland, 2000, NIH. Retrieved from http://www.consensus.nih.gov.

Parry S, Strauss J: Premature rupture of fetal membranes, *N Engl J Med* 338(10):663–670, 1998.

Roberts D, Dalziel SR: Antenatal corticosteroids for accelerating fetal lung maturation for women at risk of preterm birth, *Cochrane Database Syst Rev* Issue 3. Art. No.: CD004454, 2006.

Svigos J, Robinson J, Vigneswaran R: Prelabor rupture of membranes. In James D, and others, editors: *High risk pregnancy: management options*, ed 3, Philadelphia, 2006, Saunders.

Stringer M, and others: Nursing care of the patient with preterm premature rupture of membranes, *MCN Am J Matern Child Nurs* 29(3):142–150, 2004.

Weiner C, Buhimschi C: *Drugs for pregnant and lactating women*, ed 2, Philadelphia, Saunders.

Weitz B: Premature rupture of membranes: an update for the advanced practice nurse, *MCN Am J Matern Child Nurs* 26(2):86–92, 2001.

Wilkes P, Galan H: Premature rupture of membranes, *Emedicine.com, Inc* , 2004.

Woods J, Plessinger M, Miller R: Vitamins C and E: missing links in preventing preterm premature rupture of membranes? *Am J Obstet Gynecol* 185(1):5–10, 2001.

25

Trauma

Trauma during pregnancy varies in degree and causation. It is caused by motor vehicle collisions (MVCs), accidental injury, and domestic violence. An estimated 7% of all pregnant women suffer some type of trauma during their pregnancy (Grossman, 2004a). Trauma is a leading cause of maternal death, accounting for 46% of such cases (Chames and Pearlman, 2008). The frequency of injury increases with each trimester; therefore the highest risk for injury is in the third trimester. Trauma causes death of the fetus more often than death of the mother (Bobrowski, 2006).

When pregnancy is complicated by trauma, providers who are not routinely accustomed to managing trauma may provide emergency care in a variety of settings outside trauma units, including obstetric units and outpatient settings. In addition, trauma teams in emergency centers are often unfamiliar with some of the physiologic considerations specific to pregnancy and with caring for a second, invisible patient (the fetus).

INCIDENCE

Statistics support recognition of trauma as a significant complication in pregnancy:
- Significant trauma occurs to approximately 1 in 12 pregnant women; about two thirds of these injuries occur as a result of motor vehicle injuries (Klinich, Schneider, Moore, and others, 2000).
- Of all injuries during pregnancy, 54% result from MVCs; 70% of the major, life-threatening injuries are from MVCs (Divekar and Keith, 2004).
- Fifty percent of fetal deaths result from a life-threatening trauma (Mattox and Goetzl, 2005)
- Approximately 25% to 30% of pregnant women are physically or sexually abused (Guth and Pachter, 2000; Hedin and Janson, 2000) but only 3% to 8% of these abuses are detected (Cox, Kilpatrick, and Geller, 2004; FVPF, 2004).

ETIOLOGY

MVCs and domestic violence are the leading causes of maternal trauma during pregnancy, and MVCs lead to the most deaths (FVPF, 2004; Grossman, 2004a; Chang and others, 2005). Falls (49%); assaults (18%); burns (1%); and penetrating injuries, such as stabbing to the abdomen and gunshot wounds (4%) (Pearlman and others, 2000), are also significant causes of maternal and fetal trauma.

Battering is reported as a source of serious injury during pregnancy, but it is difficult to acquire specific statistics because these crimes are generally under-reported. Abuse can be physical, emotional, or sexual; it can also be in the form of economic abuse or isolation. The cause of domestic violence and abuse involves the need for the partner in a domestic relationship to exert power and control over the pregnant woman. Recent research indicates that between 1% and 20% of pregnant women are battered, and those asked more than once in the pregnancy reported an even higher prevalence (Shoffner, 2008).

Violent assaults and suicide are other causes of maternal death from trauma. Most of maternal deaths from trauma of this type are the result of head trauma or intraabdominal injuries.

PATHOPHYSIOLOGY

The pathophysiology to be considered depends on the type of injury, the source of injury, and the system or part of the body affected. Because head injury and abdominal hemorrhage are common lethal maternal effects, discussion of pathophysiology focuses on both. Other complications of trauma include abruption, preterm rupture of membranes (PROM), preterm delivery, fetomaternal hemorrhage, Rhesus D alloimmunization, and direct fetal injury or death (Chames and Pearlman, 2008).

HEMORRHAGE

Because of the total blood volume increase during pregnancy, trauma involving abdominal hemorrhage has profound hemodynamic consequences that place the pregnant woman at much greater risk than a nonpregnant counterpart. These consequences include the following (Grossman, 2004a; Bobrowski, 2006):

- By 32 to 34 weeks of gestation, there is an average of 50% blood volume increase. Because clinical signs of shock usually present as a function of percentage of total blood loss, the pregnant patient has a greater absolute amount of blood loss than a nonpregnant person in a similar state. Thus a larger amount of blood replacement is needed in resuscitative efforts.
- Because of the increased blood volume available to her, the pregnant woman may be able to more readily, although temporarily, maintain hemodynamic stability at the expense of the fetus. Reflex compensatory vasoconstrictive responses can significantly decrease uteroplacental perfusion, compromising the fetus.
- Although cardiac output is increased by 30% to 40% near term, supine positioning is likely to confuse the general picture of potential shock by potentiating hypotension. Supine positioning decreases cardiac output secondary to decreased cardiac return from mechanical obstruction of the inferior vena cava by the gravid uterus.
- Because the pregnant woman's heart rate is already increased by approximately 10 to 15 beats/minute and blood pressure falls in the second trimester, these two parameters may confuse the clinical picture for the provider who is unfamiliar with normal physiologic hemodynamic alterations in pregnancy.

- When the gravid abdomen sustains trauma, both the uterus, with its increased circulating volume, and the bladder are more anatomically prone to injury. Abdominal injury adds an additional risk for significant maternal hemorrhage secondary to placental abruption.
- The kidneys and ureters are relatively protected from injury by the uterus. However, normal dilation of the ureters may be misinterpreted on radiologic examination of the abdomen following injury.
- Anatomically, the bowel is pushed upward and is more prominent during pregnancy. As a result, the small and large intestines are at greater risk for injury from blunt or penetrating trauma.
- Because pregnancy is a hypercoagulable state, risks for thrombosis after injury are increased.
- Disseminated intravascular coagulopathy (DIC), a frequent complication of severe abdominal trauma, may also present atypically. The normal fibrinogen level in pregnancy is four to five times the nonpregnant level. As a result, the lower nonpregnant levels, when applied to pregnant women, may signify early DIC. (See Chapters 19 and 20 for signs and symptoms of shock, DIC, and placental abruption.)

Neurologic Injury

The neurologic exam may be confusing. For example, eclampsia can mimic head injury. Therefore to make the correct diagnosis, first identify if the patient has hyperreflexia, proteinuria, or hypertension to differentiate between eclampsia and a neurologic head injury caused by trauma. Head injury is often severe enough to result in maternal death. No significant neurophysiologic adaptations in pregnancy alter presentation of the clinical picture. However, if maternal brain death occurs, the fetus may remain viable. Therefore maternal brain death needs to be considered from an ethical perspective because of the presence of the fetus.

Brain death is the unequivocal and irreversible loss of total brain function. It is a concept used to determine when death has occurred even though Advanced Cardiac Life Support (ACLS) and life support technology may obscure the conventional criteria for diagnosis of life or death. Once the diagnosis of brain death is made, cardiopulmonary collapse may be expected within 72 hours. Continued somatic support of the mother may be possible, even for prolonged periods, to extend the pregnancy and further fetal maturation. The ICU team will need to provide nutrition, temperature regulation, and respiratory and hemodynamic support and anticipate the expected physiologic changes after brain death that may occur, such as infection (Mallampalli and Guy, 2005). If the woman has given an advance directive for removal of life support in such a situation, maternal brain death presents a case for continued artificial support for the sake of the fetus. Spinal injury is another type of neurologic injury that can have pathophysiologic consequences in the pregnant woman. When spinal cord injury occurs during the course of an established pregnancy, the following complications may occur (Carbuapoma, Tomlinson, and Levine, 2006):

- With lesions above the tenth thoracic segment, the woman will not note onset of abdominal pain or discomfort. Because of the caudal entrance of the afferent uterine nerves, the nerve supply to the uterus is interrupted. Thus the uterus can contract normally, but there is an absence of associated pain sensation with onset of labor contractions.

- Complete cord lesions above the fifth or sixth thoracic segment, above the splanchnic outflow, may cause the development of the syndrome of hyperreflexia with the onset of contractions.

- Hyperreflexia is caused by the sudden release of catecholamines. These symptoms include throbbing headache, hypertension, reflex bradycardia, sweating, nasal congestion, and vasodilation.

- Autonomic dysplasia may result from a noxious stimulus such as a full bladder, contractions, or a vaginal exam resulting in tremors. If the woman becomes a paraplegic from neurologic injury, operative assisted delivery may be necessary after passive fetal descent in second stage labor.

Chest Injury

Physiologic adaptations in respiratory functions may confuse the understanding of the pathophysiology of chest injury and confound resuscitative efforts. During pregnancy there is increased oxygen (O_2) consumption, increased tidal volume, decreased arterial carbon dioxide partial pressure (PCO_2), and decreased serum bicarbonate. Chronic, compensatory respiratory alkalosis may mislead the resuscitation team in evaluation of blood gases. Blood buffering capabilities decrease during pregnancy; therefore reestablishing acid-base homeostasis is more difficult.

Before placing a chest tube, rule out a rib injury, pneumothorax, or injury to the diaphragm. The chest tube may need to be inserted one to two interspaces higher than normal because of the decreased vertical height of the chest. Analgesia is important to prevent atelectasis (Weinberg, Steele, Pugh, and others, 2005).

Pelvic Fractures

The large, engorged pelvic vessels that surround the gravid uterus can result in massive retroperitoneal bleeding and/or placental abruption after a blunt trauma associated with pelvic fractures. The pelvis usually fractures in two places in the bony ring. If the fetal head is engaged, fetal skull fracture may occur.

Thermal (Burn) Trauma

Classification of thermal injury is according to the percentage of the body burned, the depth involved, and gestational age. If more than 60% of the body is affected, there is significant risk for maternal death. Because of the normally hypervolemic state in pregnancy, fluid resuscitation must be vigorous, with prompt evaluation and correction of electrolyte imbalance. After a severe burn, fetal survival is directly related to maternal complications such as hypoxia, hypotension, hypovolemia, and sepsis. According to Shah and Kilcline (2003), fetal mortality rate approximates the percent of total body surface (TBSA) burned. They found the mortality rate for the fetus approaches 100% when maternal burns cover more than 50% of the mother's body. Fetal survival is approximately 78% if the total body surface area (TBSA) is less than 30%. When fetal death occurs, it is usually within one week of initial injury (Shah and Kilcline, 2003).

Gunshot and Stab Wounds

The location and gestational age are crucial to the risk of fetal injury, fetal mortality, and maternal outcomes in cases of penetrating trauma injury resulting from stabbings or gunshot wounds. As the pregnancy advances to the second trimester, the gravid uterus moves out of the protective bony pelvis into the abdominal cavity. Then severity of injury is dependent on direct injury location and may precipitate a preterm delivery. According to Shah and Kilcline (2003), "Abdominal gunshot wounds can cause transient shock waves and cavitations as they impart their kinetic energy to the high-density tissues of the body, and result in more severe injuries than a low velocity knife. The fetus is at high risk with 66% of fetal injuries resulting from gunshot injuries to the uterus."

Homicide

Homicide is a leading cause of traumatic death for pregnant and postpartum women in the United States, accounting for 31% of maternal injury deaths (Campbell and Furniss, 2002).

MATERNAL EFFECTS

Trauma is the leading cause of nonobstetric maternal death from head injury, hemorrhage, shock, disseminated intravascular coagulation (DIC), respiratory compromise, cardiopulmonary arrest, or syndrome of hyperreflexia with spinal cord injury. Shock from excessive bleeding can reduce perfusion to the enlarged pituitary gland, which increases in size by 30% in pregnancy. Sheehan syndrome develops as a result of pituitary cell damage and/or necrosis, thus the production of the usual pituitary hormones will be significantly reduced. With blunt abdominal trauma, injury to the liver or spleen can occur, causing severe hemorrhage. With blunt trauma, indirect injury to the fetus may occur from rapid compression, deceleration, the contrecoup effect, or a shearing force resulting in placental abruption.

Indirect injury caused by abuse during pregnancy can have indirect adverse effects as well, including causing chronic health problems such as depression, substance abuse, delayed prenatal care, and inadequate nutrition (ANA, 2000).

FETAL EFFECTS

The fetus is extremely vulnerable to the effects of maternal trauma, especially blunt or penetrating trauma to the abdomen (Bobrowski, 2006). Fetal deaths result from MVCs (82%), gunshot wounds (6%), and falls (3%), with maternal death accounting for 11% of fetal deaths (Weiss, Songer, and Fabio, 2001). Once trauma has occurred, maternal shock is the leading cause of fetal death; the second most common cause is abruptio placentae, which can occur without a direct blow to the abdomen (Bryan and Bledsoe, 2002; Grossman, 2004a). Abruptio placentae is the most common cause of fetal death when the mother survives (Divekar and Keith, 2004). There is also a 5% risk following a minor injury. There is a 50% risk for an abruption following severe trauma or blunt abdominal trauma. In those cases of severe injuries, fetal mortality may be greater than 60% (Tsuei, 2006). Other common fetal effects include the following:
- PROM
- Premature labor and delivery

- Spontaneous abortion or stillbirth
- Fetal maternal transfusion
- Fetal skull injuries, especially when the fetal head is engaged and there is a maternal pelvic fracture
- Hypoxia secondary to maternal respiratory compromise; hypovolemic, spinal, or cardiogenic shock; DIC; thermal injury; or maternal cardiopulmonary arrest

MANAGEMENT OF THE PREGNANT TRAUMA PATIENT

Management of the pregnant woman and the fetus can be prioritized depending on gestational age of the fetus. The first group consists of women who at the time of the injury did not realize they were pregnant. All injured women of reproductive age should receive a pregnancy test. There is a potential for teratogenic injury to the fetus in the first trimester resulting from routine radiographic studies. The second group of patients consists of those women of less than 24 weeks of gestation (previability). Resuscitation is primarily aimed at the mother in this group. In the third group two patients must be considered during the assessment, monitoring, and resuscitation. Care must be focused on the mother for a life-threatening event; once the mother is stabilized the fetus can be rescued.

Minor Injury Management

A minor injury may be described as losing one's balance and falling, with or without a blow to the abdomen. It may also be described as a minor MVC with no obvious injuries or marks, but with some degree of jarring. After a minor injury, the initial assessment usually takes place in the trauma unit, emergency department, or obstetric triage unit. The following areas should be covered in the initial assessment:

- History of the circumstances surrounding the incident
- Diagnostic tests and procedures as dictated by the initial injury
- Monitoring of mother and fetus for contractions and fetal heart rate (FHR) if 20 weeks of gestation or more
- Follow-up evaluation for occult abruption with continuous fetal monitoring, usually for a minimum of 6 to 8 hours (ACOG, 1998), and a Kleihauer-Betke test for fetal to maternal hemorrhage

Major Injury Management

Immediately after major trauma, diagnosis and treatment occur almost simultaneously in three phases.

Initial Care Phase

Primary survey of a pregnant woman

The trauma healthcare team does a primary assessment and evaluation of each patient who arrives to the emergency trauma room for care using Advance Trauma Life Support (ATLS).

A - Airway: Establish an airway, provide prompt and aggressive ventilation and oxygenation, and place a cervical spine immobilizer for stabilization and to prevent further neurologic damage.

Weinberg and others (2005) suggest using cricoid pressure and preoxygenation before any intubations for airway compromise.

B - Breathing: A PaCO$_2$ of 35 to 40 mm Hg may indicate respiratory failure during pregnancy. If not recognized, it may lead to impending respiratory failure during pregnancy. Reduced functional residual capacity and increased oxygen consumption can result in rapid decline in oxygenation (Mallampalli and Guy, 2005).

C - Circulation and Control hemorrhage: Provide circulation volume and log roll the >20 week parturient on a backboard with a towel rolled under the hip to prevent supine hypotension. The pregnant patient can lose a significant amount of blood before becoming symptomatic with tachycardia and hypotension because of the increased intravascular volume. Hypovolemia may first manifest as fetal distress. The viable fetus (over 24 weeks) should be monitored to assure placental perfusion. Two large bore intravenous cannulae with a rapid infuser should be available if needed. Replace blood loss with isotonic crystalloid fluid and if the patient is clinically showing signs of anemia, a blood transfusion should be administered to support physiologic hypovolemia.

D - Disability: Perform a brief neurologic evaluation. Assign an injury severity score using the Glasgow coma scale, or assess the patient in terms of alertness (alert is measured by response to voice, response to pain, or unresponsive).

E - Expose the patient and temperature control: Inspect the entire body while preventing the patient from becoming acidotic, as it can lead to hypothermia.

F - Fetal basic assessment: Fetal ultrasound for fetal heart rate and gestational age, placenta location, and amniotic fluid volume; fetal heart rate; uterine tenderness; and contraction monitoring. When assessing for fetal heart tones, check the maternal heart rate that can be tachycardiac because of being frightened or in pain. The maternal pulse can be confused for the fetal heart rate.

Secondary assessment starts after the initial stabilization by reevaluating vital signs. The most common laboratory studies are complete blood count (CBC), blood type and Rh, lactic acid, serum alcohol level, urine drug screen, and the Kleihauer Betke test. If the patient's condition warrants, additional laboratory tests are ordered that include: comprehensive metabolic panel, urinalysis, clotting time and panel such as fibrinogen split products and fibrinogen. A sterile speculum and/or vaginal examination done by an obstetrical practitioner may be necessary to determine testing for amniotic fluid and progression of labor. Observe for vaginal bleeding.

The secondary physical assessment is a complete "head to toe" evaluation with a focus on mechanism of injury. Figure 25-1 summarizes the secondary physical assessment following trauma during pregnancy.

Cardiopulmonary Resuscitation

Standard Advanced Cardiac Life Support should be followed with a pregnant woman. There is increased likelihood that artificial ventilation will be needed because of the anatomic shift of the diaphragm.

Defibrillation. If defibrillation is necessary and a fetal spiral electrode is being used to monitor the FHR, the wires should be disconnected from the fetus.

Perimortem. If maternal resuscitation efforts are not successful after the first 5 minutes of cardiac arrest, a perimortem (agonal or postmortem) cesarean section may facilitate maternal resuscitation and preserve the life of the fetus unless the fetus is no longer viable or less than 23 weeks of gestation (Foley and Strong, 2004;

Head	__Clear __Abrasions __Swelling __Lacerations __Drainage
Face	__Clear __Abrasions __Swelling __Lacerations __Drainage __Other
Neck	__Clear __Tender __Crepitus __Abrasions __Trachea midline __Trachea deviated R__L__ __Laceration
Tympanic Membranes	__Clear __Blood Present R__L__ Central spinal fluid present R__L__
Nares	__Clear __Blood Present R__L__ Central spinal fluid present R__L__
Mouth	__Clear __Broken teeth __Lacerations __Bite deviated Foreign bodies __Tongue cut __Swollen
Chest	__Clear __Crepitus __Abrasions __Lacerations __Instability __Deformity __Symmetrical breathing __Seat belt sign on chest
Heart Tones	__Present __Deviated R__L__ __Muffled __Absent
Abdomen	__Clear __Crepitus __Abrasions __Lacerations __Abrasions __Tender __Seat belt sign on chest
Bowel Sounds	__Present __Absent __Hypoactive __Hyperactive
Genito-urinary	__Clear __Blood at meatus __Lacerations __Bruising __Drainage
Rectal Exam	__Normal Tone __Decreased Tone __Absent Tone __Guaiac Done __hemorrhoids present
Upper Extremities	__Clear __Pulses Present R__L__ __Pulses Absent R__L__ __Lacerations __Abrasions __Deformity __Motor sensory
Lower Extremities	__Clear __Pulses Present R__L__ __Pulses Absent R__L__ __Lacerations __Abrasions __Deformity __Motor sensory
Back	__Clear __Crepitus __Abrasions __Lacerations __Instability __Deformity
Emotional	__Cooperative __Crying\Upset __Anxious __Uncooperative __Sedated

Figure 25-1 Secondary physical assessment following trauma during pregnancy.

Mallampalli and Guy, 2005; Weinberg and others, 2005). The assistance of the neo-natal nursery team must be elicited because surviving infants will frequently be premature and may need extensive support immediately after delivery.

Tertiary Assessment

Not all injuries are detected by the first and secondary assessment surveys. According to Janjua, Sugrue, and Deane (1998), "between 2% and 50% of combined life-threatening and non–life-threatening injuries are missed. Centers that examined the incidence of missed injuries concur that patients who sustain blunt trauma have a higher rate of missed injuries than those who sustain penetrating trauma." The tertiary survey usually occurs within 24 hours after admission and is repeated when the patient is awake, responsive, and able to communicate any complaints. The tertiary trauma survey consists of a comprehensive review of the medical record emphasizing the cause of injury and any pertinent comorbid factors such as age. The primary and secondary surveys are repeated and all diagnostic tests reviewed. Any new physical findings require further studies to rule out missed injuries. Continuously monitor for uterine contractions and fetal wellbeing for a minimum of 4 to 6 hours or longer as indicated. (Foley and Strong, 2004) Amniocentesis may be done to assess fetal lung maturity, infection, or intrauterine bleeding.

Continued Monitoring in the Labor and Delivery or Critical Care Unit

Although initial emergency assessment and stabilization may be performed in any level trauma center, emergency department, or surgical service, continued maternal care for serious trauma commonly is delivered in critical care units.

Cesarean delivery is usually indicated when the fetus is bradycardiac and older than 24 weeks of gestation. However, other variables to consider are the length of time the cardiopulmonary resuscitation was in progress, amount of time the patient had loss of vital signs, and the patient's status when arriving to the trauma room. If the mother is brain dead, she may be kept on life support until the fetus has an opportunity to grow to maturity.

Recovery and Rehabilitation Phase

During the recovery and rehabilitation phase, assessments are directed at identification of potential long-term complications and sequelae. Interventions during this phase are focused on restoration of optimal functional capabilities.

NURSING MANAGEMENT

Prevention

All pregnant women should be made aware of their potential for injuries and trauma and ways to prevent them, especially those related to MVCs and domestic violence and abuse. Prevention of violence against women is one of the top priority health issues for the United States as identified in the *Healthy People 2010* report (USD-HHS, 2000). Association between domestic violence and 8 of the 10 leading health indicators of the federal *Healthy People 2010* initiative have been recognized (FVPF, 2003). These indicators are obesity, tobacco use, substance abuse, responsible sexual behavior, mental health, injury, immunization, and access to health care.

Motor Vehicle Collision Prevention

Efforts to teach and demonstrate safe and consistent use of car safety belts can have a major impact on the degree of injury, especially blunt trauma to the abdomen. Studies over the past 10 years state that 25% to 33% of pregnant women do not wear car seat restraints properly, in part because of the mother's fear the seat belt could harm the fetus (Metz and Abbott, 2006). Every pregnant patient should be taught that the seat belt harness should be used, no matter how short the trip. The current recommendation for seat belt use during pregnancy is for the shoulder strap to cross between the breasts and over the upper abdomen above the uterus. The lap belt should cross over the pelvis below the uterus (McGwin and others, 2004; Grossman, 2004b; Metz and Abbott, 2006).

The unrestrained pregnant patient has a higher risk of premature delivery and fetal death in comparison with the restrained parturient. The use of a lap belt alone may result in abruption and cause uterine rupture from the direct force to the uterus on impact. The use of the combined lap and shoulder seat belt reduces the direct and indirect forces to the uterus. The lap and shoulder straps used together prevent forward flexion of the mother and distributes the force or the thrusting/deceleration movement over a greater surface area. Placental abruption does not occur more frequently in MVCs with airbag deployment (Metz, and Abbott, 2006). A discussion of the pregnant woman's vulnerability should include encouragement to avoid fatigue, avoid late departures, and avoid distractions such as loud music, cell phones, and arguing children.

The major risk in an MVC is from the impact and resultant momentum, causing gross traumatic separation of the placenta from the wall of the uterus. If a small amount separates at the beginning, the signs may occur slowly with uterine tenderness, frequent contractions, and uterine tetany. Thirty percent of cases that develop an abruption will have insidious symptoms and 70% will manifest an overt massive separation, usually accompanied by obvious signs of shock and hemorrhage (ATLS, 2008; Harris, 2001). The most sensitive laboratory test indicating an abruption is a decreased fibrinogen test (Foley and Strong, 2004).

Uterine rupture is rare. If it occurs, common symptoms are abdominal tenderness, guarding, rigidity, or rebound tenderness. The uterus may have an irregular shape, palpable fetal parts, or an abnormal lie upon ultrasound. Profound shock may result.

Other Accidental Injuries

Pregnant women should be made aware of sources of injury, such as falls resulting from the displaced center of gravity or increased joint flexibility.

Intimate Partner Violence (IPV)

Intimate partner violence (IPV), more commonly known as domestic violence, is defined as the use of threats, physical, emotional, and/or sexual abuse, with the intent of instilling fear and intimidating and controlling another person (Centers for Disease Control, 2004). Approximately 5.3 million intimate partner victimizations occur every year among women over 18 years of age, particularly common during the ages 16 to 24 years, within the United States. It has been estimated that approximately 324,000 of these victimizations occur during pregnancy (Tjaden and Thoennes, 2000).

Homicide may be the result of IPV. Health care professionals see 47% of intimate partner homicide and attempted homicide in the year before their deaths (Parsons, Goodwin, and Petersen, 2000). Intimate partner violence can affect the fetus. High rates of stress can lead to illicit drug use, coping by self medicating. Physical assaults can result in higher rates of preterm labor, infections, complications, placental abruption, hemorrhage, women less likely to seek prenatal care, and low birth weight infants (Ellis, Chang, Bhandari, and others, 2008). Children raised in violent homes have both immediate and life-long adverse health outcomes as a result of their exposure to IPV (Chambliss, 2008).

Signs of intimate partner violence or abuse include the following:
• Delayed prenatal care
• Frequent visits to emergency units

- Recurrent or unexplained chronic pain or vague complaints of fatigue, depression, or difficulty swallowing without apparent etiology
- Unexplained injuries or injuries at different stages of healing
- Very low self-esteem or flattened affect
- Jealous or possessive partner
- Partner speaking for the patient, acting overprotective, or refusing to leave the room for any part of examination or interview

Intimate Partner Violence (IPV) Prevention

The American College of Obstetricians and Gynecologists (ACOG, 2006) recommends screening for abuse during every trimester of pregnancy and postpartum. Families that are known to be at risk should be observed and provided preventive intervention as needed, such as referral for stress reduction, emotional support, improving communication, and improving interpersonal relationships. If there already exists a pattern of abuse in handling conflict, it is more likely that it will continue and escalate during and after pregnancy (Kramer, 2007). Therefore an environment friendly and conducive to disclosure should be established in every obstetric care setting. Ways to accomplish this include the following:

- Place posters and brochures in accessible areas in the health care setting such as in the waiting room, in the bathrooms, and near the scales.
- Ensure privacy during the screening assessment.
- Have referral information available.

According to Dunn and Oths (2004), prenatal predictors of domestic violence are:

- Stressful life
- Depression
- Lack of spiritual values
- Lack of contraceptive use

An abuse assessment screen that can be reproduced was developed by the Nursing Research Consortium on Violence and Abuse (Parker, McFarlane, and Soeken, 1994; Christian, 1995; Norton and others, 1995). The assessment screen includes four basic questions and a scoring system for the degree of threat pertaining to specific types of abuse. The Abuse Assessment Screen (AAS) is an effective screening tool of abused pregnant women (Higgins and Hawkins, 2005). There are four questions and it takes less than a minute to complete if all the answers are no. Identification and intervention of IPV impacts both mother and infant. It is important to construct the questions in a comfortable manner and in a setting likely to encourage disclosure from the patient. You may formulate the questions below into a less formalized questionnaire or use a preprinted form with an explanation that makes the patient feel comfortable, cared about, and not singled out. For example, "This is a questionnaire we have found helpful in assessing all our patients so that we are better able to help keep you and your baby healthy." Most assessment tools include the following questions:

- Has your partner or someone important to you ever emotionally or physically abused you?
- Within the last year, have you been hit, slapped, kicked, or otherwise physically hurt by someone?

- Since you have been pregnant, have you been hit, slapped, or otherwise physically hurt by someone?
- Are you afraid of your partner or anyone else listed above?

Disclosure most often occurs when there is a trusting relationship, when the abused woman needs help, or when the emotional pain is intense. It may take as many as six interactions with a healthcare professional before a woman who is abused discloses the violence (Mayer, 2000). Pregnancy may be the catalyst for abuse. Perinatal nurses should screen all pregnant women. Box 25-1 presents an abuse assessment screening tool. At times healthcare providers do not recognize the subtle or overt signs of abuse, or choose to ignore them or accept the woman's statement that she "fell down the stairs" because of their discomfort in getting involved with helping her make decisions about how to best deal with the violent situation in which she lives (Shoffner, 2008).

Pregnant women who are battered need education, support, and intervention to break the cycle of abuse that includes an immediate risk assessment and safety plan. A Danger Assessment instrument by Campbell (2004) is available for a fee online (*http://www.dangerassessment.org*). The first portion of the measure assesses severity and frequency of battering by presenting the woman with a calendar of the past year. The second part of the Danger Assessment is a 20-item instrument that uses a weighted scoring system to count yes/no responses of risk factors associated with intimate partner homicide. Other excellent resource materials regarding documentation, intervention, and referral are available from the Family Violence Prevention Fund (FVPF, 2004) entitled *National Consensus Guidelines*. These materials can also be accessed online (*www.endabuse.org/programs/healthcare/files/Consensus.pdf*).

Box 25-1   Abuse Assessment Screen

Assessment Questionnaire

Have you ever been emotionally or physically abused by your partner or someone important to you?

☐ Yes or ☐ No

Within the last year, have you been hit, slapped, kicked, or otherwise physically hurt by someone?

☐ Yes or ☐ No

If yes, by whom? _____

Total number of times? _____

Since you have become pregnant, have you been hit, slapped, kicked, or otherwise physically hurt by someone?

☐ Yes or ☐ No

If yes, by whom? _____

Total number of times? _____

Are you afraid of your partner or anyone you have already mentioned?

☐ Yes or ☐ No

Reference: Christian A: Home care of the battered pregnant woman: one woman's battered pregnancy, *J Obstet Gynecol Neonatal Nurs* 24(9):836-842,1995; Norton L, and others: Battering in pregnancy: an assessment of tool screening methods, *Obstet Gynecol* 85(3):321-325,1995; Parker B, McFarlane J, Soeken K: Abuse during pregnancy: effects on maternal complications and birth weight in adult and teenage women, *Obstet Gynecol* 84(3):323-328, 1994.

General Nursing Interventions for Psychosocial and Physical Diagnoses Related to Intimate Partner Violence

- Provide education about battering.
- Provide information about community resources and how to use them.
- Assist in planning strategies for safety crisis intervention.
- Support and advocate for the pregnant woman when she is unable to advocate for herself.
- Encourage a problem-solving approach with the woman so that she is able to look at and evaluate various options. Support her choices whenever possible.
- Be aware of the local laws regarding reporting procedures and assist the woman if she wishes to file a report.
- Be prepared to make appropriate referrals to available resources for the family. If the woman or children are in danger of harm, refer immediately to a battered women's shelter.
- Refer the woman's partner to a resource for abusers if the opportunity presents and it does not violate issues of trust for the woman.

Specific Nursing Interventions for Intimate Partner Violence

If the woman reveals that she has been abused, respond using the ABCDEs for universal screening:

A: Acknowledge to the woman that she is not alone. "Many women are in abusive relationships."

B: Believe the woman and acknowledge her grief and pain. "No one deserves to be hurt" and "It is not your fault."

C: Confidentiality is vitally important. Reassure the woman that health care providers will keep all the information she provides confidential. Know the state laws about mandatory reporting. A few states such as California, Kentucky, New Mexico, New Hampshire, and Rhode Island currently mandate reporting. If child abuse is reported or suspected, all states require that the local child protection agency be informed. Child abuse occurs in 50% of domestic violence situations (U.S. Advisory Board on Child Abuse and Neglect, 1995).

D: Document specific details and place the patient's statements in quotation marks. Document any visual injury by using a body map or photograph with size referencing such as a coin or ruler next to the injury. If injuries are in various stages of healing, record this as well. Documentation can be helpful to the woman later during any legal encounters. Document referrals and information provided. If prenatal records are sent to the labor and delivery area, an undefined coding system might be used and the documentation written in a form separate from the chart. A documentation form is available for use from the Family Violence Prevention Fund.

E: Educate the woman regarding the cyclic nature of abuse, safety measures, importance of a safety plan, legal issues such as restraining and protection orders, and referrals. National resources are listed in Table 25-1. If social services are available, provide referral.

S: Safety is the key. Communicate concern for the woman's safety and assure her that help is available when she is ready. Assist the woman if she wishes to file a report and obtain a restraining/protective order. If the woman or children are in danger of harm, refer immediately to a battered women's shelter. Refer the woman's partner to a resource for abusers if the opportunity presents and it does not violate issues of trust for the woman. If she is not ready to report or leave the situation, support her by providing her with information about how to develop a safety plan. Many community agencies provide written materials to help the woman develop a plan. Provide her with resources as well.

There is another method for IPV assessment and intervention (Open question, Affirming, Reflecting, and Summarizing) that uses the acronym OARS (Miller and Rollnick, 2002; Kramer, 2007).

- Open questions avoid a simple no or yes answer.
- Affirming helps the abuser with feelings of self worth and courage for confiding.

Table 25-1   Domestic Violence Resouces

Agency	Phone Number or Web Address
National Domestic Violence Hotline	(800) 799-SAFE (7233)
Family Violence Prevention Fund (FVPF)	(888) RX-ABUSE http://www.endabuse.org/health
American College of Obstetricians and Gynecologist: Violence Against Women	http://www.acog.org/departments/dept_web.efm?recno=17
National Guidelines and Health Care Protocols	
National Coalition Against Domestic Violence CDC Guidelines	www.ncadv.org
CDC Guidelines	www.cdc.gov/reproductivehealth/violence/IntimatePartnerViolence/Index.htm
U.S. Department of Health and Human Services	http://www.ama-assn.org/ama/upload/mm/386/guidlines.pdf
Reporting Requirements	http://www.ndaa.org/pdf/dv_reporting_requirements.pdf
Rape Abuse & Incest National Network (RAINN)	(800) 656-HOPE (4673)
Prevent Domestic Violence Assists in developing a personalized safety plan	http://www.domesticviolence.org/plan.html
Shelter Hotline	(800) 799-7739
Legal Advocacy Hotline	(800) 782-6400
List of state domestic violence or sexual assault coalitions	http://www.ojp.usdoj.gov/vawo/state.htm

- Reflecting means listening carefully to what you understand the woman to be thinking and feeling.
- Summarizing means recapping, assessing, and focusing on what may be needed.

For resource material and guidelines, refer to the National Consensus Guidelines on Identifying and Responding to Domestic Violence Victimization in Health Care Settings (FVPF, 2004). For information on mandatory reporting of domestic violence by health care providers, contact the local District Attorney's office or health facility counsel. This information can also be accessed online (*http://www.endabuse. org/health/mandatoryreporting*).

Nursing Interventions for Minor Trauma

- Treat any area of abrasion with antibiotic ointment or oral antibiotics.
- Treat ecchymotic areas with ice applications.
- Provide mild pain relief medications such as Tylenol or nonsteroidal antiinflammatory agents. Monitor FHR and uterine contractions for 4 hours after administration of these agents.
- Provide a Kleihauer-Betke screen to detect fetomaternal hemorrhage and quantitated fetal blood loss and to determine the dosage of Rh_o (D) immune globulin for the Rh-negative woman. As little as 0.01ml of Rh-positive blood will sensitize 70% of RhD-negative patients (ATLS, 2008).
- Administer Rh_o (D) immune globulin therapy to RhD-negative woman should be instituted within 72 hours of injury.
- If FHR decelerations or uterine contractions are noted in the initial 4-hour monitoring period or if there is a positive Kleihauer-Betke test, admit for 24 hours of continuous observation, FHR and uterine contraction monitoring, evaluation for PROM, and evaluation for signs of abruptio placentae.
- Repeat nonstress test and Kleihauer-Betke in 24 hours.
- Toxicity screen for illicit drug or alcohol use may be indicated.
- Manage expectantly.

Critical Care Interventions for Acute Severe Trauma Maternal Focus

Stabilization

- Stabilize the mother first; then be concerned about the fetus.
- Keep airway patent.
- Maintain breathing and circulation.
- Control bleeding.
- Position the patient on a lateral tilt, if no spinal cord injury below the thoracic region is suspected, to prevent spine hypotension and vena cava syndrome. If spinal immobilization is indicated, the backboard can be tilted slightly to either side.
- Administer oxygen at 10 L/minute on a non-rebreather as indicated because of increased maternal oxygen consumption and high fetal sensitivity to maternal hypoxia.
- Assess level of consciousness.

- Assess and document respiratory status for rate, depth, regularity, and breath sounds.
- Assess and document peripheral pulses, skin color, and capillary bed refill.
- Monitor blood pressure frequently.
- Start an intravenous infusion with a 14-to 16-gauge needle.
- Infuse crystalloid fluids such as lactated Ringer's and blood as indicated.
- If the patient remains hypotensive, a suit of medical antishock trousers (MAST) can be applied without using the abdominal flap.
- Auscultate laterally for bowel sounds.
- Intermittent nasogastric suctioning may be ordered because of the increased risk for regurgitation and aspiration related to trauma, further decreasing gastrointestinal motility.
- Monitor urinary output. A Foley catheter may be ordered to monitor urine output and evaluate urologic injuries after some types of trauma.
- Refer to diagnostic data, such as complete blood cell count, blood type, antibody screen, and Kleihauer-Betke test to determine a fetomaternal hemorrhage, platelet count, arterial blood gases, or coagulation studies, in case signs of DIC develop; refer to a toxicity screen for illicit drug or alcohol use if indicated.
- If a computed tomography scan of the abdomen is ordered, shield the fetus if at all possible. Magnetic resonance imaging and computed tomography scans are good choices for evaluation.
- In the event of maternal cardiopulmonary arrest, be prepared to assist with a cesarean delivery within 4 minutes to enhance maternal and fetal survival.
- If placental abruption, maternal injury resulting in persistent fetal compromise, intrauterine infection, or maternal death occurs and the fetus is more than 24 weeks of gestation and alive, prepare for a cesarean birth (Divekar and Keith, 2004; Grossman, 2004a).

Continued Care

- Work together. The perinatal nurse works with the critical care nurse unless the patient is in a tertiary care center with a critical care obstetrics unit.
- Provide consultation such as physiologic changes related to pregnancy, fetal monitoring, and signs and treatment of pregnancy complications such as abruptio placentae, preterm labor, and PROM.
- Assist the physician with a quick abdominal ultrasound to evaluate fetal status and general gestational age.
- After stabilization, assess FHR and uterine contractions with an electronic fetal monitor (EFM) for 4 to 24 hours after an MVA or abdominal injury for early detection of abruptio placentae and preterm labor (Bobrowski, 2006).
- Assess for signs of abruptio placentae, such as dark vaginal bleeding, sustained abdominal pain, uterine tenderness, or increasing fundal height.
- Assess for uterine contractions, warning signs of preterm labor, and PROM.
- If placental abruption, maternal injury resulting in persistent fetal compromise, intrauterine infection, or maternal death occurs and the fetus is more than 24 weeks of gestation and alive, prepare for a cesarean birth.

- Explain any ordered test such as biophysical profile or nonstress test for fetal surveillance and amniocentesis for fetal lung maturity or intrauterine bleeding.
- Check injury areas for redness, swelling, and drainage every shift.
- Administer a prophylactic tetanus shot if there is no recent reliable history of administration.
- If the patient is RhD-negative, administer Rh_o (D) immune globulin as ordered for fetomaternal hemorrhage, which occurs in approximately 8% to 30% of patients who experience trauma.

Critical Care Interventions for Acute Severe Trauma with Fetal Focus

- Initially determine FHR.
- Assist physician with a quick abdominal ultrasound to evaluate fetal status and general gestational age.
- After stabilization, assess FHR and uterine contractions with EFM for 4 to 24 hours after an MVA or abdominal injury for early detection of abruptio placentae and preterm labor (Harris, 2001; Bobrowski, 2006).
- If signs of fetal compromise develop, prepare for emergent or postmortem cesarean birth.
- Prepare for transfer of premature or injured infant to an intensive care nursery.
- If not delivered in the initial phase or in early gestation, assess for spontaneous abortion, preterm labor, PROM, or intrauterine fetal compromise.
- If the mother needs to be positioned supine, place a small wedge under right hip if no spinal cord injury exists.
- Assist physician with a quick abdominal ultrasound to evaluate fetal status and general gestational age.
- Assess for signs of abruptio placentae, such as dark vaginal bleeding, sustained abdominal pain, uterine tenderness, or increasing fundal height.
- Assess for uterine contractions, warning signs of preterm labor, and PROM.

Recovery and Rehabilitation Nursing Interventions

- Educate the patient in self-care and self-assessment after discharge.
- Teach the patient to keep a daily fetal movement chart.
- Explain any ordered test such as biophysical profile or nonstress test for fetal surveillance and amniocentesis for fetal lung maturity or intrauterine bleeding.
- Instruct the patient about the importance of immediately reporting the development of signs of an infection, abruption, or preterm labor.
- If the mother is left physically disabled because of the trauma, physical and occupational therapy may be needed to teach skills for caring for other children and a new baby.

CONCLUSION

As a leading cause of maternal death, maternal trauma is a serious consequence of the increase in societal violence, lack of protection of pregnant women, and a general apathy to the need for maternal protection from injury. Many life-threatening injuries to mother and fetus resulting from MVAs could be prevented by safe and consistent use of car seat belts. Other injuries related to falls, burns, and acts of individual violence might be prevented by education. Pregnant women, family members, employers, and society in general need to be made more aware of the incidence of, risks for, and potential dangers of exposure of pregnant women to possible physical injury and trauma. Pregnancy provides a window of opportunity for identification and management of IPV (Lauti and Miller, 2008).

BIBLIOGRAPHY

Advanced Trauma Life Support for Doctors: *ATLS student course manual*, ed 8, Chicago, 2008, American College of Surgeons.

American College of Obstetricians and Gynecologists (ACOG): *Obstetric aspects of trauma management*, ACOG Educ Bull No. 251, Washington, DC, 1998, ACOG.

American College of Obstetricians and Gynecologists (ACOG): *Intimate partner violence and domestic violence*, Washington, DC, 2006, ACOG.

American College of Obstetricians and Gynecologists (ACOG): *Domestic violence*, ACOG Tech Bull, No. 257, Washington, DC, 1999, ACOG.

American Nurses Association (ANA): *Position statement on violence against women*, Washington, DC, 2000, Author.

Bobrowski R: Trauma in pregnancy. In James D, and others, editors: *High risk pregnancy: management options*, ed 3, Philadelphia, 2006, Saunders.

Bryan E, Bledsoe M: Trauma during pregnancy, *Merginet* 7:4, 2002.

Campbell J: *Danger assessment*, Baltimore, 2004, John Hopkins University. Retrieved from http://endabuse.org

Campbell J, Furniss K: Violence against women: identification, screening, management for intimate partner violence, *AWHONN Lifelines* 1–12, 2002.

Carbuapoma J, Tomlinson M, Levine S: Neurologic disorders. In James D, and others, editors: *High risk pregnancy: management options*, ed 3, Philadelphia, 2006, Saunders.

Centers for Disease Control and Prevention Intimate: *Partner Violence and Uniform Definitions and Recommendations Data Elements*, Atlanta, GA, 2004, National Center for Injury Prevention and Control.

Chambliss L: Intimate partner violence and its implications for pregnancy, *Clin Obstet Gynecol* 51(2):385–397, 2008.

Chames M, Pearlman M: Trauma during pregnancy: outcomes and clinical management, *Clin Obstet Gynecol* 51(2):398–408, 2008.

Chang J, and others: Homicide: a leading cause of injury deaths among pregnant postpartum women in the United States, 1991-1999, *Am J Public Health* 95(3):471–477, 2005.

Christian A: Home care of the battered pregnant woman: one woman's battered pregnancy, *J Obstet Gynecol Neonatal Nurs* 2(9):836–842, 1995.

Cox S, Kilpatrick S, Geller S: Preventing maternal deaths in America, *Contemp OB/GYN* Sept 1, 2004.

Divekar P, Keith L: Pregnancy outcome in motor vehicle accidents, *Female Patient* 29:31–35, 2004.

Dunn L, Oths K: Prenatal predictors of intimate partner abuse, *J Obstet Gynecol Neonatal Nurs* 33(1): 54–63, 2004.

Ellis K, Chang C, Bhandari S, and others: Rural mothers, the stress of intimate partner violence or not: Their newborn health concerns, *Am Coll Nurse Midwives* 93(6):556–562, 2008.

Family Violence Prevention Fund (FVPF): *Fact sheet: Intimate partner violence and Healthy People 2010 fact sheet*, San Francisco, 2003, FVPF. Retrieved from http://www.endabuse.org/userfiles/file/HealthCare/healthy_people_2010.pdf

Family Violence Prevention Fund (FVPF): *National consensus guidelines on identifying and responding to domestic violence victimization in health care settings*, ed 2, San Francisco, 2004, FVPF. Retrieved from http://www.endabuse.org/userfiles/file/HealthCare/pediatric.pdf.

Foley M, Strong T: *Obstetric intensive care*, ed 2, Philadelphia, 2004, Saunders.

Grossman N: Blunt trauma in pregnancy, *Am Fam Physician* 70(7):1303–1310, 2004a.

Grossman N: Seat belt use during pregnancy, *Am Fam Physician* 70(7):1313, 2004b.

Guth A, Pachter L: Domestic violence and the trauma surgeon, *Am J Surg* 179(2):134–140, 2000.

Harris C: *Trauma in pregnancy,* Presented at OB Challenges of the Millennium, Phoenix, AZ, April 2001.

Hedin L, Janson P: Domestic violence during pregnancy: the prevalence of physical injuries, substance use, abortions, and miscarriages, *Acta Obstet Gynecol Scand* 79(8):625–630, 2000.

Higgins L, Hawkins J: Screening for abuse during pregnancy implementing a multi-site program, *Mat Child J* 30(2):109–114, 2005.

Houshian S, Larsen M, Holm C: Missed injuries in a level one trauma center, *J Trauma Injury Infect Crit Care* 52(4):715–719, 2002.

Institute for Clinical Systems Improvement (ICSI): *Domestic violence,* Bloomington, MN, 2003, Institute for Clinical Systems Improvement.

Janjua K, Sugrue M, Deane S: Prospective evaluation of early missed injuries and the role of tertiary trauma survey, *J Trauma Injury Infect Crit Care* 44:1000–1007, 1998.

Klinich K, Schneider L, Moore J, Pearlman M: Investigation of crashes involving pregnant occupants, *Annual proceedings/Association for the advancement of automotive medicine association for the advancement of automotive medicine* 44:37–55, 2000.

Kramer A: Stages of change: Intimate partner violence during and after pregnancy, *J Perinat Neonatal Nurs* 21(4):285–295, 2007.

Lauti M, Miller D: Midwives and obstetricians' perceptions of their role in the identification and management of family violence, *N Z Coll Midwives* 38:12–16, 2008.

Mallampalli A, Guy E: Cardiac arrest in pregnancy and somatic support after brain death, *Crit Care Med* 33(10):S325–S331, 2005.

Mattox K, Goetzl L: Trauma in pregnancy, *Crit Care Med* 33(10):S385–S389, 2005.

Mayer B: Female domestic violence victims' perspective on emergency care, *Nurs Screening Q* 13: 340–346, 2000.

McGwin G, and others: A focused educational intervention can promote the proper application of seat belts during pregnancy, *J Trauma* 56(5):1016–1021, 2004.

Metz T, Abbott J: Uterine trauma in pregnancy after motor vehicle crashes with airbag deployment: a 30 case series, *J Trauma Injury Infect Crit Care* 61(3):658–661, 2006.

Miller W, Rollnick S: *Motivational interviewing: preparing people to change addictive behavior,* ed 2, New York, 2002, Guilford Press.

Norton L, and others: Battering in pregnancy: an assessment of tool screening methods, *Obstet Gynecol* 8(3):321–325, 1995.

Parker B, McFarlane J, Soeken K: Abuse during pregnancy: effects on maternal complications and birth weight in adult and teenage women, *Obstet Gynecol* 84(3):323–328, 1994.

Parsons L, Goodwin M, Petersen R: Violence against women and reproductive health: toward defining a role for reproductive healthcare services, *Matern Child Health J* 4(2):135–140, 2000.

Pearlman M, and others: A comprehensive program to improve safety for pregnant women and fetuses in motor vehicle crashes: a preliminary report, *Am J Obstet Gynecol* 182(6):1554–1564, 2000.

Plichta S, Falik M: Prevalence of violence and its implications for women's health, *Womens Health Issues* 11(3):244–258, 2001.

Shah A, Kilcline B: Trauma in pregnancy, *Emerg Med Clin North Am* 21:615–629, 2003.

Shoffner D: We don't like to think about it: intimate partner violence during pregnancy and postpartum, *J Perinat Neonatal Nurs* 22(1):39–48, 2008.

Tjaden P, Thoennes N: *Extent, nature, and consequences of intimate partner violence: findings from the National Violence Against Women Survey,* Washington, DC, 2000, The National Institute of Justice and the Centers for Disease Control and Prevention.

Tsuei B: Assessment of the pregnant trauma patient, *Injury* 37(5):367–373, 2006.

U.S. Advisory Board on Child Abuse and Neglect: *A nation's shame: fatal child abuse and neglect in the United States, 5th report,* Washington, DC, 1995, U.S. Department of Health and Human Services, Administration for Children and Families.

U.S. Department of Health and Human Services: *Healthy People 2010: Understanding and improving health,* Washington, DC, 2000, USDHHS. Retrieved from http://health.gov/healthypeople/Document/tableofcontents.htm.

Weinberg L, Steele R, Pugh P, and others: The pregnant trauma patient, *Anesthes Intensive Care* 33(2):167–180, 2005.

Weiss H, Songer T, Fabio A: Fetal deaths related to maternal injury, *J Am Med Assoc* 286:1863, 2001.

26

Sexually and Nonsexually Transmitted Genitourinary Infections

C urrently more than 20 sexually transmitted diseases (STDs) and numerous other genitourinary infections are recognized that affect the outcome of pregnancy (NIH, 2005). Because of the continuing rise in the incidence of sexually and nonsexually transmitted infections, the development of microbial resistance to antibiotics, the emergence of incurable and fatal disease types, and the risk that they pose to the fetus and expectant mother, it is imperative that nurse practitioners and nurses caring for families who are in their childbearing years have an in-depth understanding of these diseases. This chapter focuses on the seven most common STDs and the six most common nonsexually transmitted diseases and how each can affect pregnancy.

BACTERIAL VAGINOSIS

Organism
The organisms responsible for bacterial vaginosis (BV) are anaerobic bacteria, such as *Gardnerella vaginalis, Mobiluncus, Mycoplasmas hominis, Prevotella, and Atopobium vaginae* (Atashili and others, 2008).

Transmission
BV is not considered an STD. It usually results from a disturbance in normal vaginal flora initiated by sexual intercourse, hormonal changes, pregnancy, antibiotic administration, or use of nonoxynol-9 spermicidal products, which have a bactericidal effect on lactobacilli (Andrist, 2001). Douching may wash out the normal bacteria flora and increase the risk for BV (Cottrell, 2006).

Signs and Symptoms

Up to 50% of women with BV may be asymptomatic (Duff, Sweet, and Edwards, 2009). Signs and symptoms of BV follow:

- Thin, gray or white homogeneous vaginal discharge
- Increased vaginal discharge odor (fishy) after intercourse
- Alkaline pH (>4.5); BV does not cause vaginal itching or dysuria.

Screening

Patients should be screened for BV if they are symptomatic. According to ACOG's meta-analysis, there is no evidence to support the benefit of screening asymptomatic patients with a positive history for preterm labor (Okun, Gronau, and Hannah, 2005). Clinical diagnosis is made if three of the following four characteristics (Mayeaux, 2001) are present:

1. Saline wet mount showing clue cells that are characterized by 1:5 epithelial cell margins obscured by bacteria; no white blood cells
2. Whiff test (fishy odor prevalent when vaginal fluid is mixed with 10% potassium hydroxide [KOH])
3. Anterior fornix or lateral vaginal wall pH greater than 4.5
4. Homogeneous white to gray discharge that adheres to the vaginal wall

No cervical or vaginal inflammation is usually present. Smoking and douching increase the risk for developing BV.

Treatment in Pregnancy

Symptomatic

According to the Centers for Disease Control and Prevention (CDC, 2006), the recommended treatment regimen during pregnancy is metronidazole (Flagyl), 500 mg orally twice daily for 7 days or 250 mg orally three times daily for 7 days. An alternative regimen is clindamycin, 300 mg orally twice daily for 7 days. Clindamycin vaginal cream is not recommended during the second half of pregnancy because of the increased risk for low birth weight and neonatal infections (CDC, 2006). During breastfeeding, the woman should be treated with one dose of metronidazole, 2 g orally, and instructed to pump and discard breast milk for 24 hours (Lawrence and Lawrence, 2005).

In a review of fifteen studies involving 5888 women, antibiotic therapy was found effective in eradicating bacterial vaginosis; however, treatment did not reduce the risk of preterm birth before 37 weeks. There is evidence that treatment before 20 weeks of gestation may reduce the risk of preterm birth less than 37 weeks (McDonald, Brocklehurst, and Gordon, 2006).

Current treatment of the woman's sexual partner or partners is not necessary and does not improve outcome.

Asymptomatic

According to ACOG's metaanalysis, there is no benefit to treating asymptomatic pregnant patients with antibiotics for BV to prevent preterm labor (Okun, Gronau, and Hannah, 2005).

Effect on Pregnancy Outcome

BV is the most common vaginal infection (CDC, 2008) and has the following effects on pregnancy:

- Increases the risk for spontaneous abortion, premature rupture of membranes (PROM), and preterm labor (Leitich and others, 2003; Macones and others, 2004)
- Increases the risk for clinical chorioamnionitis and postpartum endometritis (Duff, Sweet, and Edwards, 2009)
- May cause neonatal septicemia

Pregnancy Considerations

BV affects up to 16% of all pregnancies (CDC, 2004). It changes the normal vaginal flora to (1) a small amount of lactobacilli, which normally produce lactic acid and protect against vaginal pathogens by maintaining an acid pH, and (2) a high concentration of anaerobes. Instruct all women regarding the risks and nonbenefits of douching, which can increase the risk for BV, chlamydia, pelvic inflammatory disease, HIV transmission, and cervical cancer (Cottrell, 2006).

CANDIDIASIS

Organism

Candida albicans is the most common cause (90% of cases) of candidiasis. *Candida tropicalis* and *Candida glabrata* are two other possible causes of candidiasis, a fungal (yeast) infection.

Transmission

Candidiasis is not considered an STD. It usually results from a disturbance in normal vaginal flora, conditions that cause vaginal pH to be more alkaline, and high estrogen levels, causing increased production of vaginal glycogen (Duff, Sweet, and Edwards, 2009).

Signs and Symptoms

Signs and symptoms of candidiasis follow:

- Vaginal and vulvar irritation (erythematous and edematous)
- Pruritic, white, curdlike vaginal discharge
- Yeasty odor
- Dysuria
- Dyspareunia

Screening

Screening for candidiasis is as follows:

- Saline or KOH wet mount microscopically examined: shows hyphae, pseudohyphae, and budding yeast
- Usually pH lower than 4.7
- Whiff test absent amine (fishy) odor

Treatment in Pregnancy

Only symptomatic women should be treated for candidiasis. Use an antifungal, intravaginal agent such as butoconazole (e.g., Femstat 3), clotrimazole (e.g., Gyne-Lotrimin and Mycelex), miconazole (e.g., Monistat), or terconazole (e.g., Terazol). These drugs come in a vaginal suppository or cream form. Duration of treatment is 7 days during pregnancy (CDC, 2006).

Sitz baths twice daily may decrease the external irritation. Instruct the patient to abstain from intercourse, avoid bubble baths, wear cotton undergarments, and practice good perineal hygiene. To treat recurrent yeast infections or to prevent yeast infections when taking antibiotics, eating yogurt or inserting a tampon dipped in plain (unsweetened) yogurt can help restore *Lactobacillus acidophilus* in the vagina (Sierpina, 2001). Echinacea has been demonstrated by research to decrease the recurrence rate of *Candida* infections as well (Freeman and Lawlis, 2001).

Pregnancy Considerations

Candidiasis is the second most common vaginal infection (Andrist, 2001). The risk for acquiring candidiasis during pregnancy is increased; the highest risk is in patients with diabetes and patients receiving antibiotic therapy because they have decreased levels of lactobacilli. Approximately 15% of pregnant women are affected because of the high levels of estrogen produced and increased concentration of vaginal glycogen. Suppression of cell-medicated immunity in pregnancy may decrease the ability to limit fungal proliferation (Duff, Sweet, and Edwards, 2009).

Candidiasis may be more resistant to treatment during pregnancy. Treat all symptomatic pregnant patients vigorously to avoid neonatal thrush.

CHLAMYDIA

Organism

Chlamydia trachomatis, an obligate-intracellular, bacteria-like parasite, is the organism responsible for chlamydia.

Transmission

Chlamydia is transmitted by close sexual contact.

Signs and Symptoms

The pregnant woman with chlamydia is asymptomatic approximately 75% of the time. However, she may exhibit some or all of the following symptoms (CDC, 2004):

- Increased, clear, white to yellowish mucous vaginal discharge
- Painful, frequent urination
- Dyspareunia
- Rectal pain, discharge, or bleeding from chlamydial infection in the rectum from anal sex
- Posterior pharyngitis from chlamydial infection in the throat from oral sex

Objective Findings

- Bartholin, urethral, and Skene glands: swelling and abnormal discharge
- External genitalia: erythema, edema, and excoriation
- Vagina: abnormal discharge
- Cervix: mucopurulent cervicitis; edematous, erythematous, and friable; cervical motion tenderness

Screening

It is estimated that 2.3 million Americans between 14 to 39 years of age have Chlamydia. This is called a "silent" sexually transmitted disease. Symptoms do not appear until 1 to 3 weeks after infections occurs (NCQA, 2008). To reduce pelvic inflammatory infections, screening for chlamydia should be offered to all women who are 25 years of age or younger who come for gynecologic care and to women over 25 who have new or multiple sex partners (AHRQ, 2001; CDC, 2006). All pregnant women should be screened on the first prenatal visit, and high risk patients should be screened again during the third trimester because the disease is asymptomatic in 70% to 85% of cases (NGC, 2005; CDC, 2006). Screening methods (Ward, 2003) follow:

- **Gene amplification molecular diagnostics**, such as polymerase chain reaction (PCR) or ligase chain reaction (LCR), are the newest screening methods that identify chlamydia and gonorrhea organisms via hybridization or nucleic acid amplification. These tests are popular because of their sensitivity, specificity, and ease of sampling (endourethral, endocervix, or noninvasive sampling of a fresh voided urine).
- **Tissue culture**, which was previously considered the screening method of choice, is only 70% to 90% sensitive related to decreased survival during transportation (Tiller, 2002).
- Two other classic diagnostics are **antigen detection enzyme immunoassay (EIA) and direct fluorescent antibody detection (DFA).**

Treatment in Pregnancy

Treatment of choice for the pregnant woman with chlamydia is one dose of azithromycin 1 g. An alternative treatment is erythromycin base, 500 mg orally four times daily for 7 days (NGC, 2005). If gastrointestinal side effects occur, erythromycin base, 250 mg four times daily for 14 days (NGC, 2005), is given. Erythromycin should be taken with 8 ounces of water 1 to 2 hours after a meal. For patients who cannot tolerate erythromycin, amoxicillin, 500 mg orally three times daily for 7 days, is an acceptable alternative (NGC, 2005). Because of the decreased effectiveness and compliance of these drugs, the National Guidelines Clearinghouse (2005) recommends follow-up testing with cultures 3 weeks after completion of therapy.

Avoid tetracycline, doxycycline, and ofloxacin during pregnancy because they have harmful effects on fetal teeth and cartilage. All sexual partners within 60 days before onset and diagnosis should be tested and treated as well.

Effect on Pregnancy Outcome

Chlamydia is an ascending infection and, if left untreated, can lead to pelvic inflammatory diseases (PIDs) up to 40% of the time (Parratt and Hay, 2003), which can later cause infertility, ectopic pregnancies, and chronic pelvic pain (Rawlins, 2001).

However, PID is unlikely during pregnancy. Women infected with chlamydia have an increased risk for acquiring human immunodeficiency virus (HIV), if exposed.

Pregnancy Considerations

Chlamydia is the most frequently reported STD in the United States and in most developed countries (CDC, 2007). If the infection is present at the time of vaginal birth, the neonate is at a 15% to 25% risk for conjunctivitis, which can lead to blindness and a 5% to 15% risk for pneumonitis (Sweet and Gibbs, 2002); therefore all neonates' eyes should be treated with either 0.5% erythromycin or 1.0% tetracycline ophthalmic ointment on delivery. This does not prevent pneumonitis caused by chlamydia infection. Any neonate who develops conjunctivitis should be screened for chlamydia.

GONORRHEA

Organism

The organism responsible for gonorrhea is *Neisseria gonorrhoeae*, a gram-negative intracellular diplococcus bacterium.

Transmission

Gonorrhea is transmitted by close sexual contact. The risk for transmission from an infected man to an uninfected woman is 50% to 90% with a single exposure. The incubation period is 3 to 5 days (Duff, Sweet, and Edwards, 2009).

Signs and Symptoms

Gonorrhea is commonly asymptomatic (Duff, Sweet, and Edwards, 2009). Signs and symptoms of gonorrhea if present are as follows:
- Vaginal discharge: may be profuse, purulent, yellow-green
- Anal discharge
- Itching or swelling of vulva
- Dysuria
- Dyspareunia
- Joint and tendon pain
- Anal discharge, discomfort, and pain with a rectal infection

Objective Findings

- Inguinal or cervical adenopathy
- Bartholin, urethral, and Skene glands tender to palpation
- External genitalia: erythematous, edematous; excoriation may be present
- Vagina: abnormal discharge; blood or pus may be seen
- Cervix: mucopurulent cervicitis indicated by erythema; friable, cervical os with cervical motion tenderness
- Rectal examination: assess for discharge, bleeding, or tenderness

Screening

Gonorrhea is the second most commonly-reported notifiable disease in the Unites States (CDC, 2007). Routine screening for gonorrhea is standard practice. All pregnant women should be screened on the first prenatal visit, and high risk patients should be screened again during the third trimester (Duff, Sweet, and Edwards, 2009) because the disease is commonly asymptomatic. Screening should also be done before procedures such as dilation and curettage and chorionic villus sampling. Screening methods follow:

- **Molecular diagnostics** are the newest screening methods that identify chlamydia and gonorrhea organisms via hybridization or nucleic acid amplification. Because of their sensitivity, specificity, and ease of sampling (endourethral, endocervix, or noninvasive sampling of a fresh voided urine sample), these tests are popular.
- **Endocervical culture** was previously considered the gold standard. To collect a culture, insert a cotton, polyester, or calcium alginate swab moistened with warm water 2 to 3 cm into the cervical canal and move it in and out with a rotary motion for 10 seconds to allow absorption of exudate. If a Pap smear is to be taken during the same examination, it should be obtained first. There is a new DNA amplification test of urine that is used for screenings (CDC, 2006).

Treatment in Pregnancy

For the pregnant woman with gonorrhea, the drug of choice is one dose of cefixime, 400 mg orally, or one dose of ceftriaxone, 125 mg intramuscularly (IM). If chlamydia is suspected, follow up with either azithromycin or amoxicillin (CDC, 2006). If the patient is allergic to cephalosporins, one dose of spectinomycin, 2 g IM, can be given (CDC, 2006).

Avoid tetracyclines and quinolones during pregnancy because of their injurious effect on fetal teeth and cartilage (CDC, 2006).

Sexual partners within the preceding 60 days should be identified, examined, cultured, and treated.

Effect on Pregnancy Outcome

Gonorrhea can affect pregnancy outcome in any trimester, causing chorioamnionitis, preterm delivery, PROM, intrauterine growth restriction, or postpartum sepsis (Duff, Sweet, and Edwards, 2009). If the organism is present at the time of delivery, the greatest neonatal risk (30% to 47%) is an eye infection called *gonococcal ophthalmia*, which can cause blindness. This is one of the reasons all newborns' eyes should be treated with either 0.5% erythromycin or 1% tetracycline ophthalmic ointment as soon as possible after birth (CDC, 2006). If the organism is known to be present in the birth canal at delivery, the infant is treated with a single 1 gram IM injection of ceftriaxone (CDC, 2006).

Pregnancy Considerations

Gonorrhea is an ascending infection. If it is left untreated, it can cause a PID (CDC, 2006). PID can in turn cause infertility. Untreated gonorrhea is a significant cause of postpartum endometritis. The risk for coexisting chlamydia infection is 20% to 40% (Parratt and Hay, 2003).

GROUP B STREPTOCOCCUS INFECTION

Organism

Streptococcus agalactiae is a gram-positive encapsulated coccus, a two-cell wall polysaccharide.

Pregnancy Considerations

Streptococcus agalactiae is present in the lower genital tract or rectum of 10% to 30% of all healthy pregnant women. These women are asymptomatic carriers of group B streptococcal (GBS) infection, which causes a 1% to 2% risk for GBS disease in the newborn (CDC, 2002). Approximately 80% of these neonates develop early-onset invasive GBS disease in the first 7 days of their life. If a newborn contracts early-onset invasive GBS, mortality is 4% (Schrag and others, 2000).

GBS has maternal morbidity implications as well. During pregnancy, there is an increased risk for urinary tract infection (UTI), chorioamnionitis, sepsis, postpartum endometritis, and rarely meningitis (CDC, 2002).

Risk Factors

The following risk factors increase the likelihood of early onset neonatal GBS infection:
- Positive prenatal culture for GBS this pregnancy
- Preterm birth of less than 37 weeks of gestation
- PROM for longer than 18 hours
- Intrapartum maternal fever greater than 38°C
- Positive history for early onset neonatal GBS

Screening

The CDC (2002), American College of Obstetricians and Gynecologists (ACOG, 2002), American Academy of Pediatrics, and The Society of Obstetricians and Gynaecologists of Canada (Money and Dobson, 2004) recommend prenatal lower vaginal and ano-rectal GBS screening (IDI-Strep B) between 35 and 37 weeks of gestation for all pregnant women. The only exceptions are cases of GBS bacteriuria during current pregnancy or a planned cesarean before labor or amniotic membrane rupture. The culture should be obtained without use of a speculum. The swabs should be placed in transport broth immediately (CDC, 2002).

Recommendations for Intrapartum Prophylaxis and Appropriate Therapy

The CDC (2002) recommends intrapartum antimicrobial prophylaxis for positive GBS screening culture, GBS bacteriuria during this pregnancy, and an unknown GBS status and any of the following:
- Preterm labor before 37 weeks of gestation
- Duration of ruptured membranes longer than 18 hours
- Intrapartum temperature greater than 100.4°F (38°C)

The antibiotic of choice is penicillin G, 5 million units by IV load and then 2.5 million units IV every 4 hours during labor. Ampicillin, 2-g loading dose and then 1 g IV every 4 hours during labor, is an alternative therapy. If the patient is allergic to penicillin, the alternative is cefazolin, 2-g IV loading dose and then 1 g IV q 8 hours. If the patient is at high risk for anaphylaxis, then clindamycin, 900 mg IV every 8 hours, or erythromycin, 500 mg IV every 6 hours, can be administered during labor (CDC, 2002). Figure 26-1 shows the algorithm for prevention of early onset GBS disease according to the 2002 CDC recommendations.

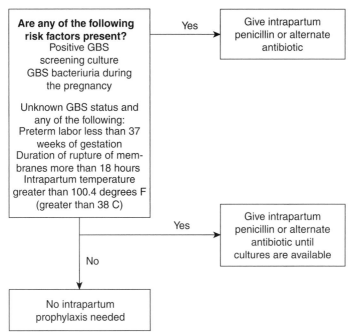

Figure 26-1 Algorithm for the prevention of early-onset group B streptococcal disease in neonates, using prenatal screening at 35 to 37 weeks of gestation.

Other Considerations

Treat all symptomatic or asymptomatic pregnant patients who have a positive urine culture for group B streptococcus with a 10-day course of antibiotics. Notify the pediatrician of any group B streptococcal infection during pregnancy.

Outcomes

In the United States, there has been an 80% decline in early-onset neonatal group B streptococcal infections since the beginning efforts to prevent GBS disease (Phares, Lynfield, Farley, and others, 2008). However, according to the CDC, early-onset neonatal GBS increased from 2003 to 2006 because of an increased incidence among black term infants (CDC, 2009). Therefore a revised perinatal GBS disease prevention guideline is being considered within the next year. Watch for information from the CDC at *http://www.cdc.gov/groupbstrep.*

HEPATITIS B

Organism

Hepatitis B virus (HBV), a hepadnavirus, is a partially double-stranded DNA virus consisting of a core antigen (HBcAg) carried in a lipoprotein envelope that contains the surface antigen (HBsAg). It carries a third antigen, the e antigen (HBeAg), which is highly infectious (Williamson and Mackillop, 2009).

Transmission

Hepatitis B is transmitted by blood and body fluids, such as semen, vaginal secretions, and saliva. The organism is extremely hardy and can survive outside the body in dried blood or body secretions for 1 week or more. Therefore the two major modes of HBV transmission are contact with contaminated blood or blood products and participation in sexual intercourse.

Signs and Symptoms

Acute HBV infection usually resolves as the body develops protective antibodies, but a chronic infection (the carrier state) may result. The risk for becoming a carrier is inversely associated with the age at which the infection is acquired. Young children have the greatest risk (Williamson and Mackillop, 2009). The pregnant woman with acute hepatitis B may be asymptomatic, or she may exhibit some or all of the following signs and symptoms:
- Chronic low-grade fever
- Anorexia
- Nausea and vomiting
- Fatigue
- Skin rashes
- Arthralgia

Screening

The Centers for Disease Control and Prevention (CDC), American College of Obstetricians and Gynecologists (ACOG), American Academy of Pediatrics (AAP), and Advisory Committee for Immunization Practice (ACIP) recommend routine prenatal HBV screening of all pregnant women at the initial visit and rescreening of all high risk women during the third trimester. Women who were not screened prenatally should be screened on admission to labor and delivery (CDC, 2005). Individuals at high risk for contracting HBV infection are the following (CDC, 2006):
- People of Africa, Asia, Middle East, Western Europe, Alaska, Central America, South America, and the Caribbean
- IV drug users
- People with multiple sexual partners
- Health care workers with blood and needlestick exposure
- Recipients of multiple blood transfusions

Screening for the presence of HBV is easily done by drawing blood and testing it for HBsAg. If HBsAg is positive, order HBeAg, anti-HBe, anti-HBc, aspartate transaminase (AST), alkaline phosphatase, and liver profile studies per consult. In the presence of an acute HBV infection, HBsAg, HBeAg, and immunoglobulin M (IgM) anti-HBc are all elevated. In chronic HBV infection (the carrier state), HBsAg remains elevated, as does the IgG anti-HBc, but IgM anti-HBc is absent (CDC, 2008). If HBsAg is positive but HBeAg is negative, this indicates a carrier state without active liver disease. If HBsAg and HBeAg are positive, it indicates a carrier state with most likely active liver disease (IAC, 2004).

Treatment in Pregnancy

If exposure occurs during pregnancy and the patient is HbsAg-negative, hepatitis B immunoglobulin (HBIG), 0.06 ml/kg IM, should be given; the HBIG dose is repeated 1 month later, followed by the hepatitis B vaccination series (CDC, 2005). If an expectant mother contracts the disease during pregnancy, symptomatic treatment only is given. This usually includes increased bedrest, a diet high in protein and low in fat, adequate hydration, and avoidance of medications that are metabolized in the liver.

Pregnancy Considerations

Acute HBV infection occurs in 1 or 2 per 1000 pregnancies. Acute HBV infection does not usually affect the course of pregnancy, except when the severe acute phase occurs during the third trimester, wherein it can increase the risk for preterm delivery (Williamson and Mackillop, 2009). The risk for transmission to the fetus during an acute HBV infection in the first and second trimester is low (10%). However, risk for transmission to the fetus during an acute HBV infection in the third trimester is 80% to 90% (CDC, 2005).

If the mother is a carrier, she is infectious and can transmit the disease to her child as well. If the mother is positive for both HbsAg and HbeAg, the child has a 70% to 90% risk for becoming infected. If she is HbsAg-positive only, the risk is less than 10% from perinatal transmission and approximately 40% from horizontal transmission (CDC, 2005). The infant rarely develops signs and symptoms, but 90% become chronic carriers if not treated (CDC, 2005). Chronic carriers have a 15% to 25% risk for developing liver cancer or cirrhosis by 50 years of age (CDC, 2005; Williamson and Mackillop, 2009). To prevent perinatal HBV infection and development of a chronic carrier state, the following care of the newborn is important.

Newborn Care if the Mother Is HbsAg-Negative

The CDC recommends routine HBV vaccination of all newborns to prevent HBV infection later in life. Vaccine for these infants is Recombivax HB 5 mcg or Engerix-B 10 mcg IM in the anterolateral thigh. The three-injection schedule recommended currently by the CDC is as follows: the first dose is given between birth and 2 months, the second dose between 1 and 4 months, and the third between 6 and 18 months.

Newborn Care if the Mother Is HbsAg-Positive

To prevent the chronic carrier state if the mother has a positive HBsAg test, the newborn is treated with HBIG 0.5 ml by 12 hours postdelivery and an initial dose of Recombivax HB 5 mcg or Engerix-B 10 mcg IM. Follow-up care includes a subsequent hepatitis B vaccination between 1-2 and 6 months of age and diagnostic studies between 9 and 18 months to determine the infant's carrier status. If anti-HB antibodies are present (greater than 10 mIU/ml), the prophylactic program was effective. Revaccinate nonresponders. However, if HBsAg is detected, the prophylactic program was ineffective and the infant is a carrier of HBV (CDC, 2005; 2008).

The prophylactic program just described is 95% effective in preventing exposed infants from becoming chronic carriers (CDC, 2005). It is ineffective in 5% to 15% of all infants and may be related to a transplacental exposure. Approximately 10%

of neonates of infected mothers fail to receive HBIG and vaccination after birth despite recommendation for both maternal screening and newborn immunoprophylaxis (Williamson and Mackillop, 2009).

Breastfeeding is not contraindicated if the infant has been immunized.

HEPATITIS C

Organism

Hepatitis C virus (HCV) is an RNA virus of the *Flaviviridae* family. It is currently the most common chronic bloodborne infection (CDC, 2006).

Transmission

The primary route of transmission of hepatitis C is parenteral, including illicit IV drug use, accidental needlesticks, and blood transfusions. Transmission by sexual contact occurs, but it is rare, the rate varying from 0% to 4.4% (Strader, Wright, Thomas, and others, 2004). The body's immunologic defenses have difficulty clearing the virus. Therefore HCV becomes chronic in 60% to 85% of acute infected people (CDC, 2006).

Signs and Symptoms

Acute cases (75%) are asymptomatic This means that approximately 25% to 30% of infected individuals are diagnosed. Data suggest that 80% of infected patients will develop chronic liver disease with biochemical evidence of liver dysfunction, 35% will develop cirrhosis, and 5% will progress to hepatocellular carcinoma (Williamson and Mackillop, 2009).

Screening

The CDC (2006) recommends screening women at risk for HCV, but they do not recommend routine prenatal screening of all pregnant women. Individuals at high risk for HCV infection are follows (NGC, 2004; CDC, 2006):
- IV drug users or women who ever injected an illegal drug
- Women who received clotting factor products before 1987
- Recipients of blood transfusions or organ transplants before July 1992
- Health care workers with blood and needlestick exposure

The EIA test for anti-HCV is the preferred screening test; if this test is positive, it is confirmed by a recombinant immunoblot assay (RIBA) (NGC, 2002). In an HCV-positive patient, a polymerase chain reaction RNA for hepatitis C may be drawn to estimate viral load, and an HIV screen is encouraged because of the increased association with this infection. In the presence of a coinfection, the maternal to fetal transmission is increased.

Treatment in Pregnancy

Routine prenatal care is recommended with baseline liver function studies including alanine transaminase (ALT). Currently no method has been found to lower vertical transmission. Cesarean delivery, unless otherwise indicated, has not proved beneficial in lowering the rate of transmission (NGC, 2004; CDC, 2006). For patients with a high viral load, avoiding artificial rupture of membranes and fetal scalp electrodes may be beneficial. Interferon-alpha and ribavirin treatment of HCV is not currently recommended during pregnancy but is reserved for the postpartum period as indicated by a liver biopsy.

Pregnancy Considerations

There does not appear to be an increased risk to the pregnancy if the woman is HCV-positive unless other behavioral influences coexist. The risk for vertical transmission can occur antepartally, intrapartally, or postpartally. According to the NIH (2002), the risk for transmission to the fetus is approximately 4% to 7%. If the patient is also HIV-positive, the risk increases to 20% (NIH, 2002). There also appears to be an increased transmission rate as the viral load increases (Thomas and others, 1998). However, there are no current data to indicate whether antiviral therapy reduces perinatal transmission. The current antiviral drugs used in the treatment of chronic hepatitis C—ribavirin and interferons—are contraindicated during pregnancy (NIH, 2002). Breastfeeding does not seem to be contraindicated because there has been no increase in transmission risk shown (NGC, 2002) unless the nipples are cracked or bleeding (CDC, 2006).

After 12 months of age, the infant born to an HCV-positive mother should be screened for HCV. Passively acquired maternal antibodies persist up to 18 months of life (Mass, Huang, and Seto, 2005).

HERPES SIMPLEX VIRUS TYPE 2

Organism

The organism responsible for genital herpes is herpes simplex virus (HSV-2), a double-stranded DNA virus.

Transmission

Transmission occurs through direct, intimate, oral-genital, or genital-genital contact (CDC, 2007).

Signs and Symptoms

HSV-2 is a chronic infection characterized by periods of remissions and exacerbations. There are three different infectious states: primary, first episode nonprimary, and recurrent infections. Signs and symptoms of primary infection are as follows:

- Prodrome: lasts 2 to 10 days
- Neuralgia
- Paresthesia
- Hypoesthesias
- Vesicle pustule: lasts approximately 6 days
- Painful vesicular lesions
- Dysuria
- Fever
- Malaise
- Cervicitis
- Wet ulcer: lasts approximately 6 days
- Dry crust: lasts approximately 8 days

Recurrent infections are usually less severe and of shorter duration.

Objective Findings with Lesions

- Papules, vesicles, ulcerations, pustules, or crusts on the vulva, vagina, or perianal area
- Cervical lesions resembling mucus patches, with central necrosis and elevated borders
- General cervicitis

Screening

The first prenatal assessment should include questions regarding a history of HSV infection of both the father and mother. If the history is positive, screen for other STDs, such as gonorrhea, chlamydia, syphilis, hepatitis B, and HIV. Status-unknown pregnant women who have atypical symptoms suggestive of atypical HSV, an HSV-positive partner, or history of another sexually transmitted disease or HIV should be screened with an FDA-approved serologic test such as a viral culture, which has previously been considered the most accurate screening method.

New polymerase chain reaction (PCR) HSV type-specific glycoprotein IgG-based type serology such as HerpeSelect ELISA or HerpeSelect immunoblot IgG for HSV-1 and HSV-2 are more cost-effective and 10 times more sensitive than viral culture (Wald and others, 2003; Clinical Effectiveness Group, 2007). Also, HSV IgG type-specific serology is effective in predicting nonspecific or asymptomatic shedding, whereas viral cultures are not (Morrow, 2004).

Treatment in Pregnancy

No therapy can eradicate HSV, and this chronic infection is noted for its frequent asymptomatic viral shedding (Leone, 2004). Oral Acyclovir is highly selective of infected cells, and the international acyclovir pregnancy registry has concluded that observed rates and types of birth defects are not significantly different for pregnancies exposed to Acyclovir and the general population (Stone and others, 2004). Therefore suppressive therapy with acyclovir is the current treatment of choice during pregnancy. Acyclovir antiviral suppressant therapy is started at 36 weeks and continued until delivery (ACOG, 2007). Sheffield and others (2003) metaanalysis of five studies indicated a five-fold decrease in genital HSV recurrence at delivery with the used of antiviral suppressant therapy during pregnancy.

At the time of delivery, if primary or recurrent active HSV lesions or prodromal symptoms are present, a cesarean delivery should be performed. All maneuvers that might cause a break in the infant's skin should be avoided, such as the following:

- Artificial rupture of membranes
- Fetal scalp electrode
- Fetal scalp pH
- Forceps and vacuum

Discordant couples (female seronegative, male seropositive) should be counseled to avoid oral and ano-genital sex and to use condoms during pregnancy. The male should also be encouraged to consider suppressive antiviral therapy once daily. Valacyclovir significantly reduces the risk for transmission among heterosexual HSV-2 discordant couples (Corey and others, 2004; Clinical Effectiveness Group, 2007).

Pregnancy Considerations

Intrauterine infection is rare and is caused by a primary maternal infection during pregnancy. If infection occurs, it may cause spontaneous abortion, birth anomalies, intrauterine growth restriction, or preterm labor (ACOG, 2007). Contact at the time of delivery is the most common mode of transmission to the baby. Primary HSV infections during pregnancy have the greatest risk for transmission to the baby (USP-STF, 2005). Exposure may lead to serious neonatal complications such as learning disabilities, psychomotor retardation, seizures, spasticity, blindness, and even death (Wald and Link, 2002).

Infected parents should be counseled regarding the importance of good handwashing and hygiene in preventing transmission to their infant. Any skin lesions present at birth should be cultured for HSV-2. The currently accepted antiviral therapy for the neonate is acyclovir IV 20 mg/kg every 8 hours for 14 to 21 days (CDC, 2006).

HUMAN IMMUNODEFICIENCY VIRUS

Organism

The HIV organism is a retrovirus of the lentivirus family that has an affinity for the T-lymphocytes (or "T helper cells"), macrophages, and monocytes.

Transmission

Transmission occurs from exposure to infected blood or body secretions of semen or vaginal fluid. The most common means is unprotected sexual activity or the sharing of contaminated needles. Pediatric HIV primarily results from perinatal or breast-feeding transmission (Pediatric HIV Working Group, 2009).

Normal Physiology of Immune System of Pregnancy

In HIV, the helper T cells (T4) are suppressed, which is important in cell-mediated immunity. The suppressor T cells (T8) are not affected. The polymorphonuclear leukocyte function is decreased. Antibody formation is not affected. The net result is that the pregnant woman is not more susceptible to an infection, but once she contracts an infection, it is harder to eradicate.

Pathophysiology

HIV is an envelope virus consisting of a p24 protein capsule (p24 antigen) containing two short strands of genetic material (RNA) and a unique reverse transcriptase enzyme encapsulated in a lipid envelope.

A virus can reproduce only inside a cell. To enter the cell, there must be an attachment molecule on the cell wall for the virus to attach to and then enter the cell. HIV attaches to the glycoprotein antigen (CD4) receptors on the T4 cells, B-lymphocytes, macrophages, and monocytes, as well as other cells in the immune system and CNS, and then enters these cells.

The virus reproduces inside the CD4 cells, such as the T4 cells, and eventually destroys them. The T4 cells are the master immune cells. They send out alerting messages, by way of hormones, to the rest of the immune system. This activates the killer T-lymphocytes that hunt down and destroy microbes, monocytes that engulf microbes, and B cells that produce antibodies. Therefore HIV weakens the immune system, causing the patient to be susceptible to opportunistic infections that can lead to death.

HIV Disease Continuum

Initial infection with HIV may manifest with mononucleosis-like symptoms, such as fever, fatigue, sore throat, lymphadenopathy, and occasionally splenomegaly. In the asymptomatic phase the patient is infectious without any signs or symptoms for months to 10 or more years. Next is persistent generalized lymphadenopathy that lasts at least 3 months.

Acquired immunodeficiency syndrome (AIDS) is the final phase. In this phase, the immune system is suppressed, making the person susceptible to opportunistic infections.

Screening

Preconception Screening for Known HIV-Positive Women

Preconception screening is being emphasized for the HIV-positive woman to discuss maternal infection status, viral load, immune status, and therapeutic regimen, perinatal transmission risks, and prevention strategies (Perinatal HIV Guidelines Working Group, 2009). Additional screening for maternal psychologic disorders and substance abuse use of alcohol, cigarette smoking, and illicit drugs are essential components of preconception counseling. Ideal nutritional status is important in optimizing the woman's health and preparing her body for a pregnancy. Use of an appropriate contraception to decrease the risk of an unintended pregnancy according to the Perinatal HIV Guidelines Working Group (2009) is an essential part of preconception counseling as well.

Screening if HIV Status is Unknown

The American College of Obstetricians and Gynecologists (ACOG), Centers for Disease Control (CDC), and U. S. Preventive Services Task Force (USPSTF) recommends all pregnant women be screened for HIV antibodies on the first prenatal visit, during the third trimester if classified as high risk for HIV, and on admission to the labor and delivery area if their HIV status is unknown and are classified as high risk for HIV (Qaseem and others, 2009). The current recommendation for health care providers is the "opt out" screening policy, which informs all pregnant women that HIV screening is a standard prenatal test unless they decline (ACOG, 2008). Recommendation is based on evidence that early recognition of HIV:

- Allows for early antiretroviral treatment that has been shown to significantly reduce mother-to-fetus transmission.
- Alerts provider so that invasive procedures are minimized to avoid the increased risk for transmission.
- Allows time for teaching regarding the increased risk for transmission with breastfeeding.

Screening Methods Currently Used

Currently there are two categories of screening methods: rapid HIV tests and confirmatory tests. The new rapid HIV tests allow for screening at the point of care, as well as the traditional laboratory, increasing compliance with the "opt out" HIV screening policy. Three currently available rapid HIV tests are FDA-approved:

- OraQuick Advance HIV-1 Antibody Test (whole blood can be used and test is CLIA-waived)
- Uni-Gold Recombigen HIV Test (whole blood can be used)
- Reveal Rapid HIV-1 Antibody Test (serum or plasma is required)

For information about the rapid testing waiver for the OraQuick test, go to the CDC's website (*http://www.cdc.gov/hiv/topics/testing/rapid*). These tests have a high sensitivity and specificity (Lampe and others, 2004). A positive result is to be followed up with one of the two confirmatory tests:

- Western blot
- Immunofluorescence assay (IFA)

A false-negative can result if the tests are done sooner than 3 months after exposure to HIV.

Risk Factors

Risk factors for HIV are as follows:

- Has multiple sex partners or has practiced serial monogamy
- Is infected with another STD
- Personally has used or sexual partner has used illicit IV drugs
- Is an emigrant from an HIV-endemic area, such as Haiti or Africa
- Has been or is employed in the sex trades (prostitution)
- Received a blood transfusion between 1977 and 1985

Pregnancy Outcome

The risk for transmission to the fetus or neonate is approximately 20% to 25% without the use of antiretroviral therapy (Cooper, Charurat, Mofenson, and others, 2002; Lampe and others, 2004). Transmission appears to occur transplacentally, likely late in pregnancy, during delivery, and through breast milk (Perinatal HIV Guidelines Working Group, 2009). In areas where breastfeeding is not the norm for HIV-positive patients, the greatest risk is during delivery; more than 60% of transmissions occur during exposure to birth canal secretions and blood (Penn and Ahmed, 2003).

With the use of antiretroviral (ARV) therapy as a regimen used to treat HIV infection or as prophylaxis to prevent HIV transmission to the fetus/neonate, the risk for perinatal transmission can be significantly lowered. Research has indicated that zidovudine (ZDV) administered during pregnancy can reduce the transmission rate to 10% (Cooper and others, 2002). With the use of combination ARV therapy, which can lower the viral loads more effectively, a number of retrospective studies have reported reduction of HIV transmission rates to below 2% (McGowan and others, 1999; Clarke and others, 2000; Cooper and others, 2002; Perinatal HIV Guidelines Working Group, 2009). Therefore mother-to-child transmission of HIV is virtually eliminated (Moodley and Wennberg, 2005). The risk was similarly reduced in women with viral loads greater than 1000 copies/ml if delivered by cesarean (Perinatal HIV Guidelines Working Group, 2009).

Pregnancy may mask the symptoms of HIV infection because clinical manifestations of HIV such as fatigue, nausea, and weight loss can be common discomforts of pregnancy. However, pregnancy does not appear to accentuate the course of HIV infection (Minkoff and others, 2003).

Treatment in Pregnancy, During Intrapartum, and of the Newborn

The treatment goals are to treat the woman's HIV infection and reduce the risk for perinatal HIV transmission by reducing and maintaining the viral load at or as close to an undetectable level as possible. Initial assessment includes the CD4+ count and HIV-1 RNA copy number, history of medication use, ARV drug resistance status, and gestational age. This is followed by serial monitoring of the CD4+ counts and HIV-1 RNA copy number. Liver function should be followed monthly when the woman is taking nevirapine during pregnancy (Perinatal HIV Guidelines Working Group, 2009). An initial assessment for opportunistic infection risk for *Pneumocystis pneumonia (PCP)* or *Mycobacterium avium complex (MAC)* is an important prophylaxis measure (Perinatal HIV Guidelines Working Group, 2009).

ARV regimens take on two forms: antiretroviral prophylaxis or antiretroviral treatment. Prophylaxis is used to prevent transmission from mother to child when the mother herself has no indication for ARV therapy. It is recommended for all pregnant women infected with HIV regardless of viral load (Perinatal HIV Guidelines Working Group, 2009). The current ART prophylaxis, according to the Perinatal HIV Guidelines Working Group (2009) and World Health Organization (2004), is as follows:

- Antepartum: Three-drug combination ARV regimen starting by 28 weeks of gestation and continued throughout pregnancy; an example of a three-drug combination ARV is triple nucleotide analogue reverse transcriptase (NRTI) (combined zidovudine (ZDV)/lamivudine (3TC)/abacavir (ABC); ZDV as a component of the regimen is recommended because of its efficient transplacental passage resulting in a higher ARV fetal level.
- Intrapartum: At onset of labor start intravenous ZDV.
- Neonate: Dose the neonate with ZDV within 6 to 12 hours of birth and continue for 6 weeks; the usually dose for the term infant is 2 mg/kg body weight orally every 6 hours. For varying situations reference the perinatal HIV Guidelines Working Group recommendations (2009).
- Postpartum: Discontinue the ARV medications postnatally for the mother if used solely for prevention of perinatal HIV transmission.

For women who are on ARV treatment before pregnancy, the current recommendation is to stay on the medications and to avoid known teratogenic drugs such as the nonnucleoside reverse transcriptase inhibitor, efavirenz (EFV) in the first trimester. ZDV may be added or substituted to the current regimen, avoiding incompatible drug combinations. Screen for therapy-associated side effects such as hyperglycemia, anemia, and hepatic toxicity (Perinatal HIV Guidelines Working Group, 2009). ARV treatment can be started anytime during pregnancy if the viral load indicates. These women should be given the option of starting their medications after the first trimester to decrease the risk for teratogenicity, while also weighing the risk for delayed therapy (Perinatal HIV Guidelines Working Group, 2009). For a complete evidence-based resource on teratogenicity of antiretroviral drugs, refer to the Public Health Service Task Force Recommendations for Use of Antiretroviral Drugs in Pregnant HIV-Infected Women for Maternal Health and Interventions to Reduce Perinatal HIV Transmission in the United States (*http://www.aidsinfo.nih.gov, http://aidsinfo. nih.gov/contentfiles/Peri_Tables.pdf*), or the World Health Organization's Guidelines (*http://www.who.int/hiv/pub/mtct/guidelines/en*).

Women with HIV infection, who are in labor and have had no prior ART therapy, should be started on intravenous ZDV immediately because of the placenta's permeability of this drug. It is recommended that the infant be treated with oral ZDV for 6 weeks. This combined intrapartum neonatal treatment regime decreases transmission of HIV from 27% to 10% (Wade, Birkhead, Warren, and others, 1998; Petra Study Team, 2002). Other regimens involve oral ZDV/lamivudine (3TC) or a single dose of nevirapine given to mother, 200 mg orally, at the onset of labor (Perinatal HIV Guidelines Working Group, 2009). More studies are needed to determine the most effective preventive treatment.

Counseling regarding scheduled cesarean at 38 weeks should take into consideration the viral load and gestational age confirmation, as well as the risk to the mother. If the viral load is less than 1000 copies/ml, given the low risk for transmission, it is unlikely that the cesarean would further reduce transmission. However, if the viral load is greater than 1000 copies/ml or if the viral load is unknown and the mother has been receiving only ZDV monotherapy, or not receiving antiretroviral therapy, a cesarean scheduled at 38 weeks further reduces the risk for transmission (Lampe and others, 2004; Perinatal HIV Guidelines Working Group, 2009). Refer to the antiretroviral clinical scenarios for varying situations to obtain specific guidelines for individualized treatment found in the Perinatal HIV Guidelines Working Group (2009) recommendations for use of antiretroviral drugs in pregnant women with HIV infection.

To enhance the treatment of HIV during pregnancy, an Antiviral Pregnancy Registry (800-258-4262; fax: 800-800-1052) is being maintained to collect data to follow the long-term safety of exposure of the fetus to antiretroviral agents. Current treatment guidelines and patient handouts are available at AIDSinfo, a service of the U.S. Department of Health and Human Services (USDHHS) (*http://www.aidsinfo. nih.gov*).

Pregnancy Considerations

Antepartum

If HIV infection is diagnosed during pregnancy, the woman needs initial and ongoing counseling for the social, emotional, and economic ramifications. She also needs education as to potential consequences of pregnancy on HIV disease progression as well as risk for transmission and consequences to her child. To facilitate health promotion, the woman needs adequate instructions in ways to enhance the immune system, such as (1) adequate sleep; (2) decreased stress; (3) adequate protein because a deficiency can cause depression of cell-mediated immunity, complement, and phagocytes; (4) balanced intake of polyunsaturated fatty acids and vitamin E because a high intake can depress the humoral-and cell-mediated immunity; (5) adequate zinc and vitamin A for overall growth and development of immune cells; (6) adequate pyridoxine, pantothenic acid, and folic acid for general cell synthesis (a deficiency in any of these nutrients can impair both humoral-and cell-mediated immunity); (7) avoidance of infections; and (8) cessation of cigarette smoking because smoking further alters immunity. Screen for other STDs. Assist in the notification plan of all sexual partners.

Intrapartum

Another current recommendation is that all women presenting in labor without documentation of HIV status be screened for HIV using one of the rapid HIV tests unless the woman declines through the "opt out" approach. Measures must be taken to protect confidentiality.

Elective cesarean delivery before rupture of membranes has been shown to further decrease the risk for mother-to-child transmission of HIV infection in women whose viral loads are greater than 1000 copies/ml (Perinatal HIV Guidelines Working Group, 2009). However, cesarean delivery increases the HIV-positive mother's risk for postpartum complications. Therefore the woman should be allowed to make the decision after receiving current information about the known and potential benefits and risks to her and her infant (Perinatal HIV Guidelines Working Group, 2009). If cesarean delivery is chosen, schedule the procedure for 38 weeks of gestation. A ZDV infusion should be started 3 hours before surgery and continued until the cord is clamped (Perinatal HIV Guidelines Working Group, 2009).

If vaginal delivery is chosen, care should be taken to decrease risk for inoculation of the virus into the neonate during labor by not using a scalp electrode for fetal monitoring or doing a scalp blood sampling for fetal pH (Penn and Ahmed, 2003). Delay amniotomy to possibly decrease the transmission rate of HIV because of the evidence that increasing duration of membrane rupture is associated with an increasing transmission risk. Avoid such invasive procedures as forceps- or vacuum-assisted delivery and episiotomy if clinically appropriate (Lampe and others, 2004).

Postpartum

According to the Perinatal HIV Guidelines Working Group (2009), comprehensive care and support services are important for the HIV-positive postpartum woman and should include the following:
- Case management coordination of care by the primary care provider, obstetrician, pediatrician, and HIV clinical specialist
- Observation for signs of clinical depression with appropriate referrals made as indicated
- Reemphasis on safe-sex practices and referral for family planning
- Counseling regarding importance of adherence to use of antiretroviral agents and prophylactic drugs against opportunistic infections, if indicated
- Review of immunization status, updating vaccines, and reviewing prevention of opportunistic infections
- Reference for substance abuse treatment, if appropriate

A recent Kenyan study added to the plethora of existing research that shows a significant transmission during breastfeeding (Nduati and others, 2000). If formula is readily available, as it is in all industrialized countries, the mother should not breastfeed her baby.

Neonate

Because the length of exposure appears to be important, bathe the infant as soon as possible after delivery (Lampe and others, 2004). Percutaneous needlesticks should be done only after the initial bath and with thorough cleansing of the skin just before the injections. Refer parents to a pediatric HIV specialist for follow-up care.

Because of the risk for anemia, a baseline complete blood count with differential should be obtained before starting antiretroviral therapy. After the 6-week antiviral prophylaxis regimen, prophylaxis antibiotic treatment for *Pneumocystis jiroveci* pneumonia should be initiated (Pediatric HIV Working Group on Antiretroviral Therapy, 2009).

Antibody screening is not reliable during infancy because maternally produced immunoglobulin G (IgG) antibodies to HIV are present in the body up to 18 months of age. However, an HIV DNA PCR and HIV RNA virologic assays are used to determine whether the neonate received the virus from the mother. The test is usually performed between 14 and 21 days of life, at age 1 to 2 months, and at age 4 to 6 months. HIV is diagnosed by two positive test results at two different times. Two negative test results, one of which must be after 14 days and one after 1 month or one negative test result after 2 months, means HIV can be reasonably ruled out (Pediatric HIV Working Group on Antiretroviral Therapy, 2009).

Health Care Workers

Use standard precautions when caring for all pregnant women during labor, during delivery, and during the postpartum period and for infants until they have had their first bath. This includes wearing gloves, protective eyewear, and water-repellent gowns.

HUMAN PAPILLOMAVIRUS

Organism

The organisms responsible for human papillomaviruses (HPVs) are human wart viruses of the papillomaviridae family of DNA viruses. Currently, more than 100 HPV types are identified, 40 of which infect the genital area (CDC, 2007). Twenty-five percent of cervical cancer cases are associated with HPV. HPV types 16, 18, 45, and 56 are found to be strongly associated with genital dysplasia and invasive cancer. HPV types 31, 33, and 35 are more commonly associated with squamous intraepithelial neoplasia (Canavan and Doshi, 2000; Thomas, 2001). HPV types 6 and 11, the most common types, have a lower but increased risk for dysplasia (CDC, 2006).

Transmission

Sexual contact is the most common form of transmission, with the highest transmission rate among sexually active adolescents and young adults. The age group between 15 and 24 years old accounts for 75% of the new HPV infections (Duff, Sweet, and

Edwards, 2009). Other risk factors associated with HPV infection are smoking and poor nutrition, which affect the immune response, and lack of male circumcision (Gerberding, 2004).

Prevention

In 2006, an HPV vaccine (a recombinant immunization) was approved against HPV types 6, 11, 16 and 18 and is between 95% and 100% effective. Therefore it protects against 70% of all cervical cancers and 90% of genital warts. The vaccine is administered in three doses with the second and third doses to be administered at 2 months and 6 months after the initial dose (Teitelman, Stringer, Averbuch, and others, 2009). It is approved for girls and women ages 9 to 26. There are two reasons to administer the vaccine between these ages. The highest risk group is ages 15 to 24 but the highest anti-HPV response to the vaccine is greatest among girls ages 9 to 15 (Dempsey, Gebremariam, Koutsky, and others, 2008).

Signs and Symptoms

Most women with HPV are asymptomatic. The virus requires magnification or acetic acid for visualization and can be transmitted before visual lesions appear. Visible warty growths are single or multiple growths called *condylomata acuminata* (genital warts); these warts may be fleshy-colored, pale pink or red, raised or flat, and small or large. If clustered together, they may have a cauliflower-shaped appearance (CDC, 2006). Mucosal warts located on nonhairy areas of the genital tract are softer. Hyperkeratotic warts located in outer hairy skin of the vulva are firm (Thomas, 2001).

Screening

Screening for HPV includes the following:
- Hybrid capture HPV DNA test with liquid-based cytology (Thin-Prep)
- Visualization
- Application of acetic acid to wart to magnify its presence
- The U. S. Food and Drug Administration has approved two new DNA tests, Cervista HPV 16/18 and Cervista HR, to identify two types of HPV that cause the majority of cervical cancers, type 16 and type 18 (USDHHS, 2009).

Treatment in Pregnancy

Most HPV infections are controlled by the body's immune system. Research studies indicate that 70% of HPV infections clear within 1 year and 90% clear within 2 years (Ho and others, 1998; Moscicki and others, 1998; Molano and others, 2003; Cox, 2006; Rodriguez, Schiffman, Herrero, and others, 2008). However, reactivation or reinfection occurs (CDC, 2006). No treatment has been shown to eradicate HPV. Therefore the goal is to remove the visible lesions and ameliorate the signs and symptoms only, not to eliminate the virus (Thomas, 2001). After removal of visible lesions, wait for the immune response to control replication of the virus. Various treatments are used to do this. A safe treatment regimen during pregnancy is the use of trichloroacetic acid (TCA), bichloroacetic acid (BcA), or cryotherapy with liquid nitrogen.

Electrocautery effectively removes small lesions throughout pregnancy. Surgical removal during pregnancy has an increased risk for hemorrhage related to the increased vascularity. Podophyllum resins and interferon are not safe treatment modalities during pregnancy because of their teratogenic potential. Safety of the patient-applied medications podofilox, imiquimod, and podophyllin is unknown and should not be used during pregnancy (CDC, 2006).

If the patient smokes, instruct her regarding the effect that smoking has on the immune system, which can decrease the effectiveness of any HPV treatment.

All sexual partners should be examined for any evidence of warts and instructed to use condoms to decrease transmission.

Effect on Pregnancy Outcome

Condylomata acuminata (genital warts) have an insignificant adverse effect on pregnancy.

Pregnancy Considerations

HPV is currently the most common viral STD in North America (Thomas, 2001) and, according to the CDC, HPV is the most common STD in young, sexually active women 25 years and under (CDC, 2006). Warts tend to proliferate and become friable during pregnancy (CDC, 2006). During delivery, condylomata can cause pelvic outlet obstruction and severe hemorrhage related to lacerations of the friable condylomatous tissue.

There is a 2% to 5% risk for HPV, especially types 6 and 11, causing laryngeal papillomas in infants and children exposed during delivery through an infected birth canal (McCance and Huether, 2006). These laryngeal papillomas usually appear between 2 and 5 years of age, causing such symptoms as an abnormal cry, voice changes, stridor, or evidence of airway obstruction.

Cesarean delivery is indicated only when warts are so large at the time of delivery that the risk for dystocia and hemorrhage is great (CDC, 2006).

There is a 25% to 33% risk for coexisting STDs such as trichomoniasis, BV, and chlamydia. Coinfection with chlamydia and herpes simplex type 2 may increase the risk for cervical cancer (Smith and others, 2002; Castle and Giuliano, 2003).

There is strong research evidence regarding the association between HPV and the development of cervical cancer (Gerberding, 2004). Therefore all patients with HPV should be instructed regarding the risk and reminded of the importance of a yearly Pap smear. Thin-Prep Pap test is the preferred test for any patient with a history of HPV or with a prior positive Pap. If the report comes back as positive for atypical squamous cells of undetermined significance (ASCUS), ask for a hybrid capture HPV DNA assay, a diagnostic test for HPV, or the Thin Prep (ACOG, 2003). If the HC_2 is positive, colposcopy is an appropriate follow-up.

A healthy lifestyle with exercise, with a healthy diet low in fat and high in vegetables and fruits, and without cigarette smoking enhances the immune system and is important in decreasing the cervical cancer risk. Smoking and deficiencies in vitamin A, vitamin C, and folic acid can increase the risk for progressive development of invasive carcinoma in the presence of HPV (Carson, 1997; Thomas, 2001).

HUMAN PARVOVIRUS B19

Organism

Human parvovirus B19 is a small, nonenveloped, single-stranded DNA virus. Lack of a lipid envelope makes B19 resistant to antiviral procedures such as detergent and heat treatments (Ramirez and Mastrobattista, 2005).

Transmission

Transmission is mainly by respiratory secretions and in some instances by blood products (Ramirez and Mastrobattista, 2005). Approximately 50% of all adults have been infected sometime during childhood or adolescence. Parvovirus B19 only infects humans. There are animal parvoviruses, but they do not infect humans. A person cannot catch parvovirus B19 from a dog or cat (CDC, 2007).

Signs and Symptoms

Human parvovirus B19 causes "fifth disease," which is a mild rash. Children typically have a "slapped-cheek" rash on the face and lacy red rash on the trunk and limbs. Other symptoms may include:

- Malaise
- Cold symptoms
- Low grade fever—101°
- Red cheekskin rash—potentially itchy
- Arms, legs, trunk skin rash—sometimes itchy

Adults may also experience joint pain and swelling, often in their hands, wrist and knees. Fifth disease is only contagious during the early part of the illness. Once the characteristic bright red rash appears, the person is no longer contagious. Fifth disease is usually a mild illness and resolves without medical treatment among children and healthy adults. Severe cases have been noted in those who have a weakened immune system (CDC, 2007).

Treatment

Under normal conditions the virus is not treated, only symptoms such as fever or itchy rash. Joint pain seen in adults may be treated with ibuprofen. In extremely severe cases in which anemia may develop, hospitalization may be necessary (CDC, 2007).

Pregnancy Considerations

The annual incidence of acute B19 infection in pregnancy has been estimated to be 1 in 400 pregnancies. Usually, an evaluation is performed after the pregnant woman has been exposed to a child diagnosed with fifth disease. Maternal infection is confirmed by serologic testing (Ramirez and Mastrobattista, 2005). Most women have been exposed and have immunity to the virus before childbearing years. There is no universally recommended approach to monitor or treat a pregnant woman who has a documented parvovirus B19 infection. Some physicians treat B19 as a low-risk condition, whereas others may increase the frequency of examinations to monitor the health of the fetus. Treatment is dependent on the severity of the disease (CDC, 2007).

Fetal Implications

The risk of vertical transmission to the fetal is estimated to be approximately 33%. Fetal B19 infection is associated with various fetal outcomes, depending on the gestational age when the infection occurs. Infection during the first trimester may result in fetal loss or miscarriage. During the second and third trimester, the infection may result in fetal anemia, myocarditis, high-output cardiac failure, fetal hydrops, and stillbirth. Health providers should always be suspicious of B19 infection in their evaluation of a fetus with nonimmune hydrops (Ramirez and Mastrobattista, 2005). A large study was conduced by the University of Bologna, Bologna, Italy, to determine the most reliable laboratory diagnosis for fetal parvovirus B19 infection in hydropic fetuses by evaluating the most appropriate clinical sample and laboratory test. The result was that diagnosis of fetal parvovirus B19 cannot always rely on maternal serological testing and should be based on virological analysis of fetal samples. Both fetal cord blood and amniotic fluid are suitable for diagnosis; however, the detection of B19 DNA in the cells of amniotic fluid samle proved to be the most reliable diagnostic system (Bonvicini and others, 2009).

The simple task of frequent hand washing is recommended as a practical and probably effective method to reduce the spread of parvovirus.

SYPHILIS

Organism

The organism responsible for syphilis is *Treponema pallidum*, an anaerobic spirochete bacterium.

Transmission

Syphilis is transmitted by way of sexual contact during the primary, secondary, and early latent stages.

Signs and Symptoms

After exposure to syphilis, there is an incubation period before the first stage of the disease. This time period can last 10 to 90 days, during which the patient is sero-nonreactive. After this incubation phase, syphilis has four distinct stages:

- **Primary syphilis.** Stage one is evidenced by a chancre, which is a highly infectious, painless, round, ulcerated sore that does not get better fast. It may last 3 to 6 weeks.
- **Secondary syphilis.** Stage two is evidenced by a maculopapular rash that typically occurs on the face, palms of the hands, or soles of the feet and is characterized by brown sores about the size of a penny. This rash is usually exhibited between 1 week and 3 months after the primary chancre. It typically clears in 2 to 6 weeks but can last up to a year. Other manifestations include wartlike genital "growth," lymphadenopathy, fever, sore throat, patchy hair loss, headaches, weight loss, muscle aches, and tiredness.
- **Latent syphilis.** Stage three is usually asymptomatic. The spirochete goes into hiding for 5 to 20 years. The patient is seroreactive during this stage. However, in about one third of patients, the infection may develop into the tertiary stage of syphilis. The other two thirds will experience no further consequences of the disease. During the first year of this stage (early latent), the patient is infectious.

- **Tertiary syphilis.** The fourth stage is a remanifestation of the disease; it slowly destroys the heart, eyes, brain, central nervous system, and occasionally, the liver, bones, and skin.

Screening

Routine screening is considered a standard of practice to be performed on the first prenatal visit and repeated at 28 weeks of gestation and at delivery if the patient is at high risk (CDC, 2006). Some states mandate syphilis screening at delivery for all pregnant women. All cord blood should be tested as well. Increased cord blood sample error occurs if the cord is milked to obtain the sample. Common screening tests for syphilis are the nontreponemal tests, that is, either the Venereal Disease Research Laboratory (VDRL) test or the rapid plasma reagin (RPR) test. Common tests used to confirm the diagnosis are the treponemal antibody titer tests, either the microhemagglutination assay for antibodies to *T. pallidum* (MHA-TP) or the fluorescent treponemal antibody absorption test (FTA-ABS).

Treatment in Pregnancy

If the patient has had the disease for less than 1 year, she is given benzathine penicillin G, 2.4 million units IM for one dose. If the patient has had the disease for more than 1 year, she is given Bicillin L-A (penicillin G benzathine), 2.4 million units IM for three doses 1 week apart for 3 consecutive weeks, for a total of 7.2 million units (CDC, 2006).

This therapy cures a maternal infection and prevents congenital syphilis (CDC, 2006). Sixty percent of women who receive this treatment experience a Jarisch-Herxheimer reaction; that is, a fever, myalgia, headache, mild hypotension, tachycardia, decreased fetal activity, and uterine contractions (CDC, 2006).

If the patient is allergic to penicillin, the CDC (2006) guidelines suggest skin testing and referral for penicillin desensitization. This is indicated because tetracycline and doxycycline are contraindicated during pregnancy and nonpenicillin drugs such as erythromycin fail to prevent congenital syphilis (CDC, 2006).

Monthly quantitative nontreponemal serologic tests for the remainder of the pregnancy should be drawn. If the titers show a four-fold rise, the pregnant woman is retreated.

All sexual partners are managed according to the CDC latest guidelines.

Effect on Pregnancy Outcome

The syphilis spirochete can cross the placenta at any time. However, treatment is very effective if given before 16 weeks of gestation; this is related to fetal immune competence before that gestational age (Duff, Sweet, and Edwards, 2009).

Untreated syphilis can profoundly affect the fetus, depending on the stage of maternal infection and the length of exposure to the organism. During the active phases of the disease, the organism load is the highest and has the gravest effect on the fetus. If the mother has untreated early latent syphilis, infection of the fetus is possible but there is significantly lower risk (Duff, Sweet, and Edwards, 2009).

Consequences of congenital syphilis include the following:

- Spontaneous abortion
- Prematurity

- Stillbirth
- Multisystem failure of the heart, lungs, spleen, liver, and pancreas, as well as structural bone damage and nervous system involvement and mental retardation.

TRICHOMONIASIS

Organism

The organism responsible for trichomoniasis is *Trichomonas vaginalis*, a flagellated protozoan that is sexually transmitted.

Transmission

Trichomoniasis generally is caused by sexual activity. However, it may be contracted by swimming in contaminated water, using contaminated towels, or sitting in contaminated hot tubs.

Signs and Symptoms

The pregnant woman with trichomoniasis may be asymptomatic, or she may exhibit some or all of the following signs and symptoms:

- Frothy, yellow-green or gray, foul-smelling discharge
- Constant perineal itching
- Erythema (strawberry spots)
- Vaginal pH alkaline (>4.5)
- Vaginal mucosa erythematous
- Cervix with punctate hemorrhages

Screening

If the pregnant woman is symptomatic for trichomoniasis, a saline wet mount shows motile trichomonads with an increased number of white blood cells. The amine odor (Whiff test) may or may not be positive for a fishy odor, and the vaginal pH is greater than 4.5 and often greater than 6.0. The routine Pap smear may detect trichomonads.

Treatment in Pregnancy

Symptomatic

Treatment of choice for trichomoniasis during pregnancy is metronidazole (Flagyl), a single oral dose of 2 g (CDC, 2006). Some health care providers prefer to avoid treatment until after the first trimester; however, according to the CDC (2006) there is no indication of teratogenicity. According to the *Cochrane Review* it is unknown whether this treatment has any adverse effect on the pregnancy (Gülmezoglu, 2004). The U.S. National Institute of Child Health and Human Development trial has shown an increased risk for preterm labor when trichomoniasis is treated with metronidazole (Kigozi and others, 2003).

No alcoholic beverages or vinegar products are allowed for 48 hours after therapy to avoid nausea, vomiting, cramping, and headaches. No intercourse is allowed for 2 weeks to allow pelvic and cervical rest.

During breastfeeding the woman could be treated with metronidazole, 2 g orally for one dose, and instructed to pump and discard breast milk for 24 hours (Lawrence and Lawrence, 2005). All sexual partners should be treated also.

Asymptomatic

According to ACOG's metaanalysis, there is an increased risk for preterm labor when asymptomatic trichomoniasis is treated with metronidazole (Okun, Gronau, and Hannah, 2005). It is speculated that the dying organisms elicits an inflammatory response that stimulates preterm contractions.

Effect on Pregnancy Outcome

Trichomonas vaginalis is diagnosed in 20% of all pregnancies and has been implicated in PROM and preterm delivery (CDC, 2006). The prevalence of *T. vaginalis* in pregnancy ranges from 10% to 50%, depending on the patient population. Consequently, it has been difficult to establish whether the incidence of this infection truly is increased in pregnant women (Duff, Sweet, and Edwards, 2009).

URINARY TRACT INFECTION

UTI is manifested by the following three clinical types:
- Asymptomatic bacteriuria
- Acute cystitis
- Acute pyelonephritis

Organism

The common causative organisms of UTIs are coliforms, particularly *Escherichia coli* gram-negative pathogenic bacteria. They account for approximately 85% of all UTIs. Other gram-negative pathogenic bacteria (*Klebsiella pneumoniae, Proteus* species) are important pathogens, especially in recurrent UTIs. Less frequent causative organisms involved in UTIs are gram-positive organisms: group B streptococci, enterococci, and staphylococci. They account for approximately 3% to 7% of the infections (Delzell and Lefevre, 2000). Two other causative organisms are *N. gonorrhoeae* and *C. trachomatis* (sexually transmitted pathogens).

Transmission

Coliform organisms are a normal part of the perineal flora and may be introduced into the urethra during intercourse or improper wiping after defecation. *N. gonorrhoeae* and *C. trachomatis* are transmitted by sexual contact.

Signs and Symptoms

Signs and symptoms of a UTI depend on the location of the infection. In 5% to 10% of cases, they are asymptomatic. In acute cystitis or lower UTI, the following symptoms are common:
- Urinary frequency
- Urinary urgency
- Dysuria

- Hesitancy or dribbling
- Suprapubic tenderness
- Gross hematuria

Accompanying symptoms with acute pyelonephritis (upper UTI) are usually chills, fever, and back pain with costovertebral angle (CVA) tenderness. Signs of a lower UTI may be present as well.

Screening

Routine screening for UTI is standard practice at the first prenatal visit and is repeated at 32 to 34 weeks of gestation. It should also be performed if there are complaints of any signs or symptoms:
- Microscopic examination shows white blood cells; bacteria may or may not be present.
- Dipstick urine may be positive for nitrites and leukocyte esterase.
- Clean-catch midstream specimen for culture and sensitivity

Treatment in Pregnancy for Asymptomatic or Acute Cystitis

According to the *Cochrane Systematic Review*, antibiotic therapy for asymptomatic bacteriuria is effective in lowering the risk for pyelonephritis and preterm labor (Smaill and Vazquez, 2007). Table 26-1 lists the most common antibiotics used in treatment of asymptomatic or acute cystitis. According to a *Cochrane Systematic Review*, there is insufficient evidence to recommend a duration of antimicrobial therapy for asymptomatic bacteriuria during pregnancy (Villar, Widmer, Lydon-Rochelle, and others, 2006). For several reasons a short 3-day course is preferred because of the decreased risk of adverse side effects and development of resistance while improving the rate of compliance and decreasing the cost. However, during pregnancy a 7-to 10-day course of treatment is usually preferred (Duff, Sweet, and Edwards, 2009). With a recurrent infection, a 7-to 10-day course of treatment is necessary.

To facilitate antibacterial action, acidify urine by having the woman take ascorbic acid (vitamin C) or cranberry tablets (Fontaine, 2000; Sierpina, 2001) has been shown to be beneficial. Other therapeutic measures are to instruct the patient to drink at least one glass of water or low sugar juice per waking hour and to void before and after intercourse to decrease the risk for recurrent UTIs. At all remaining prenatal visits, screen the urine for nitrites and leukocyte esterase. If either of these tests is positive, repeat urine culture and re-treat as culture indicates. A "test of cure" is recommended following treatment of an acute cystitis. Recurrent acute cystitis can be prevented with daily antibiotic prophylaxis.

Treatment in Pregnancy for Pyelonephritis

The incidence of acute pyelonephritis in pregnancy ranges from 1% to 2.5% with an increased risk of recurrence (Duff, Sweet, and Edwards, 2009). The patient may be treated on an outpatient basis if the disease manifestations are mild and the patient is hemodynamically stable and without evidence of preterm labor. A common outpatient treatment is amoxicillin clavulanate (Augmentin), 875/125 mg bid for 14 days, or trimethoprim and sulfamethoxazole DS (Bactrim DS), 160/800 mg bid for 14 days.

Table 26-1   Antibiotics for Asymptomatic Bacteriuria or Cystitis

Antibiotics	Organism Sensitivity	Oral Dose	Administration Considerations
Penicillin (Amoxicillin)	70%-80% of *Escherichia coli*, most *Proteus* species, group B streptococci, enterococci, some staphylococci	500 mg three times daily for 3 or 7 days	Do not use this drug unless sensitivity test indicates sensitivity Side effects: diarrhea and candidiasis
Cephalosporin (Keflex)	Most *E. coli*, *Klebsiella*, *Proteus* species, group B streptococci, staphylococci	250-500 mg four times daily for 3 or 7 days	Do not use this drug unless sensitivity test indicates sensitivity Side effects: diarrhea and candidiasis
Nitrofurantoin (Macrobid)	Most gram-negative aerobic bacilli	100 mg twice daily for 3 or 7 days	Best to use if drug-resistant *E. Coli* is suspected
Sulfonamides (Bactrim DS)	Most gram-negative aerobic bacilli	160/800 mg twice daily for 3 or 7 days	Pregnancy category C drug Avoid first trimester use and do not use near delivery date because it has a possible effect on protein binding of bilirubin, causing hemolytic anemia.

Data from Duff P, Sweet R, Edwards R: Maternal and fetal infections. In Creasy R, Resnik R, Iams J, and others, editors: *Creasy & Resnik's maternal-fetal medicine: principles and practice*, ed 6, Philadelphia, 2009, Saunders; Weiner C, Buhimschi C: *Drugs for pregnant and lactating women*, ed 2, Philadelphia, 2009, Saunders.

If the patient is hemodynamically unstable, disease manifestations are severe, including high fever, chills, and tachycardia. If the patient is experiencing uterine contractions, she must be hospitalized for treatment. Obtain a catheterized urine sample and send immediately for culture and sensitivity. Initiate parenteral antimicrobial therapy immediately as ordered. Various extended spectrum antimicrobials may be used. Possible examples are third-generation cephalosporin, such as ceftriaxone (Rocephin) 1 to 2 g IV piggyback every 8 hours, or a third-generation penicillin, such as ampicillin, 1 to 2 g IV piggyback every 6 hours plus gentamicin 3 to 5 mg/kg every 8 hours (Duff, Sweet, and Edwards, 2009). Consider changing the IV antibiotic therapy if the culture and sensitivity indicate or if the patient has not responded to therapy within 48 hours (Duff, Sweet, and Edwards, 2009). Ensure adequate hydration; usually intravenous crystalloid fluid is needed to maintain urine output at 30 to 50 ml hourly. Monitor closely for signs of impending sepsis such as tachypnea, hypotension, and oliguria. Watch for uterine contractions and fetal stress. In the presence of a high fever, cooling measures are indicated to reduce cardiovascular stress. A cool blanket and acetaminophen may be ordered.

Discontinue the IV antibiotics when the patient is afebrile for 48 hours, and continue on oral antibiotics to complete a 14-day course of therapy. Commonly used oral antibiotics are listed in Table 26-1. Repeat a urine culture and sensitivity before discharge from hospital.

Effect on Pregnancy Outcome

The endotoxins released from gram-negative bacteria may stimulate the production of prostaglandins and thus cause preterm labor (Cram and others, 2002; AAP and ACOG, 2007). If the causative organism was GBS, the woman should be treated with antibiotics during labor to decrease the risk for GBS infection in the newborn. Refer to the Group B Streptococcus section earlier in this chapter.

Pregnancy Considerations

UTI is the most common medical complication of pregnancy and occurs in up to 20% of pregnancies and accounts for 10% of antepartum hospitalizations. Left untreated, UTIs in pregnancy place the fetus and mother at risk for substantial morbidity and mortality (Duff, Sweet, and Edwards, 2009).

GENERAL NURSING MANAGEMENT FOR GENITOURINARY INFECTIONS

Prevention

Prevention is the cornerstone of nursing practice and includes three steps: primary, secondary, and tertiary prevention. Primary prevention of genitourinary infections, including sexually transmitted infections (STIs), involves health promotion and prevention activities. When primary prevention fails, secondary prevention, involving activities for early detection, is the next important step in the prevention of serious consequences. Tertiary prevention involves appropriate treatment to prevent or reduce disability once the infection is contracted.

Primary Prevention of Sexually Transmitted Infections

- Nurses should be actively involved in accurate, timely education programs that teach about the method of transmission and risk reduction behaviors.
- The only absolutely safe sexual practice is abstinence until one establishes a mutually monogamous relationship. Health care providers should not avoid mentioning this option, especially with teens (Tumolo, 2000).
- Safe sexual practice, if one chooses to have sex outside a mutually monogamous relationship, is use of condoms. Use of condoms decreases the risk but is not 100% effective. The health care provider must inform the patient that she can contract an infection, especially viral herpes or HPV, from viral shedding in the genital area not covered by the condom (Waldrop, 2001).
- Abstinence from illegal drug use, especially the sharing of needles and syringes with anyone, is important.

- Conduct a sexual history. A guide to taking a sexual history is an excellent resource provided by the CDC in the Syphilis Elimination Effort (SEE) Tool Kit. This resource can be retrieved online (*http://www.cdc.gov/std/see/description.htm*).
- Periodic examinations for STDs in the at-risk woman are beneficial.
- Expression of values and beliefs that might not follow this type of suggested lifestyle are allowed.
- Motivation seminars can increase one's reasons to delay sex, including the following examples:
  - Job training
  - Staying in school
  - Building self-esteem
  - Life planning and counseling
  - Recreational activities

Secondary Prevention of Sexually Transmitted Infections

- When women of childbearing age seek health care, a thorough history should be taken and should include the following:
  - Cultural background
  - Sexual practices
  - Drug use
- Periodic examinations for STDs in the at-risk group are beneficial.
- Further investigation of the following manifested signs should be conducted:
  - Perineal, vaginal, or cervical lesions or sores
  - Increased, abnormal, or malodorous vaginal discharge
  - Dysuria
- Teach the significant signs and symptoms to at-risk patients, and instruct them to report to health care workers to enable effective treatment to be initiated early.

Tertiary Prevention of Sexually Transmitted Infections

- Implement treatment according to the CDC guidelines.
- Inform of the requirement to report specific STDs, such as syphilis, gonorrhea, and HIV, to community health officials, and explain local follow-up procedures in this event.
- Educate as to the importance of notifying all sexual partners who could have been infected when an STD is diagnosed.
- Encourage abstinence from sex until follow-up cultures are negative.
- Educate as to the importance of using condoms lubricated with a spermicide containing nonoxynol-9 to prevent reinfection.
- Educate as to the importance of seeking immediate medical treatment if any symptoms reappear or if a sexual partner is diagnosed with an STD.
- Inform that cigarette smoking may accelerate the pathogenic course of many STIs, especially HPV.

Affect Self-Esteem When Diagnosed with an Incurable Sexually Transmitted Infection

- Provide opportunities to discuss feelings in a nonjudgmental environment.
- Provide referrals to support groups if indicated.

- Assist in planning for future with regard to sexual activity.
- Provide assistance with notification of sexual partners if applicable.
- Provide opportunities for family members to discuss feelings in a nonjudgmental environment.
- Provide appropriate referrals as needed.
- Suggest alternative methods of sexual gratification for couples who have an active STD.
- Educate regarding the importance of ongoing screening protocols and treatment regimens.
- Empower in self-care strategies.

Primary Prevention of Vaginal Infections Related to Nonsexually Transmitted Infections

- Teach behaviors to promote normal vaginal flora:
  - Wear cotton undergarments and avoid tight-fitting clothing.
  - Maintain good perineal hygiene.
  - Reduce simple sugars in the diet.
  - Refrain from douching for hygienic reasons.
  - Eat yogurt or drink milk containing active acidophilus cultures when taking an antibiotic.

CONCLUSION

Most STDs pose a risk not only to the pregnant woman but also to the fetus she carries. It is particularly important that childbearing women be free of STDs. Nurses who provide health care to childbearing families can participate in primary prevention by conducting education programs and consistently providing ongoing education about the risk and prevention of these diseases. Nurses should also be involved in secondary and tertiary prevention, which includes early diagnosis and appropriate intervention if the problem arises. Only by addressing these diseases at every level will progress be made in diminishing their prevalence and devastating effects.

BIBLIOGRAPHY

Bacterial Vaginosis

Andrist L: Vaginal health and infections, *J Obstet Gynecol Neonatal Nurs* 30(3):306–315, 2001.

Atashili J, and others: Bacterial vaginosis and HIV acquisition: a meta-analysis of published studies, *Aids* 22(12):1493–1501, 2008.

Centers for Disease Control and Prevention (CDC): *Bacterial vaginosis,* Factsheet, Rockville, Md, 2004, Author. Retrieved from http://www.cdc.gov/std/healthcomm/fact_sheets.htm.

Centers for Disease Control and Prevention (CDC): Sexually transmitted diseases treatment guidelines, 2006, *MMWR Morb Mortal Wkly Rep* 55(RR11):1–94, 2006.

Centers for Disease Control and Prevention (CDC): *Bacterial vaginosis.* Factsheet, Rockville, Md, Reviewed 2008, Author. Retrieved from http://www.cdc.gov/std/bv/STDFact-Baterial-Vaginosis.htm.

Cottrell B: Vaginal douching practices of women in eight Florida panhandle counties, *J Obstet Gynecol Neonatal Nurs* 35(1):24–33, 2006.

Duff P, Sweet R, and Edwards R: Maternal fetal infections: In Creasy R, Resnik R, Iams J, and others, editors: *Creasy and Resnik's maternal-fetal medicine: principles and practice,* ed 6, Philadelphia, 2009, Saunders.

Lawrence R, Lawrence M: *Breastfeeding: a guide for the medical profession*, ed 6, Philadelphia, 2005, Mosby.

Leitich H, and others: Bacterial vaginosis as a risk factor for preterm delivery: a meta-analysis, *Am J Obstet Gynecol* 189(1):139–147, 2003.

Macones G, and others: A polymorphism in the promoter region of TNF and bacterial vaginosis: preliminary evidence of gene-environment interaction in the etiology of spontaneous preterm birth, *Am J Obstet Gynecol* 190(6):1504–1508, 2004.

Mayeaux E: Work-up of bacterial vaginosis, *Female Patient* 26(5):21, 2001.

McDonald HM, Brocklehurst P, Gordon A: Antibiotics for treating bacterial vaginosis in pregnancy, *Cochrane Database of Systematic Reviews* (Issue 3), Art. No.: CD000262, 2006.

Okun N, Gronau K, Hannah M: Antibiotics for bacterial vaginosis or trichomonas vaginalis in pregnancy: a systematic review, *Obstet Gynecol* 105(4):857–868, 2005.

Candidiasis

Andrist L: Vaginal health and infections, *J Obstet Gynecol Neonatal Nurs* 30(3):306–315, 2001.

Centers for Disease Control and Prevention (CDC): Sexually transmitted diseases treatment guidelines, 2006, *MMWR Morb Mortal Wkly Rep* 55(RR11):1–94, 2006.

Duff P, Sweet R, Edwards R. Maternal and fetal infections. In Creasy R, Resnik R, Iams J, and others, editors: *Creasy and Resnik's maternal-fetal medicine: principles and practice*, ed 6, Philadelphia, 2009, Saunders.

Freeman L, Lawlis G: *Mosby's complementary and alternative medicine: a research-based approach*, St Louis, 2001, Mosby.

Pappas P, Kauffman C, Andes D, and others: The Expert Panel of the Infectious Diseases Society of America: Clinical practice guidelines for the management of candidiasis: 2009 update by the Infectious Diseases Society of America, *Clin Infect Dis* 48:503–535, 2009. Retrieved from http://www.uphs.upenn.edu/bugdrug/antibiotic_manual/idsacandidiasisrx2009.pdf.

Sierpina V: *Integrative health care: complementary and alternative therapies for the whole person*, Philadelphia, 2001, FA Davis.

Chlamydia

Agency for Healthcare Research and Quality (AHRQ): *U.S. Preventive Services Task Force calls for chlamydia, lipid screening among first four recommendations*, Rockville, Md, 2001, U.S. Department of Health and Human Services.

Centers for Disease Control and Prevention (CDC): *Chlamydia*, Factsheet, Rockville, Md, 2004. Author, Retrieved from http://www.cdc.gov/std/healthcomm/fact_sheets.htm.

Centers for Disease Control and Prevention (CDC): Sexually transmitted diseases treatment guidelines, 2006, *MMWR Morb Mortal Wkly Rep* 55(RR11):1–94, 2006.

Centers for Disease Control and Prevention (CDC): *Sexually transmitted disease surveillance*, 2007. Author. Retrieved from http://www.cdc.gov/std/stats07/Chlamydia.htm.

National Committee for Quality Assurance (NCQA): *The state of healthcare quality 2008*, Washington, DC, 2008.

National Guideline Clearinghouse (NGC): *Guideline synthesis: screening for and management of chlamydial infection*. Rockville, MD, 2005, NGC. Retrieved from http://www.guideline.gov.

Parratt J, Hay D: Sexually transmitted infections, *Curr Obstet Gynaecol* 13(4):224, 2003.

Rawlins S: Nonviral sexually transmitted infections, *J Obstet Gynecol Neonatal Nurs* 30(3):324–331, 2001.

Sweet R, Gibbs R: *Infectious diseases of the female genital tract*, Philadelphia, 2002, Lippincott Williams & Wilkins.

Tiller C: Chlamydia during pregnancy: implications and impact on perinatal and neonatal outcome, *J Obstet Gynecol Neonatal Nurs* 31(1):93–98, 2002.

Ward M, webmaster: *A portal to the Chlamydia literature and news*, Southampton, UK, 2003, University of Southampton. Retrieved from http://www.Chlamydiae.com.

Gonorrhea

Centers for Disease Control and Prevention (CDC): Sexually transmitted diseases treatment guidelines, 2006, *MMWR Morb Mortal Wkly Rep* 55(RR11):1–94, 2006.

Centers for Disease Control and Prevention (CDC): Sexually transmitted disease surveillance 2007, Rockville Md. Retrieved from hppt://www.cdc.gov.

Duff P, Sweet R, Edwards R. Maternal and fetal infections. In Creasy R, Resnik R, Iams J, and others, editors: *Creasy and Resnik's maternal-fetal medicine: principles and practice,* ed 6, Philadelphia, 2009, Saunders.

Parratt J, Hay D: Sexually transmitted infections, *Curr Obstet Gynaecol* 13(4):224, 2003.

Group B Streptococcus

American College of Obstetricians and Gynecologists (ACOG): *Prevention of early-onset group B Streptococcal disease in newborns,* ACOG Committee Opinion No 279, Washington, DC, 2002, Author.

Centers for Disease Control and Prevention (CDC): Prevention of perinatal group B streptococcal disease: revised guidelines from CDC, *MMWR Morb Mortal Wkly Rep* 51:RR-11, 2002. Retrieved from http://www.cdc.gov/groupbstrep/hospitals/hospitals_guidelines.htm.

Centers for Disease Control and Prevention (CDC): Trends in perinatal group B streptococcal disease United States, 2000-2006, *MMWR Morb Mortal Wkly Rep* 58(05):109–112, 2009.

Money D, Dobson S: The prevention of early-onset neonatal group B streptococcal disease, *J Obstet Gynaecol Can* 26(9):826–840, 2004.

Phares C, Lynfield R, Farley M, and others: Epidemiology of invasive group B streptococcal disease in the United States, 1999-2005, *JAMA* 299:2056–2065, 2008.

Schrag S, and others: Group B streptococcal disease in the era of intrapartum antibiotic prophylaxis, *N Engl J Med* 342(1):15–20, 2000.

Hepatitis B

Centers for Disease Control and Prevention (CDC): A comprehensive immunization strategy to eliminate transmission of hepatitis B virus infection in the United States: Recommendations of the advisory committee on immunization practice (ACIP). Part I: Immunization of infants, children, and adolescents, *MMWR Morb Mortal Wkly Rep* 54(RR16):1–33, 2005.

Centers of Disease Control and Prevention (CDC): A comprehensive immunization strategy to eliminate transmission of hepatitis B virus infection in the United States: Recommendations of the advisory committee on immunization practices (ACIP). Part II: Immunization of adults, *MMWR Morb Mortal Wkly Report* 55 (RR16):1–25, 2006.

Centers of Disease Control and Prevention (CDC): Recommendations for identification and public health management of persons with chronic hepatitis B virus infection, *MMWR Recomm Rep* 57(RR-8):1–20, 2008.

Immunization Action Coalition: *Hepatitis B facts: testing and vaccination,* St Paul, 2004, IAC. Retrieved from http://www.immunize.org/catg.d/p2110.htm.

Williamson C, Mackillop L: Diseases of the liver, biliary system, and pancreas. In Creasy R, Resnik R, Iams J, and others, editors: *Creasy and Resnik's maternal-fetal medicine: principles and practice,* ed 6, Philadelphia, 2009, Saunders.

Hepatitis C

Centers for Disease Control and Prevention (CDC): Sexually transmitted diseases treatment guidelines, 2006, *MMWR Morb Mortal Wkly Rep* 55(RR11):1–94, 2006.

Mass E, Huang I, Seto D: Risk factors for perinatal transmission of hepatitis C virus and the natural history of HCV infection acquired in infancy, *J Infect Dis* 192:1880–1889, 2005.

National Guideline Clearinghouse: *National guideline for the management of the viral hepatitides A, B, and C, 2002,* 2002. Retrieved from http://guideline.gov.

National Guideline Clearinghouse: Screening for hepatitis C virus infection in adults: recommendation statement, *Ann Intern Med* 140(6):462, 2004. Retrieved from http://guideline.gov.

National Institutes of Health (NIH): Management of hepatitis C. *NIH Consensus and State-of-the-Science Statements* 19(3), 2002. Retrieved from http://consensus.nih.gov/cons/cons.htm.

Strader D, Wright T, Thomas D, Seeff L: AASLD practice guideline: diagnosis, management and treatment of hepatitis C, *Hepatology* (39):1147–1171, 2004.

Thomas S, and others: A review of hepatitis C virus (HCV) vertical transmission: risks of transmission to infants born to mothers with and without HCV viremia or human immunodeficiency virus infection, *Int J Epidemiol* 2(1):108–117, 1998.

Williamson C, Mackillop L: Diseases of the liver, biliary system, and pancreas. In Creasy R, Resnik R, Iams J, and others, editors: *Creasy and Resnik's maternal-fetal medicine: principles and practice,* ed 6, Philadelphia, 2009, Saunders.

Herpes Simplex Virus-2

American College of Obstetricians and Gynecologists (ACOG): *Management of Herpes in Pregnancy.* ACOG Practice Bulletin, number 82, Washington, DC, June 2007, ACOG.

Centers for Disease Control and Prevention (CDC): *Genital herpes fact sheet,* December, 2007. Retrieved from http://www.edcp.org/pdf_factsheets/Herpes.pdf.

Centers for Disease Control and Prevention (CDC): Sexually transmitted diseases treatment guidelines, *MMWR Morb Mortal Wkly Rep* 55(RR11):1–94, 2006.

Clinical Effectiveness Group: 2007 national guideline for the management of genital herpes, London, 2007, British Association for Sexual Health and HIV.

Corey L, and others: Once daily valacyclovir to reduce the risk of transmission of genital herpes, *N Engl J Med* 350(1):11–20, 2004.

Leone P: Asymptomatic shedding in the transmission, prevention, and treatment of genital herpes, *Medscape Infect Dis* 6(1), 2004. Retrieved from http://www.medscape.com/viewarticle/478550.

Morrow R: Importance of testing and diagnosis in genital herpes, *Medscape Infect Dis* 6(2): 2004. Retrieved from http://www.medscape.com/viewarticle/483440.

Sheffield J, and others: Acyclovir prophylaxis to prevent herpes simplex virus recurrence at delivery: a systematic review, *Obstet Gynecol* 102(6):1396–1403, 2003.

Stone K, and others: Pregnancy outcomes following systemic prenatal acyclovir exposure: conclusions from the international acyclovir pregnancy registry, 1984-1999, *Birth Defects Res A Clin Mol Teratol* 70(4):201–207, 2004.

U.S. Preventive Services Task Force (USPSTF): Screening for genital herpes: recommendation statement, Rockville, MD, 2005, Agency for Healthcare Research and Quality.

Wald A, and others: Polymerase chain reaction for detection of herpes simplex virus (HSV) DNA on mucosal surfaces: comparison with HSV isolation in cell culture, *J Infect Dis* 188(9):1345–1351, 2003.

Wald A, Link K: Risk of human immunodeficiency virus infection in herpes simplex virus infection type 2-seropositve persons: a meta-analysis, *J Infect Dis* 185(1):45–52, 2002.

HIV

American College of Obstetricians and Gynecologists (ACOG): *Committee opinion: scheduled cesarean delivery and the prevention of vertical transmission of HIV infection,* No. 234, Washington, DC, 2000, ACOG.

American College of Obstetricians and Gynecologists (ACOG): *Prenatal and perinatal human immunodeficiency virus testing; expanded recommendations.* Committee Opinion No. 418, Washington, DC, 2008, ACOG.

Clarke S, and others: The efficacy and tolerability of combination antiretroviral therapy in pregnancy: infant and maternal outcome, *Int J STD AIDS* 11(4):220–223, 2000.

Cooper E, Charurat M, Mofenson L, and others: Combination antiretroviral strategies for the treatment of pregnant HIV-1 infected women and prevention of perinatal HIV-1 transmission, *J Acquir Immune Defic Syndr Hum Retroviral* 29(5):484–494, 2002.

Lampe M, and others: RapidHIV-1 antibody testing during labor and delivery for women of unknown HIV status. A Practical Guide and Model Protocol, Washington, DC, 2004, Centers for Disease Control and Prevention (CDC). Retrieved from http://www.cdc.gov/hiv/projects/perinatal.

McGowan J, and others: Combination antiretroviral therapy in human immunodeficiency virus-infected pregnant women, *Obstet Gynecol* 94(5 Pt 1):641–646, 1999.

Minkoff H, and others: The relationship of pregnancy to human immunodeficiency virus disease progression, *Am J Obstet Gynecol* 189(2):552–559, 2003.

Moodley J, Wennberg J: HIV in pregnancy, *Curr Obstet Gynecol* 17(2):117–121, 2005.

Nduati R, and others: Effect of breastfeeding and formula feeding on transmission of HIV-1: a randomized clinical trial, *JAMA* 283(9):1167–1174, 2000.

Pediatric HIV Working Group on Antiretroviral Therapy and Medical Management of HIV-Infected Children: *Guideline for the use of antiretroviral agents in pediatric HIV infection*, Rockville, Md, 2009, Public Health Service Task Force. Retrieved from http://aidsinfo.nih.gov/contentfiles/PediatricGuidelines.pdf.

Penn Z, Ahmed S: Human immunodeficiency virus in pregnancy, *Curr Obstet Gynaecol* 13(6):321–328, 2003.

Perinatal HIV Guidelines Working Group: Public Health Service Task Force recommendations for use of antiretroviral drugs in pregnant HIV infected women for maternal health and interventions to reduce perinatal HIV transmission in the United States, Rockville, Md, 2009, Public Health Service Task Force. Retrieved from http://aidsinfo.nih.gov/contentfiles/PerinatalGL.pdf.

Petra Study Team: Efficacy of three short-course regimens of zidovudine and lamivudine in preventing early and late transmission of HIV-1 from mother to child in Tanzania, South Africa, and Uganda (Petra study): a randomized, double-blind, placebo-controlled trial, *Lancet* 359(3913):1178–1185, 2002.

Qaseem A, Snow V, Shekelle P, Hopkins R Jr, Owens DK: Clinical Efficacy Assessment Subcommittee, American College of Physicians: Screening for HIV in health care settings: a guidance statement from the American College of Physicians and HIV Medicine Association, *Ann Intern Med* 150(2):125–131, 2009. Retrieved from http://www.guideline.gov.

Wade N, Birkhead G, Warren B, and others: Abbreviated regimens of zidovudine prophylaxis and perinatal transmission of the human immunodeficiency virus, *N Engl J Med* 339(20):1409–1414, 1998.

World Health Organization (WHO): *Antiretroviral drugs for treating pregnant women and preventing HIV infection in infants*, Geneva, 2004, Department of HIV/AIDS, Department of Reproduction Health and Research.

Human Papillomavirus

American College of Obstetricians and Gynecologists (ACOG): Cervical cytology screening: clinical management guidelines for obstetrician-gynecologists, *ACOG Practice Bulletin* 45, 2003, ACOG.

American College of Obstetricians and Gynecologists (ACOG): Human papillomavirus, *ACOG Practice Bulletin* 61, 2005.

Burk R: Pernicious papillomavirus infection, *N Engl J Med* 341(22):1687–1688, 1999.

Canavan R, Doshi N: Cervical cancer, *Am Fam Physician* 61(5):1369–1376, 2000.

Carson S: Human papillomatous virus infection update: impact on women's health, *Nurse Pract* 22(4):24–25, 1997.

Castle P, Giuliano A: Genital tract infections, cervical inflammation, and antioxidant nutrients assessing their roles as human papillomavirus cofactors, *J Natl Cancer Inst Monogr* 31:29–34, 2003.

Centers for Disease Control and Prevention (CDC): Sexually transmitted diseases treatment guidelines, 2006, *MMWR Morb Mortal Wkly Rep* 55(RR11):1–94, 2006.

Centers for Disease Control and Prevention (CDC): Quadrivalent human papillomavirus vaccine: Recommendations of the advisory committee on immunization practices, *MMWR Recommend Rep* No. 56, RR-02, 2007.

Cox J: The development of cervical cancer and its precursors: what is the role of human papillomavirus infection? *Curr Opin Obstet Gynecol* 18(Suppl 1):S5–S13, 2006.

Dempsey A, Gebremariam A, Koutsky L, Manhart L: Behavior in early adolescence and risk of human papillomavirus infection as a young adult; results from a population-based study, *Pediatrics* 122(1):1–7, 2008.

Duff P, Sweet R, Edwards R: Maternal and fetal infections. In Creasy R, Resnik R, Iams J, and others, editors: In *Creasy and Resnik's maternal-fetal medicine: principles and practice*, ed 6, Philadelphia, 2009, Saunders.

Gerberding J: Report to congress: Prevention of genital human papillomavirus infection, 2004, CDC. Retrieved from http://www.cdc.gov/std/hpv/default.htm.

Ho G, and others: Natural history of cervicovaginal papillomavirus infection in young women, *N Engl J Med* 338(7):423–428, 1998.

McCance K, Huether S: *Pathophysiology: the biologic basis for disease in adults and children*, ed 5, St Louis, 2006, Mosby.

Molano M, and others: Determinants of clearance of human papillomavirus infections in Colombian women with normal cytology: a population-based, 5 year follow-up study, *Am J Epidemiol* 158(5):486–494, 2003.

Moscicki A, and others: The natural history of human papillomavirus infection as measured by repeated DNA testing in adolescent and young women, *J Pediatr* 132(2):277–284, 1998.

Rodriguez A, Schiffman M, Herrero R, and others: Rapid clearance of human papillomavirus and implications for clinical focus on persistent infection, *J Natl Cancer Inst* 100(7):513–517, 2008.

Smith J, and others: Evidence for *Chlamydia trachomatis* as a human papillomavirus cofactor in the etiology of invasive cervical cancer in Brazil and the Philippines, *J Infect Dis* 185(3):324–331, 2002.

Thomas D: Sexually transmitted viral infections: epidemiology and treatment, *J Obstet Gynecol Neonatal Nurs* 30(3):316–323, 2001.

Teitelman A, Stringer M, Averbuch T, Witkoski A: Human papillomavirus, current vaccines, and cervical caner prevention, *J Obstet Gynecol Neonatal Nurs* 38(1):69–80, 2009.

United States Department of Health and Human Services (USDHHS): *FDA approved first DNA test for two types of human papillomavirus*, 2009. Author. Retrieved from http://www.fda.gov/NewsEvents/Newsroom/PressAnnouncements/ucm149544.htm.

Human Parvovirus B19

Bonvicini F, and others: Diagnosis of fetal parvovirus B19 infection: value of virological assays in fetal specimens, *An Int J Obstet Gynacol* 116(6):813–817, 2009.

Centers for Disease Control and Prevention (CDC): Parvovirus B19 infection and pregnancy, *Factsheet* 2007. Retrieved from http://www.cdc.gov/ncidod/dvrd/revb/respiratory/B19&preg.htm.

Ramirez M, Mastrobattista J: Diagnosis and management of human parvovirus B19 infection, *Clin Perinatol* 32(3):697–704, 2005.

Syphilis

Centers for Disease Control and Prevention (CDC): Sexually transmitted diseases treatment guidelines, 2006, *MMWR Morb Mortal Wkly Rep* 55(RR11):1–94, 2006.

Duff P, Sweet R, Edwards R: Maternal and fetal infections. In Creasy R, Resnik R, Iams J, and others, editors: *Creasy and Resnik's maternal-fetal medicine: principles and practice,* ed 6, Philadelphia, 2009, Saunders.

Trichomoniasis

Centers for Disease Control and Prevention (CDC): Sexually transmitted diseases treatment guidelines, 2006, *MMWR Morb Mortal Wkly Rep* 55(RR11):1–94, 2006.

Duff P, Sweet R, Edwards R. Maternal and fetal infections. In Creasy R, Resnik R, Iams J, and others, editors: *Creasy and Resnik's maternal-fetal medicine: principles and practice,* ed 6, Philadelphia, 2009, Saunders.

Gülmezoglu AM: Interventions for trichomoniasis in pregnancy, *Cochrane Database Syst Rev* (Issue 1), Art. No.: CD000220, 2004.

Kigozi G, and others: Treatment of trichomonas in pregnancy and adverse outcomes of pregnancy, *Am J Obstet Gynecol* 189(5):1398–1400, 2003.

Lawrence R, Lawrence M: *Breastfeeding: a guide for the medical profession*, ed 6, Philadelphia, 2005, Mosby.

Okun N, Gronau K, Hannah M: Antibiotics for bacterial vaginosis or trichomonas vaginalis in pregnancy: a systematic review, *Obstet Gynecol* 105(4):857–868, 2005.

Urinary Tract Infection

American Academy of Pediatrics and American College of Obstetricians and Gynecologists: *Guidelines for perinatal care*, ed 6, Washington, DC, 2007, Author.

Cram L, and others: Genitourinary infections and their association with preterm labor, *Am Fam Physician* 65(2):241–248, 2002.

Duff P, Sweet R, Edwards R: Maternal and fetal infections. In Creasy R, Resnik R, Iams J, and others, editors: *Creasy and Resnik's maternal-fetal medicine: principles and practice,* ed 6, Philadelphia, 2009, Saunders.

Delzell J, Lefevre M: Urinary tract infections in pregnancy, *Am Fam Physician* 61(3):713–721, 2000.

Fontaine K: *Healing practices: alternative therapies for nursing*, Upper Saddle River, NJ, 2000, Prentice Hall.

Sierpina V: *Integrative health care: complementary and alternative therapies for the whole person*, Philadelphia, 2001, FA Davis.

Smaill FM, Vazquez JC: Antibiotics for asymptomatic bacteriuria in pregnancy, *Cochrane Database Syst Rev* (Issue 1), Art. No.: CD000490, 2007.

Tolosa JE: Antibiotics for asymptomatic bacteriuria in pregnancy: RHL commentary (last revised: 14 January 2008). *The WHO Reproductive Health Library*, Geneva: World Health Organization. Retrieved from http://apps.who.int/rhl/pregnancy_childbirth/complications/infection/jtcom/en/index.html.

Villar J, Widmer M, Lydon-Rochelle M, and others: Duration of treatment for asymptomatic bacteriuria during pregnancy, *Cochrane Database Syst Rev* (Issue 3), Art. No.: CD000491, 2006.

General Nursing Management

National Institute of Health (NIH): *Sexually transmitted diseases and infections and HIV/AIDS research*, Bethesda, Md, 2005, Author. Retrieved from http://www.nichd.nih.gov/womenshealth/STDHIV.cfm.

Tumolo J: Sweet 16 and infected: sexually transmitted diseases in adolescents, *Adv Nurse Pract* 8(9):49–52, 2000.

Waldrop J: Tough lessons in STD prevention, *Clin Advis NPs* 92, June, 2001.

27

Substance Abuse

The rate of substance abuse among childbearing women continues to increase dramatically. Approximately 15% of all pregnant women have a substance abuse problem (USDHHS, 2000). Four percent use illicit drugs (SAMHSA, 2007). Abusing any kind of substance increases the risk for pregnancy complications and the risk for adverse physical and mental outcomes in the fetus. It is imperative that nurse practitioners and nurses caring for families during their childbearing years understand substance abuse and implement care in a collaborative effect to support the *Healthy People 2010* goal of increased abstinence from alcohol, cigarettes, and illicit drug use among pregnant women. This chapter focuses on six of the most commonly abused substances and provides insight into the management of care for pregnant women who are using any of these six substances.

ALCOHOL

Incidence

Currently, alcohol is the most common teratogen. According to the National Survey on Drug Use and Health (SAMHSA, 2009), 19% of childbearing women admit to drinking alcohol during the first trimester, 8% during the second trimester, and 6% during the third trimester. According to the National Survey on Drug Use and Health in 2006, 1% are heavy drinkers, consuming at least 7 drinks per week, and 3% binge-drink, consuming more than three drinks on occasion (SAMHSA, 2009). The highest incidence is in the Native American population (Gardner, 2000).

Pathophysiologic Effects

Alcohol use during pregnancy can have varied pathophysiologic effects, including the following:
- Interferes with the absorption of such nutrients as thiamin (vitamin B_1), vitamin B_{12}, folic acid, and zinc related to its irritation effect on the GI tract
- Interferes with nerve cell growth and development in various ways (USDHHS, 2000)
- Impairs neuronal differentiation and facilitates free radical damage (USDHHS, 2000)
- Induces premature death of cells that develop into facial bones and cartilage (USDHHS, 2000)

Maternal Complications

Maternal complications with alcohol use during pregnancy include increased risk for the following problems:

- Infertility
- Spontaneous abortion
- Abruptio placentae
- Preterm labor

Fetal Complications

Alcohol is the leading preventable cause of birth defects and mental retardation (Floyd, Jack, Cefalo, and others, 2008). Alcohol can have varying adverse effects on the fetus, depending on factors such as genetic sensitivity, time of exposure, and dose (Goodlett and Johnson, 1999). Fetal Alcohol Spectrum disorders (FASD) is the term used to describe the continuum for adverse fetal outcome that results from alcohol exposure during fetal life.

The most severe fetal alcohol spectrum disorder is fetal alcohol syndrome (FAS). Other fetal alcohol spectrum disorders manifest as neurobehavioral deficits without the physical characteristics of FAS.

FAS is a pattern of defects that are characterized by three clinical features. To make the diagnosis of FAS, two of the three facial abnormalities and one manifestation from each of the other deficits must be present (Table 27-1) (NCBDDD,

Table 27-1   Possible Characteristics in Each of the Three Categories for Diagnosis of Fetal Alcohol Syndrome

Categories	Characteristics
Facial anomalies	*Exhibit two of the following three:* Flattened philtrum (the groove between the nose and upper lip) Thin vermilion border (flat upper lip) Short palpebral fissures (eye openings)
Prenatal and/or postnatal growth deficits	*Exhibit one of the following:* Low birth weight for gestational age Failure to thrive
Neurodevelopmental abnormalities	*Exhibit one of the following:* Microcephaly at or below 10th percentile Impaired fine motor skills Neurosensory hearing loss Poor tandem gait Poor eye-hand coordination Attention deficit disorder Aggressiveness Mental retardation Poor short-term memory Difficulty in problem solving

Data from National Center on Birth Defects and Developmental Disabilities (NCBDDD), Centers for Disease Control and Prevention (CDC), Department of Health and Human Services (USDHHS): *Fetal alcohol syndrome: guidelines for referral and diagnosis,* Atlanta, GA, 2004, NCBDDD, CDC.

CDC, and USDHHS, 2004). Prenatal alcohol exposure can cause other alcohol-related disorders referred to as fetal alcohol spectrum disorders (FASD). The Institute of Medicine (IOM) of the National Academy of Science classifies fetal alcohol spectrum disorders into four diagnostic categories (Stratton, Howe, and Battaglia, 1996; USDHHS, 2000; Avner and Nulman, 2005). In 2005, diagnostic clarification of the various fetal alcohol spectrum disorders was published (Table 27-2) (Hoyme and others, 2005).

Table 27-2   Diagnostic Criteria for Fetal Alcohol Spectrum Disorders

Diagnosis	Criteria for Diagnosis
Fetal alcohol syndrome (FAS)	Exhibits two of the three
With confirmed maternal alcohol exposure	Facial anomalies
	Evidence of prenatal and/or postnatal growth deficits
	Neurodevelopmental abnormalities
Without confirmed maternal alcohol exposure	Evidence of one or more
Partial fetal alcohol syndrome (PFAS)	Facial anomalies
With confirmed maternal alcohol exposure	Exhibits two of the three
	Prenatal and/or postnatal growth deficits or neurodevelopmental abnormalities
Without confirmed maternal alcohol exposure	Exhibits one
Alcohol-related birth defects (ARBD)	Facial anomalies
Confirmed maternal alcohol exposure	Exhibits two of the three
	One or more congenital structural defects associated with alcohol such as congenital heart defect, skeletal anomaly, kidney defect, hearing impairment, or other characteristic anomalies
Alcohol-related neurodevelopmental disorders (ARND)	Evidence of one deficient brain growth or abnormal prenatal or postnatal growth deficit
Confirmed maternal alcohol exposure	Evidence of complex pattern of behavioral or cognitive abnormalities such as impairment of performance of complex tasks
	Higher-level receptive and expressive language deficits
	Disordered behavior

Reference: Hoyme H, and others: A practical clinical approach to diagnosis of fetal alcohol spectrum disorders: clarification of the 1996 Institute of Medicine criteria, *Pediatrics* 115(1):39–47, 2005.

Childhood Effects

Current research indicates that newborns are at increased risk for an infection if exposed to alcohol during fetal life (Gauthier and others, 2005).

Children with FAS continue to demonstrate growth deficiency, facial dysmorphic characteristics, performance deficits, and varying degrees of learning difficulties. FAS is the most common cause of mental retardation (Gardner, 2000; ACOG, 2008). The social and emotional development of these children can be affected by their lack of understanding of consequences, aggressiveness, and destructive behavior. They also have a high pain tolerance (Gardner, 2000).

Screening

The American Medical Association (AMA) has endorsed universal screening in a nonjudgmental and supportive manner (NCBDDD, CDC, and USDHHS, 2004; ACOG, 2008). The best screening method for alcohol abuse is a self-administered questionnaire given to all pregnant women on their first prenatal visit. The questions should be worded in a manner that assumes alcohol use in order to lessen defensive responses and increase honesty. Two different ways of wording the questions have been found to facilitate disclosure. The first way is a simple question such as, "Have you ever had a drink containing alcohol?" (ACOG, 2006). A second way is to use Ewing's Four Ps (yes and no questions) to assess use of alcohol or other drugs (Taylor, Zaichkin, and Bailey, 2002). The four questions are as follows (see Box 27-3):

- Have you ever used drugs or alcohol during this **P**regnancy?
- Have you had a problem with drugs or alcohol in the **P**ast?
- Does your **P**artner have a problem with drugs or alcohol?
- Do you consider one of your **P**arents to be an addict or alcoholic?

If it is determined that the pregnant woman drinks, administer a questionnaire to determine at-risk levels of drinking. The T-ACE (Table 27-3), CAGE (Table 27-4), and TWEAK (Table 27-5) questionnaires are three such instruments. According to research done by Bradley and others (1998), these questionnaires provide the most reliable screening survey for women, especially during pregnancy.

Table 27-3   T-ACE Questionnaire for At-Risk Drinking Patterns

Questions	Score
T How many drinks does it take to make you feel high (**T**olerance)?	≥6 drinks = 2
	<6 drinks = 1
A Have people **A**nnoyed you by criticizing your drinking?	No = 1
	Yes = 2
C Have you felt you ought to **C**ut down on your drinking?	No = 1
	Yes = 2
E Have you ever had a drink first thing in the morning to steady your nerves or get rid of a hangover (**E**ye opener)?	No = 1
	Yes = 2

A score of 2 on any question indicates a high probability of being a risk drinker.
Modified from Sokol R, Martier S, Ager J: The T-ACE questions: practical prenatal detection of risk drinking, *Am J Obstet Gynecol* 160(4):863–868, 1989; American College of Obstetricians and Gynecologists: *ACOG Technical Bulletin*, No. 195, 1994.

Table 27-4   CAGE Questionnaire for At-Risk Drinking Patterns

Questions	
C	Have you ever felt you ought to **C**ut down on drinking?
A	Have people **A**nnoyed you by criticizing your drinking?
G	Have you ever felt bad or **G**uilty about your drinking?
E	Have you ever had a drink first thing in the morning to steady your nerves or get rid of a hangover (**E**ye opener)?
More than one positive response suggests an alcohol at-risk problem.	

Reference: American Society of Addiction Medicine: *Questions to ask,* patient pocket card, 2001. Retrieved from http://www.asam.org/publ/CAGE.htm.

Table 27-5   TWEAK Questionnaire for At-Risk Drinking Patterns

Questions	
T	*Tolerance.* How many drinks can you hold?
W	*Worry.* Does your spouse or do your other family members ever worry or complain about your drinking?
E	*Eye opener.* Have you ever had a drink first thing in the morning to steady your nerves or get rid of a hangover?
A	*Amnesia.* Have you ever awakened the morning after drinking the night before and found that you could not remember a part of the evening before?
K	*Kut.* Have you ever felt you ought to cut down on your drinking?
Positive answers to the first two questions score 2 points each; the other three questions score 1 point each for a positive answer.	

Modified from Chan A and others: Use of the TWEAK test in screening on alcoholism/heavy drinking in three populations, *Alcohol Clin Exp Res* 17(16):188–1192, 1993.

Very carefully screen women who are particularly at risk, including the following groups:
- Single pregnant women
- Women of Native American descent
- Smokers
- Women with alcoholic husbands

American College of Obstetrics and Gynecology (ACOG) in collaboration with the Center for Disease Control and Prevention (CDC) has recently developed a Fetal Alcohol Spectrum disorders Prevention Tool Kit for women's health care providers. The Tool Kit is available at *http://www.cdc.gov/ncbddd/fas/acog_toolkit.htm.*

Pregnancy Considerations

No level of alcohol has been proved to be safe for the fetus, and alcohol should be completely avoided when planning for conception and during pregnancy (U.S. Surgeon General, 2005). Because alcohol readily passes to the infant through breast milk and research has shown that when it contains alcohol, infants consume significantly less breast milk, sleep less, and show developmental delays (Lawrence and Lawrence, 2005), drinking is not recommended during breastfeeding either. Health care providers should avoid prescribing alcohol to help with letdown.

The teratogenic effect of alcohol is dose-related, and *risk drinking* is of greatest concern. This is defined as maternal drinking that produces blood alcohol levels high enough and for long enough to produce fetal damage (Bertrand, Floyd, Weber, and others, 2004). However, the precise level of alcohol varies with each individual. Therefore no safe drinking level has been established.

Maternal nutrition is usually affected if the pregnant woman drinks. Ethanol is a source of energy; therefore a person with alcoholism usually has a low intake of nutrients. Ethanol can also interfere with intestinal absorption of certain vitamins and nutrients, such as calcium, amino acids, thiamin, vitamin B_6, vitamin B_{12}, folate, and zinc.

Women are frequently more receptive to making lifestyle changes during pregnancy than at any other time during their lives. Offering advice that can be easily remembered versus mass media education is more effective in motivating a woman to choose to stop drinking (Hankin and Sokol, 1995). Examples follow:

- You have a whole life to drink but only 9 months to grow a healthy baby.
- Although only 1 in 10 heavy drinkers has a baby with FAS, you cannot predict that you will not be the one.
- The most important thing you can do to influence the health of your baby is to cut your drinking or quit altogether.

Treatment During Pregnancy

Randomized studies demonstrate strong evidence that brief behavioral counseling interventions significantly reduce alcohol use (Chang, 2001; O'Connor and Whaley, 2007; USDHHS, 2007). Therefore when a pregnant woman identifies that she does use alcohol to some degree, classify her drinking pattern according to (1) social drinking, (2) symptom-relief drinking (drinking to relieve depression or to elevate mood), or (3) syndrome drinking (physiologic and psychologic dependence on alcohol). Then implement nursing interventions based on the woman's drinking pattern to facilitate her quitting or at least decreasing her drinking.

The social drinker just needs complete information as to the effects of alcohol on her unborn child, and she will most likely quit. Yet in a qualitative study, Barbour (1990) found that 60% of pregnant women received information that occasional drinking was not likely to be harmful. However, as stated previously, no safe drinking level during pregnancy has been established. On the other hand, to decrease undue anxiety, a woman who has had a few social drinks before the pregnancy was recognized should be reassured of a relatively low risk for fetal damage but instructed as to the importance of avoiding alcohol for the remainder of the pregnancy.

The symptom-relief drinker should receive the same education as to the effects of alcohol but needs supportive counseling as well. This can be provided effectively in the prenatal office setting by trained health care workers. The woman with alcoholism requires referral to an appropriate detoxification program, as well as support programs. However, the nurse practitioner and the prenatal nurse need to remain actively involved after making the appropriate referrals.

One technique shown to be effective in reducing excessive alcohol consumption is defined by the acronym FRAMES (Fleming and others, 1997; ACOG, 2006):

F　*Feedback* about the adverse effects of alcohol
R　*Responsibility* for change
A　*Advice* about appropriate drinking amounts
M　*Menu* of available options
E　*Empathy* for the patient
S　*Self-efficacy*

COCAINE

Cocaine can be snorted, injected, or smoked as *freebase* or *crack*. Cocaine comes in two forms: powder and crystals. Cocaine hydrochloride, cocaine sulfate, and cocaine base come in the form of a powder and are inhaled (snorted or sniffed); therefore they are readily absorbed through the mucous membranes or dissolved and taken intravenously (IV). Cocaine powders are only 15% to 25% pure and have many street names, such as *lady, snow, coke, white girl, nose candy, Cadillac,* and *gold dust.* Crack, which is 90% pure cocaine, comes in the form of crystals called *rocks* and is smoked (freebased); therefore it is absorbed through the lung tissue.

Sniffing cocaine produces a high after several minutes, and the effect lasts for more than 1 hour. Cocaine that is smoked or taken IV produces a high in seconds that causes rapid euphoria that lasts only about 30 minutes. Thus the latter two methods are usually repeated more often and are therefore more highly addicting. Many people are hooked after their first experience with it.

Pathophysiologic Effects

Cocaine interferes with the reuptake of dopamine and norepinephrine at the nerve synapses, resulting in increased circulating levels of these two neurotransmitters. Cocaine also alters the metabolism of serotonin and acetylcholine. The resulting neurotransmitter imbalance overactivates certain receptors that regulate (1) mood, causing euphoria (a feeling of confidence and sexual arousal); (2) sleep, causing a hyperaroused state; (3) motor function, causing excitation and restlessness; and (4) sympathetic nervous system stimulation, causing tachycardia, tachypnea, hyperthermia (38.8° C to 41° C [102° F to 106° F]), hypertension (increased mean arterial pressure approximately 50%), and intense, generalized vasoconstriction (Schiller and Allen, 2005). After depletion of the neurotransmitters, depression, malaise, and an extreme craving for the drug ensue.

Resulting complications that can occur from cocaine use are as follows (Wagner and others, 1998; Kuczkowski, 2003; Vidaeff and Mastrobattista, 2003):

- Decreased blood flow to the heart muscle, which predisposes to dysrhythmias, a myocardial infarction, and platelet aggregation
- Decreased blood flow to the brain, which predisposes to seizures, stroke, and cerebral infarction
- Decreased blood flow to the intestines, which can cause peristaltic stimulation but can also lead to tissue death
- Decreased uterine blood flow by 50% and increased uterine vascular resistance

- Increased levels of fetal neurotransmitters. The resulting consequences are the same as for the adult, such as increased fetal mean arterial pressure by 24%, increased FHR by 50%, and decreased fetal oxygen partial pressure [PO_2] by 30%, which may cause various teratogenic effects (Dolkart, Plessinger, and Woods, 1990; Buehler, Conover, and Andres, 1996).

Cocaine is metabolized by plasma and liver cholinesterase to water-soluble substances called *metabolites* that are excreted in the urine. Because the plasma cholinesterase is decreased during pregnancy and is much less in the fetus and neonate, cocaine is more toxic during pregnancy and to the fetus (Wagner and others, 1998).

Maternal Complications

Cocaine can stimulate uterine contractions. Therefore its use in the first trimester of pregnancy increases the risk for a spontaneous abortion. Its use in the second and third trimesters can increase the risk for preterm labor and premature rupture of membranes (Bateman and Chiriboga, 2000; Bandstra and others, 2001; Fajemirokun-Odudeyi and Lindow, 2004). It is not known whether these risks are directly related to cocaine use or to the frequent associated use of tobacco and inadequate prenatal care.

Cocaine decreases blood flow to the heart, brain, and uterus to a greater extent during pregnancy. Because of this vasoconstrictor effect of the drug, cardiovascular failure, intracerebral hemorrhage, respiratory failure, seizures, and hypertensive crises that may mimic pregnancy-induced hypertension (PIH) occur significantly more frequently (Plessinger and Woods, 1998).

Abruptio placentae and stillbirth occur more frequently in cocaine users and may be related to the effect on blood pressure (Singer and others, 2002; Fajemirokun-Odudeyi and Lindow, 2004; MOD, 2004).

Fetal and Neonatal Complications

Because of the dramatic decrease in uterine blood flow with resultant fetal hypoxia and the blocking reuptake of the neurotransmitters that occur with maternal cocaine use, complications are prevalent. Prematurity caused by a preterm delivery is related to cocaine-induced uterine contractions (Bandstra and others, 2001; Bada and others, 2002). Cocaine-exposed infants have been observed to be small-for-gestational-age, including small head circumference (Bateman and Chiriboga, 2000; Bandstra and others, 2001; Singer and others, 2002). Congenital malformations have been reported in the literature and include cardiac anomalies, urinary tract defects, segmental intestinal atresia, and central nervous system (CNS) abnormalities (Potter and others, 2000; Hepburn, 2004). However, available research data do not provide unequivocal proof.

Infants exposed to cocaine during pregnancy do not exhibit physiologic withdrawal symptoms as seen when other types of substances are abused but frequently manifest neurobehavioral abnormalities (AAP, 1998), such as the following:

- Hyperreflexia, which can be seen as an exaggerated startle response and tremulousness
- Abnormal state patterns such as difficulty sleeping and maintaining an alert, inactive state, thus spending prolonged time in the crying and alert active state

- Inappropriate interactive behaviors and inability to respond appropriately to parents, affecting parent-infant attachment
- Difficulty in habituating and therefore extreme sensitivity to environmental stimuli
- Extremely short attention to a stimulus before showing signs of agitation, such as color changes, rapid respirations, and agitated motor activity
- Deficient self-consoling abilities and poor response to comforting by care providers
- Difficulty eating because of an ineffective suck

The preceding neurobehavioral abnormalities may partially correct but frequently lead to learning difficulties caused by attention deficits and behavioral problems. In their longitudinal prospective study, Singer and associates (2002) found that prenatal cocaine exposure has a significant effect on later cognitive development. This has been especially observed in boys (Bennett, Bendersky, and Lewis, 2008). Aggressive and antisocial behavior has been noted more often in boys exposed to prenatal cocaine (Bennett, Bendersky, and Lewis, 2007).

Effect of Paternal Cocaine Use

If the man is exposed to cocaine just before the intercourse that results in conception, the offspring has an increased risk for abnormalities. Research has demonstrated that cocaine binds to the human spermatozoa (Yazigi, Odem, and Polakoski, 1991).

Screening

During the initial prenatal assessment, all pregnant women should be asked about cocaine use. Health care providers may screen prenatally for cocaine use with various biologic specimens if the history is positive, as shown by one of the following:

- No or inadequate prenatal care
- Inadequate prenatal weight gain
- Previous induced abortion
- Preterm labor
- Abruptio placentae
- History of substance abuse, such as cigarettes, alcohol, or cocaine
- Presence of a sexually transmitted disease
- Inconsistent support system
- Chronic nasal congestion

The American Medical Association recommends urine toxicology screening be performed on all pregnant women because the chances of missing drug use are significant if one screens only those with an indicating history (ACOG, 2004).

Various biologic specimens such as blood, urine, hair, meconium, saliva, amniotic fluid, and perspiration are used. Toxicology urine screen can detect cocaine use by the pregnant woman during the previous week because of its slow metabolism during pregnancy. Newborn meconium (stool of the first 3 days of life) can be analyzed by radioimmunoassay (RIA) for drug metabolites, and analysis of hair is being used as well because the drug remains embedded for the life of the hair shaft (Ursitti, Klein, and Koren, 2001; Boumba, Ziavrou, and Vougiouklakis, 2006; López, Bermejo, Tabernero, and others, 2007).

Treatment During Pregnancy

Be able to recognize the signs of possible cocaine use, such as sweatiness, tachycardia, flushed skin, tremulousness, irritability, difficulty sitting still, and being "high" or sleepy. Dispel myths, such as the misconception that recreational use is not harmful or that cocaine use will bring about a shorter, easier labor. Education as to the harmful effects of cocaine is essential because many feel it is harmless.

When it is determined that the pregnant woman is taking cocaine, she should be told that the best thing to do is to stop immediately. Then provide supportive services so that she can stop, such as referrals to drug rehabilitation programs that address women's needs, individual and family counseling, support groups such as Narcotics Anonymous, financial assistance, and home nurse visitation. A cocaine addict usually resists treatment. Therefore the health care provider must persist in all avenues appropriate for the patient, such as patient support systems and multidisciplinary resources, in attempting to help her understand and admit that cocaine is harmful to her and her fetus and that she should stop using the drug.

Compose a list of available community and state resources. A helpful national treatment referral and information service resource is 800-COCAINE. This resource can give health care providers names of local perinatal cocaine treatment centers. This same number serves as a cocaine hotline that is available for cocaine addicts and family members.

Assess for multiple risk factors, such as cigarette smoking, alcohol use, use of other drugs, and inadequate prenatal care.

Become familiar with the legislative issues related to drug testing, reporting drug use, and fetal rights for your state. Become involved, in cooperation with the risk management department of your institution, in policy development to legally manage the care of pregnant women who use cocaine.

Care of the laboring patient who has recently used cocaine should include close observations for signs of complications, oxygen by mask at 7 to 10 L/min to enhance fetal oxygenation, and notification of the intensive care nursery of a potential high risk neonate. Cocaine may induce fetal tachycardia and affect variability (Lynch and McKeon, 1990). These patients experience labor pains as much as any other patient, and withholding pain medication is not beneficial. If epidural anesthesia is necessary, the nurse should monitor closely for hypotension because it seems to occur more frequently in the cocaine-positive laboring woman (Kain and others, 1996; FIRST Consult, 2006).

If there is a chance that the mother will use cocaine after the birth of her infant, she should be counseled not to breastfeed because cocaine readily passes to the infant byway of breast milk (Lawrence and Lawrence, 2005).

HEROIN

Heroin is the most common drug injected intravenously, referred to as *mainlining*. Smoking or inhaling the drug is becoming more popular because of the fear of contracting HIV from needles. Taken by any route, heroin is extremely addicting. Street names for this drug are *snow, stuff, junk, smack, horse*, and *joy powder.*

Maternal Complications

Infertility is common because heroin frequently inhibits ovulation. A woman usually becomes pregnant only when heroin levels drop.

It is difficult to ascribe specific maternal effects to heroin because 75% of women who use heroin report using more than one drug (Little and others, 1990). A pregnant heroin addict has a three-fold to seven-fold increased risk for preterm labor, preeclampsia, and postpartum hemorrhage (Archie, 1998). Infections such as syphilis, hepatitis, tuberculosis, cellulitis, thrombophlebitis, and HIV are common complications of heroin because the route of administration is likely IV (NIDA, 2005).

Fetal and Neonatal Complications

Fetal and neonatal complications of heroin use include the following:
- Preterm birth and prematurity (Lee, 1995)
- Intrauterine growth restriction (IUGR), which is compounded by maternal abuse of other substances and malnutrition (Archie, 1998)
- Appears to accelerate fetal lung maturity but increases the risk for meconium-stained amniotic fluid and the risk for SIDS (Kendig, 1996)
- Signs of withdrawal (Box 27-1) manifested by 60% to 80% of the infants exposed to prenatal heroin; withdrawal usually occurs within the first 24 to 72 hours but may be delayed up to 10 days of life (Archie, 1998)
- Postnatal growth deficiency, mild developmental delays, and behavior problems observed in follow-up studies of children exposed to perinatal heroin; however, these problems are reported to be more related to poor maternal nutrition and inappropriate postnatal environment than to the direct effect of the perinatal heroin (Robins and Mills, 1993)

Treatment During Pregnancy

Screening for STDs is essential. Sudden withdrawal from heroin can be harmful and is not recommended during pregnancy because of heroin's significant physical and psychologic addictive properties. Methadone treatment is safe for pregnant women

Box 27-1	Signs of Drug Withdrawal
W	**W**akefulness
I	**I**rritability
T	**T**remulousness, **T**emperature variation, and **T**achypnea
H	**H**yperactivity and **H**igh-pitched or continuous cry
D	**D**iarrhea, **D**iaphoresis, and **D**isorganized suck
R	**R**ub marks, **R**estless sleeping, and **R**espiratory difficulty
A	**A**pneic attacks
W	**W**eight loss or failure to gain weight
A	**A**lkalosis (respiratory)
L	**L**acrimation (runny eye syndrome)

Modified from American Academy of Pediatrics Committee on Drugs: Neonatal drug withdrawal, *Pediatrics* 72:895, 1983; Torrence C, Horns K: Appraisal and caregiving for the drug addicted infant, *Neonatal Netw* 8(3):49-59, 1989.

and their fetus and is frequently used to help the pregnant mother stop using heroin (NIDA, 2009).

During labor, methadone may be continued and narcotics can be used to manage pain. Avoid narcotics with mixed agonist-antagonist properties because they may precipitate acute withdrawal. The newborn needs withdrawal treatment. Breastfeeding is not contraindicated during methadone maintenance therapy if the mother is not abusing other drugs.

MARIJUANA

Street names for marijuana are *grass, pot, joint, reefer,* and *weed.*

Incidence

Marijuana is the most commonly used illicit drug among childbearing women (DPNA, 2004). According to the National Survey on Drug Use and Health (SAMHSA, 2009), approximately 5% of pregnant women admitted to the use of marijuana during pregnancy.

Pathophysiologic Effects

One of the active ingredients of marijuana is delta-9-tetrahydrocannabinol, which crosses the placenta and is fat soluble. Therefore, it may take 30 days for the drug to be excreted from the fetal body (Hubbard, Franco, and Onaivi, 1999).

Marijuana interferes with the production of follicle-stimulating hormone, luteinizing hormone, and prolactin, thereby inhibiting ovulation.

Marijuana increases the carbon monoxide levels in blood five times more than tobacco smoke and therefore decreases fetal oxygenation.

Maternal Complications

- Marijuana can cause infertility problems, especially in the male.
- Marijuana does not cause physical addiction, but it can cause psychologic addiction.
- Marijuana smoke contains more cancer-causing properties than tobacco smoke. One joint affects the lungs as much as smoking 16 cigarettes (Wu and others, 1988). It also causes similar respiratory problems as does tobacco smoke (USDHHS, 2007).
- Marijuana impairs T cell immunity (USDHHS, 2007).

Fetal Complications

Research results are equivocal as to the teratogenic effects of marijuana on fetal growth, neurobehavioral activities, and length of gestation (Lee, 1998). Marijuana has been linked to low birth weight, preterm birth, and such neurobehavioral effects as attention deficit and impulsiveness (Faden and Graubard, 2000; Fried and Smith, 2001; Fergusson, Horwood, and Northstone, 2002). Significantly, executive function deficiency, causing lower scores in childhood verbal and memory abilities, poor focused attention, and self-directed responses have been associated with maternal marijuana use (Fried and Smith, 2001).

Screening

Many marijuana users, as well as substance users of most illegal drugs, go undetected if a drug toxicity screen is not done on all pregnant patients. A commonly used toxicity urine screen is the enzyme-multiplied immunoassay. It is effective in detecting marijuana use for the past 3 to 30 days (Hubbard, Franco, and Onaivi, 1999).

Meconium is a useful sample for drug screening in newborns (Maynard, Amoruso, and Oh, 1991).

Treatment During Pregnancy

Because no drug has proved safe for the unborn child, marijuana is not safe. Therefore a woman is encouraged to stop using it. She should be closely evaluated for the use of other substances as well.

METHAMPHETAMINES

Two common amphetamines are Ecstasy and methamphetamines. Methamphetamines, stimulants known as *meth, crystal meth, crack, glass, ice,* or *blue ice,* have vasoconstrictive properties like cocaine and are used in a similar manner. Methamphetamine is snorted, swallowed, injected, or smoked. In the IDEAL longitudinal study, 5% of pregnant women used methamphetamine sometime during their pregnancy (Arria, Derauf, LaGasse, and others, 2006).

Maternal Complications

The following complications are known to occur with amphetamine use:
- Abruptio placentae
- Preterm labor
- Insomnia
- Loss of appetite
- Cardiac dysrhythmias
- "Meth mouth" (gum erosion and infection)

Perinatal Effects
- Strongest correlations are IUGR and reduced brain growth (Smith and others, 2003).
- May cause neonatal withdrawal.
- Dose related neurobehavioral patterns of decreased arousal, poor quality movement, and increased fetal stress (Smith and others, 2007).
- Developmental effects occur related to prenatal exposure and postnatal environment (Medical Study News, 2004).
- Risk for SIDS is increased (DEA, 2006).

Treatment During Pregnancy

Ideal treatment is as follows:
- Cessation of use
- Optimal nutrition
- Ongoing prenatal care

TOBACCO

Incidence

According to the National Survey on Drug Use and Health, 22% of all pregnant women smoked sometime during their pregnancy (SAMHSA, 2009). The *Healthy People 2010* goal is that no more than 1% of pregnant women will smoke.

Pathophysiologic Effects

A cigarette contains more than 2500 chemicals and 200 poisonous compounds (Cleveland Clinic, 2004; MOD, 2004). One of them, carbon monoxide, readily crosses the placenta and decreases the oxygen-carrying capacity of the hemoglobin. Nicotine, another substance in cigarettes, stimulates adrenergic release, which causes generalized vasoconstriction, leading to decreased uterine perfusion and narrowing of the umbilical arteries. Compensatory signs are manifested, such as increased maternal and fetal heart rate and decreased fetal movement. Exposure to the many substances in cigarettes also disrupts the fetus' neurophysiological development.

Research indicates that cigarette smokers eat a poorer diet than nonsmokers (Haste and others, 1990). Cigarette smoking also interferes with the assimilation of various essential vitamins and minerals, resulting in an increased loss of calcium caused by mobilization from bones, decreased intestinal synthesis of vitamin B_{12}, and increased usage of vitamin C (Wardlaw and Smith, 2008).

Maternal Complications

The risk for the following complications is increased in the pregnant woman who smokes (Maloni, 2000; USDHHS, 2004):
- Infertility related to ovulatory dysfunction and alteration in sperm
- Spontaneous abortion or ectopic pregnancy
- Placenta previa
- Abruptio placentae
- Premature rupture of membranes
- Preterm delivery

Fetal and Neonatal Complications

Maternal smoking affects the oxygen pathway to the fetus leading to fetal hypoxia by increasing carboxyhemoglobin and availability of nutrients by reducing blood flow to the uterus, placenta, and fetus (ACOG, 2005). According to *Healthy People 2010* (USDHHS, 2002), 20% to 30% of low-birth-weight and very-low-birth-weight neonates may be attributed to smoking. The severity of low birth weight is in direct proportion to the number of cigarettes smoked per day or the amount of exposure to passive ("side stream") smoke (MOD, 2004).

The risk for the following complications is increased in the fetus, neonate, and infant when exposed to cigarette smoke:
- IUGR and stillbirth are increased.
- Teratogenic effects of cleft palate and lip are seen.
- Increased risk for childhood cancer related to prenatal exposure to cigarette smoking exists.

- Increased risk for Infantile colic and childhood obesity (Sondergaard, Henriksen, Obel, and others, 2001; von Kries, Toschke, Koletzko, and others, 2002)
- Lower IQ and behavioral abnormalities such as attention deficit hyperactivity disorder (ADHD), resulting in later learning difficulties, have been observed in follow-up studies (Dobson, 2005; Li and others, 2005). An association with other behavioral problems such as aggressive behavior (Cornelius, Leech, Goldschmidt, and others, 2000), impulsiveness (Brook, Brook, and Whiteman, 2000), and disruptive behaviors (Wakschlag and others, 2006; Wakschlag and others, 2007) are being indicated through research.
- Smoking can reduce breast milk and expose the infant to harmful compounds that pass freely into breast milk (Lawrence and Lawrence, 2005).
- Children exposed in utero or through second-hand smoke have an increased risk for developing asthma (Li and others, 2005).
- Postnatal exposure to passive smoke can increase the infant's risk for developing SIDS (USDHHS, 2004) and childhood respiratory illnesses such as respiratory syncytial virus (RSV), pneumonia, bronchitis, and inner ear infections (Bradley and others, 2005).

Treatment During Pregnancy

The goal of treatment for smokers during pregnancy is to convince all pregnant women and those around them to stop smoking. Quitting before conception is most beneficial. However, even quitting before 16 weeks of gestation significantly decreases the adverse risks (Maloni, 2001). According to the *Cochrane Review*, smoking cessation programs during pregnancy are effective, and it is recommended that all health care providers provide smoking cessation programs to all pregnant women in all maternity care settings (Lumley, Oliver, Chamberlain, and others, 2004).

Based on recommendations of the U.S. Department of Health and Human Services (2008), the American College of Obstetrics and Gynecology (2005) offers guidelines to help health care practitioners implement an effective smoking cessation program (Box 27-2). The outlined steps to this smoking cessation program are available from the Publications Clearinghouse (800-358-9295).

Implementing a smoking cessation program is challenging, and the counseling must be individualized. Health professionals must motivate their patients to choose to stop smoking and empower them to be successful. Some additional general guidelines follow:

- Set the right example as a health care provider by not smoking—or at least not smoking in the presence of patients. Make the health care facility a smoke-free environment.
- If the woman is reluctant to quit, assess her reasons. For example, she may be afraid of gaining too much weight or going through withdrawal symptoms. She may feel that she needs smoking as a psychologic support or may have tried and failed to quit in the past. Keep in mind that a woman may believe that smoking will not hurt her baby because it did not hurt someone else's baby or because she discovers that her health care provider smokes.
- If the woman chooses to keep smoking, encourage her to reduce the amount she smokes but remind her that quitting entirely is the best for her and her fetus.

Box 27-2   Smoking Cessation Plan for Expectant Mothers

Ask every woman about her smoking habits. Improve disclosure by using multiple-choice questions rather than yes or no type questions.

Choose the answer that best describes your pattern of cigarette smoking:
- I smoke regularly now, about the same amount as before I was pregnant.
- I smoke regularly now, but I have cut down since finding out I was pregnant.
- I smoke every once in a while.
- I quit after finding out I was pregnant.
- I do not currently smoke and was not smoking at the time I got pregnant.
- I have NEVER smoked.

Advise

Advise every smoking woman to stop smoking now. Present a clear, strong message on the need to quit. Personalize the advice to her health and to the health of her fetus. Compliment and affirm the patient who has stopped smoking.

Assess

Assess the woman's willingness to set a stop date now. You could say, "Quitting smoking is the most important thing you can do for your health and the health of your baby. If we provide you with help, are you willing to try to quit?"
- If the woman is willing to make a quit attempt, provide assistance by moving to the next step.
- If the woman is not willing at this time to make a quit attempt, provide a motivation intervention.

Assist

Assist the woman by helping her with a plan to quit smoking using the acronym
STAR:
- **S**et a quit date within 2 weeks.
- **T**ell your family, friends, and coworkers and request their support.
- **A**nticipate challenges such as withdrawal symptoms and triggers.
- **R**emove tobacco products from the environment.

Provide self-help materials that are pregnancy-specific (see Table 26-6).
Provide encouragement and help patient obtain social support.

Arrange

Arrange for immediate follow-up, within 1 week after the quit date, and provide ongoing follow-up to congratulate, support, and reinforce success—or to encourage her to try again if a relapse occurs. During the postpartum period, use relapse prevention strategies because of the high relapse rate during this time.

If the patient continues to smoke, assess smoking status at all prenatal visits and keep encouraging cessation.

Counsel her to increase her intake of calcium, vitamins B_{12} and C, and folic acid to compensate for the smoking-induced loss of these vitamins and minerals.
- Also, give family members a clear, brief message on the need to quit or at least never smoke in the presence of the expectant mother or young child because passive smoke is harmful prenatally, as well as postnatally.

- Take an active part in legislative and legal strategies to reduce cigarette smoking, such as increasing cigarette taxes, banning cigarette advertisements, or enforcing provisions to make public places smoke-free.
- Nicotine replacement therapy (NRT) such as nicotine gum, nasal spray, patch, or the inhaler and pharmacotherapy such as bupropion SR (Zyban) have not been shown to be effective in treating tobacco dependency during pregnancy and carries risks. Therefore the U.S. Department of Health and Human Services, in their 2008 updated clinical practice guideline, does not make a recommendation regarding their use during pregnancy (USDHHS, 2008).
- The new CPT coding for smoking cessation counseling for Nurse Practitioners are 99406 for smoking and tobacco use cessation counseling visit, intermediate, greater than 3 minutes and up to 10 minutes; 99407 for smoking and tobacco use cessation counseling visit, intensive, greater then 10 minutes.

NURSING MANAGEMENT

Prevention and Early Detection

Nurse practitioners and nurses should be actively involved in accurate, timely education programs that teach about the effects of practicing substance abuse on one's personal health and the potential teratogenic effects on the growing fetus.

These programs should be available in grade school, in high school, during contraceptive counseling, and on gynecologic visits.

- Develop and consistently use a matter-of-fact, nonjudgmental questionnaire to obtain a substance abuse assessment because a screening tool is the most effective method for detecting substance abuse (Morse, Gehshan, and Hutchins, 1997). Laboratory tests, urine and meconium screens, and hair analysis have been found to have major limitations in determining substance abuse (ACOG, 2008).
- Prepare the patient by introducing the screening with a statement such as "I ask all my patients these questions because it is important to their health and the health of their baby" (Morse, Gehshan, and Hutchins, 1997).
- The four Ps is one screening device often used as a way of beginning the discussion about substance abuse (Box 27-3).

Intervention for a Positive Screen[*]

- Assess for barriers such as peer pressure, socioeconomic status, psychologic stress, or other environmental factors.
- In a positive, nonjudgmental manner, motivate the woman who is considering childbearing or who is pregnant to want to make lifestyle changes to improve health-related behavior. Provide her with information about health risks and the effects of substance abuse on her fetus.
- Assess the family's need for detoxification; if they need it, determine whether outpatient, inpatient, or family treatment would be most effective. The CAGE questionnaire for at-risk drinking patterns has been adapted for general drug use as well by substituting drug use or a specific abused substance in place of drinking (Archie, 1998).

---

[*]Morse, Gehshan, and Hutchins, 1997.

Box 27-3   General Screening for Substance Abuse Using the Four Ps

Have you ever used drugs or alcohol during this **P**regnancy?
Have you had a problem with drugs or alcohol in the **P**ast?
Does your **P**artner have a problem with drugs or alcohol?
Do you consider one of your **P**arents to be an addict or alcoholic?
If the pregnant woman answers "yes" to one or more of these questions, it is
considered a positive screen for substance abuse.

From Ewing H, Medical Director, Born Free Project. Contra Costa County, 111 Allen Street, Martinez, Calif, (510) 646-1165; Morse B, Gehshan S, Hutchins E: *Screening for substance abuse during pregnancy: improving care, improving health*, Arlington, Va, 1997, National Center for Education in Maternal and Child Health.

- State the need to stop and verbalize assistance.
- Discuss possible options such as individual counseling, a 12-step program, or additional treatment programs.
- Provide supportive counseling to help the patient make changes, build self-esteem, and overcome feelings of inadequacy. Avoid using threatening statements that make her feel like a bad mother for abusing a substance.
- Make appropriate referrals to self-help groups: 12-step programs such as Alcoholics, Cocaine, or Narcotics Anonymous.
- Provide smoking cessation materials (Table 27-6).
- Refer to the cocaine hotline: 800-COCAINE
- Refer to local clinics dealing specifically with pregnant substance abusers.
- If use is related to defined problems in the woman's life, such as depression, marital discord, domestic violence, or history of abuse, make appropriate community referrals to resources that address these issues.
- Provide ongoing encouragement and support.
- If efforts to encourage total abstinence fail, provide a message of the potential benefits from reduction of use.
- Become active in legislative issues to block punitive legislation dealing with childbearing women who are substance abusers because if these women are punished legally, they will be driven away and perhaps not seek help when they need it the most.

CONCLUSION

Health care providers have a unique opportunity to help prevent birth defects by implementing the three evidence-based best practice guidelines for treating substance abuse during pregnancy. They are (1) early screening by either a self-administered questionnaire or use of a validated screening tool; (2) provide brief appropriate intervention for mild to moderate substance-related problems; and (3) refer to specialized treatment for severe dependence related substance abuse (Floyd and others, 2008). Obtaining an accurate assessment can be exceptionally complex because of the varying symptoms manifested and the need of the patient to conceal her habit. Planning appropriate nursing care for these patients is challenging.

Table 27-6   Resources for Smoking Cessation Materials

Title/Type	Resource	Website
Tobacco and Pregnancy (general reference for tobacco and pregnancy material)	Addressing Tobacco in Managed Care (313) 874-6815	http://www.ahip.org/content/default. aspx?bc=38%7C65%7C67%7C309
You Can Quit Smoking (consumer guide, 2008)	Agency for Healthcare Research and Quality	www.ahrq.gov/consumer/tobacco/quits.htm
Make Yours a Fresh Start Family (comprehensive program package for health care professionals to help counsel pregnant women to stop smoking)	American Cancer Society 1599 Clifton Road NE Atlanta, GA 30329 (800) 277-2345 or call local chapter	www.cancer.org
Freedom From Smoking for You and Your Baby (a 10-day quit smoking web program for pregnant women)	American Lung Association 1703 Broadway New York, NY 10017 (800) LUNG-USA	http://www.lungusa.org/site/ pp.asp?c=dvLUK9O0E&b=33570
Clinical Practice Guidelines: Treating Tobacco Use and Dependence	Centers for Disease Control and Prevention Office on Smoking and Health	www.cdc.gov/tobacco/how2quit.htm http://www.surgeongeneral.gov/tobacco/ treating_tobacco_use.pdf
You Can Quit Smoking Consumer Guide	Publications Clearinghouse (800) 358-9295	
You Can Quit Smoking Tear Sheet *Nurses Help Your Patients Stop Smoking* Publication No. 92-2962	National Heart, Lung, and Blood Institute 4733 Bethesda Avenue, Suite 350 Bethesda, MD 20814 (301) 951-3260	www.nhlbi.nih.gov/health/prof/lung/other/ nurssmok.txt
Smoke-Free Families	Robert Wood Johnson Foundation	http://smokefreefamilies.tobacco-cessation. org/

BIBLIOGRAPHY

Introduction, Nursing Management, and Conclusion

American College of Obstetricians and Gynecologists (ACOG): *At-risk drinking and illicit drug use: ethical issues in obstetric and gynecologic practice,* ACOG Committee Opinion, No. 422, 2008.

Archie C: Methadone in the management of narcotic addiction in pregnancy, *Curr Opin Obstet Gynecol* 10(6):435–440, 1998.

Floyd R, Jack B, Cefalo R, and others: The clinical content of preconception care: alcohol, tobacco, and illicit drug exposures, *Am J Obstet Gynecol* 199(6):S333–S339, 2008.

Morse B, Gehshan S, Hutchins E: *Screening for substance abuse during pregnancy: improving care, improving health,* Arlington, VA, 1997, National Center for Education in Maternal and Child Health. Retrieved from http://www.ncemch.org.

Substance Abuse and Mental Health Services Administration (SAMHSA): *2006 National survey on drug use and health: detailed tables,* Rockville, Md, 2007.

Substance Abuse and Mental Health Services Administration (SAMHSA): *The NSDUH report: substance use among women during pregnancy and following childbirth,* Rockville, Md, 2009.

U.S. Department of Health and Human Services (USDHHS): *Tenth special report to the U.S. Congress on alcohol and health,* Rockville, Md, 2000, USDHHS.

U.S. Department of Health and Human Services (USDHHS): *Healthy People 2010: understanding and improving health:* Maternal, Infant, and Child Health, Rockville, Md, 2001, Office of Disease Prevention and Health Promotion (ODPHP). Retrieved from http://www.health.gov/healthypeople/Document/tableofcontents.htm.

Alcohol

American College of Obstetricians and Gynecologists (ACOG): *At-risk drinking and illicit drug use: ethical issues in obstetric and gynecologic practice,* ACOG Committee Opin, No. 442, 2008.

American College of Obstetricians and Gynecologists (ACOG) in collaboration with Centers for Disease Control and Prevention (CDC): *Drinking and reproductive health: a fetal alcohol spectrum disorders prevention tool kit.* Washington, DC, 2006, Author. Retrieved from http://www.cdc.gov/ncbddd/fas/acog_toolkit.htm.

Avner M, Nulman I: Attempts at more specific and practical diagnostic criteria for fetal alcohol spectrum disorders, *JFAS Int* 3:e12, 2005.

Barbour B: Alcohol and pregnancy, *J Nurse Midwifery* 35(2):78–85, 1990.

Bertrand J, Floyd R, Weber M, and others: *Fetal alcohol syndrome: guidelines for referral and diagnosis.* Atlanta, GA, 2004, Department of Health and Human Services. Retrieved from http://www.cdc.gov/ncbddd/fasd/documents/FAS_guidelines_accessible.pdf.

Bradley K, and others: Alcohol screening questionnaires in women: a critical review, *JAMA* 280(2):166–171, 1998.

Chang G: Alcohol-screening instruments for pregnant women, *Alcohol Res Health* 25:204–209, 2001.

Ewing J: Detecting alcoholism: the CAGE questionnaire, *JAMA* 252(14):1905–1907, 1984.

Fleming M, and others: Brief physician advice for problem alcohol drinkers: a randomized controlled trial in community-based primary care practices, *JAMA* 277(13):1039–1045, 1997.

Floyd R, Jack B, Cefalo R, and others: The clinical content of preconception care: alcohol, tobacco, and illicit drug exposures, *Am J Obstet Gynecol* 199(6):S333–S339, 2008.

Gardner J: Living with a child with fetal alcohol syndrome, *MCN Am J Matern Child Nurs* 25(5):252–257, 2000.

Gauthier T, and others: Maternal alcohol abuse and neonatal infection, *Alcohol Clin Exp Res* 29(6):1035–1043, 2005.

Goodlett C, Johnson T: Temporal windows of vulnerability to alcohol during the third trimester equivalent: why 'knowing when' matters. In Hannigan J, and others, editors: *Alcohol and alcoholism,* Hillsdale, NJ, 1999, Lawrence Erlbaum Associates.

Hankin J, Sokol R: Identification and care of problems associated with alcohol ingestion in pregnancy, *Semin Perinatol* 19(4):286–292, 1995.

Hoyme H, and others: A practical clinical approach to diagnosis of fetal alcohol spectrum disorders: clarification of the 1996 Institute of Medicine criteria, *Pediatrics* 115(1):39–47, 2005.

Lawrence R, Lawrence M: *Breastfeeding: a guide for the medical profession*, ed 6, Philadelphia, 2005, Mosby.

National Center on Birth Defects and Developmental Disabilities (NCBDDD), Centers for Disease Control and Prevention (CDC), US Department of Health and Human Services (USDHHS): *Fetal alcohol syndrome: guidelines for referral and diagnosis*, Atlanta, GA, 2004, NCBDDD, CDC.

O'Connor M, Whaley S: Brief intervention for alcohol use with pregnant women in the WIC setting, *Am J Public Health* 97(2):252–258, 2007.

Sokol R, Martier S, Ager J: The T-ACE questions: practical prenatal detection of risk drinking, *Am J Obstet Gynecol* 160(4):863–868, 1989.

Stratton K, Howe C, Battaglia F: *Fetal alcohol syndrome: diagnosis, epidemiology, prevention, treatment*, Washington, DC, 1996, National Academy Press.

Substance Abuse and Mental Health Services Administration (SAMHSA): *The NSDUH report: substance use among women during pregnancy and following childbirth,* Rockville, MD, 2009.

Taylor P, Zaichkin J, Bailey D: *Substance abuse during pregnancy: guidelines for screening*, Olympia, WA, 2002, Maternal and Child Health. Retrieved from http://www.doh.wa.gov.

U.S. Department of Health and Human Services (USDHHS): *Substance Abuse and Mental Health Services Administration results from the 2006 national survey.* Publication No. SMA 07–4923, Rockville, Md, 2007, USDHHS. Retrieved from: http://sbirt.samhsa.gov.

U.S. Department of Health and Human Services (USDHHS): *Drinking and reproductive health: a fetal alcohol spectrum disorders prevention tool kit*, Rockville, MD, 2006, USDHHS.

U.S. Department of Health and Human Services (USDHHS): *Tenth special report to the U.S. Congress on alcohol and health*, Rockville, MD, 2000, USDHHS.

U.S. Surgeon General: *Advisory on alcohol use in pregnancy,* News Release, 2005, USDHHS.

Cocaine

American Academy of Pediatrics: Neonatal drug withdrawal, Committee on Drugs, *Pediatrics* 101(6):1079–1088, 1998.

American College of Obstetricians and Gynecologists: *At-risk drinking and illicit drug use: Ethical issues in obstetric and gynecologic practice,* ACOG Committee Opin No. 294, 2004.

Bada H, and others: Gestational cocaine exposure and intrauterine growth: maternal lifestyle study, *Obstet Gynecol* 100(5 Pt 1):916–924, 2002.

Bandstra E, and others: Intrauterine growth of full-term infants: impact of prenatal cocaine exposure, *Pediatrics* 108(6):1309–1319, 2001.

Bateman D, Chiriboga C: Dose-response effect of cocaine on newborn head circumference, *Pediatrics* 106(3):E33, 2000.

Bennett D, Bendersky M, Lewis M: Preadolescent health risk behavior as a function of prenatal cocaine exposure and gender, *J Dev Behav Pediatr* 28(6):467–472, 2007.

Bennett D, Bendersky M, Lewis M: Children's cognitive ability from 4 to 9 years old as a function of prenatal cocaine exposure, environmental risk, and maternal verbal intelligence, *Dev Psych* 44(4): 919–928, 2008.

Boumba V, Ziavrou K, Vougiouklakis T: Hair as a biological indicator of drug use: drug abuse or chronic exposure to environmental toxicants, *Int J Toxicol* 25(3):143–163, 2006.

Buehler B, Conover B, Andres R: Teratogenic potential of cocaine, *Semin Perinatol* 20(2):93–98, 1996.

Dolkart L, Plessinger M, Woods J: Effect of alpha receptor blockade upon maternal and fetal cardiovascular responses to cocaine, *Obstet Gynecol* 75(5):745–751, 1990.

Fajemirokun-Odudeyi O, Lindow S: Obstetric implications of cocaine use in pregnancy: a literature review, *Eur J Obstet Gynecol Reprod Biol* 112(1):2–8, 2004.

FIRST Consult: *Clinical information for quality care*, St Louis, 2006, Mosby. Retrieved from http://www. firstconsult.com.

Hepburn M: Substance abuse in pregnancy, *Clin Obstet Gynaecol* 14(6):419, 2004.

Kain Z, and others: Cocaine-abusing parturients undergoing cesarean section. A cohort study, *Anesthesiology* 85(5):1028–1035, 1996.

Kuczkowski K: Anesthetic implications of drug abuse in pregnancy, *J Clin Anesth* 15(5):382–394, 2003.

Lawrence R, Lawrence M: *Breastfeeding: a guide for the medical profession*, ed 6, Philadelphia, 2005, Mosby.

López P, Bermejo A, Tabernero M, and others: Determination of cocaine and heroin with their respective metabolites in meconium by gas chromatography-mass spectrometry, *J Applied Toxicol* 27(5):464–471, 2007.

Lynch M, McKeon V: Cocaine use during pregnancy: research findings and clinical implications, *J Obstet Gynecol Neonatal Nurs* 19(4):285–292, 1990.

March of Dimes: *Illicit drug use during pregnancy, professionals and researchers,* White Plains, NY, 2004, MOD.

Plessinger M, Woods J Jr: Cocaine in pregnancy: recent data on maternal and fetal risks, *Obstet Gynecol Clin North Am* 25(1):99–118, 1998.

Potter S, and others: Adverse effects of fetal cocaine exposure on neonatal auditory information processing, *Pediatrics* 105(3):E40, 2000.

Schiller C, Allen J: Follow-up of infants prenatally exposed to cocaine, *Pediatr Nurs* 31(5):427–436, 2005.

Singer L, and others: Cognitive and motor outcomes of cocaine-exposed infants, *JAMA* 287(15): 1952–1960, 2002.

Ursitti F, Klein J, Koren G: Confirmation of cocaine use during pregnancy: a critical review, *Ther Drug Monit* 23(4):347–353, 2001.

Vidaeff A, Mastrobattista J: In utero cocaine exposure: a thorny mix of science and mythology, *Am J Perinatol* 20(4):165–172, 2003.

Wagner C, and others: Substance abuse in pregnancy, *Obstet Gynecol* 25(1):169–194, 1998.

Yazigi R, Odem R, and Polakoski K: Demonstration of specific binding of cocaine to human spermatozoa, *JAMA* 266(14):1956–1959, 1991.

Heroin

Archie C: Methadone in the management of narcotic addiction in pregnancy, *Curr Opin Obstet Gynecol* 10(6):435–440, 1998.

Kendig S: Substance abuse in pregnancy, *Childbirth Instructor* 6(3):18, 1996.

Lee R: Drug abuse. In Burrow G, Ferris T, editors: *Medical complications during pregnancy,* ed 4, Philadelphia, 1995, Saunders.

Little B, and others: Patterns of multiple substance abuse during pregnancy: implications for mother and fetus, *South Med J* 83:507, 1990.

National Institute on Drug Abuse: *How does heroin abuse affect pregnant women?* Bethesda, Md, 2005, NIH. Retrieved from http://international.drugabuse.gov.

National Institute on Drug Abuse (NIDA): *Methadone research web guide.* Bethesda, Md, 2009, NIH. Retrieved from http://international.drugabuse.gov.

Robins L, Mills J: Effects of in utero exposure to street drugs, *Am J Public Health* 83(Suppl):1–32, 1993.

Marijuana

Drug Prevention Network of the Americas (DPNA): *Marijuana,* Washington, DC, 2004, National Institute on Drug Abuse and National Institute of Health.

Faden V, Graubard B: Maternal substance use during pregnancy and developmental outcome at age three, *J Subst Abuse* 12(4):329–340, 2000.

Fergusson D, Horwood L, Northstone K: Maternal use of cannabis and pregnancy outcome, *BJOG* 109(1):21–27, 2002.

Fried P, Smith A: A literature review of the consequences of prenatal marihuana exposure: an emerging theme of a deficiency in aspects of executive function, *Neurotoxicol Teratol* 23(1):1–11, 2001.

Hubbard J, Franco S, Onaivi E: Marijuana: Medical implications, *Am Fam Physician* 60(9):2583–2588, 1999.

Lee M: Marihuana and tobacco use in pregnancy, *Obstet Gynecol Clin North Am* 25(1):65–83, 1998.

Maynard E, Amoruso L, Oh W: Meconium for drug testing, *Am J Dis Child* 145(6):650–652, 1991.

Substance Abuse and Mental Health Services Administration (SAMHSA): *The NSDUH report: substance use among women during pregnancy and following childbirth,* Rockville, Md, 2009.

U.S. Department of Health and Human Services (USDHHS): *Marijuana facts parents need to know,* NIH Publication No. 07-4036, Washington, DC, 2007, USDHHS.

Wu T, and others: Pulmonary hazards of smoking marijuana as compared with tobacco, *N Engl J Med* 318(6):347–351, 1988.

Methamphetamines

Arria A, Derauf C, LaGasse L, and others: Methamphetamine and other substance use during pregnancy: preliminary estimates from the infant development, environment, and lifestyle (IDEAL) study, *Matern Child Health J* 10(3):293–302, 2006.

Drug Enforcement Administration (DEA): *Methamphetamine fact sheet*, Alexandria, VA, 2006, DEA. Retrieved from http://www.usdoj.gov/dea/concern/meth_factsheet.html.

Medical Study News: *Exposure to methamphetamine in the womb causes adverse developmental effects*, 2004. Available at http://www.news-medical.net/.

Smith L, and others: Effects of prenatal methamphetamine exposure on fetal growth and drug withdrawal symptoms in infants born at term, *J Dev Behav Pediatr* 24(1):17–23, 2003.

Smith M, and others: Methamphetamine use and neonatal neurobehavioral outcome, *Neurotoxicol Teratol* 30(1):20–28, 2007.

Tobacco

American College of Obstetricians and Gynecologists (ACOG): *Smoking cessation during pregnancy*, Committee Opinion, No. 316, Washington, DC: 2005, Author.

Bradley J, and others: Severity of respiratory syncytial virus bronchiolitis is affected by cigarette smoke exposure and atopy, *Pediatrics* 115(1):e7–e14, 2005.

Brook J, Brook D, Whiteman M: The influence of maternal smoking during pregnancy on the toddler's negativity, *Arch Pediatr Adolesc Med* 154(4):381–384, 2000.

Cleveland Clinic: *Smoking cessation*, Cleveland, OH, 2004, Author. Retrieved from http://www.clevelandclinic.org/emergencymedicine/smoking.htm.

Cornelius M, Leech S, Goldschmidt L, Day N: Prenatal tobacco exposure: is it a risk factor for early tobacco experimentation? *Nicotine Tob Res* 2:45–52, 2000.

Dobson R: Smoking in late pregnancy is linked to lower IQ in offspring, *BMJ* 330:499, 2005.

Haste F, and others: Nutrient intakes during pregnancy: observations on the influence of smoking and social class, *Am J Clin Nutr* 51(1):29–36, 1990.

Lawrence R, Lawrence M: *Breastfeeding: a guide for the medical profession*, ed 6, Philadelphia, 2005, Mosby.

Li Y, and others: Maternal and grandmaternal smoking patterns are associated with early childhood asthma, *Chest* 127(4):1232–1241, 2005.

Lumley J, Oliver SS, Chamberlain C, Oakley L: Interventions for promoting smoking cessation during pregnancy, *Cochrane Database Syst Rev* (Issue 4), Art. No.: CD001055, 2004.

Maloni J: *The prevention of preterm birth: research-based practice, nursing interventions, practice scenarios*, Washington, DC, 2000, AWHONN.

Maloni J: Preventing low birth weight: how smoking cessation counseling can help, *AWHONN Lifelines* 5(1):32–35, 2001.

March of Dimes (MOD): *Smoking during pregnancy, professionals and researchers*, White Plains, NY, 2004, MOD.

National Institute on Alcohol Abuse and Alcoholism (NIAAA): *A pocket guide for alcohol screening and brief intervention*, Rockville, MD, 2005, National Institute of Health. Retrieved from http://pubs.niaaa.nih.gov/publications/Practitioner/PocketGuide/pocket_guide.htm.

Sondergaard C, Henriksen T, Obel C, Wisborg K: Smoking during pregnancy and infantile colic, *Pediatrics* 108:342–346, 2001.

Substance Abuse and Mental Health Services Administration (SAMHSA): *The NSDUH report: substance use among women during pregnancy and following childbirth*, Rockville, Md, 2009.

U.S. Department of Health and Human Services (USDHHS): *Healthy People 2010: understanding and improving health: Maternal, infant, and child health*, Rockville, MD, 2002, Office of Disease Prevention and Health Promotion (ODPHP). Retrieved from http://www.health.gov/healthypeople/Document/tableofcontents.htm.

U.S. Department of Health and Human Services (USDHHS): *The health consequences of smoking: a report of the Surgeon General*, Atlanta, GA, 2004, CDC, Office on Smoking and Health.

U.S. Department of Health and Human Services (USDHHS): *Substance use during pregnancy: 2002 and 2003, update*, Rockville, Md, 2005, USDHHS.

U.S. Department of Health and Human Services (USDHHS): *Treating tobacco use and dependence 2008 update,* Clinical Practice Guideline, Rockville, MD, 2008, USDHHS. Retrieved from http://www.ahrq. gov/consumer/tobacco/quits.htm.

Von Kries R, Toschke A, Koletzko B, Slikker W Jr: Maternal smoking during pregnancy and childhood obesity, *Am J Epidemiol* 156:954–961, 2002.

Wakschlag L, and others: Elucidating early mechanisms of development psychopathology: the case of prenatal smoking and disruption behavior, *Child Dev* 77(4):893–906, 2006.

Wakschlag L, and others: A developmental framework for distinguishing disruptive behavior from normative misbehavior in preschool children. *J Child Psychol Psychiatry* 48(10; Special Issue on Preschool Psychopathology):976–987, 2007.

Wardlaw G, Smith A: *Contemporary nutrition,* ed 7, Boston, 2008, McGraw Hill.

28

Labor Stimulation

There are two classifications of labor stimulation: induction and augmentation. *Induction of labor* is any attempt to initiate uterine contractions before their spontaneous onset to facilitate a vaginal delivery. Before an induction, the ability of the cervix to be induced is determined. Artificial ripening of an unripe cervix is usually beneficial.

Augmentation of labor is any attempt to stimulate uterine contractions during the course of labor to facilitate a vaginal delivery. It is frequently used for certain types of uterine dysfunction. A labor should not be augmented until noninvasive interventions have been attempted, such as the following:

- Assurance the bladder is empty
- Encouraging ambulation if possible or changing of position
- Allaying anxiety because epinephrine decreases uterine efficiency
- Ensuring the patient is properly nourished and hydrated

Labor stimulant methods considered in this chapter include pharmacologic and mechanical cervical ripening methods and natural methods of labor induction and augmentation. Pharmacologic methods include using oxytocin; physiologic means include using amniotomy and stripping of fetal membranes.

INCIDENCE

Use of a labor stimulant for either inducing or augmenting labor varies among countries, cities, and hospitals. Rates between 10% and 25% are common in industrialized countries (RCOG, 2008). Current data from the United States National Center for Health Statistics for 2006 reveal that approximately 22% of all labors are stimulated, or 225 per thousand (Martin, Hamilton, Sutton, and others, 2009). Additionally, the data reveal an induction rate that has doubled since 1990 as it was 9.5 percent of births (Martin, Hamilton, Sutton, and others, 2007). Since 1999, induction rates have shown that one in five births has been induced (Zhang, Yancey, and Henderson, 2002; Martin and others, 2009).

INDICATIONS

Common indications for induction of labor follow (Simpson, 2008; ACOG, 2009):
- Postterm
- Maternal conditions such as hypertension, diabetes, cardiac disease, pulmonary disease, or antiphospholipid syndrome
- Gestational hypertension
- Fetal stress or compromise such as severe fetal growth restriction, oligohydramnios, or isoimmunization
- Premature rupture of membranes (PROM)
- Abruptio placentae
- Chorioamnionitis
- Fetal demise

Labor induction may also be done for nonmedical or elective reasons, such as a history of rapid labor, distance from hospital, or psychosocial reasons (Simpson, 2008; ACOG, 2009). According to Martin and others (2009), 25% of all labor inductions are elective or nonmedical, whereas others estimate one half to one third of all labor inductions are for nonmedical indications (Moore and Rayburn, 2006). According to AHRQ (2009), a key finding is that women who undergo an elective induction of labor have the same or lower rates of cesarean delivery compared with women who were expectantly managed.

Prior to elective induction, fetal maturity must be confirmed to avoid the risk of iatrogenic prematurity (National Institute of Child Health and Human Development [NICHD], 2005; ACOG, 2009). If one of the American College of Obstetricians and Gynecologists (ACOG, 2009) confirmation of term gestation (as outlined in Box 28-1) is met, amniocentesis to determine fetal lung maturity is not necessary.

CRITERIA

Criteria for an induction of labor are listed:
- Engaged presenting part
- No previous classic uterine incision
- No fetopelvic disproportion
- No Category II or III fetal heart rate (FHR) patterns
- No major bleeding from an abruptio placentae

Box 28-1   ACOG Confirmation of Term Gestation

- Ultrasound measurement at less than 20 weeks of gestation supports gestational age of 39 weeks or greater.
- Fetal heart tones have been documented as present for 30 weeks by Doppler ultrasonography.
- It has been 36 weeks since a positive serum or urine human chorionic gonadotropin pregnancy test result.

Modified from American College of Obstetricians and Gynecologists: Induction of labor, *ACOG Practice Bulletin*, No. 107, Washington, DC, 2009, ACOG.

- No placenta previa or vasa previa
- No active genital herpes infection
- Staff competency on the effects of uterine stimulants on mother and fetus (Simpson, 2008)
- Uterine contractions and fetal heart rate should be monitored during induction or augmentation similar to any high-risk patient in active labor (ACOG, 2009).
- Registered Nurse-to-patient ratio during induction is one nurse to two patients (AAP and ACOG, 2007).
- Cervical ripening, induction of labor, and augmentation of labor are currently being questioned for a vaginal birth after previous cesarean.

Criteria for augmentation of labor are the same as for induction. There must also be definite signs that the progress of labor is slowing down.

Labor is seldom induced or augmented (1) on a grand multipara more than five parity, (2) on a multiple pregnancy, or (3) in the presence of polyhydramnios because of the increased risk for uterine rupture related to uterine overdistention.

PREDICTORS OF SUCCESS

The success of the induction or augmentation usually depends on a ripe cervix. A cervix is considered ripe when it is soft, anterior, effaced more than 50%, and dilated 2 cm or more. Bishop (1964) developed a 13-point scoring system to predict the responsiveness of a patient to an induction. When the pelvic score totals 8 or more, induction is similar to that after spontaneous labor (Table 28-1) (ACOG, 2009). However, when the score is unfavorable as defined as 6 or less, cervical ripening is usually considered prior to induction as reported in randomized trials (ACOG, 2009).

According to Crane (2006), the patient's parity, age, weight, height, and body mass index (BMI) are associated with the success of induction. The younger, taller woman with a low BMI has a higher rate of induction success. Several tools were researched as predictors of induction success including transvaginal ultrasound (TVUS) and biochemical markers (including fetal fibronectin [fFn]) (Crane, 2006). As reported by Crane (2006), TVUS and fFn demonstrated positive predictive measure of induction; however, Bishop scoring remains superior.

Table 28-1   Bishop Prelabor Scoring System

	Score			
	0	**1**	**2**	**3**
Dilation (cm)	0	1-2	3-4	5-6
Effacement (%)	0-30	40-50	60-70	80
Station	-3	-2	-1/0	+1/+2
Consistency of cervix	Firm	Medium	Soft	
Cervical position	Posterior	Medium	Anterior	

Reference: Bishop E: Pelvic scoring for elective induction, *Obstet Gynecol* 24:266–268, 1964.

RISKS

The need for other interventions increases with inductions (Simpson and Atterbury, 2003) such as:

- Intravenous line
- Activity limitation
- More frequent monitoring
- Increased need for epidural analgesia related to more painful contractions
- Increased need for other interventions such as instrumental or cesarean delivery

CONTRAINDICATIONS

The contraindications for labor induction (Simpson, 2008; ACOG, 2009) are similar to those for spontaneous labor and include, but are not limited to:

- Transverse fetal lie
- Umbilical cord prolapse
- Previous transfundal uterine incision
- Vasa previa or complete placenta previa
- Active genital herpes infection
- Previous classical cesarean delivery

PHYSIOLOGY OF UTEROTROPINS AND UTEROTONINS

Many substances interplay to prepare for and promote labor. Prostaglandins are formed enzymatically from phospholipids and arachidonic acid in most tissues of the body. They act as a local hormone by exerting their action primarily at the site of production. The biosynthesis of reproductive tissue prostaglandins varies among tissue. The myometrium is the primary source of prostacyclin (PGI_2) (PGE_2), and the decidua is the primary source of prostaglandin F_2a (PGF_2a).

During pregnancy, PGI_2 helps the uterus remain quiet by inhibiting the formation of gap junctions and the release of phospholipase A, and blocks calcium movement into cells. Progesterone further regulates the myometrial activity throughout pregnancy by inhibiting the formation of oxytocin receptors and gap junctions (Havelock, Keller, Muleba, and others, 2005). Estrogen promotes this process (Hertelendy and Zakar, 2004).

During the prelabor phase or preparation phase just before true labor, production of PGE_2 by the amnion increases; this increase is normally induced by the fetus (Olson, Mijovic, and Sadowsky, 1995). Cervical ripening involves the regulation of estrogen and progesterone through a complex biochemical relationship with the cervical epithelium and stroma (Andersson, Minjarez, Yost, and others, 2008). During this phase, the body is prepared for labor by the following occurrences:

- Increasing myometrial receptors for estrogen but not progesterone (Olson, Mijovic, and Sadowsky, 1995)
- Softening and ripening of the cervix caused by enzymatic rearrangement of the collagen fibers into smaller, more flexible fibers and increasing synthesis of

hyaluronic acid, thereby facilitating water absorption by the cervix (Leppert, 1995; Winkler and Rath, 1999; Iwahashi, Muragaki, Ooshima, and others, 2003), leading to a softer, more stretchable cervix

- A study conducted by Schlembach, MacKay, Shi, and others (2009) found cervical collagen plays a significant role in influencing cervical ripening as evident by their findings utilizing a light-induced fluorescence (LIF).
- Increasing elastin in the cervix, which gives the cervix its ability to recoil and regain its shape after birth
- Increasing the frequency of Braxton-Hicks contractions
- Developing gap junctions in the myometrium that are cell-to-cell contact areas to coordinated myometrium contractions
- Cervical dilatation incorporates leukocytes and the release of proteases and collagenases (Word, Xiang-Hong, Hnat, and others, 2007).
- Increasing the number of oxytocin receptors in the myometrium and decidua; myometrium receptors gradually increase during the latter part of pregnancy peaking at the end of the first stage of labor, whereas decidua receptors increase during labor and peak at birth (Simpson, 2008).

As true labor is initiated, PGF_2a production increases significantly by the decidua, which continues to promote the responses that PGE_2 initiated, as well as increasing the contractile responsiveness of the myometrium by moving calcium into the cells. Production of prostacyclin is suppressed during labor because of high levels of cortisol (MacKenzie and others, 1988). The timing and transformation of the cervical ripening is thought to be a slow process. Studies propose a biochemical model or explanation that outlines the changes in the cervix during active labor (Leppert, 1995; Winkler and Rath, 1999).

Oxytocin levels in the plasma may not increase significantly until labor begins with a significant increase during the second stage of labor, when oxytocin appears to maximize uterine contractions (Arias, 2000). Oxytocin is ineffective in promoting myometrial contractions until oxytocin receptors are present in the myometrium and then the decidua. High levels of estrogen, PGF_2a, and PGE_2 (Olson, Mijovic, and Sadowsky, 1995) stimulate these receptors, thus playing an important role in the effectiveness of myometrial contractions (Cunningham, Leveno, Bloom, and others, 2005).

According to Clayworth (2000), there are three important variables that influence the body's response to oxytocin:

1. Oxygen status of the uterus
2. Availability of glucose for uterine energy
3. Number of oxytocin receptors present in the uterus

PHARMACOLOGIC METHODS FOR CERVICAL RIPENING: PROSTAGLANDINS E_2-DINOPROSTONE

Dinoprostone is the most commonly used medication for ripening the cervix, the first step in labor induction. It causes dissolution of the cervical collagen bundles and increases cervical submucosal water content, stimulates smooth muscle contraction of the cervix and uterus, and increases gap junction formation (Rayburn and others, 1994; Witter, 2000; Sanchez-Ramos and Delke, 2006). Cervidil and Prepidil are U.S. Food and Drug Administration (FDA)-approved for labor stimulation.

Dosages
Table 28-2 presents a comparison of the most commonly used forms of PGE_2.

Advantages
The advantages of prostaglandin-initiated cervical ripening as demonstrated by research reviewed in the *Cochrane Review* (Kelly, Malik, Smith, and others, 2009) follow:
- Enhanced cervical ripening
- Decreased need for oxytocin for induction
- Decreased oxytocin induction time, when used
- Reduced amount of oxytocin needed for a successful induction

The effectiveness of cervical ripening before labor induction with prostaglandins has been compared with low-dose oxytocin. According to Pollnow and Broekhuizen (1996), prostaglandin was superior to low-dose oxytocin. This was demonstrated by the incidence of higher Bishop scores, a higher rate of successful inductions, and shorter labors. Morbidity and cesarean delivery rates were similar in both groups.

Risks

Uterine Tachysystole
The National Institute of Child Health and Human Development (NICHD) workshop produced the following recommendation that the terms hyperstimulation and hypercontractility not be used to define contraction activity and the practice be abandoned (Macones, Hankins, Spong, and others, 2008). Uterine tachysystole, previously referred to as hyperstimulation, is associated with approximately 1% to 5% of patients, with the greatest risk following administration of prostaglandins through the intravaginal route or vaginal insert (Hofmeyr and Gülmezoglu, 2004; ACOG, 2009). Uterine contractions are qualified as the number of contractions identified in a 10-minute period, averaged over 30 minutes (Macones and others, 2008). Thus, *uterine tachysystole* is defined as five or more contractions in 10 minutes, or a single contraction lasting more than 2 minutes either with or without signs of fetal stress such as late decelerations or fetal bradycardia. When uterine tachysystole occurs, it is effectively reversed with the use of beta$_2$-adrenergic tocolytic therapy, such as intravenous or subcutaneous terbutaline, 250 mcg or 0.25 mg (ACOG, 2009). When a vaginal insert is being used, removal helps reverse the effect of uterine tachysystole.

Category II or III Fetal Heart Rate Pattern Changes
A category II or III FHR pattern, such as severe variable decelerations or bradycardia, is very uncommon in patients during prostaglandin labor stimulation. When associated FHR changes occur because of uterine tachysystole, they are responsive to

Table 28-2   Comparison of Commonly Used Pharmacologic Cervical Ripening Products

Drug	Route	Dosage	Considerations
Dinoprostone (Cervidil) Vaginal insert: a thin, flat, polymer chip in a polyester mesh net with attached cord Prostaglandin E₂ agent	Insert into vaginal posterior fornix	10 mg, which is released slowly (approximately 0.3 mg/hr for maximum of 12 hr)	Can be inserted by a perinatal nurse Stored at -20° C but does not require warming Oxytocin can be administered 30-60 min after removal of insert Can be removed when labor starts or when tachysystole occurs FDA-approved Not messy
Dinoprostone (Prepidil) Prostaglandin E₂ gel Prefilled syringe applicator with 10-mm or 20-mm endocervical catheter	Intracervical: one syringe application inserted into cervical canal	2.5 ml gel with 0.5 mg dinoprostone May repeat every 6 hr Maximum of three doses per 24 hr (1.5 mg)	Inserted by physician or midwife FDA-approved Requires refrigeration and must be warmed to room temperature before catheter administration Prompts minimal uterine activity Product reliable Quite expensive Efficiency decreased with rupture of membranes Must wait 6-12 hr to start oxytocin induction per package insert Has been used for outpatient management
Misoprostol (Cytotec) Synthetic PGE₁ analog tablet	Posterior vaginal fornix	25 mcg (¼ of a 100-mcg tablet) (ACOG, 2003) May repeat in 3-6 hr for a maximum of 6 doses Comes in 100- or 200- mcg tablet	FDA-approved in 2002 Inexpensive Stable at room temperature Effective in presence of rupture of membranes Not to be used in patients with a history of previous cesarean or prior uterine surgery because of the increased risk for uterine rupture Oxytocin can be administered 4 or more hr after the last dose

FDA, Food and Drug Administration; *PGE₁,* prostaglandin E₁.

the standard treatment protocol, such as position change, increasing intravenous (IV) fluids, and administering oxygen at 10 L/min.

Other Side Effects

Gastrointestinal side effects such as nausea, vomiting, and diarrhea are negligible for patients being treated with low-dose prostaglandins (Sanchez-Ramos and Delke, 2006). Rarely, an infection, a fever, or headache occurs.

Nursing Interventions

Preadministration

- Obtain an informed consent following an informative discussion as to the procedure, reasons for the procedure, what it means to the patient, and potential side effects and risks.
- Determine the cervical Bishop score (see Table 28-1), which is a standard of predicting inducibility. A score of 4 or less indicates an unfavorable cervix that could benefit from prostaglandin softening.
- Assess for any contraindications of prostaglandin use such as an active pelvic infection, vaginal bleeding, active cardiopulmonary disease, known hepatic or renal disease, or an allergy to the drug (Weiner and Buhimschi, 2009).
- Evaluate for maternal conditions warranting caution such as asthma, glaucoma, intraocular pressure, hepatic or renal dysfunction (Weiner and Buhimschi, 2009).
- Assess amniotic membrane status because the intravaginal route is usually used after rupture of membranes (ROM).
- Obtain a baseline FHR tracing per institution policy or protocol.
- Analyze the tracing for category II or III FHR patterns, such as bradycardia or late decelerations.
- Obtain baseline readings of blood pressure, temperature, pulse, and respiration rate.
- Assess for uterine activity.

Administration

- Assess blood pressure, temperature, pulse, and respiratory rate before each PGE_2 gel application.
- Prepare medication and equipment for insertion.
- Instill gel per protocol with patient in a dorsal lithotomy position.
- Provide ongoing emotional support, and encourage relaxation.
- Turn the patient on her side and rest in bed for 30 to 60 minutes after each PGE_2 gel application.
- Monitor for tachysystole uterine activity and category II or III FHR changes per protocol.
- Prepare to treat uterine tachysystole and any category II or III FHR changes with the standard treatment protocol, such as changing the patient's position, increasing IV fluids, and administering oxygen at 10 L/min. Have a beta$_2$-adrenergic tocolytic drug readily available to give on physician's order. The dosage is usually 250 mcg or 0.25 mg of terbutaline administered subcutaneously or IV (ACOG, 2009).

- Assess for the development of any side effects, such as diarrhea, nausea, or vomiting, which occur most often during the first 30 minutes after administration.
- Permit ambulation after the assessment phase until the next dose, in most cases.
- Reassess the Bishop score after completion of the prostaglandin protocol.

PHARMACOLOGIC METHODS FOR CERVICAL RIPENING: PROSTAGLANDIN E_1-MISOPROSTOL

Misoprostol (Cytotec) is a synthetic PGE_1 analog that is FDA-approved for the prevention and treatment of gastric and duodenal ulcers. Although it is not FDA-approved for obstetric use, it is widely used for cervical ripening and induction of labor. Various research studies (Buser and others, 1997; Sanchez-Ramos and others, 1997; Sanchez-Ramos and others, 1998; Blanchette, Nayak, and Erasmus, 1999; Nunes, Rodrigues, and Meirinho, 1999) have demonstrated benefits to misoprostol, such as increased cervical ripening, decreased oxytocin use, shortened labor, and decreased cost. These studies did show an increased risk for uterine tachysystole, which can cause uterine rupture and meconium-stained amniotic fluid. According to ACOG (2000), it is a safe, effective agent for cervical ripening and labor induction except in vaginal births after previous cesarean. There is an increased risk for uterine rupture in women with a prior cesarean or major uterine surgery.

However, according to the *Cochrane Review* (Hofmeyr and Gülmezoglu, 2004), the increase in uterine tachysystole is of concern and the studies did not exclude the possibility of serious adverse effects such as uterine rupture with or without previous cesarean. These researchers concluded that further research is needed to establish safety, and therefore some health care providers do not prescribe its use because of the concern about its effect.

If misoprostol is prescribed, see Table 28-2 for administration protocols.

MECHANICAL METHODS FOR CERVICAL RIPENING: LAMINARIA, SYNTHETIC DILATORS, OR BALLOON CATHETERS

Laminaria tents, such as *Laminaria digitata* or *Laminaria japonica*, are natural cervical dilators made from seaweed. Synthetic alternatives are currently being used more frequently. Two common synthetic dilators are Dilapan, a hygroscopic cervical dilator, and Lamicel, an alcohol polymer sponge impregnated with 450 mg of magnesium sulfate and compressed into a tent. A 30-ml Foley catheter placed in the cervical canal prior to inflation may also be used.

Physiology
The dilators are inserted into the full length of the cervical canal, where they absorb cervical fluids and swell, dilating the cervix slowly (Sanchez-Ramos and Delka, 2006).

Advantages
Dilators are used primarily for labor induction in the presence of minimal cervical effacement.

Risks

Chorioamnionitis

Infection is a risk of using dilators. It is caused primarily by beta-hemolytic strep-tococci. Because of the faster expansion time (4 hours as compared with 12 to 16 hours), the synthetic dilators pose less of a risk for an infection than the *Laminaria* dilators, but the presence of any foreign body may allow vaginal flora to ascend into the uterus (Chua and others, 1997; Sanchez-Ramos, 2005).

Premature Rupture of Membranes

There is a risk for PROM if the cervix is short. For this reason, the tents must be placed into the full length of the cervical canal, including the internal os.

Cervical Trauma

Cervical trauma is related to insertion technique.

Nursing Interventions

- Prepare the patient and assist the physician with the preinsertion assessment, which includes ruling out ruptured membranes; inspecting the cervix and vagina for an infection, especially for beta-streptococcus or *Neisseria gonorrhoeae*; assessing fetal size, position, amniotic fluid volume, and placental position with ultrasound; and assessing for fetal well-being with a biophysical profile or a con-traction stress test.
- Prepare the patient, and assist the physician with the insertion procedure, which includes a vaginal examination to assess cervical anatomy and cervical status; insertion of a sterile speculum so that the cervix can be visualized, stabilized with a ring forceps, and painted with povidone-iodine (Betadine); lubricate with a bacteriostatic cream or jelly; insert four to nine tents to fill the cervix; and pack the upper vagina with 4- × 4-inch sponges to hold the tents in place.
- Instruct the patient that she might experience mild cramping during the insertion.
- Document the number of dilators and sponges placed.
- Continue to assess urinary output following insertion because pressure on the bladder may cause urinary retention.
- Continually assess for ROM, uterine tenderness or pain, or uterine bleeding. If any of these signs occur, assess for signs of fetal compromise and notify the physician so that tents can be removed.

BALLOON CATHETERS AND EXTRA-AMNIOTIC SALINE INFUSION

Embrey and Mollison (1967) described the use of a transvaginal Foley catheter used for labor induction. The balloon catheters are made of silicone and are used for mechanical dilation of the cervical canal prior to labor induction. Cervical ripening or dilatation is accomplished through a gentle and constant pressure at the level of the cervix from both the internal and external ostia. The balloon may be the appropriate alternative for patients for whom pharmacologic agents are contraindicated (Simpson, 2008).

Extra-amniotic saline infusion used in conjunction with a balloon catheter has not been found to enhance the process when compared with the use of balloon catheter alone. The extra-amniotic saline infusion is administered through the balloon catheter with normal saline at 1 ml/min into extra-amniotic space (Simpson, 2008).

Physiology
The balloon catheter places direct pressure causing an overstretching of the lower uterine segment and cervix as well as local prostaglandin release (Simpson, 2008).

Advantages
According to Gelber and Sciscione (2006), a review of studies revealed that balloon catheters change the mean Bishop score of between 3.3 and 5.3 following cervical ripening with the catheter. There are minimal side effects associated with balloon catheter placement (Gelber and Sciscione, 2006). Results are usually seen within 8 to 12 hours following insertion (Simpson, 2008).

Risks
These include PROM, bleeding, displacement of the presenting part, or chorioamnionitis (Gelber and Sciscione, 2006).

Nursing Interventions
- Obtain an informed consent following an informative discussion as to the procedure, reasons for the procedure, what it means to the patient, and potential side effects and risks.
- Provide ongoing emotional support, and encourage relaxation. Instruct the patient that she might experience mild cramping during the insertion.
- Monitor for tachysystole uterine activity and category II or III FHR changes per protocol.
- Prepare the patient and assist the physician or nurse midwife with the preinsertion assessment, which includes ruling out ruptured membranes; inspecting the cervix and assessing fetal size, position, amniotic fluid volume, and placental position with ultrasound; and assessing for fetal well-being with a biophysical profile or a contraction stress test.
- Placement of the balloon catheter with patient in a dorsal lithotomy position
- Prep the perineum and vagina with an antiseptic prior to insertion.
- Assemble supplies utilized by providers such as sterile speculum and antiseptic to decrease local bacterial density. The uterine balloon is inserted through the cervix until both balloons have entered the cervical canal, then the cervical balloon is inflated with 40 ml of saline.
- Observation: Following the insertion the device is pulled back until the balloon is adjacent to the internal cervical os. The vaginal balloon is visible outside the external cervical os and is inflated with 20 ml of saline. When both balloons are situated on either side of the cervix, saline is added to a maximum of 80 ml per balloon. Balloon catheters: 14-26 gauge Foley catheter balloon inflated above internal os with 30 to 50 ml of sterile water.

PHARMACOLOGIC LABOR INDUCTION METHOD: OXYTOCIN

Oxytocin, a normal hormone secreted from the posterior pituitary gland, is chemically related to vasopressin antidiuretic hormone (ADH). By promoting smooth muscle contractions of the uterus, oxytocin activates the myometrium. The effect of oxytocin is enhanced in the presence of high levels of estrogen. This is why oxytocin has little effect on the pregnant uterus until near term; this is when estrogen levels are high and adequate oxytocin receptors are present in the myometrium.

Oxytocin is administered in synthetic form as Pitocin. Oxytocin is available in IV preparations or intramuscular injections. However, oxytocin cannot be administered orally because the digestive enzyme trypsin inactivates the hormone. The IV administration of dilute oxytocin is the preferred route because the absorption rate is predictable and the absorption of the drug can be stopped at any time by discontinuing the IV infusion. Additionally, the effect on the body usually ceases quickly after the drug is discontinued; the pregnant woman's plasma, near term, contains a high concentration of the enzyme pitocinase.

Physiology

Labor initiated by oxytocin bypasses the preparation for labor that normally takes place during the prelabor phase. Therefore, the initial oxytocin-induced uterine contractions must promote these activities by causing a myometrial cell inflammatory response that frees arachidonic acid so that it is converted to prostaglandins. Once enough prostaglandins have been synthesized and myometrial gap junctions formed so that the uterus can respond in a coordinated manner, the active phase of labor begins.

By the middle of the active phase of labor, adequate oxytocin receptors are formed so that the dosage of oxytocin may be decreased. It can frequently be discontinued when 7 to 8 cm of dilation is reached because of adequate endogenous prostaglandins and oxytocin production.

Pharmacologic Characteristics

Individualized Uterine Response to Oxytocin

The uterine response to oxytocin is individualized (Perry and others, 1996).

Sensitivity to Oxytocin Changes During Various Phases of Labor

Sensitivity to oxytocin increases as labor advances related to the development of gap junctions and oxytocin receptors (Dawood, 1995), peaking during the second stage of labor (Shyken and Petrie, 1995).

Oxytocin Secretion in Pulses and by the Fetus

During normal labor, oxytocin has been found to be secreted in pulses or spurts (Shyken and Petrie, 1995). The fetus is thought to secrete oxytocin in response to maternal oxytocin at a rate of 3 mU/min (Simpson, 2008).

Maximum Uterine Contractile Effect of Oxytocin

A uterine response occurs to oxytocin in 3 to 5 minutes with a half-life of approximately 10 minutes. It takes approximately 40 minutes for a steady serum plasma state to be reached after oxytocin administration (Gonser, 1995; Shyken and Petrie, 1995). However, according to Perry and others (1996), serum plasma levels of oxytocin may not be important in determining dosing of the drug.

Uterine Response to Oxytocin

A triphasic uterine response to oxytocin occurs. During the incremental phase, the uterine response increases evenly as oxytocin dose increases. In the stable phase, the uterine response is unchanged even when oxytocin doses are increased. During the third phase, uterine contractions increase in frequency but intensity decreases, leading to an ineffective uterine contraction pattern. This change in uterine response may be gradual or abrupt (Dawood, 1995).

Dosages

There is a wide discrepancy among health care providers as to the most effective protocol for administering oxytocin. Currently, there are three schools of thought.

Low-Dose Management: Physiologic Approach

Low-dose management in oxytocin administration is based on research by Seitchik and others (1982, 1985), who recommended starting oxytocin at 1 mU/min and increasing the dosage by 0.5 to 1 mU/min every 30 to 60 minutes. The effects that conservative management have on outcome variables of labor have been studied by Blakemore and others (1990), Chua and others (1991), Mercer, Pilgrim, and Sibai (1991), Muller, Stubbs, and Laurent (1992), and Shyken and Petrie (1995). The findings of these four studies include decreased tachysystole, decreased fetal compromise, and significantly less oxytocin needed without affecting the duration of labor or cesarean rate. Table 28-3 lists examples of current low-dose oxytocin management.

High-Dose (Active) Management: Pharmacologic Approach

Current high-dose oxytocin protocols are based on the active management approach by O'Driscoll, Meagher, and Robson (2004), who recommended starting oxytocin at 6 mU/min and increasing the dosage by 6 mU/min every 15 minutes. The goal is

---

Table 28-3   Examples of Low-Dose and High-Dose Oxytocin Management for Labor Stimulation

Oxytocin	Starting Dose (mU/min)	Incremental Increase (mU/min)	Dosage Interval (in minutes)	Maximum Dose (mU/min)
Low dose	0.5-1.0	1	30-40	20
	1-2	2	15	40
High dose	6	6, 3, 1	20-40	42
	6	6	15	40

Modified from American College of Obstetricians and Gynecologists: Induction of labor, *ACOG Practice Bulletin*, No. 107, Washington, DC, 2009, ACOG.

strong uterine contractions leading to shortened labor and delivery. The effect that active management has on outcome variables of labor has been studied by Lopez-Zeno and others (1992), Xenakis and others (1995), Peaceman and Socol (1996), Crane and Young (1998), and Merrill and Zlatnik (1999). The findings of these studies include decreased length of labor, rate of forceps delivery, and rate of cesarean birth for dystocia, with increased tachysystole and cesarean birth for fetal stress. However, Frigoletto and others (1995) found active management to shorten labor to some degree and decrease risk for maternal fever but not to decrease cesarean delivery rate.

According to O'Driscoll and others (2004), there are other components to the active management protocol beyond just high-dose oxytocin. Most American obstetricians emphasize the high-dose oxytocin and fail to incorporate all other components.

Components of active management (O'Driscoll and others, 2004) are:

- *Childbirth education.* The patient is taught what to expect in labor and that it will not last more than 12 hours.
- *Criterion for diagnosis of labor.* The Dublin criterion is complete effacement. The healthy primigravida is not admitted until this criterion is met.
- *Amniotomy.* On admission, the membranes are artificially ruptured if still intact. If the amniotic fluid is clear, FHR is auscultated. If the amniotic fluid is meconium-stained, a continuous electronic monitor is used.
- *Criterion for early diagnosis and treatment of dystocia.* The Dublin criterion is 1 cm of progress per hour. If the patient's progress is slower than the standard, high-dose oxytocin (6 mU) is started immediately. It is increased every 15 minutes by 6 mU until the patient dilates 1 cm/hour. In their patients in 2000, 24% were induced (O'Driscoll and others, 2004). If the patient's contraction pattern cannot be stimulated to accomplish a dilation rate of 1 cm/hour in a reasonable time, a cesarean delivery is done. The cesarean birth rate in Dublin was 14% in 2000 (O'Driscoll and others, 2004).
- *Continual presence of a personal nurse.* One nurse is assigned to one patient, and the nurse remains with the patient until her delivery. According to a review and meta-analysis (Thorton and Lilford, 1994) of published studies on active labor management, the personal nurse who provides constant emotional and physical support is the only component associated with shorter labors and lower cesarean rates (see Table 28-3 for examples of current high-dose oxytocin management in the United States.)

Pulsatile Oxytocin Management

Oxytocin is administered by some health care providers in 10-minute pulsed infusions as opposed to a continuous IV infusion. According to Willcourt and others (1994), significantly less oxytocin and infusion fluid is used without loss of effectiveness.

Maternal Side Effects

Uterine Tachysystole

Uterine tachysystole can cause strong tetanic contractions that occur more often than four times in a 10-minute period, last longer than 90 seconds without a period of relaxation, or have an increased uterine resting tone above 20 mm Hg. This type of uterine contraction pattern can cause abruptio placentae or uterine rupture, as well as fetal stress. This is seen more often with high-dose regimens and more frequent dose increases. According to a study conducted by Bakker, Kurver, Kuik, and others (2007), tachysystole during the first and second stage of labor demonstrated an increased incidence of lower pH values in the umbilical artery.

Uncoordinated, Unproductive Uterine Activity

Unproductive uterine activity may be defined as an increase in frequency with a decrease in intensity of the contractions. This type of activity is related to the cessation of uterine blood flow during a contraction, causing accumulation of metabolites and hypoxia, which renders the muscle ineffective.

Antidiuretic Effect: Water Intoxication

Because oxytocin has a weak antidiuretic property, large doses can cause the kidneys to increase the reabsorption of water, decreasing urinary output (Smith and Merrill, 2006). Antidiuretic effect is seen more frequently when the oxytocin infusion rate is 40 mU/min or more. This condition is enhanced if large amounts of electrolyte-free dextrose solution are used to administer the oxytocin (Sanchez-Ramos, 2005; Smith and Merrill, 2006). Possible signs of water intoxication are decreased urine output, hypotension, tachycardia, headache, and nausea and vomiting. Additionally, if a patient exhibits symptoms consistent with water intoxication oxytocin should be discontinued; notify the provider, and expect to initiate steps to correct the electrolyte imbalance (Smith and Merrill, 2006).

Cesarean Birth

Cesarean birth rate is increased for nonreassuring fetal status or failed induction. A study by Cammu, Martens, Ruyssinck, and others (2002) revealed that elective induction in nulliparous patients had a 9.9% cesarean section rate versus the 6.5% cesarean section rate in those in spontaneous labor. Additionally, Vahratian, Zhang, Troendle, and others (2005) analyzed delivery data from January 2002 through March 2004 that illustrated a cesarean section delivery rate that was above 40% of term, nulliparous patients. Additionally, according to Martin and others (2007) a cesarean section delivery resulting from an induction may be followed by a repeat cesarean delivery in subsequent pregnancy.

Failed Induction

According to Stubbs (2000), failed induction is the most common risk and is directly related to the degree of cervical ripening.

Fetal and Neonatal Effects

Iatrogenic Prematurity

Any time labor is induced, there is a risk for prematurity. Therefore fetal maturity should always be assessed before an induction unless it is being performed because of medical indications when the benefits of delivery outweigh the risks of prematurity.

Fetal Stressors

Labor contractions normally impede uterine blood flow. A healthy fetus that has an adequate oxygen reserve can withstand this stress. However, if the frequency, intensity, duration, or resting tone of the contractions is increased by a labor stimulant, this can further impede the uterine blood flow and can cause fetal compromise, resulting in a category II or III FHR pattern. Thus, oxytocin must be administered with careful monitoring and prompt recognition and interventions of tachysystole to assist in prevention of fetal acidemia (Bakker and van Geijn, 2008).

Intrauterine Fetal Demise

The induction of those patients suffering an intrauterine fetal demise present challenges to both the patient and the clinicians. Because of the emotional stress of the patient an expedient method of delivery may be pursued (Smith and Merrill, 2006).

High-Alert Medication

In 2007, the Institute for Safe Medication Practices (ISMP) identified IV oxytocin as a high-alert medication. Those identified as high-alert medications have a heightened risk of causing significant patient harm when they are used in error. Errors with high-alert medications may or may not be more common than other medications (ISMP, 2007), yet patient injury or consequences associated with the error may be more devastating (ISMP, 2007). Note that the ISMP has 18 categories or classes of medications designated as high alert and 12 medications are identified, including IV oxytocin (ISMP, 2007).

According to Clark and others (2008), errors involving IV oxytocin administration during labor are most commonly related to dosage; however, the lack of timely recognition and appropriate treatment of tachysystole is commonly the cause of administration errors. Additionally, other types of IV oxytocin errors include mistaken administration of IV fluids with IV oxytocin for IV fluid resuscitation, inappropriate timing of increases in oxytocin infusion rate, or excessive doses of IV oxytocin (Clark, Simpson, Knox, and others, 2008). Thus, IV oxytocin errors resulting in maternal and fetal harm are preventable through the adherence to principles of safe care, development of standard care processes to prevent errors and harm, methodology of error identification, and methods to minimize the harm resulting from the error (AHA and ISMP, 2002; JCAHO, 2003; Clark, and others, 2007; ISMP, 2007; Simpson and Knox, 2009).

Nursing Interventions

Because of the individualized response to oxytocin, the variations of practice philosophy supported by research, and variable resources unique to each institution, the following oxytocin protocol is generic:

- Ensure an informed consent has been obtained by providing information about the indication, the agents and methods, alternative options, and risks such as repeat induction and cesarean delivery (JCAHO, 2003).
- Initiate oxytocin induction or augmentation only after a physician who can perform a cesarean delivery and who is readily available has evaluated the patient, determined a medical indication, provided documentation of fetal maturity, and obtained an informed consent from the patient. The consent must include indication for, risks, and methods to be used and possible alternatives.

- Have an appropriate nurse-to-patient ratio on the unit, 1:1 or 1:2 (AAP and ACOG, 2007).
- Have a unit- or hospital-based validation program established for the registered labor nurse to prepare the nurse to safely administer and monitor labor stimulants (Simpson and Atterbury, 2003).
- Explain the procedure and what to expect to the patient and her coach.
- Assess the response of the patient and her coach to labor stimulation. Often, they feel as if they have failed when such an intervention is needed. An explanation as to the reason can help to alleviate these feelings.
- Assess the patient's level of fear associated with labor-induced contractions. Many patients have heard alarming reports about oxytocin. The nurse should inform the patient and her coach that stimulated contractions are usually very similar to normal, active labor contractions. An induced labor usually has a shorter latent phase, with contractions that may be more uncomfortable than those occurring with a spontaneous latent phase do, but the active phase is not usually altered.
- Apply an external fetal monitor or assist with the placement of an internal fetal monitor, and determine a baseline for maternal vital signs, FHR, and uterine activity for 10 to 20 minutes before initiation.
- Perform a vaginal examination to determine cervical effacement and dilation, fetal presentation, and station.
- Prepare the oxytocin solution according to institutional policy, and label properly. Usually, 10 units of oxytocin are mixed with 1000 ml of an IV isotonic electrolyte solution.
- Position the patient on her side or sitting up to avoid the vena cava syndrome.
- Administer the solution by way of a continuous infusion device to ensure precise control over the amount of medication administered.
- Piggyback the oxytocin solution into a well-functioning infusion line next to the infusion site so that oxytocin can be discontinued and restarted as necessary while maintaining an open vein for any emergency.
- Start the pump, usually at a low setting, per institutional protocol or physician's order and patient response. Frequency of uterine contractions, progression of labor, and fetal tolerance are all part of the patient response (Clayworth, 2000).
- The dose is gradually increased per institutional protocol or physician's orders until a desired contraction pattern is established or the instituted maximum dose is reached. The licensed maximum dose is 20 mU/min, but some controlled trial studies are evaluating regimens up to 32 mU/min. In the majority of cases, an adequate contraction pattern is usually achieved at around 12 mU/min (RCOG, 2008).
- When labor has progressed to 5 to 6 cm of dilation, oxytocin may be reduced by 1 to 2 mU/min every 30 to 60 minutes.
- The goal of oxytocin is to establish an adequate uterine contraction pattern that promotes cervical dilation of approximately 1 cm per hour once active labor is established. Usually, this contraction pattern consists of three contractions every 10 minutes, each lasting 40 to 60 seconds with an intensity of 25 to 75 mm Hg intrauterine pressure. This produces between 150 and 350 Montevideo units, in

which the uterus returns to baseline (resting tone, which does not exceed 20 mm Hg) for at least 1 minute between each contraction.

- Check the patency of the IV infusion frequently so that backup of the oxytocin solution into the IV tubing does not result in a bolus of oxytocin.
- Assess the FHR and uterine contractions for resting tone, intensity, frequency, and duration according to the institution's policy. According to the Association of Women's Health, Obstetric, and Neonatal Nurses (Simpson and Atterbury, 2003), the frequency of FHR and uterine contractions assessment is based on the condition of the mother and the fetus' response to labor with a minimum standard of assessment before every dose increase. The American Academy of Pediatrics and the American College of Obstetricians and Gynecologists (2007) recommend monitoring for low risk patients during the first stage of labor at least every 30 minutes and during the second stage of labor at least every 15 minutes, preferably just following a contraction. When risk factors are present or the fetus response to labor indicates, the FHR should be assessed every 15 minutes during the first stage and every 5 minutes during the second stage. However, the Royal College of Obstetricians and Gynaecologists (2008) recommends continuous monitoring similar to that for any high risk pregnancy.
- Assess vital signs per institution policy.
- Perform periodic vaginal examinations to determine cervical dilation and fetal descent. To evaluate the progress of labor, check cervical dilation and descent of the presenting part (station). A 1-cm/hour cervical dilation indicates sufficient progress and adequate oxytocin.
- Drug doses, times of increase, maternal vital signs, and FHR should be charted on a flow sheet.
- Assess the patient's level of pain frequently. Determine the effectiveness of distraction tools. If the distraction tools are ineffective for her level of discomfort, the physician should be notified. An analgesic may decrease the pain so that distraction tools are effective and the patient can stay in control. Allow the patient a choice in this regard.
- Encourage the patient and her coach by giving them frequent positive reinforcement. This can help alleviate some of the negative feelings associated with a stimulated labor.
- Ensure adequate hydration to enhance effective contractions and avoid dehydration and exhaustion. A fluid bolus may be requested before initiating oxytocin, and fluid should usually infuse at a minimum of 125 ml/hour.
- IV hydration or fluid bolus amounts may vary with preeclampsia or eclamptic patients.
- Keep an accurate intake and output record.
- Assess for signs of fluid retention such as decreased urine output, bounding pulse, peripheral edema, increasing blood pressure, shortness of breath, or crackles.
- Decrease or discontinue oxytocin if a tachysystole contraction pattern is noted, and notify the attending physician. Tachysystole contractions (1) occur more often than four every 10 minutes, (2) last 90 seconds or more without a period

of relaxation, and (3) have an increased uterine resting tone above 20 mm Hg pressure.

- Discontinue oxytocin, administer oxygen, position patient on her side, and notify the attending physician if category II or III FHR pattern is noted, such as late or variable decelerations, loss of long- or short-term variability, tachycardia, or bradycardia. The oxytocin infusion may be restarted after careful assessment by the attending physician of the uterine contraction pattern and the FHR. It may be advantageous to lower the dose and lengthen the dose interval. If oxytocin has been stopped for longer than 30 minutes, it may be necessary to restart from the initial ordered dose (Clayworth, 2000).
- If uterine tachysystole persists, be prepared to give terbutaline or another tocolytic as order by the attending physician.
- Ensure the attending physician is close to the labor and delivery area to manage any complication that might arise.
- Discontinuation of the induction may occur if labor has not started or if no progress is made within 2 to 3 hours as directed by the attending physician.
- Follow the institution's chain of command if nursing disagrees with the plan of care developed by the attending physician.

PHYSIOLOGIC METHODS OF LABOR INDUCTION: AMNIOTOMY

An *amniotomy* is an artificial rupture of membranes with an amniohook to induce or augment labor. As reported by a *Cochrane Review*, Smyth, Alldred, and Markham, (2007) suggest the utilization of amniotomy demonstrates a reduction in the incidences of dysfunctional labor and a reduction in the length of the first and second stages of labor. However amniotomy is associated with birth risks and should not be performed routinely.

Physiology

Arachidonic acid release increases with its conversion into prostaglandins following amniotomy (Tenore, 2003). Before 4-cm dilation, amniotomy may modestly shorten labor if the cervix is ripe. There is an increased risk for chorioamnionitis and cord compression (Mercer and others, 1995). After 4 cm, amniotomy may improve an uncoordinated uterine contraction pattern related to increased prostaglandin release or enhance a normal uterine contraction pattern because of the dilating wedge of the fetal head on the cervix with no adverse fetal or neonatal effect (Fraser and others, 1993; Garite and others, 1993; Rouse and others, 1994). However, according to *The Cochrane Review*, inadequate data prevents a conclusion as to its safeness and effectiveness (Howarth and Botha, 2001).

Advantages

Amniotomy has two advantages. First, it decreases the length of some labors without the use of oxytocin. Second, it allows for amniotic fluid assessment for meconium and permits internal fetal and uterine contraction monitoring.

Risks

One risk of amniotomy is that once the fetal membranes are ruptured, delivery is expected within a reasonable and safe period of time. Unresolved variable decelerations may progress to a category II or III pattern, are more likely to occur at an early stage of labor, and are more likely to be unresponsive to position change. This is the most common risk and can be treated with amnioinfusion.

The risk for an intraamniotic infection increases with the duration of the rupture. Umbilical cord prolapse and change in fetal presentation are two additional risks that can occur with amniotomy.

Fetal stressors can be related to decreased amniotic fluid that results from the rupture in amniotomy or from a prolapsed cord.

If the fetal vessels transfuse through the membranes that lie over the cervix (vasa previa), these may rupture when the membranes are ruptured. If there is an undiagnosed placenta previa, membrane rupture can also cause bleeding.

Caput succedaneum related to direct pressure on the presenting part as it acts as a dilating wedge may occur with amniotomy.

Nursing Interventions

- Amniotomy should be done only where an emergency delivery can be performed nearby.
- The provider should assess for engagement of the presenting part before an amniotomy (ROM). (The presenting part must be engaged for an amniotomy to be done.) The health care provider who is rupturing the membranes should assess for fetal blood vessels under fetal membranes before rupture is carried out.
- Assess FHR before ROM.
- Assist health care provider with rupture. According to AWHONN, an amniotomy is to be performed by a physician or midwife. If it is performed by a perinatal nurse, the institution must have a policy and protocol that meets the criteria of the respective state's scope of practice (Simpson, 2008). The institution policy or protocol should outline the competency requirements, the circumstances under which the perinatal nurse may place a fetal scalp electrode if membranes are intact, and the nurse to provider communication process (Simpson, 2008). Additionally, if the perinatal nurses perform amniotomy, the individual nurse must demonstrate and maintain competency in the procedure (Simpson, 2008).
- During the amniotomy, gentle fundal and suprapubic pressure may be applied, if needed, to decrease risk for cord prolapse.
- Check FHR immediately following ROM. If FHR change or a category II or III pattern occurs, rule out cord prolapse, cord obstruction, or fetal bleeding.
- Assess amniotic fluid (amount, color [clear or meconium-stained]), and odor.
- Monitor the uterine contraction pattern following rupture. Oxytocin may be ordered if normal labor does not follow rupture.
- Assess maternal temperature after rupture every 4 hours, or more frequently if signs and symptoms of infection occur.

- If fetal compromise develops from a prolapsed cord, apply and maintain pressure to the presenting part; with other hand, push abdomen up; call for help; notify physician; instruct helper to put bed in a Trendelenburg position; evaluate FHR; start oxygen by mask at 10 L/min; and start an IV line with an 18-gauge intra-catheter if not already started.

PHYSIOLOGIC METHODS OF LABOR INDUCTION: STRIPPING OF FETAL MEMBRANES

During membrane stripping, the chorionic fetal membrane is separated from the decidua of the lower uterine segment.

Physiology

When the membrane is stripped from the decidua, a local deciduitis results, caus-ing the local release of phospholipase A_2 and prostaglandins in the area and may increase the systemic release of oxytocin (Sanchez-Ramos and Delke, 2006). Mem-brane stripping has been shown to increase spontaneous labor, decrease the incidence of postdate gestations, and reduce the need for other induction methods without increasing complications (McColgin and others, 1990; El-Torkey and Grant, 1992; Allott and Palmer, 1993; Krammer and O'Brien, 1995). However, according to the *Cochrane Review* (Boulvain, Stan, and Irion, 2004), the decreased use of other induc-tion methods needs to be balanced against the discomfort and other risks of the procedure.

Risks

Risks with stripping the fetal membranes include (1) increased maternal discomfort during the examination, (2) PROM at the time they are stripped, and (3) bleeding if there is an undiagnosed placenta previa.

Interventions

- Firm documentation must be made that the fetus is at or older than 37 weeks of gestation.
- No medical contraindications such as an abnormal fetal presentation or a low-lying placenta may exist.
- During the procedure, the health care provider digitally separates 1 to 2 cm of the chorionic membrane from the decidua of the lower uterine segment.

COMPLEMENTARY THERAPIES: BREAST STIMULATION

Breast stimulation is a physiologic labor stimulant method that offers an alterna-tive method to pharmacologic induction or augmentation. It has been demonstrated through research to initiate or enhance labor and to shorten, especially the latent phase of labor (Chayen, Tejani, and Verma, 1986; Mastrogiannis and Knuppel, 1995; Kavanagh, Kelly, and Thomas, 2007a).

Physiology

Nipple stimulation causes the spontaneous release of oxytocin by the posterior pituitary gland.

Procedure

Manual or Warm Compress Breast Stimulation

- The patient gently rolls or brushes one nipple through her clothes or with a warm moist cloth for 10 minutes with a 5-minute rest. She then gently rolls or brushes the other nipple for 10 minutes.
- Discontinue stimulation during a contraction or after no observable effect occurs after 1 hour (Curtis and others, 1999).

Breast Pump Stimulation

- The patient stimulates one breast at a time for 10 minutes with the electric breast pump on moderate suction.
- The patient stops pumping for 10 minutes following one cycle of stimulation.
- The cycle just described may be repeated up to five times (Young and Poppe, 1987).

Risks

Uterine Tachysystole

Research has documented the risk for tachysystole from breast stimulation (Adair, 2000).

Nipple Soreness and Engorgement

Nipple soreness and engorgement occur in approximately 25% to 30% of cases of breast stimulation (Young and Poppe, 1987).

Fetal Compromise

Research has documented the risk for fetal compromise from breast stimulation to be comparable to oxytocin (Curtis and others, 1999; Kavanagh and others, 2007a).

Nursing Interventions

- Discuss the benefits of breast stimulation such as increased patient control, early milk production for the breastfeeding mother, lack of expense, and avoidance of invasive measures. Discuss the possible adverse side effects listed earlier.
- Explain the appropriate technique to the patient and her coach.
- Assess the response of the patient and her family to the procedure.
- Determine a baseline for maternal vital signs, FHR, and uterine activity for 10 to 20 minutes before having the patient begin.
- Perform a vaginal examination to determine cervical effacement and dilation, fetal presentation, and station.

- Have the patient lie on her side or sit to avoid supine hypotension from obstruction of the vena cava.
- Evaluate uterine contractions for quality, frequency, duration, and resting tone every 15 to 30 minutes.
- Assess FHR response to uterine contractions every 15 to 30 minutes.
- During periods of no stimulation, encourage patient to void, ambulate, and drink fluid unless contraindicated.
- Have the patient discontinue stimulation if a tachysystole contraction pattern occurs. Notify the attending physician, and be prepared to administer a tocolytic. Tachysystole contractions are contractions that (1) occur more often than four every 10 minutes, (2) last 90 seconds or more without a period of relaxation, or (3) have a suspected increased uterine resting tone above 20 mm Hg pressure.
- Have the patient discontinue stimulation, administer oxygen, and lie on her side; notify the attending physician if a category II or III FHR pattern is noted, such as late or variable decelerations, loss of long or short-term variability, tachycardia, or bradycardia.
- Have the patient discontinue stimulation, and notify the physician if labor has not started after five cycles of stimulation.

OTHER COMPLEMENTARY THERAPIES

Various complementary measures have been shown to enhance cervical ripening of a thick, unripe cervix or to induce labor if the cervix is ripe. A few such measures are as follows:

- *Herbal preparations.* Blue cohosh, black cohosh, evening primrose oil, raspberry leaves, or another safe herbal preparation taken orally may promote prostaglandin or oxytocin production (Hunter and Chern-Hughes, 1996; Woolven, 1997; Belew, 1999; McFarlin and others, 1999). Evening primrose oil is usually taken in the form of three capsules every day for 1 week or more (Adair, 2000). The dosage of blue cohosh tincture is 3 to 8 drops in a glass of warm water or tea; it may be repeated every 30 minutes for several hours until regular contractions occur (Hunter and Chern-Hughes, 1996). Black cohosh tincture dosage is 10 drops sublingually hourly until cervical changes occur, usually within 3 to 4 hours (Adair, 2000).
- *Orgasm.* Associated oxytocin or prostaglandin release stimulates uterine contractions.
- *Sexual intercourse.* Semen contains prostaglandin, which may hasten cervical ripening and orgasm stimulates the uterine as well. There is inadequate clinical evidence at this time to support or refute the belief that sexual intercourse enhances ripening of the cervix (Kavanagh, Kelly, and Thomas, 2007b; Howarth and Halligan, 2000). This method would be contraindicated in the presence of ROM.
- *Acupuncture or electric transcutaneous electrical nerve stimulation (TENS).* Stimulation of the nerve loci of the uterus with needles or TENS has been demonstrated to initiate labor (Adair, 2000). The issues of efficacy and safety need to be studied before their general use (Smith and Crowther, 2004).

- *Bowel stimulation.* Stimulation of the bowel with castor oil, bath, and/or enema increases prostaglandin production, which may facilitate cervical ripening. According to the *Cochrane Review* (Kelly, Kavanagh, and Thomas, 2003), further research is needed to determine the effectiveness of bowel stimulation in facilitating induction of labor. According to the AHRQ evidence report (2002), castor oil given at term has a positive effect in promoting labor but consistently causes maternal nausea.

CONCLUSION

The rate of labor inductions has risen dramatically over the past decade. Although the use of labor stimulants enables many patients to have a vaginal delivery, there are risks associated with their use. The primary role of the nurse is to closely monitor the labor progress, the uterine contraction pattern, and fetal well-being. Developing complications can then be recognized early so that the labor stimulant can be stopped before a negative development occurs. Additionally, nurses gaining knowledge and understanding of all labor stimulants is essential to patient safety. Lastly, a labor stimulant should never be used simply to speed up labor or to initiate a labor for convenience.

BIBLIOGRAPHY

Adair C: Nonpharmacologic approaches to cervical priming and labor induction, *Clin Obstet Gynecol* 43(3):447–454, 2000.

Agency for Healthcare Research and Quality (AHRQ): *Management of prolonged pregnancy*, Evidence Report/Technology Assessment, No 23, Durham, NC, 2002, AHRQ. Retrieved from http://www.ahrq.gov.

Agency for Healthcare Research and Quality (AHRQ): *Maternal and neonatal outcomes of elective induction of labor*, Evidence Report/Technology Assessment, No 176, Durham, NC, 2009, AHRQ. Retrived from http://www.ahrq.gov.

Allott H, Palmer C: Sweeping the membranes: a valid procedure in stimulating the onset of labour? *Br J Obstet Gynaecol* 100(10):898–903, 1993.

American Academy of Pediatrics (AAP) and American College of Obstetricians and Gynecologists (ACOG): *Guidelines for perinatal care*, ed 6, Elk Grove Village, Ill, 2007, AAP/ACOG.

American College of Obstetricians and Gynecologists(ACOG): Response to Searle's drug warning on misoprostol, *ACOG Committee Opinion*, Washington, DC, 2000, ACOG.

American College of Obstetricians and Gynecologists(ACOG): New U.S. Food and Drug Administration labeling on cytotec (Misoprostol) use and pregnancy, *ACOG Committee Opinion*, No 283, Washington, DC, 2003, ACOG.

American College of Obstetricians and Gynecologists (ACOG): Induction of labor for vaginal birth after cesarean delivery, *ACOG Committee Opinion,* No 342, Washington, DC, 2006, ACOG.

American College of Obstetricians and Gynecologists (ACOG): Induction of labor, *ACOG Practice Bulletin*, No 107, Washington, DC, 2009, ACOG.

American Hospital Association and Institute for Safe Medication Practices (AHA and ISMP): *Pathways to medication safety*, Chicago, 2002, Authors.

Andersson S, Minjarez, Yost N, Word R: Estrogen and progesterone metabolism in the cervix during pregnancy and parturition, *J Clin Endocrinol Metabol* 93(6):2366–2374, 2008.

Arias F: Pharmacology of oxytocin and prostaglandins, *Clin Obstet Gynecol* 43(3):455–468, 2000.

Bakker P, Kurver P, Kuik D, and others: Elevated uterine activity increases the risk of fetal acidosis at birth, *Am J Obstet Gynecol* 196:313.e1–313.e6, 2007.

Bakker P, van Geijn H: Uterine activity: Implications for the condition of the fetus, *J Perinat Med* 36:30–47, 2008.

Belew C: Herbs and the childbearing woman: guidelines for midwives, *J Nurse Midwifery* 44(3): 231–252, 1999.

Bishop E: Pelvic scoring for elective induction, *Obstet Gynecol* 24:266, 1964.

Blakemore K, and others: A prospective comparison of hourly and quarter-hourly oxytocin dose increase intervals for the induction of labor at term, *Obstet Gynecol* 75(5):757–761, 1990.

Blanchette H, Nayak S, Erasmus S: Comparison of the safety and efficacy of intravaginal misoprostol (prostaglandin E_1) with those of dinoprostone (prostaglandin E_2) for cervical ripening and induction of labor in a community hospital, *Am J Obstet Gynecol* 180(6 Pt 1):1551–1559, 1999.

Boulvain M, Stan CM, Irion O: Membrane sweeping for induction of labour, *Cochrane Database Syst Rev* (Issue 4), Art. No.: CD000451, 2004.

Buser D, and others: A randomized comparison between misoprostol and dinoprostone for cervical ripening and labor induction in patients with unfavorable cervices, *Obstet Gynecol* 89(4):581–585, 1997.

Cammu H, Martens G, Ruyssinck G, Amy JJ: Outcome after elective labor induction in nulliparous women: a matched cohort study, *Am J Obstet Gynecol* 186(2):240–244, 2002.

Chayen B, Tejani N, Verma U: Induction of labor with an electric breast pump, *J Reprod Med* 31(2): 116–118, 1986.

Chua S, and others: Oxytocin titration for induction of labour: a prospective randomized study of 15 versus 30 minute dose increment schedules, *Aust N Z J Obstet Gynaecol* 31(2):134–137, 1991.

Chua S, and others: Preinduction cervical ripening: prostaglandin E_2 gel vs. hygroscopic mechanical dilator, *J Obstet Gynaecol Res* 23(2):171–177, 1997.

Clark S, Belfort M, Saade G, and others: Implementation of a conservative checklist-based protocol for oxytocin administration: maternal and newborn outcomes, *Am J Obstet Gynecol* 197:480e1-480e5, 2007.

Clark SL, Simpson KR, Knox GE, Garite TJ: Oxytocin: New perspective on an old drug, *Am J Obstet Gynecol* 200(1):35e1-35e6, 2008.

Clayworth S: The nurse's role during oxytocin administration, *MCN Am J Matern Child Nurs* 25(2): 80–84, 2000.

Crane JM: Factors predicting labor induction success: a critical analysis, *Clin Obstet Gynecol* 49(3): 573–584, 2006.

Crane J, Young D: Meta-analysis of low-dose versus high-dose oxytocin for labour induction, *J Soc Obstet Gynaecol Can* 20:1215, 1998.

Cunningham F, Leveno K, Bloom S, Rouse D, Spong C: *Williams obstetrics*, ed 23, New York, 2005, McGraw-Hill Medical.

Curtis P, and others: A comparison of breast stimulation and intravenous oxytocin for the augmentation of labor, *Birth* 26(2):115–122, 1999.

Dawood M: Pharmacologic stimulation of uterine contraction, *Semin Perinatol* 19(1):73–83, 1995.

El-Torkey M, Grant J: Sweeping of the membranes is an effective method of induction of labour in prolonged pregnancy: a report of a randomized trial, *Br J Obstet Gynaecol* 99(6):455–458, 1992.

Embrey MP, Mollison BG: The unfavourable cervix and induction of labour using a cervical balloon, *J Obstet Gynaecol Br Commonw* 74:44–48, 1967.

Engle WA, Tomashek KM, Wallman C: Committee on Fetus and Newborn: 'Late preterm' infants: a population at risk, *Pediatrics* 120:1390–1401, 2007.

Fraser W, and others: Effect of early amniotomy on the risk of dystocia in nulliparous women, *N Engl J Med* 328(16):1145–1149, 1993.

Frigoletto F, and others: A clinical trial of active management of labor, *N Engl J Med* 333(12):745–750, 1995.

Garite T, and others: The influence of elective amniotomy on fetal heart rate patterns and the course of labor in term patients: a randomized study, *Am J Obstet Gynecol* 168(6 Pt 1):1827–1831, 1993.

Gelber S, Sciscione A: Mechanical methods of cervical ripening and labor induction, *Clin Obstet Gynecol* 49(3):642–657, 2006.

Gonser M: Labor induction and augmentation with oxytocin: pharmacokinetic considerations, *Arch Gynecol Obstet* 256(2):63–66, 1995.

Havelock F, Keller P, Muleba N, and others: Human myometrial gene expression before and during parturition, *Biol Reprod* 72:707–719, 2005.

Hertelendy F, Zakar T: Prostaglandins and the myometrium and cervix, *Prostaglandins Leukot Essent Fatty Acids* 70:207–222, 2004.

Hofmeyr GJ, Gülmezoglu AM: Vaginal misoprostol for cervical ripening and induction of labour, *Cochrane Database Syst Rev* (Issue 1), Art. No.: CD000941, 2004.

Howarth E, Halligan A: Induction of labor. In Kean L, Baker P, Edelstone D, editors: *Best practice in labor ward management*, Philadelphia, 2000, Saunders.

Howarth G, Botha D: Amniotomy plus intravenous oxytocin for induction of labour, *Cochrane Database Syst Rev* (Issue 3), 2001.

Hunter L, Chern-Hughes B: Management of prolonged latent phase labor, *J Nurse Midwifery* 41(5):383–388, 1996.

Institute for Safe Medication Practices (ISMP): *High-alert medications*, Huntingdon Valley, PA, 2007, Author.

Iwahashi M, Muragaki Y, Ooshima A, Umesaki N: Decreased type I collagen expression in human uterine cervix during pregnancy, *J Clin Endocrinol Metabol* 88(5):2231–2235, 2003.

Joint Commission on Accreditation of Healthcare Organizations: *High-alert medication and patient safety*, Sentinel Event Alert No. 11 Oakbrook Terrace, IL, 1999, Author.

Joint Commission on Accreditation of Healthcare Organizations: *Comprehensive accreditation manual for hospitals*, Oakbrook Terrace, IL, 2003, Author.

Kavanagh J, Kelly AJ, Thomas J: Breast stimulation for cervical ripening and induction of labour, *Cochrane Database Syst Rev* (Issue 2), Art. No.: CD003392, 2007a.

Kavanagh J, Kelly AJ, Thomas J: Sexual intercourse for cervical ripening and induction of labour, *Cochrane Database Syst Rev* (Issue 2), Art. No.: CD003093, 2007b.

Kelly AJ, Kavanagh J, Thomas J: Castor oil, bath and/or enema for cervical priming and induction of labour, *Cochrane Database Syst Rev* (Issue 2), Art. No.: CD003099, 2007c.

Kelly AJ, Malik S, Smith L, and others: Vaginal prostaglandin (PGE2 and PGF2a) for induction of labour at term, *Cochrane Database Syst Rev* (Issue 2), Art. No.: CD003101, 2009.

Krammer J, O'Brien W: Mechanical methods of cervical ripening, *Clin Obstet Gynecol* 38(2):280–286, 1995.

Leppert P: Anatomy and physiology of cervical ripening, *Clin Obstet Gynecol* 38(2):267–279, 1995.

Lopez-Zeno J, and others: A controlled trial of a program for the active management of labor, *N Engl J Med* 326(7):450–454, 1992.

MacKenzie L, and others: Prostacyclin biosynthesis by cultured human myometrial smooth muscle cells: dependency on arachidonic or linoleic acid in the culture medium, *Am J Obstet Gynecol* 159(6): 1365–1372, 1988.

Macones GA, Hankins GDV, Spong CY, and others: The 2008 National Institute of Child Health and Human Development Workshop Report on Electronic Fetal Monitoring, *Obstet Gynecol* 11:661–666, 2008.

Martin J, Hamilton BE, Sutton PD, and others: Births: final data for 2005, *Natl Vital Stat Rep* 56(6):1–104, 2007.

Martin JA, Hamilton BE, Sutton PD, and others: Births: final data for 2006, *Natl Vital Stat Rep* 57(7):1–102, 2009.

Mastrogiannis D, Knuppel R: Labor induced using methods that do not involve oxytocin, *Clin Obstet Gynecol* 38(2):259–266, 1995.

McColgin S, and others: Stripping membranes at term: can it safely reduce the incidence of postterm pregnancies? *Obstet Gynecol* 76(4):678–680, 1990.

McFarlin B, and others: A national survey of herbal preparation use by nurse-midwives for labor stimulation, *J Nurse Midwifery* 44(3):205–216, 1999.

McIntire D, Leveno K: Neonatal mortality and morbidity rates in late preterm births compared with births at term, *Obstet Gynecol* 111:35–41, 2008.

Mercer B, and others: Early versus late amniotomy for labor induction: a randomized trial, *Am J Obstet Gynecol* 173(4):1321–1325, 1995.

Mercer B, Pilgrim P, Sibai B: Labor induction with continuous low dose oxytocin infusion: a randomized trial, *Obstet Gynecol* 77(5):659–663, 1991.

Merrill D, Zlatnik F: Randomized, double-masked comparison of oxytocin dosage in induction and augmentation of labor, *Obstet Gynecol* 94(3):455–463, 1999.

Moore LE, Rayburn WF: Elective induction of labor, *Clin Obstet Gynecol* 49:698–704, 2006.

Muller P, Stubbs T, Laurent S: A prospective randomized clinical trial comparing two oxytocin induction protocols, *Am J Obstet Gynecol* 167(2):373–380, 1992.

National Institute of Child Health and Human Development (NICHD): *Optimizing care and long-term outcomes of near-term pregnancy and near-term newborn infants*, Bethesda, MD, 2005, Author.

National Institute of Child Health and Human Development (NICHD): *State of the science conference statement: Cesarean delivery on maternal request*, Bethesda, MD, 2006, Author.

Nunes F, Rodrigues R, Meirinho M: Randomized comparison between intravaginal misoprostol and dinoprostone for cervical ripening and induction of labor, *Am J Obstet Gynecol* 181(3):626–629, 1999.

O'Driscoll K, Meagher D, Robson M: *Active management of labor*, ed 4, St Louis, 2004, Mosby.

Olson D, Mijovic J, Sadowsky D: Control of human parturition, *Semin Perinatol* 19(1):52–63, 1995.

Peaceman A, Socol M: Active management of labor, *Am J Obstet Gynecol* 175(2):363–368, 1996.

Perry R, and others: The pharmacokinetics of oxytocin as they apply to labor induction, *Am J Obstet Gynecol* 174(5):1590–1593, 1996.

Pollnow D, Broekhuizen F: Randomized, double-blind trial of prostaglandin E_2 gel versus low-dose oxytocin for cervical ripening before induction of labor, *Am J Obstet Gynecol* 174(6):1910–1913, 1996.

Rayburn W, and others: A model for investigating microscopic changes induced by prostaglandin E_2 in the term cervix, *J Matern Fetal Investig* 4:137, 1994.

Rouse D, and others: Active-phase labor arrest: a randomized trial of chorioamnion management, *Obstet Gynecol* 83(6):937–940, 1994.

Royal College of Obstetricians and Gynaecologists (RCOG): *Clinical guideline: induction of labor*, Regents Park, London, 2008, RCOG Press, Retrieved from http://guidance.nice.org.uk/CG70.

Sanchez-Ramos L: Induction of labor, *Obstet Gynecol Clin North Am* 32(2):181–200, 2005.

Sanchez-Ramos L, and others: Misoprostol for cervical ripening and labor induction: a metaanalysis, *Obstet Gynecol* 89(4):633–642, 1997.

Sanchez-Ramos L, and others: Labor induction with prostaglandin E_1 misoprostol compared with dinoprostone vaginal insert: a randomized trial, *Obstet Gynecol* 91(3):401–405, 1998.

Sanchez-Ramos L, Delke I: Induction of labor pregnancy termination for fetal abnormality. In James D, and others, editors: *High risk pregnancy: management options,* ed 3, Philadelphia, 2006, Saunders.

Seitchik J, Amico J, Castillo M: Oxytocin augmentation of dysfunctional labor, V: an alternative oxytocin regimen, *Am J Obstet Gynecol* 151(6):757–761, 1985.

Seitchik J, Castillo M: Oxytocin augmentation of dysfunctional labor. I. Clinical data, *Am J Obstet Gynecol* 144(8):899–905, 1982.

Schlembach D, MacKay L, Shi L, and others: Cervical ripening and insufficiency: from biochemical and molecular studies to in vivo clinical examination, *Eur J Obstet Gynecol Reprod Biol* 144S:S70–S76, 2009.

Shyken J, Petrie R: Oxytocin to induce labor, *Clin Obstet Gynecol* 38(2):232–245, 1995.

Simpson K: *Cervical ripening and induction and augmentation labor*, ed 3, Washington, DC, 2008, AWHONN.

Simpson K, Atterbury J: Trends and issues in labor induction in the United States: implications for clinical practice, *J Obstet Gynecol Neonatal Nurs* 32(6):767–779, 2003.

Simpson K, James D: Efficacy of intrauterine resuscitation techniques in improving fetal oxygen status during labor, *Obstet Gynecol* 105:1362–1368, 2005.

Simpson K, James D: Effects of oxytocin-induced uterine hyperstimulation on fetal oxygen status and fetal heart rate patterns during labor, *Am J Obstet Gynecol* 199:34.e1–34.e5, 2008.

Simpson K, Knox G: Oxytocin as a high-alert medication: implications for perinatal patient safety, *MCN Am J Matern Child Nurs* 34(1):8–15, 2009.

Smith CA, Crowther CA: Acupuncture for induction of labour, *Cochrane Database Syst Rev* (Issue 1), Art. No.: CD002962, 2004.

Smith JG, Merrill DC: Oxytocin for induction of labor, *Clin Obstet Gynecol* 49(3):594–608, 2006.

Smyth R, Alldred SK, Markham C: Amniotomy for shortening spontaneous labour, *Cochrane Database Syst Rev* 2007, (Issue 4), Art. No.: CD006167.

Stubbs T: Oxytocin for labor induction, *Clin Obstet Gynecol* 43(3):489–494, 2000.

Tenore J: Methods for cervical ripening and induction of labor, *Am Fam Physician* 67(10):2123–2128, 2003.

Thorton JG, Lilford RJ: Active management of labour: current knowledge and research issues, *BMJ* 309:366–369, 1994.

Vahratian A, Zhang J, Troendle JF, and others: Labor progression and risk of cesarean delivery in electively induced nulliparas, *Obstet Gynecol* 105(4):698–704, 2005.

Weiner C, Buhimschi C: *Drugs for pregnant and lactating women*, ed 2, Philadelphia, 2009, Saunders.

Willcourt R, and others: Induction of labor with pulsatile oxytocin by a computer-controlled pump, *Am J Obstet Gynecol* 170(2):603–608, 1994.

Winkler M, Rath W: Changes in the cervical extracellular matrix during pregnancy and parturition, *J Perinatal Med* 27(1):45–61, 1999.

Witter F: Prostaglandin E_2 preparations for preinduction cervical ripening, *Clin Obstet Gynecol* 43(3):469–474, 2000.

Woolven L: Alternative therapies for pregnancy, labor and delivery, *Childbirth Instructor* 7(2):40, 1997.

Word A, Xiang-Hong L, Hnat M, Carrick K: Dynamics of cervical remodeling during pregnancy and parturition: mechanisms and current concepts, *Sem Reprod Med* 25(1):69–79, 2007.

Xenakis E, and others: Low-dose versus high-dose oxytocin augmentation of labor—a randomized trial, *Am J Obstet Gynecol* 173(6):1874–1878, 1995.

Young J, Poppe C: Breast pump stimulation to promote labor, *MCN Am J Matern Child Nurs* 12(2): 124–126, 1987.

Zhang J, Yancey MK, Henderson CE: U.S. national trends in labor induction, 1989-1998, *J Reprod Med* 47:120, 2002.

29

Dysfunctional Labor

onditions can exist or develop that interfere with normal labor progress. An abnormal or difficult labor is usually termed *dysfunctional labor* or *dystocia*. Management of labor based on evidence and best practice can significantly reduce the incidence of dysfunctional labor and thereby decrease the incidence of preventable cesarean and instrument-assisted deliveries. Nurses must be willing to make a paradigm shift away from a routine, familiar, task-oriented labor care approach to an open-minded, individualized, evidence-based research approach to care (Kardong-Edgren, 2001; Sakala, 2005). This chapter presents evidence-based practices when available.

INCIDENCE

Dysfunctional labor occurs in approximately 8% to 11% of all deliveries and is the leading cause of cesarean deliveries (Ness, Goldberg, and Berghella, 2004; Zhu and others, 2006). In 2007 in the United States, 31.8% of all deliveries were by cesarean, up from 26.1% in 2002 (Hamilton, Martin, and Ventura, 2009). Repeat cesarean delivery rate is up to 92%, and primary cesarean birth rate is at 23.5% (Martin and others, 2008). Fetal malpresentation accounted for approximately 12% of all cesarean deliveries, and only 16% of cesarean births were done for fetal compromise (Dickinson, 2006).

The continual rise in cesarean deliveries is related to the following:
- Increasing trend in the restrictive use of vaginal birth after cesarean (VBAC)
- Current trend in the substantial use of induction as a means of timing delivery
- A lower decision threshold to perform a cesarean delivery
- Underuse of care that promotes the natural progress of labor
- Fear of litigation
- Casual attitude toward cesarean birth as a major surgery
- Maternal choice; according to Wax and others (2004), maternal choice influences 4% to 18% of cesarean deliveries worldwide; according to Declercq, Menacker, and MacDorman (2005), maternal choice influences approximately 3%-5.5% of cesarean deliveries in the United States; however, a national United States survey by Childbirth Connection (Declercq, Sakala, Corry, and others, 2006) found only 1 out of 1600 women surveyed requested a cesarean delivery.

Dysfunctional labor that occurs in stage two often leads to delivery with vacuum extractor or forceps. The incidence of instrument-assisted delivery is 10% to 15% (Patel and Murphy, 2004).

ETIOLOGY

Dysfunctional labor is influenced by 13 essential labor forces (VandeVusse, 1999). These forces, commonly referred to as the 13 Ps, are the original internal involuntary body processes listed below:

- *Power or uterine contractions.* Ineffective uterine activity or contractions can lead to uterine dystocia. Some issues that appear to increase one's risk for developing uterine dystocia include overweight, short stature, advanced maternal age, infertility difficulties, prior version, masculine characteristics, congenitally abnormal uterus, overdistended uterus as in multiple pregnancy or polyhydramnios, lack of reflex stimulation of the myometrium related to malpresentations (e.g., posterior positions; face, brow, or breech presentations; or transverse lie), fetopelvic disproportion (FPD), overstimulation of the uterus with oxytocin, extreme maternal fear or exhaustion causing the adrenal medulla to secrete catecholamines that interfere with uterine contractility, dehydration, electrolyte imbalance, administration of an analgesic too early in labor, or use of continuous epidural analgesia (Thorp and others, 1993; Morton and others, 1994; Lau and others, 1997; Fraser and others, 2002; Sheiner and others, 2002; Lowe, 2007).
- *Passenger or the fetus.* An abnormal fetal presentation or position, such as face, brow, or breech; posterior occiput presentation; or transverse lie can lead to fetal dystocia. Fetal anomalies, such as hydrocephalus, abdominal enlargement, tumors, conjoined twins, or excessive fetal size, usually greater than 4000 g (9 lb), can cause fetal dystocia as well.
- *Passageway or pelvis.* A small pelvic inlet, midpelvis, or pelvic outlet as the result of heredity, previous pelvic fracture, or disease can lead to pelvic dystocia.
- Physiologic involuntary experience by the mother.
- Psychologic state of the mother who wants to control her labor and delivery experience.
- Preparation of the mother for the birth.
- Position during labor.
- Professional providers' (especially the nurse's) attitudes, helpfulness, flexibility, support, consideration of individualized needs, communication skills in providing information and explanations, and comfort measures provided.
- Place of birth.
- Procedures performed such as electronic fetal monitoring (EFM), intravenous (IV) infusions, episiotomies, and internal examinations.
- People present other than the professional team such as office staff, family members, friends, and other patients.
- Politics defined as societal influences or expectations of appropriate labor behavior.
- Pressure interface regarding decision making.

NORMAL PHYSIOLOGY

Normal uterine contractions have two phases: contraction (systole) and relaxation (diastole). A pacemaker situated at the uterine end of the right fallopian tube initiates the contraction phase. The contraction phase, like a wave, moves downward to the cervix and upward to the fundus of the uterus. At the acme (peak) of the contraction, the entire uterus is contracting, with the greatest intensity in the fundal area. The relaxation phase follows and occurs simultaneously in all parts of the uterus. The round ligaments contain muscle and are stimulated to contract as the uterus contracts, thereby anchoring the uterus and promoting a downward force on the presenting part.

Uterine contractions of an intensity of 30 mm Hg or greater initiate cervical dilation. During active labor, the intensity usually reaches 50 to 80 mm Hg. During the second stage of labor, the intensity can peak at 100 mm Hg. Resting tone is normally between 5 and 10 mm Hg in early labor and between 12 and 18 mm Hg in active labor.

Normal labor usually begins with a latent phase, which is characterized by the cervix slowly dilating to about 4 cm. The duration of this phase is extremely variable. An active phase follows and is identified as the time when dilation takes place more rapidly and ends when the cervix is completely dilated and effaced. Historically the normal rate of cervical dilation during the active phase was at least 1.2 cm/hr in nulliparas and 1.5 cm/hr in multiparas (Friedman, 1995). More recent research indicates that the active phase of labor normally progresses more slowly related to regional anesthesia and oxytocin use (Rouse and others, 2001; Zhang, Troendle, and Yancey, 2002; Cesario, 2004). Their findings indicate a current labor pattern:

- A more gradual transition from latent to active phase labor
- No deceleration phase at the end of stage one of labor
- A wider normal range in the length of the first stage of active labor
- A longer second-stage labor

PATHOPHYSIOLOGY

Uterine Dystocia

Two types of abnormal uterine activity lead to uterine dystocia. First, there is hypotonic uterine activity, in which the rise in uterine pressure during a contraction is insufficient (<25 mm Hg) to promote cervical effacement and dilation. The force provided by voluntary contractions of the abdominal musculature, facilitated by the urge to push, may be insufficient to facilitate fetal descent and delivery. Second, there is hypertonic or uncoordinated uterine activity, in which the contractions are frequent and painfully strong but ineffective in promoting effacement and dilation. They can be ineffective because the uterine pacemakers arise in other areas of the uterus. This causes the myometrium to contract spasmodically and frequently but ineffectively, and the presenting part is not forced downward.

Fetal Dystocia

Several factors may influence the progress of labor, such as fetal lie, size, presentation, and number. The presence of anomalies may interfere with labor progress as well.

The fetus can move through the birth canal with the greatest ease when the head is sharply flexed so that the chin rests on the thorax and the occipital area of the skull (vertex) is presenting anterior to the mother's pelvis. Thus the smallest diameter of the fetal head enters the mother's pelvis, and the most flexible part of the fetal body, the back of the neck, adapts to the curve of the birth canal. At times, the fetus assumes other presentations, making labor difficult or impossible. These presentations are discussed in the following sections.

Occiput Posterior Presentation

Occiput posterior presentation occurs in approximately 15% of labors in the latent phase, and 5% are in this position at delivery (Stitely and Gherman, 2005). This form of presentation can develop during labor related to regional analgesia/anesthesia (Lieberman and others, 2005). In an occiput posterior presentation, the occiput of the fetus is in the posterior portion of the pelvis instead of in the anterior portion (Fig. 29-1). As the fetus moves through the birth canal, the occiput bone presses on the mother's sacrum. Severe back pain usually results from this presentation. The occiput must also rotate 135 degrees. This rotation can occur during fetal descent, causing slow progress in the active phase or a persistent anterior cervical lip. Most often, it does not occur until the occiput reaches the pelvic floor. Therefore the second stage of labor is usually prolonged.

Face Presentation

Face presentation, or mentum, occurs approximately once in every 500 to 600 deliveries (Simm and Woods, 2004; Thorp, 2009) when the fetal head is in extension instead of flexion as it enters the pelvic inlet (Fig. 29-2). If the mentum is in an anterior position, the labor usually progresses very close to normal and vaginal delivery results without much difficulty. This is because the widest diameter of the presenting part is similar in size to an occiput presentation and the neck can glide around

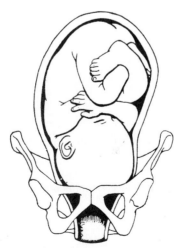

Figure 29-1 Occiput posterior presentation. (From *The normal female pelvis: clinical education aid*, No. 8, Columbus, OH, Ross Laboratories.)

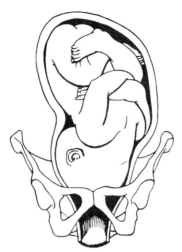

Figure 29-2 Face presentation. (From *The normal female pelvis: clinical education aid,* No. 8, Columbus, OH, Ross Laboratories.)

the short symphysis pubis with ease. When the mentum is in a posterior position, approximately 70% of the time it rotates to an anterior face presentation, making vaginal delivery possible but causing the labor to be prolonged. If the posterior position persists, cesarean delivery is necessary because the neck is too short to stretch the long distance of the sacrum.

Brow Presentation

A brow presentation occurs approximately once in every 500 deliveries (Simm and Woods, 2004; Thorp, 2009) when the fetal head presents in a position midway between full flexion and extreme extension (Fig. 29-3). This causes the largest diameter of the fetal head to engage. Vaginal delivery depends on the successful conversion to an occiput or a face presentation by varying degrees of flexion or extension, which occurs in 70% to 90% of cases. A brow presentation may be present when descent of the presenting part is prolonged or a long second-stage labor develops. Cesarean birth is indicated if this malpresentation fails to convert.

Shoulder Presentation

Shoulder presentation occurs approximately once in every 300 deliveries (Simm and Woods, 2004; Thorp, 2009) when the fetal spine is lying vertical to the mother's spine (Fig. 29-4). Because of the high mortality risk from prolapsed cord, cesarean delivery is usually the best management. However, if placenta previa and FPD are not present, external cephalic version has been successful in controlled circumstances.

Compound Presentation

Compound presentation occurs approximately once in every 1000 deliveries (Simm and Woods, 2004; Thorp, 2009) when one or more of the fetal extremities accompany the presenting part. An arm presenting along with the head is the most common

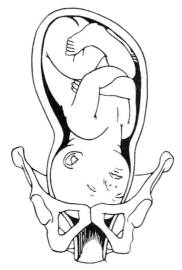

Figure 29-3 Brow presentation. (From *The normal female pelvis: clinical education aid*, No. 8, Columbus, OH, Ross Laboratories.)

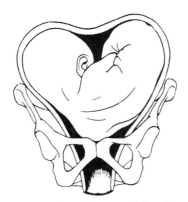

Figure 29-4 Shoulder presentation. (From *The normal female pelvis: clinical education aid*, No. 8, Columbus, OH, Ross Laboratories.)

compound presentation. Vaginal delivery is usually possible unless cord prolapse occurs or labor fails to progress. Then, an emergency cesarean delivery is done. Attempts should not be made to replace the prolapsed fetal part.

Breech Presentation

Breech presentation occurs in approximately 4% of all deliveries (Hofmeyr and Kulier, 2005) when the buttocks of the fetus present. The breech can present in three different attitudes. It is termed a *frank breech* when the thighs are flexed and the legs lie alongside the fetal body; a *complete breech* when the legs are flexed at the thighs, allowing the feet to present with the buttocks; and a footling breech when one foot (single footling) or both feet (double footling) present before the buttocks (Fig. 29-5).

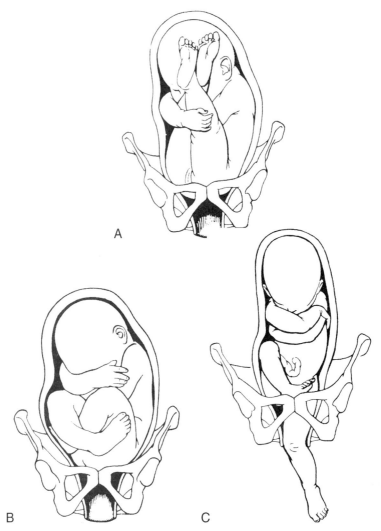

Figure 29-5 Breech presentation. **A,** Frank breech. **B,** Complete breech. **C,** Single footling breech. (From *The normal female pelvis: clinical education aid*, No. 8, Columbus, OH, Ross Laboratories.)

Prematurity, multiple gestation, and advancing maternal age are causes of breech presentation (Simm and Woods, 2004). Other causes are uterine relaxation associated with parity greater than 5 and decreased fetal capability to move within the uterus associated with diminished muscle tone of the fetus, neuromuscular disorders, or decreased uterine space. Infrequent causes are placenta previa, polyhydramnios, and hydrocephalus.

A breech presentation is considered high risk for the following reasons:

- Prolapse of the cord is more likely to occur, especially in a footling breech, because the buttocks do not fit as snugly into the cervix as does the fetal head.

- Dysfunctional labor is much more likely to result because the buttocks are soft and make a poor dilating wedge against the cervix.
- Birth trauma is more likely to occur because the head does not have time to mold and it must pass through the birth canal quickly. The premature fetus is even more prone to birth trauma from an incompletely dilated cervix.

Today's trend, based on the Term Breech Trial (Hannah and others, 2000), is to attempt external version. Currently a large pragmatic trial (Early ECV 2 Trial) is ongoing to determine the safest time to perform the external version (between 34 0/7 and 35 6/7 weeks or after 37 0/7 weeks) (*http://clinicaltrials.gov/ct2/show/NCT00141687*). If the version is unsuccessful, a scheduled cesarean delivery is discussed. Scheduled cesarean birth can decrease perinatal and neonatal mortality with modest increased morbidity risk to the mother according to a *Cochrane Review* (Hofmeyr and Hannah, 2004). Once labor is established, cesarean birth further increases maternal morbidity. The American College of Obstetricians and Gynecologists recommends cesarean delivery for all women with persistent term breech presentation (ACOG, 2001). However, the woman's preferences should be considered in the plan of management once risks and benefits have been shared. Vaginal delivery is the safest if it is a frank or complete breech with adequate neck flexion, symmetric fetal body proportions, normal gynecoid or clinically adequate pelvis, as indicated by pelvic radiography or prior delivery, and an estimated fetal weight 3800 g or less (Edelstone, 2000; Thorp, 2009).

Pelvic Dystocia

The shape and dimensions of the pelvis influence the progress of labor. The bony pelvis is composed of the inlet, midcavity (or canal), and the outlet. Pelvic dystocia is related to a contraction of one or more of the three planes of the pelvis.

Inlet Contraction

The pelvic inlet normally has a larger transverse diameter than anteroposterior diameter. No matter what the pelvic size measures, most obstetricians allow the patient to go into labor. Descent and engagement of the fetal head would indicate an adequate pelvic inlet.

Midcavity Contraction

Contraction of the midcavity is more common than an inlet contraction and often causes an arrest of descent. It is more difficult to determine manually. Possible indicators are (1) prominent ischial spines, (2) convergent pelvic side walls, and (3) a narrow sacrosciatic notch.

Outlet Contraction

The outlet of the pelvis normally has a larger anteroposterior diameter than transverse.

The final outcome of any labor depends on the interrelation of the size and shape of the pelvis; the size, presentation, and position of the fetus; and the quality of uterine contractions. Therefore dystocia can rarely be diagnosed until labor has progressed for a time. If the fetus is too large to pass through the pelvis or the pelvis is too small for the fetus to pass through, the condition is usually referred to as *fetopelvic disproportion* (FPD) or *cephalopelvic disproportion* (CPD).

SIGNS AND SYMPTOMS

Cervical dilation, effacement, and fetal descent occur progressively during labor. In an abnormal labor (1) contractions slow or fail to advance in frequency, duration, or intensity; (2) the cervix fails to respond to the uterine contractions by dilating and effacing; or (3) the fetus fails to move downward. Thus labor does not progress normally.

MATERNAL EFFECTS

Any time the birth canal is too small to accommodate the presentation of the fetus, uterine rupture can result. This can lead to maternal death related to hemorrhage. However, the incidence is rare; an obstructed labor is not usually allowed to continue. The greatest risk to the mother with a dysfunctional labor is associated with maternal exhaustion and a cesarean delivery.

Cesarean birth is associated with a 7 times higher maternal mortality rate and 5 to 10 times more maternal risks than is vaginal birth (Clark and others, 2008; Collard and others, 2008). These risks include postoperative complications of hemorrhage, endomyometrial and incision infections, urinary tract infection, aspiration pneumonitis, amniotic fluid embolism, anesthesia complications, thromboembolism, bowel and bladder trauma, and anemia (Edelstone, 2000; Enkin and others, 2000; Bernstein, 2005; Liu and others, 2007). More than 75% of postpartum deaths caused by a thromboembolism were associated with cesarean delivery (National Institute for Clinical Excellence, 2003). Infertility issues occur more often following a cesarean (Lobel and DeLuca, 2007). In a pregnancy following a cesarean birth, the risk for placenta previa is increased three times (Ananth, Smulian, and Vintzileos, 1997; Menacker, Declercq, and Macdorman, 2005). In the presence of a placenta previa, the risk for an invasive placenta is 35 times higher in those with a uterine scar from a prior cesarean than in those with an unscarred uterus (Miller, Chollet, and Goodwin, 1997; Rosen, 2008). There is a longer recovery period following the birth and a potential for incisional scarring and adhesions (Lobel and DeLuca, 2007). Negative psychologic effects that adversely influence maternal-neonatal attachment occur more often (Porter and others, 2007). Costs are doubled (Collard and others, 2008).

FETAL AND NEONATAL EFFECTS

Fetal and infant mortality are usually related to hypoxia or birth trauma. Hypoxia is often the result of intense uterine contractions that lead to uteroplacental insufficiency or cord prolapse related to malpresentation. A malpresentation can also cause such birth traumas as cranial or neck compression; fracture of the trachea, larynx, or shoulder; and spinal cord injury during an attempted vaginal delivery. The various interventions to facilitate delivery also increase the risk to the fetus of hypoxia and trauma.

According to an extensive review of literature, increased cesarean rate has not decreased the rate of neurologic disorders or cerebral palsy (Paneth, Hong, and

Korzeniewski, 2006). Cesarean birth does increase the risk for respiratory difficulties related to failed transition (Lobel and DeLuca, 2007; Ramachandrappa and Jain, 2008; Tita, Landon, and others, 2009), trauma related to surgical cuts (Dessole and others, 2004), breastfeeding problems (Towner and others, 1999), and later risk for developing asthma (Bager and others, 2003; Hakansson and Kallen, 2003; Lobel and DeLuca, 2007). Neonatal mortality rate is three times greater following a cesarean rather than a vaginal birth (Lobel and DeLuca, 2007).

DIAGNOSTIC TESTING

During the prenatal period, the health care provider determines general pelvic size and configuration and fetal position and presentation. This is done by abdominal palpation and vaginal examination. The Leopold maneuver is an effective way to screen for a fetal malpresentation.

Diagnostic prediction of the outcome of labor is rarely possible before labor. This is because it depends not only on the size and shape of the pelvis, but also on the size, presentation, and position of the fetus and the quality of uterine contractions. Therefore dystocia can rarely be diagnosed until labor has progressed for a time. The diagnosis is then based on clinical findings during labor, such as the uterine contraction pattern or the progression of labor as indicated by cervical dilation and effacement and fetal descent.

Labor progress historically was evaluated according to Friedman normal labor curves or the labor line of active labor. These evaluation tools provide a visual picture of some basic labor patterns, but are less relevant today. This is because of the changing demographics of childbearing women, which include maternal body mass, interracial and mixed ethnicity, and wider age range and the different patterns of labor management that include increased use of regional analgesia/anesthesia and oxytocin.

Current evidence supports categorizing dysfunction labor disorders as protracted or arrest disorders occurring in the first or second stages of labor. Protracted disorders involve slower than normal labor progress for that stage of labor. Arrest disorders are the result of cessation of labor progress. Proposed diagnostic guidelines for each disorder are summarized in Table 29-1.

USUAL MEDICAL MANAGEMENT AND PROTOCOLS FOR NURSE PRACTITIONERS

Labor Management to Decrease Cesarean Rate

The current focus is on managing labor more effectively to decrease primary cesarean rate. In the presence of a dysfunctional labor without FPD or other contraindication for labor augmentation, oxytocin should be used. Cesarean delivery has great potential benefits if indicated. However, it should be the last option because it is of higher maternal risk. Cesarean delivery also has increased risks for the newborn such as respiratory distress and lower breastfeeding rates. The timing of a planned cesarean should be based on fetal lung maturity.

Table 29-1 Summary of Abnormal Labor Patterns

Type	Definition	Etiology	Management
Protracted latent phase or "prelabor" Arrested latent phase	*Current Evidence-based Standard* Wide variation in length *Traditional Standard:* Nullipara: Latent phase of labor continues for longer than 20 hr (Friedman, 1995) Multipara: Latent phase of labor continues for longer than 14 hr (Friedman, 1995)	May be false labor Unfavorable cervical status Early administration of regional anesthesia Abnormal position of fetus Emotional concerns "Longing to complete the pregnancy" "Having difficulty managing the uncertainty" "Having difficulty with the slow progress of labor" (Carlsson, Hallberg, and Odberg, 2009)	Perform initial maternal and fetal assessment. Best place for latent phase labor is at home. Best treated by explanation, reassurance, alleviating anxiety, and allowing time for cervical changes to occur at home (Gee, 2006). Encourage adequate fluid and small, frequent meals. If analgesia or anesthetic has been used, let it wear off. Therapeutic rest has value; give oral zolpidem 5-10 mg or morphine 15-20 mg (80% will awake in active phase labor) Administer labor stimulant if delivery is indicated and start low dose epidural if requested.
Protraction active-phase Arrest of active-phase	*Current Evidence-based Standard:* Active phase not reached with 12 hours of oxytocin Rate of dilation in active phase: *Current Evidence-based Standard* Nullipara/Multipara: <0.6 cm/hr (Mancuso and Rouse, 2008; Zhang, Troendle, and Yancey, 2002) *Traditional Standard:* Multipara: <1.5 cm/hr (Friedman, 1995)	No specific cause Ineffective uterine contractions FPD Excessive sedation Fetal malpresentation Early conduction anesthesia ROM before onset of labor Inadequate nutrition Maternal exhaustion Extreme anxiety	Rule out obvious FPD; if FPD, prepare for cesarean delivery Amniotomy Augmentation with oxytocin to achieve 3-5 contractions/10 min Assess for uterine tachysystole Ongoing fetal assessment Initiate or continue the following nursing interventions to enhance uterine activity:

Nullipara: <1.2 cm/hr (Friedman, 1995)

Current Evidence-based Standard:
Without cervical change for
-4 hr with adequate uterine activity using oxytocin or
-6 hr without adequate uterine contraction using oxytocin (Mancuso and Rouse, 2008; Thorp, 2009)

Traditional Standard
Progressive dilation during active labor stops before full dilation occurs and continues for 2 hr or longer (Friedman, 1995)

- Continue to inform patient of progress and reassure regarding possible reasons for slow progress
- Encourage patient to keep bladder empty
- Provide physical and emotional support
- Let patient know you are there for her and that you have confidence in her ability
- Allay anxiety
- Encourage position change
- Assess fluid and electrolyte needs and administer IV as ordered

Precipitous labor

Nullipara: Cervix dilates faster than 5 cm/hr or descent faster than 1 cm per 12 min
Multipara: Cervix dilates faster than 10 cm/hr or descent faster than 1 cm per 6 min

Abnormally low cervical resistance
Abnormally strong uterine or abdominal muscular contractions

Tocolytic agents, such as magnesium sulfate or terbutaline, may be used in attempt to slow down progress of labor.

Reference: Carlsson I, Hallberg L, Odberg P: Swedish women's experiences of seeking care and being admitted during the latent phase of labour: a grounded theory study, *Midwifery* 25(2):172-180, 2009.
FPD, Fetopelvic disproportion.

The most common medical indications for a planned cesarean follow:
- Fetus with known meningomyelocele: cesarean may improve later motor function
- Macrocephaly for improved later mechanical function
- Active herpes and positive HIV status in certain situations
- Known placenta previa
- Previous classic uterine incision
- Family preference in the case of a prior cesarean

To reduce the number of preventable primary cesarean deliveries, labor protocols should be based on the best available evidence. The best practice factors include the following:
- View and treat labor as a normal physiologic event in low risk patients.
- Decrease the overuse of technology.
- Avoid elective inductions and manage inductions more effectively. Evidence suggests that elective inductions increase the risk of cesarean delivery by 1.5 to 2.5 times in the healthy nulliparous woman (Johnson, Davis, and Brown, 2003; Vronenraets and others, 2005; Caughey and others, 2006).
- Provide information to obtain a complete informed consent.
- Provide realistic expectations by teaching parents that it is not possible to have a perfect outcome with every pregnancy (Lowe, 2007).
- Consider alternatives to cesarean delivery for breech presentation, such as external version and possible vaginal delivery.
- Consider the time of admission; unless maternal or fetal status indicates, delay admission of low-risk patients until they are dilated 4 cm or more. This policy prevents misdiagnosis of the preparatory status of prelabor versus true labor and thus decreases unnecessary interventions, including cesarean delivery. Instead of admission, encourage ambulation with periods of rest and reevaluate in several hours (DeMott, 2000; Ness, Goldberg, and Berghella, 2004; Lowe, 2007).
- Remember that prolonged latent phase of labor, according to ACOG (2003), is not indicative of dystocia, and failure to progress should not be diagnosed until the cervix has dilated to a least 4 cm (Rouse and others, 2001).
- Use forceps or vacuum delivery carefully, when appropriate (Patel and Murphy, 2004).
- Revise the 2-hour limit for stage two of labor, as recommended by Association of Women's Health, Obstetric, and Neonatal Nurses (Sampselle and others, 2005; Simpson and James, 2005a; AWHONN, 2008), thus allowing the second stage of labor to continue as long as there is progress in descent without fetal compromise (Hansen, Clark, and Foster, 2002).
- When epidural pain management is considered, instruct the patient regarding benefits and associated risks. According to a *Cochrane Review* (Anim-Somuah, Smyth, and Howell, 2005), epidurals are effective in relieving pain, and have no effect on cesarean birth rates or long-term backache. However, they do increase the need for oxytocin augmentation and instrumental delivery, increase the risk of hypotension, the length of second stage labor but not the first stage, and increase both the incidence of intrapartum fever and the incidence of the fetus developing an OP position (Anim-Somuah and others, 2005; Lieberman and others, 2005).

- Use one-to-one labor support, when possible, which has been shown by research to decrease the length of labor, rate of cesarean birth, and the rate of instrument-assisted vaginal delivery (Hodnett and others, 2007).

VBAC is still an appropriate way to decrease the repeat cesarean delivery rate. Both repeat cesarean delivery and VBAC are associated with maternal and fetal risks (ACOG, 2004; Landon, 2008). Uterine rupture is the greatest risk for VBAC but occurs in less than 1% (0.69%) of VBAC attempts (Mozurkewich and Hutton, 2000; Kieser and Baskett, 2002; Landon and others, 2004). Variables that increase the success rate of VBAC are prior vaginal delivery, nonrecurring prior cesarean birth indication, and admission cervical dilation of 4 cm or greater (Landon, 2008). Failed VBAC trial of labor carries the greatest risk for operative complications, hysterectomy, and increased neonatal mortality (Kieser and Baskett, 2002; Chauhan and others, 2003). Factors that increase this risk are need for oxytocin, maternal obesity, gestational age greater than 40 weeks, birth weight greater than 4000 g, and time since prior delivery less than 19 months (ACOG, 2004; Goodall and others, 2005; SOGC, 2005; Poobalan and others, 2009). Multiple cesarean births cause cumulative increased maternal risks (Mankuta and others, 2003). Epidural is safe to use in a VBAC labor (ACOG, 2004). Therefore according to ACOG (2004b), women with a history of one previous low-transverse cesarean may be offered VBAC after discussion of the risks and benefits. Immediate availability of a physician and anesthesia during the trial of labor are essential to the labor care.

To further lower the primary cesarean delivery rate, consideration should be given to external version as an appropriate treatment of a breech presentation. More than 50% of all attempted external versions are successful, with a very small (2%) reversion rate (Grootscholten and others, 2008).

Instrument-assisted delivery with either vacuum extraction or forceps is indicated for shortening second-stage labor caused by factors such as the following (O'Grady, Pope, and Patel, 2000):

- Maternal paralysis
- Heavy motor block epidural
- Indication of fetal stress
- Maternal exhaustion

According to the *Cochrane Review* (Johanson and Menon, 1999), the use of a vacuum extractor as compared with forceps reduces maternal morbidity, but a forceps delivery is less likely to cause newborn cephalohematoma, hyperbilirubinemia, and retinal hemorrhages. A forceps, however, is more likely to cause facial and cranial injuries as well as maternal soft tissue injury.

Dysfunctional Labor Disorders

Significant slowing of any phase of labor should be individually evaluated as to the possible cause or causes. Table 29-1 summarizes the types, possible causes, and suggests evidence-based management plans for each dysfunctional labor pattern.

Fetal Malpresentations

The manner in which the fetus presents also influences the outcome and manner of treatment. Table 29-2 outlines the various fetal malpresentations and the appropriate treatment.

Table 29-2 Fetal Malpresentations

	Occiput Posterior	Face	Brow	Shoulder	Compound Presentation	Breech
Definition	Fetal occiput lies in either right or left posterior quadrant of mother's pelvis	Presenting head completely extended	Presenting head midway between full flexion and extreme extension	Fetal spine lies vertical to mother's spine	One or more fetal art extremities accompany presenting part	Buttocks of fetus present in one of three attitudes: • *Frank:* thighs flexed and legs lie along side fetal body • *Complete:* legs flexed at thighs, allowing feet to present with buttocks • *Footling:* one or both thighs extended and present before buttocks
Presenting part	Occiput	Chin (mentum)	Brow	Scapula		Sacrum
Incidence	10%-25%	0.2%	0.2%	0.33%	0.01%	4%
Diagnosis Leopold maneuver	Patient will often complain of severe back or suprapubic pain; differentiation by Leopold maneuver is difficult	Absence of smooth, flexed spine; prominent extremities and head	No differentiation	Abdomen may look wider than long; head can be palpated on one side of mother's abdomen and buttocks on other	No differentiation	Fetal heart tones heard best above umbilicus; fetal head palpated in upper part of uterus

Vaginal examination	Anterior fontanel can be felt in anterior quadrant of mother's pelvis and posterior fontanel in posterior quadrant	Nose, eyes, and mouth can be felt	Anterior fontanel can be felt in center of cervical opening with eyes on one side	Scapula can be felt or no presenting part reached since it is often high	Fetal extremity felt alongside presenting part	Soft presenting part felt
Treatment	Almost all fetuses rotate spontaneously to anterior position and are delivered vaginally; in 10% that do not rotate completely, rotation usually done with forceps or vacuum extraction	Vaginal delivery if anterior rotation of chin occurs Cesarean delivery if chin is directed posteriorly and progress stops	Vaginal delivery if brow presentation converts by flexion to occiput presentation or extension to face presentation Cesarean delivery if brow presentation persists	Increased risk for cord prolapse with ROM during labor	Vaginal delivery unless cord prolapses or labor fails to progress	Ultrasound scan at 36 weeks to assess amniotic fluid volume, placental site, position of fetal extremities and neck in relation to the umbilical cord External version may be attempted after 37 weeks If external version fails, a planned cesarean birth is recommended by the *Term Breech Trial* (Hannah and others, 2000) and ACOG (2001)

Continued

Table 29-2   Fetal Malpresentations—cont'd

Presenting part Incidence	Occiput 10%-25%	Chin (mentum) 0.2%	Brow 0.2%	Scapula 0.33%	Sacrum 4%
	If posterior position persists without progress, cesarean delivery is done			Cesarean delivery if version fails; external cephalic version can be attempted under very controlled circumstances if placenta previa or FPD not present after 37 weeks	Immediate cesarean delivery if prolapsed cord develops or progress stops	If mother requests, vaginal delivery for a frank or complete breech, with adequate neck flexion, gestational age greater than 36 weeks, and estimated fetal weight between 2000 and 4000 g Vaginal birth increases risk for perinatal mortality and morbidity by 3%

FPD, Fetopelvic disproportion *ROM,* rupture of membranes.

NURSING MANAGEMENT

Prevention

Managing labor by considering all of the 13 Ps is the art and science of labor nursing. The nurse can have a significant positive influence on the progress and outcome of labor when evidence-based clinical practice is followed. More emphasis needs to be on the nursing assessment and therapeutic interventions to facilitate labor and instilling confidence in the laboring patient, and providing support can make a significant difference as outlined under the following section. This is also true for women who have a regional analgesia/anesthesia as well (Bianchi and Adams, 2009). Once pain is managed, these patients have more concerns about the baby's well-being and their labor's progress.

Interventions to Enhance Labor Progress through Each of the Eleven Functional Health Patterns to Decrease Risk for Dystocia, Epidural Anesthesia, and Instrumental Delivery

Health-Perception and Health-Management Pattern

- Assess the woman's risk for dystocia.
- Assess the woman's progress in labor.
- Ask the patient and her coach about their birth plan. Parents have varying needs and expectations of care. As long as it does not affect the health of the mother or baby, to promote and carryout the plan is therapeutic. Birth plans can decrease the family's anxiety and increase their feeling of control while facilitating communication with the health care team (Springer, 1996). However, during the prenatal care, families must be instructed that although a birth plan is a manner in which they sort out what will make their birth experience satisfying, it must be open to change when unexpected events develop (Jannke, 1995).
- Perineal Massage: According to the *Cochrane Review* (Beckmann and Garrett, 2008), perineal massage during pregnancy decreases the likelihood of perineal trauma during delivery. However, no evidence supports its benefit during the second stage of labor (Albers and others, 2005).

Nutritional and Metabolic Pattern (Preconception)

- Educate women about the importance of attaining an appropriate body weight before conception.
- Educate underweight women about the importance of eating appropriate nutritional foods in each of the food groups and avoiding empty-calorie foods that are high in fat and refined sugar, before and during pregnancy. (Being underweight increases the risk for a small-for-gestational-age fetus and preterm labor, which increases the risk for a breech presentation and cesarean delivery.)
- Educate women who are overweight before conception about the importance of a nutritious, weight-control, lifestyle diet change as opposed to an extreme quick weight loss program that usually leads to weight gain and depletes the nutritional stores needed for a healthy pregnancy. Weight reduction is contraindicated

during pregnancy. (Being overweight is related to an increased risk for gestational diabetes and fetal macrosomia, fetal intolerance, prolonged labor and soft tissue dystocia, which increases the risk for cesarean birth.) Less than 15% of women over 300 pounds will be able to deliver vaginally.

- Educate women with diabetes about the importance of achieving normal blood sugar levels before conception and maintaining this control throughout conception with diet, exercise, insulin if needed, and self-monitoring of blood glucose. This decreases the risk for congenital anomalies and a large- or small-for-gestational-age fetus, which increases the risk for a cesarean delivery.

Nutritional and Metabolic Pattern (Intrapartum)

According to the 2007 American Society of Anesthesiologist guidelines for obstetric anesthesia, during labor, allow the patient to drink clear liquids unless there is a medical or obstetric contraindication. According to the guidelines, clear liquids include water, fruit juice without pulp, clear tea, black coffee, and sports drinks. Such fluids can prevent ketosis and promote maternal comfort (Kubli and others, 2002; O'Sullivan, Liu, and Shennan, 2007). During exercise, fasting leads to accelerated fatigue. There is some evidence to suggest that dehydration, ketosis, and fatigue can turn a normal labor into a dysfunctional one in some women (Roberts and Ludka, 1994; Newton and Raynor, 2000; Scheepers and others, 2001).

Because of the rare but possibly devastating consequences of gastric aspiration in the event of general anesthesia, many labor and delivery units have a policy that the laboring patient should take nothing by mouth except sips of water or ice chips. Maternal mortality risk related to aspiration is small, and fasting has not been shown to be an effective preventive strategy. According to an analysis by the British Department of Health following their investigation of two maternal deaths from aspiration, fasting during labor was ineffective in prevention of these deaths (Sharp, 1997). Data from developing countries indicate that a more liberal policy on food and fluids during labor does not result in greater maternal risk (Scheepers and others, 2001; O'Sullivan and others, 2007).

Question a hospital or birthing center labor policy that requires routine use of IV fluids. Ringer's lactate, a non-glucose-based solution, provides no energy. IV dextrose during labor has been shown to increase the risk for hypoglycemia, hyperbilirubinemia, lactic acid, and hyponatremia in the newborn (Hazle, 1986; Ludka and Roberts, 1993; Tourangeau and others, 1999; Enkin and others, 2000). Lactated Ringer's solution has been shown to cause fewer problems if it is used when IV fluids are indicated during labor (Sleutel and Golden, 1999). If dehydrated, intravenous fluid has been shown to shorten labor (Garite and others, 2000; Eslamian, Marsoosi, and Parkneeyat, 2006). If IV fluids are ordered only to keep a vein open, determine whether a heparin lock could be used instead.

If opiate analgesic medication becomes necessary, the patient is at high risk for requiring general anesthesia, or she is experiencing gastric upset, fluids may need to be limited. IV fluids may then be therapeutic. However, there appears to be no association between delayed gastric emptying and epidural opioids (Zimmerman, Breen, and Fick, 1996; Kelly and others, 1997). Intrathecal, spinal, and systemic narcotics decrease gastric emptying.

Elimination Pattern

Encourage the patient to void every 2 hours. A full bladder interferes with fetal descent and may lead to a dysfunctional labor pattern. The sense of a full bladder is depressed related to pressure by the fetus or regional analgesia/anesthesia (Sprague and others, 2006). If a urinary catheter is indicated, intermittent catheterization and continuous Foley catheterization both increase the risk of a urinary tract infection (Rigini and others, 2006).

Activity and Position Pattern

Experimental studies clearly show that position and frequency of position change have a profound effect on uterine activity and efficiency. The maternal pelvic joints are flexible, and the baby's head will mold if given time, decreasing the risk for dystocia.

Antepartum

Educate pregnant women as to the benefits of a consistent, low-impact exercise program, such as walking, swimming, bicycling, or low-impact aerobics. Fitness during pregnancy reduces such discomforts as back pain and fatigue and fosters a more normal labor and delivery (Wong and McKenzie, 1987; Clapp, 1990). Varrassi, Bazzano, and Edwards (1989) found that plasma beta-endorphin levels are elevated in women who exercise during pregnancy as compared with expectant women who do not exercise. A higher endorphin level means a higher pain threshold.

Intrapartum: stage one

During labor, provide opportunities and encourage position changes every 30 minutes. Choice of position change should be based on maternal preference, safety, comfort, effective progress, and knowledge of hemodynamics (Romond and Baker, 1985; Rossi and Lindell, 1986; Fenwick and Simkin, 1987; ACOG, 2003; Ness, Goldberg, and Berghella, 2004). Malpresentations are frequently associated with increased pain. Allowing the mother to obtain a position she finds more comfortable frequently facilitates a favorable fetal rotation by altering the alignment of the presenting part with the pelvis. As the mother continues to change position based on comfort, the optimum presentation is maintained (Ness and others, 2004; Stremler and others, 2005; Ragnar and others, 2006; Ridley, 2007).

Supine positions are avoided because they cause compression of the vena cava and decrease blood return to the heart.

During stage one of labor, the lateral recumbent and upright positions such as 30 degrees upright, kneeling forward, or doing the lunge on a birth ball (Fig. 29-6, *A-F*) increase uterine intensity, shorten the first and second stages of labor, decrease frequency, and decrease vena caval compression (Roberts and others, 1983; McKay and Roberts, 1989; Adachi, Shimada, and Usui, 2003; Bodner-Adler and others, 2003; Ragnar and others, 2006; Terry and others, 2006). Therefore the uterine contractions are more effective because the upright position permits relaxation of the abdominal wall, allowing the fundus to fall forward. This facilitates engagement of the fetal head and descent. As the fetal head is pushed against the cervix, the uterus receives increased stimulation to contract (McKay and Roberts, 1989).

The recumbent and lithotomy positions interfere with labor progress and fetal descent, decrease uterine intensity and frequency, and increase analgesic needs

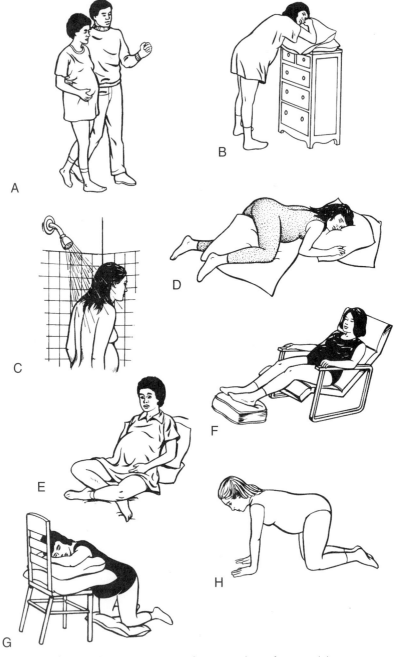

Figure 29-6 Various maternal positions during first-stage labor.

and malpresentation of the fetus (Roberts and others, 1983; Chen and others, 1987; McKay and Roberts, 1989; Wong and others, 2003; AWHONN, 2008). Therefore uterine contractions are not as effective. These positions may cause poor alignment of the fetal presenting part to the pelvic inlet as well (Fenwick and Simkin, 1987).

Intrapartum: occiput posterior presentation

When the fetus is in an occiput posterior presentation, research indicates that both an "all four" or kneeling (Fig. 29-6, *G*) and leaning-forward position (Fig. 29-6, *H*) or the Sim's lateral position on the side same as the fetal spine can facilitate anterior rotation (Stremler and others, 2005; Ridley, 2007). There is an increased risk of developing a fetal malpresentation when regional anesthesia or analgesia is used (Lieberman and others, 2005). If a low concentration of local anesthetic/analgesic lumbar epidural or combined spinal-epidural (CSE) is used, hands-and-knees position is an option (Stremler and others, 2009).

Intrapartum: stage two

Provide care for second-stage labor based on understanding of the two phases of the second stage of labor: (1) *latent phase*, a time to rest when there is a lull in the contractions; (2) *active phase*, when fetal descent takes place facilitated by maternal pushing (Roberts 2002, 2003).

According to the *Cochrane Review Group* (Gupta, Hofmeyr, and Smyth, 2005), comfort, should guide the woman's position, which is usually upright. An upright, slightly curled forward position (Fig. 29-7, *A* and *B*), squatting (Fig. 29-7, *C*), or sitting in bed curled forward (Fig. 29-7, *D-E*) or use the birth ball (Fig. 29-7, *H*) increases satisfaction with the birth experience; decreases the length of second-stage labor, FHR abnormalities, instrument-assisted births, and episiotomies; and decreases pain with only a small increase in second degree perineal tears and blood loss (Adachi and others, 2003; Roberts, 2003; DeJonge, Teunissen, and Lagro-Janssen, 2004; Ragnar and others, 2006). If the woman prefers to be lying down, left or right lateral position is preferable (Fig. 29-7, *F* and *G*) (Simpson and James, 2005b).

Squatting is the best upright position and can be achieved by using the squatting bar (Fig. 29-7, *C*). Squatting increases the pelvis size 0.5 to 2.0 cm (Fenwick and Simkin, 1987; Golay, Vedam, and Sorger, 1993). Squatting may increase the bearing-down sensation and enhance effective pushing as well (Kurokawa and Zilkoski, 1985). Therefore it has been shown to shorten second-stage labor, lessen the need for oxytocin, decrease the need for mechanical-assisted deliveries, and decrease the need for episiotomy (Bodner-Adler and others, 2003; Downe, Gerrett, and Renfrew, 2004; Roberts and others, 2005; Schiessl and others, 2005; Ragnar and others, 2006), while improving fetal oxygenation (Simpson and James, 2005b).

Positions that are best avoided:

- The reclining-back, sitting position puts pressure on the sacrum, restricting posterior movement and reducing the pelvic size (Fig. 29-7, *E*) (Fenwick and Simkin, 1987; Paciornik, 1990).
- The supine position during the second stage of labor because in this position, gravity works against the woman's pushing efforts (Fenwick and Simkin, 1987; Johnson, Johnson, and Gupta, 1991). Also, this position has been shown to decrease fetal artery pH (Johnstone, Aboelmagd, and Harouny, 1987).

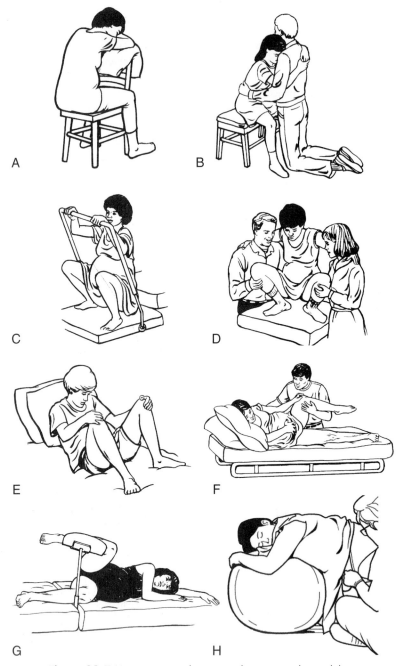

Figure 29-7 Various maternal positions during second-stage labor.

- There is an increased risk of spine and lower extremity injury as well as perineal lacerations with the use of the lithotomy position during pushing (Wong and others, 2003; Simpson and James, 2005a).

Positions for regional analgesia and anesthesia

Mobility is limited to various degrees related to the type of regional analgesia/anesthesia used. Position change and upright positions are possible and promote fetal rotation and descent, especially if a low concentration of local anesthetic lumbar epidural or combined spinal-epidural (CSE) with an opioid is used. Assist the patient in changing positions or adopting an upright position to facilitate progress based on her preference and assessed ability to assume different positions (Gilder and others, 2002; Mayberry and others, 2003). Two effective upright positions for women with epidurals presented by Bianchi and Adams (2009) are modified squatting using a squatting bar and towel pull when assuming a semi-reclining or squatting position. The towel pull encourages use of the abdominal muscles and assists with effective pushing.

Research in Arizona is in progress to determine the benefit of a peanut-shaped ball used between the legs to promote increased pelvic dimension if the mother needs to be in a Sims' lateral position related to the level of anesthesia. Other indications for Sims' lateral position are a rapid second stage labor when less bearing-down force is needed to help control the speed of delivery and decrease the risk for perineal laceration (Albers, 2003; Simkin and Bolding, 2004) or occiput posterior fetal presentation to encourage rotation (Stremler and others, 2005; Ridley, 2007).

Pushing methods

Encourage the woman to push in response to her body's urges (spontaneous, open glottis pushing) for 6 to 8 seconds; repeating this pattern for three to four times during each contraction. Discourage sustained bearing-down efforts, prolonged breath-holding, and counting to 10 (Sampselle and others, 2005; Simpson and James, 2005a; Bloom and others, 2006; Roberts and Hanson, 2007; AWHONN, 2008; Brancato, Church, and Stone, 2008). This type of pushing initiated by the woman in response to an irresistible sensation (Ferguson reflex) is usually accompanied by expiratory grunting or vocalization and is less fatiguing to the mother and has less effect on umbilical cord blood gases (Nordstrom and others, 2001; Sampselle and others, 2005; Simpson and James, 2005a). The patient with a regional anesthesia/analgesia may not feel this reflex but can be encouraged to push in this manner. Sustained, breath-holding bearing down can impose a hypoxic environment for the fetus and increase the risk for perineal trauma (Roberts and others, 2004; Bloom and others, 2006; Bianchi and Adams, 2009).

When to initiate pushing

Active pushing should be initiated when the cervix is fully dilated, the fetal head is rotating to transverse or anterior position, and station is at least one. Manage complete dilation before fetal rotation and descent by encouraging *laboring down*, meaning rest without active pushing until fetal rotation and descent has occurred (Hansen and others, 2002; Mayberry, Clemmens, and De, 2002; AWHONN, 2008). At this time, the mother may feel the urge to push, which is the result of the presenting part stimulating the stretch receptors of the pelvic floor (Roberts and others, 2004). However, if regional analgesia or anesthesia has blocked the urge to push, this can be determined by assessing fetal position and station by vaginal examination. The positive benefits of delayed pushing are fewer operative vaginal births, fewer episiotomies, fewer perineal lacerations, less fatigue, less active pushing time, and improved fetal oxygen saturation (Hansen and others, 2002; Simpson and James, 2005b).

Manage the urge to push before full dilation by assessing if (1) cervix is dilated 8 to 9 cm, (2) cervix is soft and retracting with contractions, (3) fetal head is rotating to transverse or anterior position, and (4) station is at least one. Then allow the patient to push at the peak of the contraction if she is experiencing an irresistible urge to push (Roberts and Woolley, 1996; Vause, Congdon, and Thornton, 1998; Fraser and others, 2000; Petrou, Coyle, and Fraser, 2000).

Length of second stage of labor

An arbitrary time limit such as 2 hours for the length of the second stage of labor is discouraged, as long as there is evidence of fetal descent and reassuring fetal heart rate (ACOG, 2003; Cheng, Hopkins, and Caughey, 2004; AWHONN, 2008). According to ACOG (2000), instrumental vaginal delivery may be indicated for nulliparous women without regional anesthesia when there is lack of fetal descent for 2 hours or 3 hours in nulliparous women with regional anesthesia. For multiparous women, an evaluation is recommended when there is lack of fetal descent for 1 hour without regional anesthesia or 2 hours with regional anesthesia (AWHONN, 2008).

Rest and Relaxation Pattern

Encourage use of visualization, patterned breathing, attention focusing, quiet voice, and music in active labor. These stimuli affect the thalamus in the brain and influence the limbic system, which governs emotional responses as well as inhibition of pain transmission (Simkin, 1987; Di Franco, 1988; Pugh and others, 1998; Hottenstein and Brit Pipe, 2005). The limbic system has been shown to increase pain tolerance by reducing anxiety, decreasing catecholamine response, and decreasing muscle tension. It enhances blood flow to the uterus as well (Watson, 1999).

According to a *Cochrane Review* (Laopaiboon and others, 2009), music played during a cesarean delivery under regional anesthesia may increase patient satisfaction with the birth.

Cognitive Pattern

- If involved with childbirth education, provide not only realistic information about the birth process, but also activities that will instill confidence to control pain and deal with childbirth-related fears.
- Assess the patient's and her coach's understanding of labor, delivery, and effective tools. Determine which childbirth education method the couple plans to use, if any.
- Provide honest, ongoing information during the birth experience to lessen stress and improve satisfaction (Bowers, 2002; Nerum and others, 2006). Health care consumers need to be reassured that labor is progressing safely and within normal parameters.
- Fill in the patient and coach's knowledge gaps between contractions.
- Teach the patient and coach to pace themselves as if in a race, and not to use all their tools at first.

- Keep the patient and her coach informed of the progress.
- Allow participation in decision making, and encourage questions.

Perceptual Pattern

- Assess the patient's level of pain, location of pain, and degree of coping or level of comfort. An algorithm to assess how effective the laboring patient is coping with her pain has been found to be more effective than a 10-point scale. Both non-pharmacologic and pharmacologic coping methods can be evaluated in this manner. Verbal as well as non-verbal clues are used in the pain assessment algorithm (Gulliver, Fisher, and Roberts, 2008).
- Assess for other variables that may cause discomfort, such as leg cramps or back discomfort.
- Assess how the patient and her coach feel they should respond to pain because of any cultural or personal values.
- Support the mother in her choice of pain management.
- Epidural analgesia is an effective and commonly preferred pain relief method. Another regional analgesic/anesthetic form of pain management is intrathecal narcotics (injection of narcotics into the subarachnoid space) or a CSE. As with all procedures, there are accompanying risks that should be discussed regarding any regional analgesic/anesthetic form of pain management with the expectant mother, ideally during a prenatal visit. Refer to the section later in this chapter on management of intrapartum epidural and combined spinal-epidural analgesia/anesthesia. Regional analgesics/anesthetics may increase the incidence of oxytocin use, instrumental delivery, episiotomy and antibiotic use because of fever (Newman, Lindsay, and Graves, 2001; Goetzl and others, 2003; Anim-Somuah and others, 2005).
- Encourage appropriate comfort measures no matter what method of pain relief is chosen.
- Provide back rubs and counterpressure for back labor.
- Apply cool washcloth to the forehead if feeling hot or nauseated.
- Offer hydrotherapy through baths and showers. This activates body-wide tactile receptors, which transport pleasant stimuli over the pathways that pain stimuli must travel, thus closing the gate to pain and reversing the fight-or-flight responses that frequently occur during labor while increasing uterine activity (Simkin, 1995).
- Suggest a whirlpool bath. According to the *Cochrane Review* (Cluett and Burns, 2008), this decreases analgesia needs and the rate of instrument-assisted delivery while enhancing maternal satisfaction and confidence with no increased risk for infection. However, it is contraindicated in the presence of thick meconium, oxytocin infusion, bleeding, or heavy bloody show (Rush and others, 1996). No conclusive evidence can be made related to limited research at this time (Cluett and Burns, 2008), but no significant adverse affects have been detected.
- Apply superficial heat and cold with packs, which activate local tactile receptors, thus closing the gate to some pain stimuli.
- Offer massage, which facilitates relaxation and bombards the brain with another stimulus, decreasing the amount of pain sensation being perceived.

- Provide acupressure at acupoints. This facilitates pain control when done by a professional trained in acupressure. One example is to apply intense pressure during contractions by wrapping four fingers around the balls of the feet, the quarter-moon area from the place where the toes join the foot to the furthest end of the ball of the foot (Stephens, 1997). Cook and Wilcox (1997) and Gentz (2001) provided more acupoints that can be located by trained labor nurses.
- Allow self-hypnosis; research suggests it is effective in lessening the pain of labor (Cyna, McAuliffe, and Andrews, 2004; Brown and Hammond, 2007).
- Apply double hip squeeze, knee press, and counterpressure. These can decrease back pain (Simkin, 1995).
- Encourage moaning because it decreases pain and medication need by releasing endorphins (Threlfall-Mase, 1997).
- Provide lip balm for dry lips, and keep the linen clean and dry to decrease extraneous uncomfortable sensations, thereby reducing the total amount of pain experienced.
- Provide effleurage of the abdomen to promote relaxation of the abdominal muscle, allowing the uterine muscle to be unrestrained.
- Allow the use of transcutaneous electrical nerve stimulation (TENS) in labor if the patient believes it will be helpful, according to a *Cochrane Review* (Dowswell and others, 2009). TENS is thought to stimulate peripheral nerve endings, thereby decreasing the transmission of painful impulses and stimulating the production of natural endorphins.
- Alleviate leg cramps by stretching the cramping muscle instead of massaging it.
- Value the doula, if present, as an important member of the health care team.
- Keep the patient clean and dry to promote comfort and decrease infection risk.
- Portray to her a deep sense of empathy and caring that transmits confidence so that she is enabled to trust her own body and relax more completely (Bianchi and Adams, 2009).
- Help her use appropriate techniques so that her need for anesthesia or analgesia is less.
- Know when pharmacologic interventions are needed and use them effectively.
- Administer narcotic analgesic, narcotic agonist-antagonist, or analgesic potentiates during the peak of a contraction and titrate them to desired effects, not a specific dose.

Self-Perception and Self-Concept Pattern

To give the woman more control over labor practices, treating with respect and affirmation, providing positive encouragement, and supporting the woman's natural abilities is the art of nursing that empowers the laboring woman to give birth, decreasing dystocia and improving satisfaction with the birth experience (Jackson and others, 2003; Matthews and Callister, 2004; Sampselle and others, 2005).

Role-Relationship Pattern

- Assess role expectations of all participants during the birth process.
- Assess economic needs and concerns.
- Assess cultural practices that influence the various roles of the participants.

- Promote family members' involvement, according to their birth plan, if possible.
- Provide therapeutic interventions for the support person or persons by evaluating their comfort in the labor situation, orienting them to the environment and equipment being used, asking whether they have any special requests, acknowledging their physical and psychological needs, providing times for nutritional snacks, encouraging them to actively participate, and providing a welcome environment.

Coping and Stress-Tolerance Pattern

Continuous professional labor support is an important function of the intrapartum nurse in improving both the patient's coping and satisfaction (Miltner, 2000; Jackson and others, 2003; Campbell and others, 2006; Hodnett and others, 2007) and is probably the most important aspect of effective care (ACOG, 2003). According to the *Cochrane Review* (Hodnett and others, 2007), the Cochrane Pregnancy and Childbirth Group (Enkin and others, 2000), and AWHONN (2008), continuous labor support has been demonstrated to shorten labors, decrease the need for analgesia and anesthesia, reduce the cesarean birth rate, reduce the rate of instrumental deliveries, reduce the need for oxytocin, decrease oxytocin use, and decrease the number of infants with Apgar scores lower than 7 at 5 minutes. Maternal labor satisfaction is also increased.

There are four dimensions to labor support: emotional, instructional or informational support, physical comfort, and advocacy in decision making (Bowers, 2002; Bianchi and Adams, 2004; Sauls, 2006). According to the survey results from *Listening to Mothers II,* women report a more positive labor and delivery experience when their needs are met through supportive care (Declercq and others, 2006). Classes to certify nurses in labor support as they do in EFM are worthwhile for patient and nurse satisfaction.

Interventions to Accomplish Early Detection and Treatment of Dysfunctional Labor

- Determine onset of true labor.
- Evaluate the uterine contraction pattern every 30 to 60 minutes, or more often if needed, for frequency, duration, intensity, and resting tone.
- Assess state of cervix as to soft or hard, effaced or long, dilatable or resistant, and amount of dilation as indicated (depending on phase of labor). Use the Bishop system or a comparable scoring system.
- Assess fetal position, station, and status of the presenting part.
- Assess for a malpresentation by doing the Leopold maneuver to help decide maternal positioning.
- Evaluate the woman's labor progress in active labor through observation and periodic vaginal exams.
- Assess for discomfort and tension.
- Assess for signs of dehydration and electrolyte imbalance.
- Assess for signs of hypoglycemia. A prolonged difficult labor depletes the mother's energy and glucose stores.
- Encourage patient to void every 1 to 2 hours.

- Catheterize for distended bladder if unable to void.
- Encourage patient to verbalize anxieties and fears.
- Encourage patient to try various position changes to facilitate labor progress (see Figs. 29-6 and 29-7).
- Monitor for effective use of breathing and relaxation techniques.
- Provide continuous support. Be supportive of coping methods and provide help with new ones as needed.
- Provide support to the labor coach.
- Encourage rest between contractions.
- If labor begins to progress slower than normal, encourage ambulation and alternative positioning if not contraindicated.
- Be prepared to administer a labor stimulant as ordered (see Chapter 27).
- If it is necessary to withhold analgesia or anesthesia, explain the need to the patient and her coach.
- Keep the attending physician informed of labor progress.
- If a dysfunctional labor pattern develops, outline the treatment plan so that the patient and her coach are prepared for what might occur. Stress the normalcy of patient's physiologic response to labor.

Management of Shoulder Dystocia

- Be familiar with the management plan of shoulder dystocia. Shoulder dystocia is unpredictable (Nocon, 2000; Minkin, 2004), and there are no reliable indicators according to research. It is often suspected in macrosomia, but the majority of the time when shoulder dystocia occurs, the fetus weighs less than 4000 g (Ouzounian and Gherman, 2005).
- Assess labor progress closely and use the squatting method when appropriate to increase pelvic capacity.
- An early indication of shoulder dystocia is when the fetal head retracts against the mother's perineum as soon as the head is delivered (Baxley and Gobbo, 2004). The most common risk factor for shoulder dystocia is instrumental delivery (ACOG, 2002).
- When shoulder dystocia is diagnosed, the nurse can be prepared to assist by staying calm and calling for added assistance (an anesthesiologist or nurse anesthetist and a pediatrician or intensive care nursing team).
- Be prepared to catheterize the patient to ensure a completely emptied bladder.
- Be prepared to assist in the recommended shoulder dystocia manipulations as the health care provider instructs. Refer to Table 29-3 for various sequential maneuvers. Initially the head of the bed is lowered, the end of the bed is removed, and the patient's legs are elevated and pulled back to tilt the pelvis (McRoberts maneuver).
- Fundal pressure alone is to be avoided because of the potential neurologic complications (Nocon, 2000; Simpson and Knox, 2001; Minkin, 2004).
- Superpubic pressure may be applied over the fetal shoulder.
- Be prepared to assist the patient to roll to all-fours (on her hands and knees) position if instructed. This is believed to increase pelvic size and make use of the forces of gravity (Bruner and others, 1998; Jukelevics, 2000).

Table 29-3   Sequential Shoulder Dystocia Maneuvers

Name	Benefits and Risks	Maneuver
McRoberts maneuver (Fig. 29-8)	Noninvasive; safe Straightens sacrum and decreases angle of incline of symphysis pubis Dislodges impacted shoulder 90% of time (Gonik, Allen, and Sorab, 1989)	Assist by grasping mother's posterior thighs and flexing them against her abdomen Fundal pressure is usually inappropriate because it may further affect anterior shoulder against symphysis pubis and increase risk of a brachial plexus injury (Gonik and others, 1989; Gherman and Goodwin, 1998; Simpson and Knox, 2001)
Suprapubic pressure (Figs. 29-9 and 29-10)	Noninvasive Second maneuver to be used because it may cause a clavicular fracture	Assist by exerting firm downward or oblique pressure on anterior shoulder just above symphysis pubis Instruct mother to push during this maneuver
Woods screw maneuver (Fig. 29-11)	Invasive technique Thought to attempt to unscrew fetus like a bolt is unscrewed from a nut (Horger, 1995)	Health care deliverer intravaginally applies pressure against posterior shoulder, rotating it to an anterior position Health care deliverer may request suprapubic pressure during maneuver to help keep anterior shoulder adducted (Naef and Martin, 1995)
Rubin rotational maneuver or reverse Woods screw maneuver (Fig. 29-12)	Invasive technique	Health care deliverer intravaginally applies pressure against scapula of anterior shoulder and rotates it forward 180° Health care deliverer may request suprapubic pressure during maneuver to help keep anterior shoulder adducted (O'Leary, 1992)
Delivery of posterior arm (Fig. 29-13)	Invasive Requires a large episiotomy Risk of humerus fracture	Health care deliverer intravaginally applies pressure at antecubital fossa, which causes fetal arm to flex, at which time it is grasped and drawn across chest and toward opposite side of fetal face
Cephalic replacement	Last resort	Health care deliverer returns fetal head to maternal pelvis, followed by an emergency cesarean birth

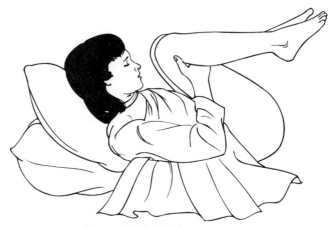

Figure 29-8 McRoberts maneuver.

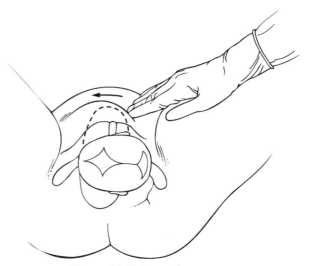

Figure 29-9 Suprapubic pressure.

- Document the event carefully.
- Following the delivery, assess the baby's Moro reflex, check for a fractured clavicle or humerus, and if ordered, obtain cord blood for pH. A complete symmetric Moro response usually indicates no brachial plexus injury, which is the most common serious resulting injury (Benedetti, 1991; Nocon, 2000). Increased intracranial pressure and hypoxia occur less often.
- If an injury occurred, be prepared to discuss the possible outcomes with the parents after the pediatrician has spoken with them. Approximately 80% of these injuries resolve and cause no permanent damage with appropriate treatment (Baxley and Gobbo, 2004).

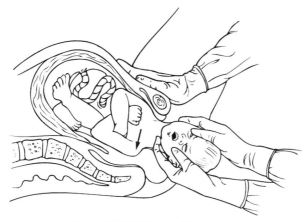

Figure 29-10 Suprapubic pressure.

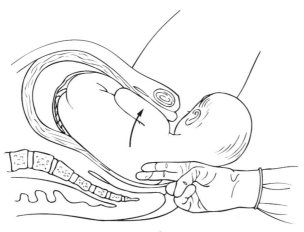

Figure 29-11 Woods screw maneuver.

- Assess for postpartum hemorrhage because this is the greatest risk to the mother from a shoulder dystocia. The hemorrhage is usually related to uterine atony or vaginal or cervical lacerations (Gherman, 2006). Other maternal trauma can include bladder injury, vaginal hematoma, uterine rupture, or endometritis.
- A shoulder dystocia drill is an ideal way to prepare for this emergency (Curtis and Guillien, 2009).

Management of External Version

Preprocedural

- Evaluate the patient's and her coach's understanding of the procedure. Greater than 50% of all attempted external versions are successful with a very low reversion rate (Grootscholten and others, 2008).

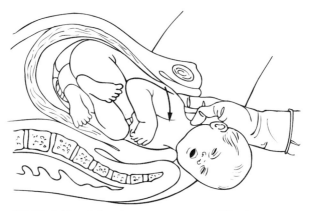

Figure 29-12 Rubin rotational maneuver or reverse Woods screw maneuver.

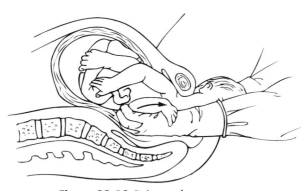

Figure 29-13 Delivery of posterior arm.

- Evaluate the patient's and her coach's understanding of the advantage and the risks of version. The advantage is decreased cesarean birth rate. Potential risks include failed version, reversion, fetal stress related to cord entanglement/prolapse or abruption, ruptured uterus, and abruptio placentae (Grootscholten and others, 2008).
- Various alternatives to version have been discussed. Postural exercises, visualization, and taped music or voices, and assuming an upright, forward leaning position at times during the day and sleeping with pillows behind the back and the top leg resting forward may facilitate occiput anterior (OA) fetal presentation (Sutton and Scott, 1996; Founds, 2005). Music played on the lower abdomen has been proposed to encourage the baby to turn. Without any random controlled trial studies, the effectiveness of these alternative practices is unknown (Hunter, Hofmeyr, and Kulier, 2007). Moxibustion, a form of Chinese medicine that involves burning herbs close to the skin, has shown some possibility of converting a breech presentation to cephalic. According to a *Cochrane Review*, further study is needed (Coyle, Smith, and Peat, 2005).

- Advise the parents that even if the version is successful, the fetus is more likely to develop signs of fetal stress during labor and there is a greater risk for labor dystocia and need for a cesarean delivery (Thorp, 2009). This may be related to factors that caused the fetus to present breech.

Intraprocedural

- Obtain a baseline FHR strip for 15 to 30 minutes before the procedure.
- Assist with a preliminary ultrasound examination to locate placenta, fetal lie, estimated size, volume of amniotic fluid, and presence of fetal anomalies. In the presence of a nuchal cord, version is not attempted.
- Start an IV infusion, as ordered, with an 18-gauge intracatheter.
- Be prepared to administer piggyback tocolytic agent before and continuously throughout the procedure. The solution usually is prepared in the same manner and concentration as that used for tocolysis in premature labor (see Chapter 23). Tocolytics have been shown to improve success (Hofmeyr and Gyte, 2004).
- Monitor the FHR every few minutes during the procedure with a Doppler instrument.
- If fetal compromise develops, be prepared to assist with an emergency cesarean delivery.

Postprocedural

- After the procedure, discontinue the tocolytic agent and reapply FHR and contraction monitors. Monitor FHR and uterine contraction pattern approximately 30 to 60 minutes after the version.
- Be prepared to administer Rh_o (D) immune globulin (RhoGAM; HypRho-D) following the procedure if the mother is RhD-negative.

Intrapartum Care

- Consider the patient high risk and monitor carefully for dystocia and fetal stress following a version.

Antepartum Management of Vaginal Birth after Cesarean (VBAC)

- Discuss the risks and benefits of a VBAC with every pregnant woman who had a previous lower segment transverse incision cesarean delivery to attempt a vaginal delivery (ACOG, 2004b; Dodd and Crowther, 2006; Montgomery and Emmett, 2007).
- Teach the pregnant woman who had prior cesarean delivery and her family early in the current pregnancy regarding the positive chances of a vaginal delivery (70% to 75%) (Landon and others, 2005).
- Help the woman and her partner weigh their options, identify the reasons for their choice, and then support their choice (Roberts and others, 1997; Zwelling, 2001; ACOG, 2004b).
- Participate in the formation of support groups and childbirth classes for couples planning a VBAC.

- Be involved with childbirth education training to increase childbirth educators' awareness and knowledge regarding VBAC; emphasize the importance of appropriate adequate nutrition; and improve the outcome of the pregnancy, labor, and delivery.

Intrapartum Management of Vaginal Birth after Cesarean—Trial of Labor

- Note that VBAC-TOL standards are to include an available physician immediately and to respond to acute emergency by performing a cesarean within a short time (ACOG, 2004b).
- Individualize the management of care based on a family assessment of physical and psychologic factors.
- Determine the family's birth plan for vaginal delivery and a contingency plan in the event that complications arise.
- Use effective physiologic techniques for promoting labor.
- Use effective psychologic techniques to promote labor. Determine first what the family's perception of the previous cesarean birth experience is, their concerns, and their expectations. Determine whether their expectations of themselves are realistic. It is important to prevent the patient from feeling like she failed or is less of a woman if she is unable to deliver vaginally.
- Evaluate the terminology used, such as "successful VBAC" or "failed trial of labor," when talking to the patient and her family.
- Assess FHR according to ACOG's standard of practice for a normal labor patient (see Chapter 3).
- Create IV access and make blood products available if that is the protocol for the institution and the status of the patient requires it.
- Assess for signs of scar separation. The most common sign is a variable FHR deceleration that evolves into a late deceleration or bradycardia and blood-stained amniotic fluid (ICSI, 2009). Other less common signs are hematuria, vaginal bleeding, alterations in uterine contractions, and abdominal pain that continues between contractions.
- Use epidural anesthesia, if needed; it has not been found to be contraindicated (ACOG, 2004a; ICSI, 2009).
- Notify the attending physician immediately of any signs of fetal compromise or uterine scar separation.
- Use a labor stimulant if there is an obstetric indication for it; it is not contraindicated, as once thought, in the patient attempting a VBAC. Close monitoring, however, is important to prevent tachysystole, which can increase the risk for uterine rupture (ACOG, 2004b; ICEA, 2009). Because of the increased risk for uterine rupture with sequential prostaglandin-oxytocin use, the combination is not recommended (Macones and others, 2005). Intracervical Foley bulb catheter ripening method does not stimulate uterine contractions; therefore, this method carries less risk of uterine rupture (ICSI, 2009).
- Progress of labor during the trial of labor should progress according to the norm of 1 cm/hr in active labor and second-stage labor not to last longer than 2 hours. A delay indicates a more aggressive intervention than for a normal low risk patient (Gee, 2000, 2006).

- Repeat cesarean may become necessary for failure to progress, fetal distress, maternal complication, or uterine rupture.

Management of Instrumental Delivery with Forceps or a Vacuum Extractor

- Promote preventive nursing management during labor to lower the need for assisted vaginal delivery. This includes the following:
  - Provide continuous labor support.
  - Encourage use of the upright position.
  - Encourage delay in initiating pushing during second-stage labor unless there is an urge to push (Cargill and others, 2004).
  - Revise the 2-hour limit for stage two to longer if there is no indication of fetal stress.
  - Epidural anesthesia/analgesia increases the frequency of instrument-assisted delivery (Thorp and Breedlove, 1996; Anim-Somuah and others, 2005) related to the degree of impaired motor mobility and abnormal fetal position. Combined local anesthetics and narcotics in the epidural provide excellent pain control with less motor blockade. The more mobile the laboring patient can be, the less likely she is to need an instrument-assisted delivery.
  - When delayed progress in second stage or decreased head rotation is noted, (1) encourage the patient to try various positions such as "all fours" or modified squatting making adjustments based on her mobility, (2) check for maternal hydration, (3) check for a full bladder, and (4) assess pushing techniques, to decrease the need for forceps or vacuum use (Bianchi and Adams, 2009).
- Provide educational opportunities for expectant parents to learn about the technique of forceps or vacuum extraction and reasons for their use to decrease anxiety in the event either is needed. The most common reasons for instrument use are delayed progress in second-stage labor, a nonreassuring FHR pattern in late second-stage labor, or medical factors prohibiting effective maternal pushing.
- Provide supportive care in the event that instrument assistance is needed by encouraging the mother to remain active in the birth process by continuing to push with each contraction unless there is a medical contraindication.
- Encourage the patient to continue to feel in control by verbally reassuring her that she is continuing to facilitate the delivery by her pushing efforts.
- Assist with appropriate anesthesia for forceps delivery. Anesthesia may not be necessary for a vacuum extraction.
- Following the delivery, encourage parents to express their feelings about the procedure to resolve any negative feelings.
- Following forceps delivery, observe the infant for facial nerve trauma, ecchymoses, and forceps marks. Assure the parents that these are only temporary effects and tell them when they can expect them to disappear. Other more serious birth injuries may include brachial plexus injury, intracranial hemorrhage, or spinal cord injury. The risk is lowest with low-outlet forceps and increases with midforceps deliveries.

- After a vacuum delivery, assess the infant for caput succedaneum or cephalohematoma. If either is present, reassure the parents that it usually disappears in 3 to 5 days. After a cephalohematoma, teach the parents to observe their infant for hyperbilirubinemia, signs of infection, and cerebral irritation and to report any signs to their pediatrician. Discuss signs of cerebral irritation: vomiting, high-pitched cry, and neck and spine rigidity.
- Assess for a clavicle fracture during the infant's routine physical examination. Positive findings are edema, crepitus, and lack of movement of the affected limb.
- After an instrumental delivery, observe the mother for soft tissue trauma such as birth canal and perineal lacerations, bladder dysfunction, and vaginal hematoma (Evans and Edelstone, 2000; Gimovsky and Han, 2007).
- If the neonate is sleepy and sucks poorly, explain to the parents that this is a normal response following a difficult delivery and does not indicate any problem.

Management of Intrapartum Epidural or Combined Spinal/Epidural (CSE)

Preprocedural

- Ensure an informed consent by providing information, preferably before labor, regarding the procedural steps of administration, maternal and fetal risks and benefits, implications for their labor, and alternative methods of pain relief. According to the *Cochrane Review* (Anim-Somuah and others, 2005), epidural anesthesia is the most highly effective method of pain relief for labor and delivery but it is not without potentially adverse side effects.
- Intrapartum regional analgesia can be provided as an epidural or a combined spinal-epidural (CSE). With an epidural, high concentrations of local anesthetic drugs or combined low-dose local anesthetic drugs with opioid drugs are used depending on the level of the sensory block required. Currently the combined low-dose epidural is most commonly used during labor to facilitate maternal mobility and perception of fetal descent decreasing the risk of instrumental vaginal births.
- According to the *Cochrane Review* by Simmons and others (2007), both the low-dose epidural and CSE are similar in relation to patient satisfaction, mobility level, risk to postdural puncture headache, obstetric outcome, and neonatal outcome. However, when compared with a low-dose epidural, CSE has a slightly faster pain relief onset but has an increased risk of pruritus, urinary retention, and the need for rescue interventions.
- Potential side effects of regional analgesia are hypotension and increased length of first and second stages of a normal labor, increasing the need for oxytocin. They may also decrease the bearing-down reflex, thereby increasing the need for episiotomy or forceps or vacuum extraction. There is an increased incidence of maternal fever as well (Newman and others, 2001; Alexander and others, 2002; Goetzl and others, 2003; Anim-Somuah and others, 2005). Other rare side effects are local anesthetic toxicity, allergic reaction, high or total spinal anesthesia, and spinal headache.

- When an opioid is used, the effects on the newborn include short-term respiratory depression and drowsiness. These effects have been shown to interfere with the newborn's spontaneous breastseeking and breastfeeding behaviors (Ransjo-Arvidson and others, 2001; Baumgarder and others, 2003).
- Provide information regarding other medical interventions that often accompany use of regional analgesia. Those that are always necessary include IV therapy, continuous FHR monitoring, and frequent blood pressure monitoring. Medical interventions that are frequently needed are oxytocin to augment labor contractions and urinary catheterization.
- Intravenous access should always be available. Preloading and maintenance fluid infusion need not be routinely administered unless a high-dose epidural block is being used. According to a *Cochrane Review*, there is a reduced need for preloading when low-dose epidural and CSE analgesia are used (Hofmeyr, Cyna, and Middleton, 2004).
- Obtain baseline maternal vital signs and an FHR tracing.
- Have the patient empty her bladder just before the procedure.
- Prepare emergency equipment at the bedside, such as oxygen and suction equipment.
- Make sure that a resuscitation bag and mask and resuscitation drugs are readily available (AWHONN, 2007).

Procedure

- Position the patient in either a lateral or a sitting position, with the head and hips flexed and shoulders and hips squared to facilitate the insertion by a licensed anesthesia provider (AWHONN, 2001).
- Provide ongoing emotional support and information to the patient.

Postinjection

- Position the patient on her side with the head of the bed elevated 30 degrees. Encourage a position change at least every 30 minutes.
- According to AWHONN (2007), the role of the registered nurse is to monitor the laboring patient with a regional analgesia/anesthesia, replace empty infusion containers with new pre-filled solutions containing the same medication and concentration, and discontinue the infusion if a safety concern arises or following the delivery of the placenta.
- Monitoring should include:
  - Check ongoing perception of pain control and level of sensory block.
  - Continuously monitor FHR.
  - Check for signs of respiratory depression related to a high spinal when anesthesia rises too high resulting in paralysis of the respiratory muscles and diaphragm (C3-C5).
  - Check blood pressure per institutional policy until delivery, because maternal hypotension can occur, resulting from vasodilatation. If hypotension develops, turn the patient on her left side, elevate her legs, increase the IV fluid, administer oxygen, notify the anesthesiologist or nurse anesthetist, and be prepared to administer ephedrine if ordered.

- Assess the patient's temperature.
- Keep an accurate intake and output record. Encourage the laboring patient to void every 2 to 4 hours. (Regional anesthesia blocks sensations of a full bladder.)
  - Assess for other side effects, such as toxicity to the drugs, breakthrough pain, and dural puncture, which can cause a postdural headache.
- Encourage position change at least every 30 minutes, to move, and adopt whatever upright positions are comfortable (NHS, 2007; AWHONN, 2008).
- If ambulatory epidural or intrathecal analgesia is used, evaluate for ambulation safety that includes no postural hypotension, normal leg strength as demonstrated by performance of a partial knee bend while standing, and assistance with ambulation at all times.
- Delay pushing after full dilation if fetal descent is less than +1 and there is a lack of the Ferguson or bearing-down reflex. This delay will lower the need for instrumental deliveries (Hansen and others, 2002; Simpson and James, 2005b).

Management of Postpartum Epidural Analgesia

Preprocedural

- Evaluate the patient's understanding of postpartum epidural analgesia if it is to be used in the event of a cesarean birth or fourth-degree laceration during vaginal delivery. The usual procedure is 4 or 5 mg of morphine analgesic injected through the epidural catheter at the close of the surgical repair. Maternal benefits include prolonged pain relief for 24 hours, ambulation, interaction with infant with minimal discomfort, and earlier recovery. Some patients experience side effects of respiratory depression, itching, nausea, vomiting, or urinary retention, but these side effects are generally mild.
- Assist in obtaining an informed consent.

Postprocedural

- Assess respiratory rate often. A typical assessment routine may be every 15 minutes for 2 hours, every 30 minutes for 6 hours (total of 8 hours after injection), and every 1 hour for 16 hours (total of 24 hours after injection).
- Assess for itching and nausea or vomiting per observational check while the patient is awake.
- Keep accurate intake and output record.
- If a Foley catheter is present, do not remove it for 14 to 16 hours after delivery. If urinary retention occurs, it usually develops early and is resolved by 14 to 16 hours after administration of medication.
- Be prepared to administer naloxone (Narcan), 0.04 to 0.40 mg, as ordered, if side effects develop.
- A low naloxone dose of 0.04 mg frequently alleviates mild side effects and does not diminish the analgesic effect.
- Notify the physician of the development of side effects and responsiveness to ordered treatment.

Management of Cesarean Birth

Preoperative

In accordance with *Healthy People 2010* objectives (USDHHS, 2000), decrease the incidence of primary cesarean delivery among low risk full-term singleton vertex presentations by maintaining a positive attitude toward the laboring woman, supporting normal physiologic processes of labor, and implementing a variety of nonpharmacologic nursing interventions. (See nursing diagnosis on interventions to enhance labor progress through each of the 11 functional health patterns.)

- Be prepared to ethically manage the family that refuses a cesarean delivery in the presence of fetal or maternal medical indicators and the family that demands a cesarean without any medical indication. To be a patient advocate, be prepared to discuss the short- and long-term risks and benefits to assist the patient in making an informed choice. The most common cited benefit for elective cesarean is prevention of pelvic floor disorders; however, the systematic review of the current research does not statistically support this benefit (Williams, 2008; Wohlrab and Rardin, 2008).
- If cesarean delivery becomes medically or obstetrically necessary, assess the couple's understanding of the reason for the cesarean and advocate for a complete informed consent.
- Involve the couple in as much of the decision-making process as possible to increase feeling of control.
- Support the coach in being able to provide support during the cesarean delivery.
- Emphasize that cesarean delivery is an "alternative birth method," and encourage "family-centered options" where possible.
- Start an IV infusion with an 18-gauge intracatheter.
- Shave the abdomen from the xiphoid process to about 5 cm (2 in) below the pubic hairline.
- Insert a Foley catheter, and connect it to continuous drainage to decrease the risk for bladder trauma during surgery. This frequently can be inserted after the administration of the anesthetic to decrease the discomfort of the procedure.
- Check to see whether laboratory work has been done, such as complete blood count, blood typed and cross-matched for two units, and urinalysis.
- Preferred anesthesia is regional.
- Have equipment available for monitoring pulse oximetry.

Postoperative

- Be prepared to administer prophylactic antibiotics to reduce the risk of a surgical site infection (SSI). An extended spectrum antibiotic regimen is frequently started just after the clamping of the umbilical cord or a narrow-spectrum antibiotic such as cefazolin is given before the surgical incision (Tita, Rouse, and others, 2009). Endomyometritis and bacteriuria are the two most common SSIs following a cesarean delivery.
- Keep in mind that the patient is foremost a new mother. Help her find success in her mothering role within postsurgical limits.

- Assess for signs of hemorrhage by recording blood pressure, pulse, and respirations according to protocol. A typical assessment routine may be every 15 minutes for 2 hrs, every 30 minutes for 1 hr, every 4 hours for 8 hrs, and then routinely. Check firmness of uterus and vaginal flow with each vital signs check. Keep a pad count.
- Manually massage a relaxed, boggy fundus very gently until firm, and maintain oxytocin and IV fluids as ordered.
- Assess for signs of an infection by checking temperature every 4 hours for 48 hours; if higher than 38° C (100.4° F), check every 2 hours. Check lochia every shift for odor.
- Encourage abdominal tightening exercises and early ambulation to decrease the risk for gas pains.
- Give the patient nothing to eat or drink until bowel sounds are present; then give the patient full liquids until she passes flatus; then a soft or regular diet can be given.
- Encourage coughing and deep breathing to decrease the risk for respiratory infection.
- Measure the first two voidings after the Foley catheter is removed. Assess for burning on urination and blood in the urine.
- Initiate prophylaxis against thromboembolism by early ambulation and adequate hydration. According to the Royal College of Obstetricians and Gynaecologists and the American College of Chest Physicians, if the woman is at increased risk, she should wear graduated compression stockings/pneumatic compression devices or be on prophylactic heparin therapy. If she is at high risk, she should be on prophylactic heparin and also wear graduated compression stockings/pneumatic compression devices (Bates and others, 2008).
- Notify the physician if the uterus fails to contract or stay contracted with massage, the patient's temperature is over 38° C, lochia develops an odor, the incision site shows signs of an infection, or the patient complains of burning on urination.
- During the woman's postpartum hospital stay, encourage the couple to verbalize their feelings about the cesarean delivery. The mother who experiences an unexpected cesarean delivery often relates a feeling of guilt or failure because she was unable to achieve a vaginal delivery (Murphy and others, 2003).
- Reassure the couple that they did not fail, and reiterate the reason for the alternative birth method.
- If the couple expresses extreme failure, refer them to a local cesarean birth support group or therapy.

CONCLUSION

The ultimate goal for any patient during labor is normal labor progression with absence of nonreassuring fetal responses. The nurse can have a significant influence on the progress of labor by using evidence-based practice, imparting confidence in the patient's ability to deliver vaginally and using a variety of therapeutic, nonpharmacologic techniques to facilitate labor. Other factors beyond the nurse's control, however, can impede labor. The nurse must assess these factors and report them to the attending health care provider immediately. The medical team should then work together to facilitate the labor and delivery for the best maternal and neonatal outcome.

BIBLIOGRAPHY

Adachi K, Shimada M, Usui A: The relationship between the parturient's positions and perception of labor pain intensity, *Nurs Res* 52:47–51, 2003.

Albers L: Reducing genital tract trauma at birth: launching a clinical trial in midwifery, *J Midwifery Womens Health* 48(2):105–110, 2003.

Albers L, Sedler K, Bedrick E, and others: Midwifery care measures in second stage of labor and reduction of genital tract trauma at birth: a randomized trial, *J Midwifery Womens Health* 192: 1692–1696, 2005.

Alexander J, and others: Epidural analgesia lengthens the Friedman active phase of labor, *Obstet Gynecol* 100(1):46–50, 2002.

American College of Obstetricians and Gynecologists (ACOG): Operative vaginal delivery, *ACOG Practice Bulletin,* No. 17, Washington, DC, 2000, ACOG.

American College of Obstetricians and Gynecologists (ACOG): Mode of term singleton breech delivery, *ACOG Committee Opinion,* No. 265, Washington, DC, 2001, ACOG.

American College of Obstetricians and Gynecologists (ACOG): Shoulder dystocia, *ACOG Practice,* Bulletin, No. 40, Washington, DC, 2002, ACOG.

American College of Obstetricians and Gynecologists (ACOG): Dystocia and the augmentation of labor, *ACOG Practice Bulletin,* No. 49, Washington, DC, 2003, ACOG.

American College of Obstetricians and Gynecologists (ACOG): Pain relief during labor, *ACOG Committee Opinion,* No. 295, Washington, DC, 2004, ACOG.

American College of Obstetricians and Gynecologists (ACOG): Vaginal delivery after previous cesarean birth, *ACOG Practice Bulletin,* No. 54, Washington, DC, 2004b, ACOG.

American Society of Anesthesiologist Task Force: Practice guidelines for obstetric anesthesia, *Anesthesiology* 106(4):843–863, 2007.

Ananth C, Smulian J, Vintzileos A: The association of placenta previa with history of cesarean delivery and abortion: a meta-analysis, *Am J Obstet Gynecol* 177:1071–1078, 1997.

Anim-Somuah M, Smyth RMD, Howell CJ: Epidural versus non-epidural or no analgesia in labour, *Cochrane Database Syst Rev* (Issue 3), Art. No.: CD000331, 2005.

Association of Women's Health, Obstetric, and Neonatal Nurses (AWHONN): *Evidence-based clinical practice guideline: nursing care of the woman receiving analgesia/anesthesia in labor,* Washington, DC, 2001, AWHONN.

Association of Women's Health, Obstetric, and Neonatal Nurses (AWHONN): Role of the registered nurse (RN) in the care of the pregnant woman receiving analgesia/anesthesia by catheter techniques, *AWHONN Epidural Statement,* Washington, DC, 2007, AWHONN.

Association of Women's Health, Obstetric, and Neonatal Nurses (AWHONN): *Evidence-based clinical practice guideline: nursing care and management of the second stage of labor,* ed 2, Washington, DC, 2008, AWHONN.

Bager, and others: Mode of delivery and risk of allergic rhinitis and asthma, *J Allergy Clin Immunol* 111(1):51–56, 2003.

Bates S, Greer I, Pabinger I, and others: Venous thromboembolism, thrombophilia, antithrombotic therapy, and pregnancy: American College of Chest Physicians evidence-based practice guidelines, ed 8, *Chest* 133(Suppl):844S–886S, 2008.

Baumgarder D, and others: Effect of labor epidural anesthesia on breast-feeding of healthy full-term newborns delivered vaginally, *J Am Board Fam Pract* 16(1):7–13, 2003.

Baxley E, Gobbo R: Shoulder dystocia, *Am Fam Physician* 69:1707–1714, 2004.

Beckmann MM, Garrett AJ: Antenatal perineal massage for reducing perineal trauma, *Cochrane Database Syst Rev* (Issue 2), Art. No.: CD005123, 2008.

Benedetti T: Dystocia: causes, consequences, correct response, *Contemp Ob Gyn* 36(Special issue):37, 1991.

Bernstein P: Complications of cesarean deliveries, *Medscape* , September 15, 2005.

Bianchi A, Adams E: Doulas, labor support, and nurses, *Int J Childbirth Educ* 19(4):24–30, 2004.

Bianchi A, Adams E: Labor support during second stage labor for women with epidurals, *Nurs Womens Health* 13(1):39–47, 2009.

Bloom S, Casey B, Schaffer J, and others: A randomized trial of coached versus uncoached maternal pushing during the second stage of labor, *Am J Obstet Gynecol* 194:10–13, 2006.

Bodner-Adler B, Bodner K, Kimberger O, and others: Women's position during labour: influence on maternal and neonatal outcomes, *Wiener Klinische Wochenschrift* 115:720–723, 2003.

Bowers B: Mothers' experiences of labor support: exploration of qualitative research, *J Obstet Gynecol Neonatal Nurs* 31(6):742–752, 2002.

Brancato R, Church S, Stone P: A meta-analysis of passive descent versus immediate pushing in nulliparous women with epidural analgesia in the second stage of labor, *J Obstet Gynecol Neonatal Nurs* 37(1):4–12, 2008.

Brown D, Hammond D: Evidence-based clinical hypnosis for obstetrics, labor and delivery, and preterm labor, *Int J Clin Exp Hypn* 55:355–371, 2007.

Bruner J, and others: All fours maneuver for reducing shoulder dystocia during labor, *J Reprod Med* 43(5):439–443, 1998.

Campbell D, Lake M, Falk M, Backstrand J: A randomized control trial of continuous support in labor by a lay doula, *J Obstet Gynecol Neonatal Nurs* 35:456–464, 2006.

Cargill YM, and others: Clinical Practice Obstetrics Committee. Guidelines for operative vaginal birth, *J Obstet Gynaecol Can* 26(8):747–761, 2004.

Caughey A, Nicholson J, Cheng Y, and others: Induction of labor and cesarean delivery by gestational age, *Am J Obstet Gynecol* 195:700–705, 2006.

Cesario S: Reevaluation of Friedman's labor curve: a pilot study, *J Obstet Gynecol Neonatal Nurs* 33(6):713–722, 2004.

Chauhan S, and others: Maternal and perinatal complications with uterine rupture in 142, 075 patients who attempted vaginal birth after cesarean delivery: a review of the literature, *Am J Obstet Gynecol* 189:408–417, 2003.

Chen S, and others: Effects of sitting position on uterine activity during labor, *Obstet Gynecol* 69(1): 67–73, 1987.

Cheng Y, Hopkins L, Caughey A: How long is too long: does a prolonged second stage of labor in nulliparous women affect maternal and neonatal outcomes? *Am J Obstet Gynecol* 191:933–938, 2004.

Clapp J: The course of labor after endurance exercise during pregnancy, *Am J Obstet Gynecol* 163 (6 Pt 1):1799–1805, 1990.

Clark S, Belfort M, Dildy G, and others: Maternal death in the 21st century causes, prevention, and relationship to cesarean delivery, *Am J Obstet Gynecol* 199(1), 36.e1-5, 2008.

Cluett ER, Burns E: Immersion in water in labour and birth, *Cochrane Database Syst Rev* (Issue 4), Art. No.: CD000111, 2008.

CNM Data Group: Oral intake in labor: trends in midwifery practice, *J Nurse Midwifery* 44(2):135–138, 1999.

Collard T, Diallo H, Habinsky A, and others: Elective cesarean section; why women choose it and what nurses need to know, *Nursing Womens Health* 12(6):481–488, 2008.

Cook A, Wilcox G: Pressuring pain: alternative therapies for labor pain management, *AWHONN Lifelines* 1(2):36–41, 1997.

Coyle ME, Smith CA, Peat B: Cephalic version by moxibustion for breech presentation, *Cochrane Database Syst Rev* 2005, (Issue 2), Art. No.: CD003928.

Curtis K, Guillien L: Shoulder dystocia drills: how one unit prepares for potential obstetric emergencies, *Nurs Womens Health* 13(1):65–69, 2009.

Cyna A, McAuliffe G, Andrews M: Hypnosis for pain relief in labour and childbirth: a systematic review, *Br J Anaesth* 93:505–511, 2004.

Declercq E, Menacker F, MacDorman M: Rise in "no indicated risk" primary cesareans in the United States, 1991-2001; cross sectional analysis, *BMJ* 330:71–72, 2005.

Declercq E, Sakala C, Corry M, Applebaum S: Executive Summary. In *Listening to mothers II: Report of the second national U.S. survey of women's childbearing experiences*, New York, 2006, Childbirth Connection. Retrieved from http://www.childbirthconnection.org/article.asp?ck=10401.

DeJonge A, Teunissen T, Lagro-Janssen A: Supine position compared to other positions during the second stage of labor: a meta analytic review, *J Psychosom Obstet Gynaecol* 25:35–45, 2004.

DeMott R: Cesarean birth. In Kean L, Baker P, Edelstone D, editors: *Best practice in labor ward management*, Philadelphia, 2000, Saunders.

Dessole S, and others: Accidental fetal lacerations during cesarean delivery: experience in an Italian level III university hospital, *Am J Obstet Gynecol* 191(5):1673–1677, 2004.

Dickinson J: Cesarean section. In James D and others, editors: *High risk pregnancy: management options*, ed 3, Philadelphia, 2006, Saunders.

Di Franco J: Music for childbirth, *Childbirth Educator*, Fall, 1988, p 36.

Dodd JM, Crowther CA: Elective repeat caesarean section versus induction of labour for women with a previous caesarean birth, *Cochrane Database Syst Rev* 2006, (Issue 4), Art. No.: CD004906.

Downe S, Gerrett D, Renfrew M: A prospective randomized trial on the effect of position in the passive second stage of labour on birth outcome in nulliparous women using epidural analgesia, *Midwifery* 20:157–168, 2004.

Dowswell T, Bedwell C, Lavender T, Neilson JP: Transcutaneous electrical nerve stimulation (TENS) for pain relief in labour, *Cochrane Database Syst Rev* (Issue 2), Art. No.: CD007214, 2009.

Edelstone D: Breech presentation. In Kean L, Baker P, Edelstone D, editors: *Best practice in labor ward management*, Philadelphia, 2000, Saunders.

Enkin M, and others: *A guide to effective care in pregnancy and childbirth*, ed 3, New York, 2000, Oxford University Press.

Eslamian L, Marsoosi V, Pakneeyat Y: Increased intravenous fluid intake and the course of labor in nulliparous women, *Obstet Gynecol Surv* 61(10):623–625, 2006.

Evans W, Edelstone D: Instrumental delivery. In Kean L, Baker P, Edelstone D, editors: *Best practice in labor ward management*, Philadelphia, 2000, Saunders.

Fenwick L, Simkin P: Maternal positioning to prevent or alleviate dystocia in labor, *Clin Obstet Gynecol* 30(1):83–89, 1987.

Founds S: Maternal posture for cephalic version of breech presentation: a review of the evidence, *Birth* 32(2):137–144, 2005.

Fraser W, and others: Multicenter, randomized, controlled trial of delayed pushing for nulliparous women in the second stage of labor with continuous epidural analgesia: the PEOPLE study group, *Am J Obstet Gynecol* 182(5):1165–1172, 2000.

Fraser W, and others: Risk factors for difficult delivery in nulliparas with epidural analgesia in the second stage of labor, *Am J Obstet Gynecol* 99:409–418, 2002.

Friedman E: Dystocia failure to progress in labor. In Flamm B, Quilligan E, editors: *Cesarean section: guidelines for appropriate utilization*, New York, 1995, Springer-Verlag.

Garite T, and others: A randomized controlled trial of the effect of increased intravenous hydration on the course of labor in nulliparous women, *Am J Obstet Gynecol* 183(16):1544–1548, 2000.

Gee H: Abnormal patterns of labor prolonged labor. In Kean L, Baker P, Edelstone D, editors: *Best practice in labor ward management*, Philadelphia, 2000, Saunders.

Gee H: Poor progress in labor. In James D and others, editors: *High risk pregnancy: management options*, ed 3, Philadelphia, 2006, Saunders.

Gentz B: Alternative therapies for the management of pain in labor and delivery, *Clin Obstet Gynecol* 44(4):704–732, 2001.

Gherman R: Shoulder dystocia. In James D and others, editors: *High risk pregnancy: management options*, ed 3, Philadelphia, 2006, Saunders.

Gherman R, Goodwin T: Shoulder dystocia, *Curr Opin Obstet Gynecol* 10:459, 1998.

Gilder K, and others: Maternal positioning in labor with epidural anesthesia: results from a multisite survey, *AWHONN Lifelines* 6(1):40–45, 2002.

Gimovsky M, Han J: Reducing the medicolegal risk of vacuum extraction, *OBG Management* 19(6): 1–15, 2007. Retrieved from http://www.obgmanagement.com/article_pages.asp?ref=1906OBGM_Article1.

Goetzl L, and others: Maternal epidural analgesia and rates of maternal antibiotic treatment in a low-risk nulliparous population, *J Perinatol* 23(6):457–461, 2003.

Golay J, Vedam S, Sorger L: The squatting position for the second stage of labor: effects on labor and on maternal and fetal well-being, *Birth* 20(2):73–78, 1993.

Gonik B, Allen R, Sorab J: Objective evaluation of the shoulder dystocia phenomenon: effect of maternal pelvic orientation on force reduction, *Obstet Gynecol* 74:44–48, 1989.

Goodall P, and others: Obesity as a risk factor for failed trial of labor in patients with previous cesarean delivery, *Am J Obstet Gynecol* 192(5):1423–1426, 2005.

Grootscholten K, Kok M, Oei S, and others: External cephalic version-related risks: a meta analysis, *Obstet Gynecol* 112:1143–1151, 2008.

Gulliver B, Fisher J, Roberts L: A new way to assess pain in laboring women, *Nurs Women's Health* 12(5):405–406, 2008.

Gupta JK, Hofmeyr GJ, Smyth RMD: Position in the second stage of labour for women without epidural anaesthesia, *Cochrane Database Syst Rev* 2005, (Issue 3), Art. No.: CD002006.

Hakansson S, Kallen K: Caesarean section increases the risk of hospital care in childhood for asthma and gastroenteritis, *Clin Exp Allergy* 33(6):757–764, 2003.

Hamilton B, Martin J, Ventura S: Births: preliminary data for 2007, *National Vital Statistics Reports* 57(12):1–23, 2009. Retrieved from http://www.cdc.gov/nchs/data/nvsr/nvsr57/nvsr57_12.pdf.

Hannah M, and others: Planned caesarean section versus planned vaginal birth for breech presentation at term: a randomized multicentre trail, *Lancet* 356(9239):1375–1383, 2000.

Hansen S, Clark S, Foster J: Active pushing versus passive fetal descent in the second stage of labor: a randomized controlled trial, *Obstet Gynecol* 99(1):29–34, 2002.

Hazle N: Hydration in labor: is routine intravenous hydration necessary? *J Nurse Midwifery* 31(4): 171–176, 1986.

Hodnett ED, Gates S, Hofmeyr GJ, Sakala C: Continuous support for women during childbirth, *Cochrane Database Syst Rev* (Issue 2), Art. No.: CD003766, 2007.

Hofmeyr GJ, Cyna AM, Middleton P: Prophylactic intravenous preloading for regional analgesia in labour, *Cochrane Database Syst Rev* (Issue 2), Art. No.: CD000175, 2004.

Hofmeyr GJ, Gyte GML: Interventions to help external cephalic version for breech presentation at term, *Cochrane Database Syst Rev* (Issue 1), Art. No.: CD000184, 2004.

Hofmeyr GJ, Hannah M: Planned caesarean section for term breech delivery, *Cochrane Database Syst Rev* (Issue 4), Art. No.: CD000166, 2004.

Hofmeyr GJ, Kulier R: External cephalic version for breech presentation at term, *Cochrane Database Syst Rev* 2005, (Issue 2), Art. No.: CD000083.

Horger E: Shoulder dystocia, *Female Patient* 20(12):12, 1995.

Hottenstein S, Brit Pipe T: Continuous labor support, *AWHONN Lifelines* 9(3):242–247, 2005.

Hunter S, Hofmeyr GJ, Kulier R: Hands and knees posture in late pregnancy or labour for fetal malposition (lateral or posterior), *Cochrane Database Syst Rev* (Issue 3), Art. No.: CD001063, 2007.

Institute for Clinical Systems Improvement: *Health care guideline: Management of labor*, ed 3, 2009, ICSI. Retrieved from http://www.icsi.org

Jackson D, and others: Outcomes, safety, and resource utilization in a collaborative care birth center program compared with traditional physician-based perinatal care, *Am J Public Health* 93(6): 999–1006, 2003.

Jannke S: Birth plans, *Childbirth Instructor* 5(3):26, 1995.

Johanson R, Menon V: Vacuum extraction versus forceps for assisted vaginal delivery, *Cochrane Database Syst Rev* (Issue 1), Art. No.: CD000224, 1999.

Johnson D, Davis N, Brown A: Risk of cesarean delivery after induction at term in nulliparous women, *Am J Obstet Gynecol* 188(6):1565–1572, 2003.

Johnson N, Johnson V, Gupta J: Maternal positions during labor, *Obstet Gynecol Surv* 46(7):428–434, 1991.

Johnstone F, Aboelmagd M, Harouny A: Maternal posture in second stage and fetal acid base status, *Br J Obstet Gynaecol* 94(8):753–757, 1987.

Jukelevics N: Big myths about big babies, *Childbirth Instructor* May/June, 18–23, 2000.

Kardong-Edgren S: Using evidence-based practice to improve intrapartum care, *J Obstet Gynecol Neonatal Nurs* 30(4):371–375, 2001.

Kelly M, and others: A comparison of the effect of intrathecal and extradural Fentanyl on gastric emptying in laboring women, *Anesth Analg* 85(4):834–838, 1997.

Kieser K, Baskett T: 10-year population-based study of uterine rupture, *Obstet Gynecol* 100(4):749–753, 2002.

Kubli M, and others: An evaluation of isotonic sport drinks during labor, *Anesth Analg* 94(2):404–408, 2002.

Kurokawa J, Zilkoski M: Adapting hospital obstetrics to birth in the squatting position, *Birth* 12(2): 87–90, 1985.

Landon M: Vaginal birth after cesarean delivery, *Clin Perinatol* 35(3):491–504, 2008.

Landon M, Hauth J, Leveno K, and others: For the National Institute of Child-Health and Human Development Maternal-Fetal Medicine Units Network: The MFMU cesarean registry: factors affecting the success and trial of labor following prior cesarean delivery, *N Engl J Med* 351: 2581–2589, 2004.

Landon M, Leindecker S, Spong C: For the National Institute of Child-Health and Human Development Maternal-Fetal Medicine Units Network: The MFMU cesarean registry: factors affecting the success and trial of labor following prior cesarean delivery, *Am J Obstet Gynecol* 193:1016–1023, 2005.

Laopaiboon M, Lumbiganon P, Martis R, and others: Music during caesarean section under regional anaesthesia for improving maternal and infant outcomes, *Cochrane Database Syst Rev* (Issue 2), Art. No.: CD006914, 2009.

Lau T, and others: Predictors of successful ECV at term, *Br J Obstet Gynaecol* 104:798–802, 1997.

Lieberman E, Kavidson K, Lee-Parritz A, Shearer E: Changes in fetal position during labor and their association with epidural analgesia, *Obstet Gynecol* 105:974–982, 2005.

Liu S, Liston R, Joseph K, and others: Maternal mortality and severe morbidity associated with low-risk planned cesarean delivery versus planned vaginal delivery at term, *Can Med Assoc J* 176(4):455–460, 2007.

Lobel M, DeLuca R: Psychosocial sequelae of cesarean delivery: review and analysis of their causes and implications, *Soc Sci Med* 64(11):2272–2284, 2007.

Lowe N: A review of factors associated with dystocia and cesarean section in nulliparous women, *J Midwifery Womens Health* 52(3):216–228, 2007.

Ludka L, Roberts C: Eating and drinking in labor: a literature review, *J Nurse Midwifery* 38(4):199–207, 1993.

Macones G, Peipert J, Nelson D, and others: Maternal complications with vaginal birth after Cesarean delivery: a multicenter study, *Am J Obstet Gynecol* 193:1656–1662, 2005.

Mancuso M, Rouse D: Cesarean delivery for abnormal labor, *Clin Perinatol* 35(3):479–490, 2008.

Mankuta D, and others: Vaginal birth after cesarean section: trial of labor or repeat cesarean section? A decision analysis, *Am J Obstet Gynecol* 189(3):714–719, 2003.

Martin W, Hutchon S: Mechanism and management of normal labour, *Curr Obstet Gynaecol* 14(5): 301–308, 2004.

Martin J, Kung H, Mathews T, and others: Annual summary of vital statistics: 2006, *Pediatrics* 121:788–801, 2008. Retrieved from http://pediatrics.aappublications.org/cgi/content/abstract/121/4/788?etoc.

Matthews R, Callister L: Childbearing women's perceptions of nursing care that promotes dignity, *J Obstet Gynecol Neonatal Nurs* 33:498–507, 2004.

Mayberry L, Clemmens D, De A: Epidural analgesia side effects, co-interventions, and care of women during childbirth: a systematic review, *Am J Obstet Gynecol* 186:S81–S93, 2002.

Mayberry L, Strange L, Suplee P, Gennaro S: Use of upright positioning with epidural analgesia: findings from an observational study, *Am J Matern Child Nurs* 28:152–159, 2003.

McKay S, Roberts J: Maternal position during labor and birth: What have we learned? *IJCE* 13(2):9, 1989.

Menacker F, Declercq E, Macdorman M: Cesarean delivery: background, trends and epidemiology, *Semin Perinatol* 30(5):235–241, 2005.

Miller D, Chollet J, Goodwin T: Clinical risk factors for placenta previa-placenta accreta, *Am J Obstet Gynecol* 177(1):210–214, 1997.

Miltner R: Identifying labor support actions of intrapartum nurses, *J Obstet Gynecol Neonatal Nurs* 29(5):491–499, 2000.

Minkin M: A no-fault approach to shoulder dystocia, *Contemp Ob Gyn* 49(12):11–12, 2004.

Montgomery A, Emmett C: Two decision aids for mode of delivery among women with previous caesarean section; randomized control trial, *BMJ* 334(7607):1305, 2007.

Morton S, Williams M, Keeler E, and others: Effect of epidural analgesia for labor on the cesarean delivery rate, *Obstet Gynecol* 83(6):1045–1052, 1994.

Mozurkewich E, Hutton E: Elective repeat cesarean delivery versus trial of labor: a meta-analysis of the literature from 1989-1999, *Am J Obstet Gynecol* 183(5):1187–1197, 2000.

Murphy D, and others: Women's views on the impact of operative delivery in the second stage of labour: qualitative interview study, *BMJ* 327(7424):1132, 2003.

Naef R, Martin J: Emergent management of shoulder dystocia, *Obstet Gynecol Clin North Am* 22:247, 1995.

National Institute of Clinical Excellence: *Why mothers die 2000-2002: report on confidential enquires into maternal deaths in the United Kingdom*, London, 2003, Royal College of Obstetrician and Gynaecologists Press.

National Institute for Health and Clinical Excellence (NHS): Intrapartum care, *NICE clinical guideline 55*, London, 2007, NHS. Retrieved from http://www.nice.org.uk.

National Institutes of Health (NIH): State of the science conference statement: cesarean delivery on maternal request, *Obstet Gynecol* 107:1386–1397, 2006.

Nerum B, Halvorsen L, Sorlie T, Oian P: Maternal request for cesarean section due to fear of birth: can it be changed through crisis-oriented counseling? *Birth* 33(3):221–228, 2006.

Ness A, Goldberg J, Berghella V: Abnormalities of the first and second stages of labor, *Obstet Gynecol Clin North Am* 32(2):201–220, 2004.

Newman M, Lindsay M, Graves W: The effect of epidural analgesia on rates of episiotomy use and episiotomy extension in an inner-city hospital, *J Matern Fetal Med* 10(2):97–101, 2001.

Newton C, Raynor M: Routine intrapartum care. In Kean L, Baker P, Edelstone D, editors: *Best practice in labor ward management*, Philadelphia, 2000, Saunders.

Newton N, Newton M, Broach J: Psychologic, physical, nutritional, and technologic aspects of intravenous infusion during labor, *Birth* 15(2):67–72, 1988.

Nocon J: Shoulder dystocia: managing risk to avoid negligence, *Contemp Ob Gyn* 36(special issue):15, 1991.

Nocon J: Shoulder dystocia macrosomia. In Kean L, Baker P, Edelstone D, editors: *Best practice in labor ward management*, Philadelphia, 2000, Saunders.

Nordstrom L, Achanna S, Naka K, Arulkumaran S: Fetal and maternal lactate increase during active second stage of labour, *Br J Obstet Gynecol* 108:263–268, 2001.

O'Grady J, Pope C, Patel S: Vacuum extraction in modern obstetric practice: a review and critique, *Curr Opin Obstet Gynecol* 12(6):475–480, 2000.

O'Leary J: *Shoulder dystocia and birth injury: Prevention and treatment*, Boston, 1992, McGraw-Hill.

O'Sullivan G, Liu B, Shennan A: Oral intake during labor, *Int Anesth* 45(1):133–147, 2007.

Ouzounian J, Gherman R: Shoulder dystocia: are historic risk factors reliable predictors? *Am J Obstet Gynecol* 192(6):1933–1935, 2005.

Paciornik M: Commentary: arguments against episiotomy and in favor of squatting for birth, *Birth* 17(2):104–105, 1990.

Paneth N, Hong T, Korzeniewski S: The descriptive epidemiology of cerebral palsy, *Clin Perinatol* 33:251–267, 2006.

Patel R, Murphy D: Forceps delivery in modern obstetric practice, *BMJ* 328(7454):1302–1305, 2004.

Petrou S, Coyle D, Fraser W: Cost-effectiveness of a delayed pushing policy for patients with epidural anesthesia: the PEOPLE study group, *Am J Obstet Gynecol* 182(5):1158–1164, 2000.

Poobalan A, Aucott S, Gurung T, and others: Obesity as an independent risk factor for elective and emergency caesarean delivery in nulliparous women: systematic review and meta-analysis of cohort studies, *Obes Rev* 10:28–35, 2009.

Porter M, Van Teijlingen E, Chi Ying Yip L, Bhattacharya S: Satisfaction with cesarean section: qualitative analysis of open-ended questions in a large postal survey, *Birth* 34(2):148–154, 2007.

Pugh L, and others: First stage labor management: an examination of patterned breathing and fatigue, *Birth* 25(4):241, 1998.

Ragnar I, Altman D, Tyden T, Olsson S: Comparison of the maternal experience and duration of labour in two upright delivery positions: a randomized controlled trial, *Br J Obstet Gynaecol* 113:165–170, 2006.

Ramachandrappa A, Jain L: Elective cesarean section; its impact on neonatal respiratory outcome, *Clin Perinatol* 35(2):373–393, 2008.

Ransjo-Arvidson A, and others: Maternal analgesia during labor disturbs newborn behavior: effects on breastfeeding, temperature, and crying, *Birth* 28(1):5–12, 2001.

Ridley R: diagnosis and intervention for occiput posterior malposition, *J Obstet Gynecol Neonatal Nurs* 36(2):135–143, 2007.

Rigini N, Evron S, Sadan O, and others: Intermittent versus continuous bladder catheterization and labor epidural, *Anesthesiology* 105:A907, 2006.

Roberts C, Algert C, Cameron C, Torvaldsen S: A meta-analysis of upright positions in the second stage to reduce instrumental deliveries in women with epidural analgesia, *Acta Obstet Gynecol Scand* 84:794–798, 2005.

Roberts C, Ludka L: Food for thought: the debate over eating and drinking in labor, *Childbirth Instructor* 4(2):24, 1994.

Roberts C, Torvaldsen S, Cameron C, Olive E: Delayed versus early pushing in women with epidural analgesia: a systemic review and meta-analysis, *Br J Obstet Gynaecol* 111:1333–1340, 2004.

Roberts J: The "push" for evidence: management of the second stage, *J Midwifery Womens Health* 47:2–15, 2002.

Roberts J: A new understanding of the second stage of labor: implications for nursing care, *J Obstet Gynecol Neonatal Nurs* 32:794–801, 2003.

Roberts J, Hanson L: Best practices in second stage labor care: Maternal bearing down and positioning, *Journal of Midwifery & Women's Health* 52(3):238–245, 2007.

Roberts J, Mendez-Bauer C, Wodell D: The effects of maternal position on uterine contractility and efficiency, *Birth* 10(4):243–249, 1983.

Roberts J, Woolley D: A second look at the second stage of labor, *J Obstet Gynecol Neonatal Nurs* 25(5):415–423, 1996.

Roberts R, and others: Trial of labor or repeated cesarean section: the woman's choice, *Arch Fam Med* 6(2):120–125, 1997.

Romond J, Baker I: Squatting in childbirth: a new look at an old tradition, *J Obstet Gynecol Neonatal Nurs* 14(5):406–411, 1985.

Rosen T: Placenta accrete and cesarean scar pregnancy: overlooked costs of the rising cesarean section rate, *Clin Perinatol* 35(3):519–529, 2008.

Rossi M, Lindell S: Maternal positions and pushing techniques in a nonprescriptive environment, *J Obstet Gynecol Neonatal Nurs* 15(3):203–208, 1986.

Rouse D, and others: Active phase labor arrest: revisiting the 2 hour minimum, *Obstet Gynecol* 98(4):550–554, 2001.

Rush J, and others: The effects of whirlpool baths in labor: a randomized, controlled trial, *Birth* 23(3):136–143, 1996.

Sakala C: Current resources for evidence-based practice, *J Obstet Gynecol Neonatal Nurs* 34(5):625–628, 2005.

Sampselle C, and others: Provider support of spontaneous pushing during the second stage of labor, *J Obstet Gynecol Neonatal Nurs* 34(6):695–702, 2005.

Sauls D: Dimensions of professional labor support for intrapartum practice, *Image J Nurs Sch* 38(1):36–41, 2006.

Scheepers H, and others: Eating and drinking in labor: the influence of caregiver advice on women's behavior, *Birth* 28(2):119–123, 2001.

Schiessl B, Janni W, Jundt K, and others: Obstetrical parameters influencing the duration of the second stage of labor, *Eur J Obstet Gynecol Reprod Biol* 118:17–20, 2005.

Sharp D: Restrictions of oral intake for women in labour, *Br J Midwifery* 5:408, 1997.

Sheiner E, and others: Risk factors and outcome of failure to progress during the first stage of labor: a population based study, *Acta Obstet Gynecol Scand* 81(3):222–226, 2002.

Simkin P: Comfort measures for labor and how they work, *IJCE* 11(1):57, 1987.

Simkin P: Reducing pain enhancing progress in labor: a guide to nonpharmacologic methods for maternity caregivers, *Birth* 22(3):161–171, 1995.

Simkin P, Bolding A: Update on nonpharmacologic approach to relieve labor pain and prevent suffering, *J Midwifery Womens Health* 49(6):489–504, 2004.

Simm A, Woods A: Fetal malpresentation, *Curr Obstet Gynecol* 14(4):231–238, 2004.

Simmons SW, Cyna AM, Dennis AT, Hughes D: Combined spinal-epidural versus epidural analgesia in labour, *Cochrane Database Syst Rev* (Issue 2), Art. No.: CD003401, 2007.

Simpson K, James D: Effects of immediate versus delayed pushing during second-stage labor on fetal well-being: a randomized clinical trial, *Nurs Res* 54(3):149–157, 2005a.

Simpson K, James D: Efficacy of intrauterine resuscitation techniques in improving fetal oxygen status during labor, *Obstet Gynecol* 105:1362–1368, 2005b.

Simpson K, Knox G: Fundal pressure during the second stage of labor, *MCN Am J Matern Child Nurs* 26(2):64–70, 2001.

Sleutel M, Golden S: Fasting in labor: relic or requirement, *J Obstet Gynecol Neonatal Nurs* 28(5): 507–512, 1999.

Society of Obstetricians and Gynaecologists of Canada (SOGC): Guidelines for vaginal birth after previous caesarean birth, *Clin Prac Guidel*, No 155, 2005.

Sprague A, Oppenheimer L, McCabe L, and others: The Ottawa Hospital's clinical practice guideline for the second stage of labour, *J Obstet Gynaecol Can* 28:769–779, 2006.

Springer D: Birth plans: the effect on anxiety in pregnant women, *IJCE* 11(3):20, 1996.

Stephens S: Body work and childbirth, proven wonders, *IJCE* 12(4):20, 1997.

Stitely M, Gherman R: Labor with abnormal presentation and position, *Obstet Gynecol Clin North Am* 32(2):165–179, 2005.

Stremler R, Halpern S, Weston J, and others: Hands and knees positioning during labor with epidural analgesia, *J Obstet Gynecol Neonatal Nurs* 38(4):391–398, 2009.

Stremler R, Hodnett E, Petryshen P, and others: Randomized controlled trial of hands-and-knees positioning for occipitoposterior position in labor, *Birth* 32:243–251, 2005.

Sutton J, Scott P: *Understanding teaching optional fetal positioning*, Tauranga, New Zealand, 1996, Birth Concepts.

Terry R, Westcott J, O'Shea L, Kelly F: Postpartum outcomes in supine delivery by physicians vs nonsupine delivery by midwives, *J Am Osteopathic Assoc* 106:199–202, 2006.

Thorp J: Clinical aspects of normal and abnormal labor. In Creasy R, Resnik R, Iams J, Lockwood C, Moore T, editors: *Creasy and Resnik's maternal-fetal medicine: principles and practice*, ed 6, Philadelphia, 2009, Saunders.

Thorp J, and others: The effect of intrapartum epidural analgesia on nulliparous labor: a randomized, controlled, prospective trial, *Am J Obstet Gynecol* 169:851, 1993.

Thorp J, Breedlove G: Epidural analgesia in labor: an evaluation of risk and benefits, *Birth* 23:63, 1996.

Threlfall-Mase A: The moaning option, *Childbirth Instructor* 7(2):43, 1997.

Tita A, Landon M, Spong C, and others: Timing of elective repeat cesarean delivery at term and neonatal out comes, *N Engl J Med* 360(2):111–120, 2009.

Tita A, Rouse D, Blackwell S, and others: Emerging concepts in antibiotic prophylaxis for cesarean delivery, *Obstet Gynecol* 113(3):675–682, 2009.

Tourangeau A, and others: Intravenous therapy for women in labor: implementation of a practice change, *Birth* 26(1):31–36, 1999.

Towner D, and others: Effect of mode of delivery in nulliparous women on neonatal intracranial injury, *N Engl J Med* 341(23):1709–1714, 1999.

Tranmer J, and others: The effect of unrestricted oral carbohydrate intake on labor progress, *J Obstet Gynecol Neonatal Nurs* 34(3):319–328, 2005.

U.S. Department of Health and Human Services: *Healthy People 2010: understanding and improving health*, Washington, DC, 2000, USDHHS.

U.S. Department of Health and Human Services: *Women's health USA 2005*, Rockville, MD, 2005, USDHHS.

VandeVusse L: The essential forces of labor revisited: 13 P's reported in women's stories, *MCN Am J Matern Child Nurs* 24(4):176–184, 1999.

Varrassi G, Bazzano C, Edwards W: Effects of physical activity on maternal plasma B-endorphin levels and perception of labor pain, *Am J Obstet Gynecol* 160(3):707–712, 1989.

Vause S, Congdon H, Thornton J: Immediate and delayed pushing in the second stage of labour for nulliparous women with epidural analgesia: a randomized controlled trial, *Br J Obstet Gynaecol* 105(2):186–188, 1998.

Vronenraets F, Roumen F, Dehing C, and others: Bishop score and risk of cesarean delivery after induction of labor in nulliparous women, *Obstet Gynecol* 105:690–697, 2005.

Watson J: *Postmodern nursing beyond*, Edinburgh, 1999, Churchill Livingstone.

Wax JR, Cartin A, Pinette MG, and others: Patient choice cesarean: an evidence-based review, *Obstet Gynecol Surv* 59:601, 2004.

Wen S, and others: Comparison of maternal mortality and morbidity between trial of labor and elective cesarean section among women with previous cesarean delivery, *Am J Obstet Gynecol* 191(4): 1263–1269, 2004.

Williams H: The ethical debate of maternal choice and autonomy in cesarean delivery, *Clin Perinatol* 35(2):455–462, 2008.

Wohlrab K, Rardin C: Impact of rout of delivery on continence and sexual function, *Clin Perinatol* 35(3):582–590, 2008.

Wong C, Scavone B, Dugan S, and others: Incidence of postpartum lumbosacral spine and lower extremity nerve injuries, *Obstet Gynecol* 101:279–288, 2003.

Wong S, McKenzie D: Cardiorespiratory fitness during pregnancy and its effect on outcome, *Int J Sports Med* 8(2):79–83, 1987.

World Health Organization: *Managing complications in pregnancy and childbirth: a guide for midwives and doctors*, Switzerland, 2002, Department of Reproductive Health and Research (RHR).

Zhang J, Troendle J, Yancey M: Reassessing the labor curve in nulliparous women, *Am J Obstet Gynecol* 187(4):824–828, 2002.

Zhu B, Grigorescu V, Le T, and others: Labor dystocia and its association with inter-pregnancy interval, *Am J Obstet Gynecol* 195(1):121–128, 2006.

Zimmerman D, Breen T, Fick G: Adding fentanyl 0.002% to epidural bupivacaine 0.125% does not delay gastric emptying in parturients, *Anesth Analg* 82(6):612–616, 1996.

Zwelling E: VBAC revisited: a declining trend? *Childbirth Forum* Spring/Summer, p 1, 2001.

30

Prolonged Pregnancy

*P*ost-term or *prolonged pregnancy* is pregnancy that lasts a gestational period of 42 completed weeks (294 days) or more from the first day of the last menses, if the menstrual cycle is 28 days. *Postmaturity* refers to the abnormal condition of the fetus or newborn resulting from a prolonged pregnancy.

INCIDENCE

The incidence of prolonged pregnancy depends upon the patient population and local practice patterns. Such factors include the percentage of primigravid women within the population, the frequency of spontaneous preterm birth, the prevalence of ultrasound equipment and trained personnel to determine gestational age, the percentage of women with pregnancy complications, rates of scheduled cesarean delivery, and routine labor induction. Within the United States, approximately 18% of singleton pregnancies extend beyond 41 weeks, 10% beyond 42 weeks, and 4% beyond 43 completed weeks in the absence of obstetric intervention (Norwitz, Snegnovskikh, and Caughey, 2007). However, when first trimester ultrasound dating is used to determine gestational age, the incidence of prolonged pregnancy is less than 3% (Bennett and others, 2004).

ETIOLOGY

The actual physiologic cause of prolonged pregnancy is still obscure. There is some evidence that the initiation of labor is triggered by sequential changes beginning within the fetal brain and influencing the fetal hypothalamus, pituitary gland, and adrenal gland, extending to the maternal myometrium and cervix, resulting in hormonal changes in the placenta and amniotic fetal membranes (Norwitz and Lye, 2009). A placental estrogen deficiency or decreased release of prostaglandins by the decidua and fetal membranes are also possible causes of prolonged pregnancy.

When there is insufficient estrogen, there is decreased production and storage of prostaglandin precursors and decreased stimulation to form oxytocin receptors in the myometrium. These physiologic processes are important in the initiation of labor. (Refer to the Normal Physiology section of Chapter 23.) Occasionally, estrogen deficiency can result from fetal adrenal hypoplasia and placental sulfatase deficiency, which may cause delay in the onset of labor and failure of normal cervical ripening (Norwitz and Lye, 2009).

NORMAL PHYSIOLOGY

Amniotic Fluid

The normal physiology of amniotic fluid (its volume and functions) is relevant to understanding the pathologic complications in prolonged pregnancy.

Volume

Amniotic fluid is derived from the following sources:
- Maternal circulation, primarily from placental sufficiency
- Amniotic membrane
- Fetal plasma via lungs and kidneys

The volume changes by (1) the fetal contribution through excretion of urine and fetal lungs, (2) fetal use of the fluid for nourishment by swallowing the fluid and sending it into the gastrointestinal tract, (3) movement of water and solutes back into fetal blood across fetal membranes and placenta, and (4) movement of water and solutes directly into maternal blood.

The volume of amniotic fluid gradually increases until it reaches its maximal level of 800 to 1200 ml at approximately 34 weeks of gestation, at which time it begins to decrease normally. By 40 weeks, the level is approximately 800 ml. In contrast, by 42 weeks, the levels are 200 ml (Cunningham and others, 2010).

Functions

The following functions of amniotic fluid are relevant to prolonged pregnancy:
- Cushions the fetus and umbilical cord from direct pressure and injury
- Allows the fetus to move and exercise freely
- Assists the fetus in respiratory efforts
- Facilitates fetal lung development and surfactant production

Placenta

Exchange

The placenta provides a large surface area through which materials can be exchanged across the placental membrane between the fetal and maternal circulations. From the maternal blood, the fetus obtains nutrients and oxygen. Waste products formed by the fetus are transferred back across the placental membrane into the intervillous space.

Functions

The placenta has an optimal functional period of about 40 to 42 weeks. There appear to be no significant morphologic changes in the post-term placenta until about 42 weeks (Cunningham and others, 2010). After 43 to 44 weeks, the placenta begins aging, as noted by the increased size of areas of infarction and deposition of calcium and fibrin within its tissue, decreasing its reserve (Gribbin and Thornton, 2006).

PATHOPHYSIOLOGY

Amniotic Fluid

Decreased Amniotic Fluid

Decreased amniotic fluid, or *oligohydramnios,* is the factor most frequently associated with prolonged pregnancy (Cunningham and others, 2010). Decreased amniotic fluid below 400 ml can reduce the cushioning effect of the fluid. As a result, it becomes far more likely that the fetus will entrap or compress its own cord, shutting off blood flow to and from itself for intermittent intervals.

Meconium Contamination

Meconium in the amniotic fluid occurs more frequently in prolonged pregnancy (Cunningham and others, 2010). When the fetus is post-term, the expulsion of meconium into the already diminished volume of amniotic fluid causes the meconium to thicken the amniotic fluid, inhibits the normal antibacterial properties of the amniotic fluid, and pulls fluid from Wharton jelly, promoting stiffening of the cord.

Placenta and Umbilical Cord

Placental Dysfunction

When the placenta ages, depositing fibrin and calcium, intervillous hemorrhagic infarcts occur and the basal membrane of the placental blood vessels thickens and degenerates, affecting diffusion of oxygen. These changes have been noted in the post-term placenta. Whether or not these placental changes affect the fetal outcome in the prolonged pregnancy is unknown at this time because most fetuses continue to grow.

Decreased Wharton Jelly

As aging takes place, water content is lost from the Wharton jelly encasing the umbilical cord, decreasing the amount of Wharton jelly. As the amount of Wharton jelly decreases, the cord stiffens and becomes firm rather than remaining flexible and pliable.

Decreased Umbilical Cord Blood Flow

As a result of umbilical cord stiffening, susceptibility to pressure on the cord and to bending of the cord is increased. If the cord bends or kinks, much like a sun-baked garden hose, increased resistance to fetal blood flow can result in serious neurologic damage or sudden intrauterine fetal death.

SIGNS AND SYMPTOMS

A number of obstetric warning signs, in conjunction with a pregnancy continuing past the estimated due date (EDD), including the following, can alert caregivers to potential problems.

Maternal Weight Loss

In the last weeks of pregnancy, a weight loss in excess of 3 pounds per week caused by a decreased amount of amniotic fluid may warn of a prolonged pregnancy.

Decreased Uterine Size

Decreased amniotic fluid (<400 ml) frequently correlates with maternal weight loss and a decrease in uterine size.

Meconium-Stained Amniotic Fluid

Meconium in the amniotic fluid can represent a normal physiologic event in the maturation of the fetal gastrointestinal tract, can be the result of vagal stimulation from transient umbilical cord compression that results in increased peristalsis, or can be the direct result of fetal hypoxia (Cunningham and others, 2010).

Advanced Bone Maturation

Advanced bone maturation can be detected by palpation of an excessively hard fetal head. It can lead to a lack of cephalic molding and a high arrest of the fetal head with potential for failure to progress, prolongation of the active phase of labor, and failure to complete the transitional phase of labor.

Prolonged Labor

A macrosomic fetus, failure of cephalic molding, or decreased uterine sensitivity to oxytocin can cause prolonged labor.

MATERNAL EFFECTS

Physical Exhaustion

Many women report extreme fatigue if their pregnancy is prolonged.

Psychologic Depression

Women express a great deal of frustration with the prolongation of the pregnancy and a feeling of total lack of personal control in ending the pregnancy. Feelings of inadequacy emerge because of their inability to complete the process of the pregnancy "like everyone else." Women often blame themselves for prolonging the pregnancy by working too hard, working too long into the pregnancy, or not seeking adequate help with everyday tasks.

Relationships with people closest to the pregnant woman become strained. Resentment and anxiety is often expressed because friends and relatives repeatedly check on the woman's progress and condition. Physical discomfort becomes an intolerable burden, which in turn decreases the ability to continue caring for the home and other family members in the accustomed manner. Women describe feeling awkward, big, and ugly. They comment that they have lost their "glow" and feel generally unattractive. A woman's negative feelings about herself may be projected as feelings of resentment toward the baby for not cooperating or for being a "stubborn" child.

Realistic fears are commonly shared about the continued well-being of the baby. Women report fears that the baby is "stuck" and will somehow be harmed or that something is very wrong and that the baby has decided not to be born.

Other Maternal Risks

Most other risks are related to labor dystocia such as increased risk for perineal injury related to macrosomia or treatment to prevent prolonged pregnancy, such as complications related to induction or cesarean delivery (Grant, 2006).

FETAL AND NEONATAL EFFECTS

When 42 weeks of gestation is exceeded, oligohydramnios increases substantially, and intrapartum perinatal risk is increased (Cunningham and others, 2010). This is related to a wide range of features.

Macrosomia

Macrosomia is defined as a birth weight greater than 4000 to 4500 g (Baschat, 2006). In the United States about 10% of newborns weigh more than 4000 g, and 1.5% weigh more than 4500 g. The risk for macrosomia increases from 8.5% at term to 11.2% if gestational age exceeds 42 weeks (Martin and others, 2009). Macrosomia poses a risk to the postdate fetus because it can lead to shoulder dystocia and birth trauma.

Postmaturity Syndrome

Postmaturity syndrome occurs in approximately 20% of postdate fetuses (Resnik and Resnik, 2009) because of a compromised environment. This syndrome is characterized by degrees of skin change, with or without loss of subcutaneous fat and muscle mass, and meconium staining, dependent on severity of cord compression and placental dysfunction. Postmaturity syndrome was initially defined by J W. Ballantyne in 1902, classified by Clifford (1954) and was later revised by Vorherr (1975). However, macrosomia is a more common complication because fetal growth continues in utero (Resnik and Resnik, 2009).

First Stage

In the first stage of postmaturity syndrome, the skin becomes desquamated because of the loss of the protective effects of vernix caseosa. It is characterized by a dry, cracked, parchment-like peeling, with or without loss of subcutaneous fat and muscle mass. The nails are usually long.

Second Stage

The second stage of postmaturity syndrome includes first-stage characteristics and also green meconium-stained fetal skin and umbilical cord.

Third Stage

The third stage of postmaturity syndrome includes the first two stages plus yellow staining of the skin and the umbilical cord. This yellow staining is related to meconium being passed several days before. The bile in the meconium, as it breaks down, turns the fluid yellow.

Fetal Hypoxia

Fetal hypoxia can be caused by placental deprivation or oligohydramnios (decreased amniotic fluid) that leads to cord compression (Resnik and Resnik, 2009).

Meconium Aspiration Syndrome

Studies of post-term gestation report a markedly higher incidence of meconium-stained amniotic fluid, compared with term pregnancies (Resnik and Resnik, 2009). There is a greater risk of meconium aspiration syndrome in these infants (Clausson, Cnattingius, and Axelsson, 1999). If amniotic fluid is diminished, the risk of meconium aspiration is greater (Resnik and Resnik, 2009).

The fetus normally moves fluids into and out of the lungs in utero by two breathing patterns. Shallow, regular breathing comprises 90% of fetal respirations, and deep, irregular breathing comprises the other 10%. An abnormal pattern of breathing may be stimulated in the presence of hypoxia, which is characterized by compensatory gasping respirations. Aspiration of meconium from the amniotic fluid into the lungs occurs if gasping respirations are stimulated by asphyxia, and a small amount may occur during the normal deep respiration breathing. If meconium aspiration occurs, it is normally cleared through the pulmonary circulation in the same manner as amniotic fluid is normally cleared from the lungs. If pulmonary vascular damage has occurred because of asphyxia, the mechanism of clearing the lung fields of fluid is affected and meconium aspiration syndrome results (Steer and Danielian, 2006).

Hypoglycemia

Acute episodes of hypoxia related to cord compression result in anaerobic glycolysis, which exhausts carbohydrate reserves. Placental deterioration can lead to chronic fetal nutritional deficiency and further depletion of the carbohydrate reserves.

Polycythemia

The fetus increases production of red blood cells as a compensatory response to hypoxia. Polycythemia can be a significant problem in the newborn period, contributing to hyperbilirubinemia from destruction of no longer needed red blood cells.

DIAGNOSTIC TESTING

When a pregnancy extends beyond 7 days past the EDD, the prenatal chart should be reviewed for confirmation of the due date. Parameters for review include the following aspects.

Gestational Length Variables

Based on the Nägele rule, the length of gestation is 280 days. However, the length of gestation has been shown to vary among women. Parity may influence gestational length. One study has shown that 287 days is the mean gestation for the primigravida and 281 days is the mean for the multigravida (Nichols, 1985). Other studies have shown that there may be ethnic variances (Mittendorf and others, 1990). The average length of gestation for white primiparas is 288 days; for white multiparas it is 283 days; for Japanese women it is 278 days; and for African-American women it is 277½ days.

Menstrual Cycle Length

If the woman has a prolonged preovulatory phase, the EDD should be appropriately adjusted to a later date.

Contraceptive Use

Oral contraceptives may delay ovulation.

Quickening

Pregnant women should be asked prospectively to note the date they felt their fetus move for the first time (quickening). For the primigravida, this usually occurs when the fetus is approximately 18 to 20 weeks of gestational age. For the multigravida, it usually occurs around 16 to 18 weeks of gestation.

Audible Fetal Heart Sounds

The fetal heart sounds can be heard with the Doppler ultrasound at around 10 to 12 weeks of gestation and with the fetoscope at 16 to 18 weeks.

Fundal Growth

Between 20 and 32 weeks of gestation, fundal height measurement, assessed with the mother's bladder empty, from the symphysis pubis to the top of the fundus, should approximate gestational age within 2 weeks.

Diagnostic Ultrasound Findings

According to the National Guideline, ultrasound performed between 11 and 14 weeks of gestation provides the most accurate gestational age assessment (Clinical Practice Obstetrics Committee, Maternal Fetal Medicine Committee, and others, 2008). Ultrasound done in the second trimester is less accurate for dating.

In estimating fetal weight, Leopold's maneuver, with fundal height measurements have similar accuracy to ultrasound measurements. However, both methods are subject to significant errors (Liao, Buhimschi, and Norwitz, 2004).

USUAL MEDICAL MANAGEMENT AND PROTOCOLS FOR NURSE PRACTITIONERS

According to a *Cochrane Review* and the National Guideline, at 41 weeks of gestation pregnant women should be offered induction. The evidence suggests a small decrease in perinatal mortality without an increase in cesarean birth risk (Gülmezoglu, Crowther, and Middleton, 2006; Clinical Practice Obstetrics Committee, Maternal Fetal Medicine Committee, and others, 2008).

However, because the absolute perinatal risk is small, women should be informed of the benefits and risks for induction of labor and expectant management (Heimstad and others, 2007). The woman's preferences should be considered in the plan of management as well as the local resources (Gülmezoglu, Crowther, and Middleton, 2006; Clinical Practice Obstetrics Committee, Maternal Fetal Medicine Committee, and others, 2008). Individualize the plan of care with the goal of not pushing nature too soon, but do not allow variables to develop that will decrease tolerance to labor, such as decreased or meconium-stained amniotic fluid, a hard fetal head, and macrosomia.

Active Management with Induction of Labor

Any of the interventions of labor stimulation outlined in Chapter 28 can be used to induce a prolonged pregnancy. Stripping fetal membranes has been shown to decrease the incidence of postdate gestations without increasing complications (Clinical Practice Obstetrics Committee, Maternal Fetal Medicine Committee, and others, 2008). Cervical ripening, with a cervical ripening agent, is usually attempted before oxytocin induction is started. If the cervix is ripe, with a Bishop score of 8 or greater, labor induction with oxytocin is usually initiated.

Expectant Management with Fetal Surveillance

If expectant management is chosen, fetal surveillance should include at least a non-stress test and amniotic fluid volume assessment according to the National Guideline (Clinical Practice Obstetrics Committee, Maternal Fetal Medicine Committee, and others, 2008). Antenatal fetal surveillance should continue until the cervix becomes ripe, spontaneous labor starts, an antepartum fetal test becomes abnormal, or labor is induced at the completion of 42 weeks (Cunningham and others, 2010).

Labor Management

Because of the increased risk for fetal hypoxia when the pregnancy is prolonged, it is ideal to do a nonstress test on admission to labor. If accelerations are absent with the use of acoustic stimulation, even if the fetal heart rate (FHR) strip is otherwise normal, this may indicate a fetus that is maintaining antenatal oxygenation but not adequate oxygen levels during the stress of uterine contractions. Close FHR monitoring is indicated.

Continuous intrapartum electronic fetal monitoring is preferable along with close monitoring of the labor progress related to the possibility of a large-for-gestational-age infant. If baseline variability is less than 5 amplitudes, if baseline FHR is less than 100 beats/min or greater than 150 beats per minute, or if late decelerations are noted, immediate cesarean delivery is considered (Steer and Danielian, 2006).

According to two randomized controlled trials when amnioinfusion is used during intrapartum to treat recurrent severe variable decelerations, it reduces the incidence of cesarean delivery for fetal distress (Pitt and others, 2000; Regi and others, 2009). Amnioinfusion was used at one time during intrapartum in the presence of meconium-stained amniotic fluid to decrease the incidence of meconium aspiration. However, a recent large randomized control trial showed no benefit with the treatment of amnioinfusion to prevent meconium aspiration syndrome (Fraser and others, 2005, 2006).

NURSING MANAGEMENT

Antepartum Nursing Interventions if Pregnancy Goes Beyond the Due Date

- Encourage the patient and her family to openly express their frustrations, feelings regarding the extreme fatigue and unattractiveness, and fears related to fetal well-being with professional health care providers and each other.
- Discuss the meaning of the EDD with the patient and her family. The EDD is merely a midpoint in a 1-month range between 38 and 42 weeks of gestation during which 90% of women will deliver (Nichols, 1987; Rehns, 2004).

- Provide opportunities for the patient to listen to the FHR and see evidence of FHR reactivity during fetal surveillance studies.
- Assist in planning alternative arrangements for help in the home for the present and postpartum periods because of fatigue.
- Discuss the benefits and risks of induction of labor and expectant management using antepartum fetal testing with selective labor induction. Consider the woman's preferences in the management plan.
- Instruct the patient about the importance of noting fetal movement. Give the patient instructions on how to assess daily fetal activity.
- Prepare the patient for weekly cervical examinations to determine cervical ripening.
- Prepare the patient for potential medical interventions, such as fetal surveillance studies, induction of labor, instrument-assisted delivery, and cesarean birth.
- Refer to available and appropriate support services, such as social services, high risk pregnancy support groups, home health aides, visiting nurses, and church or other supportive community resources.

Intrapartum Nursing Management

- Admit patient when she is in early labor or when she is due for induction of labor.
- Use pain medications and sedatives cautiously and only after other alternative methods of coping have been determined to be inadequate.
- Use continuous fetal monitoring to recognize early evidence of a category II or III FHR change.
- Manage the labor in a facility that can provide a cesarean birth or instrument-assisted delivery, if needed. Also, make sure qualified personnel for infant resuscitation are readily available.
- When rupture of membranes occurs, assess FHR and note the amount and color of amniotic fluid.
- Be prepared to collect cord pH sample from the umbilical artery immediately after delivery.
- Be prepared to manage a saline amnioinfusion if multiple variable decelerations occur related to decreased amniotic fluid.
- Notify the physician at the first signs of a category II or III FHR change.

Intrapartum Nursing Interventions for Amnioinfusion

- Chart the purpose for an amnioinfusion, if used.
- Rule out cord prolapse by performing a sterile vaginal exam.
  - An intrauterine pressure catheter must be in place.
- Educate the patient regarding the reasons for the amnioinfusion, the steps of the procedure, and obtain her consent.
- Assess baseline maternal vital signs, FHR, and uterine activity.
- Obtain a 1000-ml bag of normal saline or lactated Ringer's solution that has been stored in a heating unit or warm fluid with a blood warmer.
- Connect the warmed solution to the intrauterine pressure catheter (IUPC) using intravenous tubing. Remove air out of the tubing before infusion.

- Free flow an initial bolus of 500 to 800 ml or per protocol by hanging the IV bag 3 to 4 feet above the uterus. Monitor fluid return from the vagina. Note the amount and color of fluid.
- Cautiously continue infusing 150 to 180 ml/hour through the IUPC, monitoring the amount of fluid that continues to leak onto the pad.
- Continue infusion until variable decelerations resolve or untoward side effects develop, including an increasing uterine resting tone, non-reassuring signs of fetal compromise, uterine tenderness, or retained fluid. In any of these events, discontinue the amnioinfusion and notify the health care provider.
- Monitor uterine activity continuously with a separate or solid multiple-lumen intrauterine pressure catheter. Monitor fetal heart tones and fetal response.
- Check the temperature every 2 hours.
- Measure and mark the fundal height and reassess every hour.
- Monitor the patient's pain level.
- Keep the patient as dry and comfortable as possible by changing the pads often and providing pericare.
- Document the amount of IV fluid infused, the amount and character of the vaginal drainage, the uterine activity including resting tone, FHR, and maternal vital signs.
- Notify pediatric personnel for presence at delivery if meconium is noted in the amniotic fluid so appropriate resuscitation and oxygenation can be administered as needed. Research evidence suggests non-suctioning at the perineum in the presence of meconium-stained amniotic fluid is just as safe for the neonate as routine suctioning of the oropharynx and nasopharynx (ACOG, 2007; SOGC, 2009). If meconium is present, postnatal tracheal suction is indicated for respiratory depressed infants only according to the American Heart Association (2005) Neonatal Resuscitation Program guidelines.

CONCLUSION

The etiology and pathophysiology of prolonged pregnancy are not completely understood, but early and ongoing prenatal care is essential, and the importance of assignment of an accurate EDD is clearly evident. When prolonged pregnancy can be reasonably diagnosed, the nurse can then collaborate with the other health care team members in developing an effective plan of care to prevent undue maternal anxiety, reduce sources of fears, and lower infant mortality and morbidity.

BIBLIOGRAPHY

Agency for Healthcare Research and Quality: *Management of prolonged pregnancy, Evidence Report/Technology Assessment*, No. 53, Durham, NC, 2002, Duke Evidence-Based Practice Center.

American College of Obstetricians and Gynecologists (ACOG): Management of postterm pregnancy, *ACOG Practice Bulletin*, No. 55, Washington, DC, 2004, ACOG.

American College of Obstetricians and Gynecologists (ACOG): Management of delivery of a newborn with meconium-stained amniotic fluid, *ACOG Committee opinion*, No 379, Washington, DC, 2007, ACOG.

American Heart Association (AHA): American Heart Association guidelines for cardiopulmonary resuscitation and emergency cardiovascular care: Part 13 National Resuscitation Guidelines, *Circulation* 112(24Suppl):IV188–IV196, 2005. Retrieved from http://circ.ahajournals.org/content/vol112/24_suppl/.

Ballantyne J: The problem of the postmature infant, *J Obstet Gynaecol Br Empire* 2:512–554, 1902.

Baschat A: Fetal growth disorders. In James D, and others, editors: *High risk pregnancy: management options,* ed 3, Philadelphia, 2006, Saunders.

Bennett K, Crane J, O'Shea P, and others: First trimester ultrasound screening is effective in reducing post-term labor induction rates: a randomized control trial, *Am J Obstet Gynecol* 190:1077–1081, 2004.

Clausson B, Cnattingius S, Axelsson O: Outcomes of post-term births: the role of fetal growth restriction and malformations, *Obstet Gynecol* 94:758, 1999.

Clifford S: Postmaturity with placental dysfunction: clinical syndrome and pathologic findings, *J Pediatr* 44(1):1–13, 1954.

Clinical Practice Obstetrics Committee, Maternal Fetal Medicine Committee, Delaney M, and others: Guidelines for the management of pregnancy at 41+0 to 42+0 weeks, *J Obstet Gynaecol Can*: Retrieved from http://www.guideline.gov 2008 sep 30(9):800–810.

Cunningham F, Leveno K, Bloom S, Hauth J, Rouse D, Spong C: *Williams' obstetrics,* ed 23, New York, 2010, McGraw-Hill Medical.

Fraser W, and others: Amnioinfusion for the prevention of the meconium aspiration syndrome, *N Engl J Med* 353(9):909–917, 2005.

Fraser W, and others: Amnioinfusion for the prevention of the meconium aspiration syndrome, *Obstet Gynecol* 61(2):80–81, 2006.

Grant J: Prolonged pregnancy. In James D, and others, editors: *High risk pregnancy: management options,* ed 3, Philadelphia, 2006, Saunders.

Gribbin C, Thornton J: Critical evaluation of fetal assessment methods. In James D, and others, editors: *High risk pregnancy: management options,* ed 3, Philadelphia, 2006, Saunders.

Gülmezoglu AM, Crowther CA, Middleton P: Induction of labour for improving birth outcomes for women at or beyond term, *Cochrane Database Syst Rev,* (Issue 4), Art. No.: CD004945, 2006.

Heimstad R, Skogvoll E, Mattsson L, and others: Induction of labor or serial antenatal fetal monitoring in the post-term pregnancy: a randomized controlled trial, *Obetet Gynecol* 109:609–617, 2007.

Liao J, Buhimschi C, Norwitz E: Normal labor: mechanism and duration, *Obstet Gynecol Clin North Am* 32(2):145–164, 2004.

Martin JA, Hamilton BE, Sutton PD, et al: Births: final data for 2006. National Vital Statistics Reports, Vol 57, No 7. Hyttsville, Md, National Center for Health Statisstics, 2009.

Mittendorf R, and others: The length of uncomplicated human gestation, *Obstet Gynecol* 75(6):929–932, 1990.

Nichols C: The Yale Nurse-Midwifery Practice: addressing the outcomes, *J Nurse Midwifery* 30(3): 159–165, 1985.

Nichols C: Dating pregnancy: gathering and using a reliable data base, *J Nurse Midwifery* 32(4):195–204, 1987.

Norwitz E, Snegnovskikh V, Caughey A: Prolonged pregnancy: when should we intervene? *Clin Obstet Gynecol* 50(2), 2007.

Norwitz E, Lye S: Biology of parturition. In Creasy R, Resnik R, and others, editors: *Creasy and Resnik's maternal-fetal medicine: principles and practice,* ed 6, Philadelphia, 2009, Saunders.

Pitt C, and others: Prophylactic amnioinfusion for intrapartum oligohydramnios: a meta-analysis of randomized controlled trials, *Obstet Gynecol* 96(5 Pt 1):861–866, 2000.

Regi A, Alexander N, Jose R, and others: Amnioinfusion for relief of recurrent severe and moderate variable decelerations in labor, *J Reprod Med* 54(5):295–302, 2009.

Rehns M: The trouble with due dates, *CBE reporter* 3:1–2, 2004.

Resnik J, Resnik R: Posterm pregnancy. In Creasy R, Resnik R, Iams J, and others, editors: *Creasy & Resnik's maternal-fetal medicine: principles and practice,* ed 6, Philadelphia, 2009, Saunders.

Society of Obstetricians and Gynaecologists of Canada (SOGC): Management of meconium at birth. SOGC Technical update, No 224, *J Obstet Gynecol Can* 31(4):353–354, 2009.

Steer P, Danielian P: Fetal distress in labor. In James D and others, editors: *High risk pregnancy: management options,* ed 3, Philadelphia, 2006, Saunders.

Vorherr H: Placental insufficiency in relation to postterm pregnancy fetal postmaturity: evaluation of fetoplacental function; management of the postterm gravida, *Am J Obstet Gynecol* 123(1):67–103, 1975.

Index

A

ABCDEs for intimate partner violence
    screening, 512
Abdomen of diabetic mother, 224
Abdominal chorionic villus sampling, 94
Abdominal ectopic pregnancy, 331, 332f,
    336, 345
Abdominal hemorrhage, trauma-related,
    501
Abdominal hysterectomy
    in hydatidiform mole, 355
    in placenta cretas, 381
Abdominal pain
    in abruptio placentae, 367
    after tubal rupture, 337
    in ectopic pregnancy, 336–337
    in spontaneous abortion, 315
Abdominal surgery in preterm labor, 473
Abduction exercises during therapeutic
    bedrest, 9b–10b
Abnormal labor patterns, 620t–621t
Abnormal uterine bleeding in
    hydatidiform mole, 353
ABO and Rho (D) blood typing, 33
ABO blood group system, 405
ABO incompatibility, 402
Abortion, spontaneous; See Spontaneous
    abortion
Abruptio placentae, 364–376
    classifications of, 365t, 366f
    cocaine use and, 565
    complications of, 368–369, 370t
    delivery in, 372–376
    diagnostic testing in, 371
    eclampsia and, 449
    emergency management in, 372,
        373t–375t
    etiology of, 366

Abruptio placentae (Continued)
    expectant management in, 371–372
    fetal and neonatal effects of, 370–371
    incidence of, 364
    maternal effects of, 369
    normal physiology and, 366
    pathophysiology of, 366
    placenta previa versus, 382t–384t
    preeclampsia and, 439
    premature rupture of membranes and,
        490
    signs and symptoms of, 367–368
    trauma-related, 504
Absent variability of fetal heart rate, 61t, 62f
Abuse as high risk factor, 41
Abuse assessment screen, 510, 511b
Accelerations of fetal heart rate, 65t–67t,
    68f
Accolate. See Zafirlukast
Accreditation, 188t–189t
Acetylcholine, cocaine and, 564
Acid-base balance, 260
Acidemia in eclampsia, 449
ACOG confirmation of term gestation, 583b
Acting, process of valuing and, 171
Active transport, 45
Activity and exercise pattern, 27b–33b
    diabetic mother and, 231
    in psychologic assessment for high-risk
        pregnancy, 135b–136b
Activity and position pattern,
    dysfunctional labor and, 629–634,
    630f, 632f
Activity restriction in preeclampsia, 432
Acupressure
    for hyperemesis gravidarum, 18
    for induction of labor, 123
    for pain control during labor, 636

Page numbers followed by f, t, or b indicate figures, tables, or boxes, respectively.

Acupuncture, 108–110
  for analgesia in labor, 123
  for depression, 119–120
  for detoxification, 125
  for hyperemesis, 116
  for hyperemesis gravidarum, 18
  for induction of labor, 123, 604
  for low back pain, 121
Acute cholecystitis during pregnancy, 3
Acute fatty liver of pregnancy, 446–447
Acute pulmonary edema, 307–308
Acute pyelonephritis, 546–549
Acute renal failure
  critical care for, 269
  diagnostic testing in, 264, 264t
  etiology of, 259
  general management of, 265–266
  incidence of, 258
  maternal effects of, 263
  signs and symptoms of, 262
Acute respiratory distress syndrome
  incidence of, 290
  maternal effects of, 294
Acute tubular necrosis, 259
Acute venous thromboembolism,
    284–286
Acyclovir for herpes simplex virus type 2,
    532
Addiction, integrative therapies for, 125
Advance directive, 177–178
Advanced practice nurse, 185
Advanced Trauma Life Support, 505
After-death care in home, 164–165
Afterload, 246
Age, maternal; See Maternal age
Agonal cesarean delivery, 506–507
Albuterol, 300t–301t
  for acute exacerbation of asthma, 306
  for respiratory infection, 303–304
Alcohol-related birth defects, 560t
Alcohol-related neurodevelopmental
    disorders, 560t
Alcohol use during pregnancy
  childhood effects of, 561
  fetal complications in, 559–560,
    559t–560t
  maternal complications in, 559
  pathophysiologic effects of, 558
  screening for, 561–562, 561t–562t
  treatment of, 563–564
Aldomet; See Methyldopa
Aldosterone, 261
Alloimmunization, 406
Allow natural death, palliative care for
    dying infant and, 164

Alpha-adrenergic blockers for diabetes
    mellitus-related hypertension, 212
Alpha-fetoprotein, 90
  diabetic mother and, 220
Alpha-linolenic acid, 11
Alternative medical systems, 108–110
  homeopathy in, 110
  traditional Chinese medicine in,
    108–110
American College of Obstetricians and
    Gynecologists confirmation of term
    gestation, 583b
American Nurses Association
  code of ethics, 177b
  definition of nurse role, 25
  source of standards, 192t
Amino acids
  nutritional therapy and, 113
  renal excretion of, 261
Ammonia excretion in urine, 260
Amniocentesis, 93t, 95–96
  diabetic mother and, 206, 220
  in hemolytic incompatibility, 409–411
  in hydatidiform mole, 356
  in placenta previa, 379
  in premature rupture of membranes,
    492–493
Amnioinfusion in prolonged pregnancy,
    667–669
Amnion, 5, 489
Amniotic band syndrome, 491
Amniotic cavity, 5
Amniotic fluid, 489
  development of, 5–6
  evaluation of fetal heart rate and, 45
  normal physiology of, 661
  prolonged pregnancy and, 662
  volume evaluation of, 81b
Amniotic fluid embolism; See
    Anaphylactoid syndrome of
    pregnancy
Amniotic fluid index in premature rupture
    of membranes, 493
Amniotomy
  for induction of labor, 600–602
  oxytocin-induced labor and, 595
AmniSure Assay, 492
Amoxicillin
  for acute pyelonephritis, 547
  for gonorrhea, 525
  for premature rupture of membranes,
    494
  for urinary tract infection, 548t
Ampicillin for urinary tract infection,
    548–549

Ampullar tubal pregnancy, 331, 334t
Analgesia
    epidural
        in dysfunctional labor, 646–648
        instrumental delivery and, 645
        interventions to decrease risk for,
            627–637
        postpartum, 648
        risks of, 622
    for labor
        integrative therapies in, 123–125
        preeclampsia and, 452–453
    for renal calculi, 265
Anaphylactoid syndrome of pregnancy
    critical care in, 308–309
    diagnostic testing in, 297
    disseminated intravascular coagulation
        and, 397
    fetal effects of, 294–295
    incidence of, 290
    signs of, 293
Anemia
    fetal
        in hemolysis of fetal erythrocytes, 408
        placenta previa and, 379
    maternal
        in chronic kidney disease, 266
        hemoglobin levels in, 26
        iron deficiency and, 11
        risk after abruptio placentae, 369
Angiotensin-converting enzyme inhibitors
    for diabetes mellitus-related
        hypertension, 212
    for hypertension in chronic kidney
        disease, 266
Angiotensin II, 420–421
Angiotensin II receptor blockers
    for diabetes mellitus-related
        hypertension, 212
    for hypertension in chronic kidney
        disease, 266
Ankle circle exercises, 9b–10b
Anniversary phenomenon, spontaneous
    abortion and, 327
Announcement phase of pregnancy,
    130–131
Antepartum period
    diagnostic assessment in, 26–36
        laboratory studies in, 26–35
        ultrasound in, 35–36
    exercise during, 629
    fetal surveillance in, 65–80, 83
    glycemic management in, 213–220,
        225–234
        blood glucose monitoring in, 214, 233

Antepartum period (Continued)
        diet and, 219, 226–230, 228t–230t
        early morning hyperglycemia and,
            217t
        exercise and, 219, 231
        fetal surveillance and, 220, 232–233
        hypoglycemia management and, 233
        insulin management in, 215–218,
            215t–216t
        insulin therapy for gestational
            diabetes mellitus and, 219
        maternal surveillance and, 219–220
        sick-day rule in, 234
        urine testing in, 214
    human immunodeficiency virus
        infection and, 537–538
    management of vaginal birth after
        cesarean in, 643–644
    nursing assessment in, 25–26
    nursing interventions in
        for alloimmunization, 413–414
        for asthma, 304–305
    nutrition in, 10–21
        assessment of, 13–16
        food groups and, 15–16, 16t–17t
        hyperemesis gravidarum and, 18–21,
            19b–20b, 20t
        hyperphenylalanemia and, 18
        nutrient needs in, 10–13
        prepregnancy weight status and,
            13–14
        weight gain in multifetal pregnancy
            and, 15, 16t
        weight gain in singleton pregnancy
            and, 14–15, 14t
    physical assessment in, 36–37
    ultrasound in, 35–36
Antibiotics
    for acute pyelonephritis, 547
    for bacterial vaginosis, 520
    for chlamydial infection, 523
    for gonorrhea, 525
    for group B streptococcal infection, 526,
        527f
    for pneumonia, 302
    for renal disease, 263
    for syphilis, 544
    for urinary tract infection, 265, 548t
Antibody screen, 34
    in hemolytic incompatibility, 408
Anticipatory grieving
    in ectopic pregnancy, 348
    in gestational trophoblastic disease, 361
    in maternal cardiac disease, 253
    in spontaneous abortion, 327

Anticoagulation therapy
   for acute venous thromboembolism,
      284
   for disseminated intravascular
      coagulation, 400
   nursing interventions for, 286
Anticonvulsants for preeclampsia, 433,
      442–445, 442b–443b, 444t, 446b
Antidepressants for postpartum
      depression, 144–145
Antidiuretic effect of oxytocin, 596
Antidiuretic hormone, 260
Antidysrhythmics for maternal cardiac
      disease, 251
Antiemetics for hyperemesis gravidarum,
      19
Antifungals for candidiasis, 522
Antigen detection enzyme immunoassay
      for *Chlamydia,* 523
Antihistamines, 298
   for hyperemesis gravidarum, 21
Antihypertensives
   for chronic hypertension during
      pregnancy, 419t
   for preeclampsia, 433
   for renal disease, 267
Antimalarials for systemic lupus
      erythematosus, 277
Antiphospholipid syndrome, 271
   critical care interventions for, 280
   etiology of, 272
   fetal and neonatal effects of, 275
   general management of, 277
   incidence of, 271
   intrapartum nursing interventions for,
      279
   maternal effects of, 274
   medical diagnosis of, 276
   pathophysiology of, 272
   postpartum nursing interventions for,
      280
   prenatal nursing interventions for, 279
   recurrent spontaneous abortions and,
      312–313, 324
   signs and symptoms of, 272–273
   thromboprophylaxis in, 284, 285t
Antiretroviral therapy, 535–536
Antithrombin III
   clot formation and, 396–397
   deficiency of, 283
   for disseminated intravascular
      coagulation, 399
Antiviral drugs
   for hepatitis C, 531
   for herpes simplex virus type2, 532

Anxiety
   in adaptation to high risk pregnancy,
      132
   in placental abnormalities, 392
   in preeclampsia, 452
   in premature rupture of membranes, 497
Apparent abruptio placentae, 364, 366f
Appendicitis, 338t–341t
Apresoline; *See* Hydralazine
ARDS; *See* Acute respiratory distress
      syndrome
ARF; *See* Acute renal failure
Arm lift exercises, 9b–10b
Arnica, 121
Aromatherapy, 110–111, 111b
   for analgesia in labor, 124
   for constipation, 118–119
   for mental and emotional problems, 120
Arrhythmias, fetal, 59–62, 63f, 64t
Arterial blood gases, 295t–296t, 296–297
Arterial thrombosis, antiphospholipid
      syndrome and, 274
Artifact in fetal arrhythmias monitoring,
      60–62, 63f, 64t
Aspart, 215
Aspirin
   for antiphospholipid syndrome,
      277, 324
   to decrease risk of preeclampsia, 266,
      435–436
   for platelet aggregation in diabetic
      mother, 212
   for systemic lupus erythematosus, 277
Assisted reproduction, ectopic pregnancy
      and, 332
Association of Women's Health, Obstetric
      and Neonatal Nurses, 192t
Asthma
   acute exacerbation of, 306–307
   antepartum nursing interventions for,
      304–305
   diagnostic testing in, 295
   exacerbation signs in, 293
   fetal effects of, 294–295
   incidence of, 289–290
   intrapartum nursing interventions for,
      305
   maternal effects of, 293–294
   medical management of, 298, 299t–301t
   pathophysiology of, 292
Asymptomatic bacteriuria, 258, 546–549,
      548t
Atenolol for chronic hypertension during
      pregnancy, 418–419
Augmentation of labor, 582

Auricular stimulation therapy, 118
Autoimmune rheumatic diseases, 271
   etiology of, 272
   fetal and neonatal effects of, 274–275
   general management of, 276–277
   incidence of, 271
   intrapartum critical care interventions
      for, 280
   maternal effects of, 274
   medical diagnosis of, 275–276
   nursing management of, 277–280
   pathophysiology of, 272
   secondary and tertiary prevention in,
      277–278
   signs and symptoms of, 272–273, 273t
Autonomic dysplasia, 503
Autonomic nervous system
   in control of fetal heart rate, 46
   fetal oxygenation and, 43
   influence on blood flow, 244
   influence on uterine activity, 466t–467t
Autonomic neuropathy
   in diabetes mellitus, 213
   physical evaluation of, 224
Autonomy, 174t
Avalon FM30 transducer, 50f
Azathioprine for systemic lupus
   erythematosus, 277
Azithromycin
   for chlamydial infection, 523
   for gonorrhea, 525

B
B vitamins
   deficiency in hyperemesis gravidarum,
      18
   in intravenous formula, 20t
Baby blues, 138–140; *See also* Postpartum
      depression
Back pain in occiput posterior
   presentation, 613
Bacteremia, sporadic abortions and, 312
Bacterial infections
   chlamydial, 522–524
   gonorrhea in, 524–525
   group B streptococcus in, 525–527
   Laminaria dilator-related, 591
   premature rupture of membranes and,
      488
   preterm labor and, 461
   sporadic abortions and, 312
   syphilis in, 543–545
   of urinary tract, 546–549, 548t
Bacterial vaginosis, 519–521
Bacteriuria, 258

Balloon catheter for induction of labor,
   591–592
Bariatric surgery, pregnancy after, 14
Baseline fetal heart rate, 58–62, 58f, 59t
   baseline variability and, 58–59, 60f, 61t,
      62f
   fetal arrhythmia and artifact and,
      59–62, 63f, 64t
Battering, 501
Bearing-down effort, 633
Bedrest, 6–8
   in cardiac disease, 249
   isometric exercises during, 9b–10b
   negative physical and psychosocial
      effects of, 8
   in placental abnormalities, 392–393
   in preeclampsia, 432, 435
   in premature rupture of membranes,
      497–498
   for preterm labor in multiple gestation,
      474
Behavioral characteristics, high risk factors
   and, 39–41
Beneficence, 174t
Benzathine penicillin G
   for group B streptococcal infection, 526
   for syphilis, 544
Bereavement care, 149
   after-death care in home and, 164–165
   contact with infant's body and, 153,
      154b
   continuing development of, 151–152
   grieving process and, 151–152
   historical background of, 149–150
   palliative care for dying infant and, 164
   perinatal hospice care after diagnosis
      of life-limiting condition and,
      163–164
   Pregnancy Loss and Infant Death
      Alliance guidelines in, 155b–162b,
      165
   support during subsequent pregnancy
      and, 153–163
Beta-adrenergic blockers for maternal
   cardiac disease, 251
Beta-human chorionic gonadotropin
   in ectopic pregnancy, 342, 343t
   in hydatidiform mole, 351
   in metastatic gestational trophoblastic
      neoplasia, 359
   in spontaneous abortion, 318
Betamethasone
   for fetal lung maturity
      in placenta previa, 380
      in preeclampsia, 441b

Betamethasone *(Continued)*
  for premature rupture of membranes,
    494–495
Bicarbonate
  deficit in acute renal failure, 262
  diabetic ketoacidosis and, 235
  kidney regulation of, 260
  pregnant verus nonpregnant values of,
    295t
Biochemical markers
  in predicting success in induction of
    labor, 584
  in preeclampsia, 430, 430t–431t
Biologic-based therapies, 108, 112–113
  herbal medicine in, 112, 113b
  nutritional therapy in, 112–113
Biologic high risk factors, 40t
Biophysical profile
  diabetic mother and, 220
  in fetal surveillance, 81b–82b
  in premature rupture of membranes, 493
Biopsy
  fetal
    kidney, 98
    muscle, 97–98
    skin, 97
  renal, 264
Birth defects
  maternal alcohol use and, 559, 560t
  maternal cocaine use and, 565
Birth trauma, 618
Bishop Prelabor Scoring System, 584t
Bisphenol A exposure, 40t
Black cohosh for induction of labor, 123,
    604
Bladder infection, 546–549, 548t
  diagnostic testing in, 263–264
  signs and symptoms of, 261
Blastocyst, 4, 313
  ectopic pregnancy and, 331
  uterus and, 333
Bleeding
  in disseminated intravascular
    coagulation, 398
  in ectopic pregnancy, 337
  in placental abnormalities, 364
    abruptio placentae and, 364–376; *See
      also* Abruptio placentae
    antepartum fetal surveillance in,
      391
    assessment of blood loss in, 387
    bedrest in, 392–393
    critical care in, 389–390
    disseminated intravascular
      coagulation and, 390–391

Bleeding *(Continued)*
    fear and, 392
    hospitalization in, 392
    hypovolemic shock in, 389–390
    invasive placenta and, 381–385
    mild, 388
    moderate to severe, 388–389
    placenta accreta and, 381–385
    placenta previa and, 376–381; *See also*
      Placenta previa
    prevention of, 386–387
    RhD alloimmunization and, 393
    vasa previa and, 385–386, 385f
  postpartum
    integrative therapies for, 125
    in placental abnormalities, 389
    premature rupture of membranes and,
      490
    risk after abruptio placentae, 369
  in spontaneous abortion, 315, 321,
    325–326
  trauma-related, 501–504
Blood component therapy
  in abruptio placentae, 372, 373t–375t
  in disseminated intravascular
    coagulation, 399–400
  fetal intrauterine, 101–102
  in placenta previa, 380
  in preeclampsia-related
    thrombocytopenia, 434
  in spontaneous abortion, 321–322,
    325–326
Blood flow
  autonomic nervous system and, 244
  cocaine use and, 565
Blood glucose monitoring in diabetes
    mellitus, 214, 233
Blood pressure
  blood loss and, 370t
  chronic hypertension and, 418–419
  in disseminated intravascular
    coagulation, 398
  measurement during prenatal visit, 36
  preeclampsia and, 429
  spontaneous abortion and,
    319b–320b
Blood supply to kidney, 260
Blood transfusion; *See* Blood component
    therapy
Blood type genetics, 402–405,
    403f–405f
Blood typing, 33
Blood urea nitrogen
  in acute renal failure, 265–266
  changes during pregnancy, 3

Blood volume
    in antepartum period, 244
    changes during pregnancy, 1, 420
    fetal oxygenation and, 43
Blue cohosh for induction of labor, 123,
    604
BMI; *See* Body mass index
Body fat, diabetic mother and, 226
Body mass index, prepregnancy weight
    status and, 13
Bodywork for low back pain, 121
Bone, prolonged pregnancy and, 663
Bowel stimulation for induction of labor,
    605
BPP; *See* Biophysical profile
Brachial plexus injury, 640
Bradycardia, fetal, 59t, 60f
Brain death, 502
Breach of duty, 187
Breads
    exchange list for meal planning and,
        229t–230t
    menu guidelines for, 17t
Breast stimulation for induction of labor,
    602–604
Breastfeeding
    alcohol use and, 562–563
    antituberculous drugs and, 303
    chronic hypertension during pregnancy
        and, 419–420
    cocaine use and, 567
    diabetic mother and, 237–238
    effects on insulin, 233
    hepatitis C and, 531
    methadone and, 569
    metronidazole and, 520
Breathing changes during pregnancy, 2
Breech presentation, 615–617, 616f,
    624t–626t
    integrative therapies for, 117–118
Broad ligament pregnancy, 335
Bronchitis
    incidence of, 290
    maternal effects of, 294
    medical management of, 298
Brow presentation, 614, 615f,
    624t–626t
Budesonide, 300t–301t
BUN; *See* Blood urea nitrogen
Burn, 503
Butoconazole for candidiasis, 522

C
CAGE questionnaire for at-risk drinking
    patterns, 561, 562t

Calcium
    deficit in acute renal failure, 262
    influence on uterine activity, 466t–467t
    labor contractions and, 461
    needs during pregnancy, 12–13
    preeclampsia and, 432
    supplementation of
        in heparin therapy, 285
        in multifetal pregnancy, 15
Calcium channel blockers
    for chronic hypertension during
        pregnancy, 418–419
    for diabetes mellitus-related
        hypertension, 212
    for preterm labor, 477b–480b
Calcium chloride for magnesium sulfate
    toxicity, 445
Caloric intake
    diabetic mother and, 226–227
    dietary requirements and, 16t
    exercise and, 7
Cancer
    cervical, 541
    marijuana and, 569
Candidiasis, 521–522
Caput succedaneum
    amniotomy and, 601
    instrumental delivery and, 646
Carbohydrate counting, 228–230
Carbohydrates
    diabetic mother and, 227
    exchange list for meal planning and,
        228t
    intolerance in gestational diabetes
        mellitus, 204
    needs during pregnancy, 11, 16t
Carboprost, 389
Cardiac decompensation in maternal
    cardiac disease, 252–253
Cardiac disease, 243
    anticipatory grieving and, 253
    critical care nursing interventions in,
        253–255
    diabetic mother and, 224
    diagnostic testing in, 248
    drug therapy for, 249–251
    early detection of preterm labor in,
        253
    etiology of, 243–244
    fetal and neonatal effects of, 248
    general management of, 248–249
    hemodynamic pressure readings in,
        255t
    incidence of, 243
    maternal effects of, 247–248

Cardiac disease *(Continued)*
  maternal risk subgroups in, 247b
  normal antepartal cardiac physiology
      and, 244–245
  postpartum nursing interventions in,
      256
  prevention of cardiac decompensation
      in, 252–253
  signs and symptoms of, 246
  tertiary prevention in, 251–252
Cardiac output
  in antepartum period, 244
  changes during pregnancy, 2
  in disseminated intravascular
      coagulation, 400
  fetal oxygenation and, 44
  multiple gestation and, 464
  uterine contractions and, 245
Cardiopulmonary resuscitation,
    506–507
Cardiovascular system
  fetal oxygenation and, 43–44
  normal physiology of, 244–245
  preeclampsia and, 437–438, 437t
  pregnancy-related changes in, 1–4, 420
  systemic lupus erythematosus and, 273t
Caring, 175, 176b
  legal issues in, 192–195, 192t
Case law, 188t–189t
Caulophyllum, 124–125
Cayenne, 125
CDE (RH) blood group system and, 405
Cefazolin
  for group B streptococcal infection, 526
  for urinary tract infection, 265
Cefixime, 525
Ceftriaxone
  for gonorrhea, 525
  for pyelonephritis, 548–549
  for urinary tract infection, 265
Celestone; *See* Betamethasone
Central abruptio placentae, 364, 366f
Central fetal monitor display, 55
Central nervous system
  in control of fetal heart rate, 46
  preeclampsia and, 424, 438–439, 438t
  systemic lupus erythematosus and,
      273t
Central venous pressure
  during labor in cardiac disease, 249
  ranges in maternal cardiac disease, 255t
Cephalexin, 265
Cephalhematoma, 646
Cephalic replacement, 639t
Cephalopelvic disproportion, 617

Cephalosporins
  for pneumonia, 302
  for urinary tract infection, 548–549,
      548t
Cereals, exchange list for meal planning
    and, 229t–230t
Cerebral palsy
  abruptio placentae and, 371
  electronic fetal heart rate monitoring
      and, 47
Certified nurse midwife, 185–186
Cervical cancer, 541
Cervical ectopic pregnancy, 331, 332f, 336,
    345
Cervical incompetence
  diagnostic testing in, 318
  medical management of, 324
  pathophysiology of, 315
  recurrent abortions and, 313
  signs and symptoms of, 316
Cervical ripening
  balloon catheters and extra-amniotic
      saline infusion in, 591–592
  dinoprostone in, 586–590
  laminaria and synthetic dilators in,
      590–591
  misoprostol in, 590
  physiology of, 585
Cervidil; *See* Dinoprostone
Cervix
  anatomy during pregnancy, 461
  cervical incompetence following trauma
      to, 315
  genital warts and, 531–533
  influence on uterine activity, 466t–467t
  Laminaria dilator-related trauma to, 591
  preterm labor and, 461, 469
  structural changes with pregnancy, 314
Cesarean delivery
  in abruptio placentae, 372–376
  after maternal trauma, 508
  breech presentation and, 617
  diabetes mellitus and, 207
    insulin therapy and, 222
    nursing interventions in, 237
  in dysfunctional labor, 649–650
  electronic fetal heart rate monitoring
      and, 47–48
  heparin therapy after, 287
  in human immunodeficiency virus
      infection, 537–538
  in human papillomavirus infection, 541
  labor management to decrease risk of,
      619–623
  maternal risks in, 618

Cesarean delivery *(Continued)*
  oxytocin-induced labor and, 596
  perimortem, 506–507
  in placenta previa, 381
  in preeclampsia, 450
  in vasa previa, 386
Chamomile, 120
Chemical exposure as high risk factor, 40t
Chemotherapy
  in gestational trophoblastic neoplasia, 357, 359
  as high risk factor, 40t
Chest injury, 503
Chest tube, 503
Childhood effects
  of maternal alcohol use during pregnancy, 561
  of maternal smoking during pregnancy, 572
  of maternal use of marijuana, 569
Childhood obesity, maternal diabetes mellitus and, 209
Chinese medicine, 108–110
  for addictions, 125
  for analgesia in labor, 123–124
  for breech presentation, 117–118
  for constipation, 118
  for hyperemesis, 116
  for hypertensive disorders, 122
  for induction of labor, 123
  for low back pain, 121–122
  for mental and emotional problems, 119–120
  for postpartum bleeding, 125
  for preterm labor, 122–123
Chinese nutritional therapy, 109
Chiropractic, 113–114
  for low back pain, 121
Chlamydial infection, 522–524, 546
Chloramphenicol, 267
Chlorpheniramine, 298
Cholecystitis during pregnancy, 3
Cholelithiasis, 338t–341t
Choosing, process of valuing and, 170
Chorioamnionitis, 525
  Laminaria dilator-related, 591
Chorion, 5, 489
Chorion frondosum, 5
Chorionic villi, 333, 353, 366
  types of, 377
Chorionic villus sampling, 93–94, 93t
Chromosomal abnormality
  in recurrent abortions, 312, 323
  in sporadic abortions, 311

Chronic abruption-oligohydramnios sequence, 368
Chronic hypertension, 417t, 418–420
  abruptio placentae and, 366
  antihypertensive medications for, 419t
  preeclampsia and, 212
  stages of, 418t
Chronic kidney disease
  diagnostic testing in, 265
  etiology of, 259
  general management of, 266
  incidence of, 258
  maternal effects of, 263
  signs and symptoms of, 262
Cimicifuga, 124–125
Cinnamon, 125
Civil law, 187
CKD; *See* Chronic kidney disease
Clary sage, 124
Clavicle fracture, 646
Clindamycin
  for bacterial vaginosis, 520
  for group B streptococcal infection, 526
Clinical nurse specialist, 185
Clomiphene citrate, ectopic pregnancy and, 332
Closing capacity, 291
Clot formation, 396–397, 396f–397f
Clotrimazole, 522
Clove bud oil, 124
Coagulation factors
  changes during pregnancy, 2–3
  clot formation and, 396–397
  for disseminated intravascular coagulation, 399
Coarctation of aorta, 247
Cocaine, 564–567
  abruptio placentae and, 366, 386–387
Code of ethics of American Nurses Association, 177b
Cognitive and perceptual pattern, 27b–33b
  diabetic mother and, 232–233
  dysfunctional labor and, 634–635
  in psychologic assessment for high-risk pregnancy, 135b–136b
Collecting duct, 260
Colloid osmotic pressure, 1
Combined abruptio placentae, 364, 366f
Combined health information database, 126t
Combined spinal/epidural analgesia in dysfunctional labor, 633, 646–648
Common cold, 298

Communication
  bereavement care and, 155b–162b, 165
  litigation risk and, 184–185
Community standards, 192t
Compensatory respiratory alkalosis, 2
Complaint, legal term, 188t–189t
Complementary and alternative therapies,
    107
  for addictions, 125
  alternative medical systems in, 108–110
    homeopathy in, 110
    traditional Chinese medicine in,
      108–110
  for analgesia in labor, 123–125
  biologic-based therapies in, 112–113
    herbal medicine in, 112, 113b
    nutritional therapy in, 112–113
  for breech presentation, 117–118
  for constipation, 118–119
  energy therapies in, 115
    cranial sacral therapy in, 115
    polarity in, 115
  evidence-based databases for, 126t
  for hyperemesis, 116–117
  for hypertensive disorders, 122
  for induction of labor, 123, 602–605
  for low back pain, 121–122
  manipulative and body-based methods
    in, 113–115
    chiropractic in, 113–114
    massage therapy in, 114
    osteopathy in, 114–115
  for mental and emotional problems,
    119–120
  mind-body interventions in, 110–112
    aromatherapy in, 110–111, 111b
    hypnotherapy in, 111
    spiritual healing and prayer in, 111
    yoga in, 112
  for postpartum bleeding, 125
  for preterm labor, 122–123
Complete abortion, 316f, 317t
  medical management of, 321–322, 323f
Complete blood count, prenatal, 26
Complete breech, 615, 616f
Complete hydatidiform mole, 351, 353–354
Compound presentation, 614–615,
    624t–626t
Computer retrieval of information on
    scientific projects, 126t
Concealed abruptio placentae, 364, 366f
Condylomata acuminata, 540
Confidentiality, 174t
  in intimate partner violence screening,
    512

Conflict, adaptation to high risk pregnancy
    and, 133
Congenital disorders
  fetal
    fetal intrauterine surgery for, 103
    lower urinary tract obstruction in, 99
    maternal cocaine use and, 565
  maternal
    cervical incompetence and, 315
    diabetes mellitus and, 208
Congenital heart block, fetal, 62, 64t, 275
Conscience clauses, 175–176
Constipation, 118–119
Continuous Glucose Monitor, 214
Continuous insulin infusion during labor
    and delivery, 221–222, 236t
Continuous quality assurance, 194b–195b
Contraception
  diabetic mother and, 225
  ectopic pregnancy and, 332
  for hypertensive woman, 454
  maternal cardiac disease and, 252
  prolonged pregnancy and, 666
Contractility, 245–246
Contraction stress test, 76b–77b, 78f–80f
Contractions, uterine; See Uterine
    contractions
Conventional level of moral judgment
    development, 171–172
COP; See Colloid osmotic pressure
Coping and stress-tolerance pattern,
    27b–33b
  diabetic mother and, 232
  dysfunctional labor and, 637
  in psychologic assessment for high-risk
    pregnancy, 135b–136b
Copper supplementation in multifetal
    pregnancy, 15
Cord prolapse, breech presentation and,
    616
Cordocentesis, 409
Corometrics Model 129 maternal/fetal
    monitor, 50f
Corpus luteum cyst, 342
Corticosteroids
  for fetal lung maturity
    in HELLP syndrome, 447
    in placenta previa, 380
    in preeclampsia, 434, 441b
  for premature rupture of membranes,
    494–495
  for preterm labor in diabetic mother,
    221, 235–236
  for respiratory infection, 304
  for systemic lupus erythematosus, 277

Corticotropin-releasing hormone, preterm labor and, 465
Cotyledon, 5, 33
Cough, 292
Coumadin; *See* Warfarin
Court trial, 188t–189t
Crack cocaine, 564
Cranial sacral therapy, 115
  for hyperemesis, 117
  for mental and emotional problems, 120
Creatinine, 265–266
Creatinine clearance
  changes during pregnancy, 3
  in preeclampsia, 438
Credentialing, 188t–189t
Criminal law, 186
Crisis, adaptation to high risk pregnancy and, 133
Critical care
  in acute pulmonary edema and pulmonary embolism, 307–308
  in acute renal failure, 269
  in anaphylactoid syndrome of pregnancy, 308–309
  in autoimmune rheumatic diseases, 280
  in cardiac disease, 253–255
  in disseminated intravascular coagulation, 390–391, 400–401
  in eclampsia, 447–449
  in hypovolemic shock in placental abnormalities, 389–390
  in maternal trauma, 514–516
  in perinatal diabetic ketoacidosis, 234–235
  in preeclampsia
    anticonvulsant therapy and, 442–445, 442b–443b, 444t
    antihypertensive therapy and, 445, 446b
    HELLP syndrome and, 445–447
    invasive hemodynamic monitoring and, 450, 451t–452t
  in pulmonary edema, 481–482
  in respiratory emergencies, 307
Cromolyn sodium, 300t–301t
Cryoprecipitate for disseminated intravascular coagulation, 399
Crystal meth, 570
Crystalloids
  for abruptio placentae, 372
  for hemorrhage in uterine evacuation in spontaneous abortion, 322
Cupping, 109
Curl-ups exercise, 9b–10b

CVS; *See* Chorionic villus sampling
Cyclosporine, 277
Cystic fibrosis
  diagnostic testing in, 295–297
  fetal effects of, 294–295
  incidence of, 289
  maternal effects of, 293–294
  medical management of, 297–303
  pathophysiology of, 292
Cystic fibrosis transmembrane regulator gene, 289
Cystitis, 546–549, 548t
Cytokines
  endothelial cell dysfunction in preeclampsia and, 423
  fetal membranes and, 489
  immunosuppressive activity of gestational tissue and, 314
  influence on uterine activity, 466t–467t
  preterm labor and, 464
Cytotec; *See* Misoprostol
Cytotrophoblast, 314

D
D-dimer test, 390–391
Dairy
  daily food choices and, 16t
  menu guidelines for, 17t
Damages, legal term, 187
Dandelion root tea, 117
Danger Assessment instrument, 511
DASH diet, 418
Dawn phenomenon, 217t
Dead space, 291
Death
  fetal
    in abruptio placentae, 370–371
    after induction of labor, 597
    antiphospholipid syndrome and, 275
    in disseminated intravascular coagulation, 398
    in ectopic pregnancy, 337
    in end-stage renal disease, 266–267
    in fetal intrauterine transfusion, 101
    in maternal burn injury, 503
    maternal diabetes mellitus and, 208
    percutaneous umbilical blood sampling and, 96
    trauma-related, 500
    in vasa previa, 386
  maternal
    in abruptio placentae, 369
    diabetic ketoacidosis and, 207
    in disseminated intravascular coagulation, 398

Death *(Continued)*
　　ectopic pregnancy and, 335, 337
　　gestational trophoblastic neoplasia
　　　　and, 357
　　maternal risk subgroups and, 247b
　　in placenta cretas, 385
　　in placenta previa, 378
　　pneumonia and, 294
　　preeclampsia and, 427
　　premature rupture of membranes and,
　　　　490
　　pulmonary embolism and, 283, 294
　　spontaneous abortion and, 316
　　trauma-related, 500, 504
　perinatal, 149
　　after-death care in home and,
　　　　164–165
　　contact with infant's body and, 153,
　　　　154b
　　continuing development of
　　　　bereavement care and, 151–152
　　grieving process and, 151–152
　　historical background of perinatal
　　　　bereavement care and, 149–150
　　palliative care for dying infant and,
　　　　164
　　perinatal hospice care after diagnosis
　　　　of life-limiting condition and,
　　　　163–164
　　Pregnancy Loss and Infant Death
　　　　Alliance guidelines in,
　　　　155b–162b, 165
　　support during subsequent pregnancy
　　　　and, 153–163
Decelerations of fetal heart rate, 65t–67t, 69f
Decidua, 4, 313, 366
Decidua basalis, 5, 313
　abruptio placentae and, 367
　placenta cretas and, 381
Decidua capsularis, 313
Decidua vera, 313
Decision making, 170
　advance directive and, 177–178
　American Nurses Association code of
　　　ethics and, 177b
　clinical examples of, 178, 179b
　definitions of ethical principles and, 174t
　ethics committee and, 178
　framework for ethics and, 173
　model for, 173–176
　moral judgment development and,
　　　171–172
　Patient Self-Determination Act and, 176
　steps in, 176b
　values clarification and, 170–171

Deep tendon reflexes in preeclampsia, 438,
　　　438t
Deep vein thrombosis, 282
　acute, 284–286, 285t
　anticoagulation therapy for, 286
　diagnostic testing in, 283
　etiology of, 282
　fetal and neonatal effects of, 283
　incidence of, 282
　intrapartum and postpartum
　　　management of heparin and, 287
　maternal effects of, 283
　normal physiology and, 283
　signs and symptoms of, 283
　thromboprophylaxis and, 284
Defective placentation, 421
Defendant, 188t–189t
Defibrillation, 506
Dehydration
　in diabetes mellitus, 204–206
　in hyperemesis gravidarum, 18
Delayed menses, ectopic pregnancy and,
　　　336
Delivery
　in abruptio placentae, 372–376
　breech presentation and, 617
　cardiac disease and, 249
　cesarean; *See* Cesarean delivery
　in disseminated intravascular
　　　coagulation, 400
　eclampsia and, 449
　HELLP syndrome and, 447
　heparin therapy after, 287
　human immunodeficiency virus
　　　infection and, 538
　in placenta previa, 380–381, 382t–384t
　in preeclampsia, 431, 434, 450
Delivery of posterior arm, 639t, 642f
Demographic characteristics, high risk
　　　factors and, 38–39
Dental hygiene as high risk factor, 39
Deontology, 175
Deposition, 188t–189t, 190–191
Depression
　postpartum, 138–140
　　criteria for major depressive syndrome
　　　　and, 143b
　　diagnosis of, 140–143
　　differential diagnosis of, 139
　　Edinburgh Postnatal Depression
　　　　Scale and, 141b–142b
　　neonatal effects of, 140
　　screening for, 140
　　treatment of, 143–145
　prenatal, 138

Depression *(Continued)*
  prolonged pregnancy and, 663–664
  traditional Chinese medicine for,
    119–120
Detemir, 216
Detoxification, acupuncture for, 125
Developmental anomalies, premature
    rupture of membranes and, 491
Dexamethasone for premature rupture of
    membranes, 494–495
Diabetes mellitus, 200
  antepartum glycemic management of,
    213–220, 225–234
    blood glucose monitoring in, 214, 233
    diet and, 219, 226–230, 228t–230t
    early morning hyperglycemia and, 217t
    exercise and, 219, 231
    fetal surveillance and, 220, 232–233
    hypoglycemia management and, 233
    insulin management in, 215–218,
      215t–216t
    insulin therapy for gestational
      diabetes mellitus and, 219
    maternal surveillance and, 219–220
    sick-day rule in, 234
    urine testing in, 214
  causes of, 202
  coping with, 232
  diabetic ketoacidosis and, 234–235
  diagnostic testing in, 210–211, 211t
  fetal and neonatal effects of, 207–209
  gestational, 200
    diagnostic testing in, 210–211, 211t
    dietary guidelines for, 227
    glucose test for, 34
    insulin therapy in, 219
    pathophysiology of, 204
    postpartum nursing interventions for,
      222, 238, 239b
    signs and symptoms of, 204
  incidence of, 201
  intrapartum management of, 221–222,
    235–237, 236t
  ketoacidosis management and, 220–221
  maternal effects of, 204–207
  normal pregnancy physiology and, 202
  pathophysiology of, 203–204, 203t
  postpartum management of, 222,
    237–238
  preconception management of, 212–213,
    223–225
  preterm labor management and, 221
  Revised White's Classification of
    perinatal diabetes and, 201t
  signs and symptoms of, 204, 205t

Diabetic ketoacidosis, 207
  critical care interventions for, 234–235
  fetal mortality and, 209
  management of, 220–221
Diabetic retinopathy, 207, 213
Diagnostic testing
  in abruptio placentae, 371
  in cardiac disease, 248
  in diabetes mellitus, 210–211, 211t
  in disseminated intravascular
    coagulation, 399
  in dysfunctional labor, 619, 620t–621t
  in ectopic pregnancy, 337–344,
    338t–341t, 343t
  in gestational diabetes mellitus, 210–
    211, 211t
  in gestational trophoblastic neoplasia,
    357
  in hemolytic incompatibility, 408–409
  in hydatidiform mole, 354–355
  in placenta previa, 379
  in preeclampsia, 429–431, 430t–431t
  in premature rupture of membranes,
    491–492
  in preterm labor, 468–470
  in prolonged pregnancy, 665–666
  in pulmonary disease, 295–297,
    295t–296t
  in renal disease, 263–265, 264t
  in spontaneous abortion, 317–318
  in venous thromboembolic disease, 283
Diastolic filling pressure, 246
Diazepam for evacuation of uterus in
    spontaneous abortion, 321–322
DIC; *See* Disseminated intravascular
    coagulation
Diet
  diabetes mellitus and, 219, 226–230,
    228t–230t
  gestational diabetes and, 227
  phenylketonuria and, 18
  preeclampsia and, 432–433
Dietary Approaches to Stop Hypertension
    diet, 418
Dietary history of diabetic mother, 226
Digitalis, 250
Dilapan, 322, 590
Dinoprostone, 586–590, 588t
Direct fluorescent antibody detection for
    Chlamydia, 523
Direct monitoring of fetus, 52–54,
    53f, 54b
Discovery, legal term, 189
Disopyramide phosphate, 251
Dissecting aneurysm, 247

Disseminated intravascular coagulation, 395
  in abruptio placentae, 365t, 369
  anticoagulants for, 400
  blood replacement in, 399–400
  diagnostic testing in, 399
  eclampsia and, 449
  etiology of, 395–396
  fetal and neonatal effects of, 398
  incidence of, 395
  maternal effects of, 398
  normal process of clot formation and, 396–397, 396f–397f
  nursing management in, 400–401
  pathophysiology of, 397–398
  in placental abnormalities, 390–391
  in preeclampsia, 425
  signs and symptoms of, 398
  trauma-related, 502
Diuretics
  for acute renal failure, 265–266
  for chronic hypertension during pregnancy, 418–419
  for chronic kidney disease, 266
  for renal disease, 267
Diversional activity interventions
  in high risk pregnancy, 137–138
  in therapeutic bedrest, 392–393
Dizygotic multiple fetus, 460
DNR, palliative care for dying infant and, 164
Documentation
  of fetal age in premature rupture of membranes, 492
  guidelines for, 196b
  in intimate partner violence screening, 512
  legal issues in, 196b
  risk management and, 194b–195b
Domestic violence, 41, 509–510, 511b, 513t
Dopamine
  for acute renal failure, 265–266
  cocaine and, 564
  for hypovolemic shock in placental abnormalities, 390
Doppler flow studies
  in fetal surveillance, 83b
  in hemolytic incompatibility, 409
Doppler ultrasound in preeclampsia, 430–431
Drug abuse, 558
  alcohol in, 558–564
    childhood effects of, 561

Drug abuse (Continued)
    fetal complications in, 559–560, 559t–560t
    maternal complications in, 559
    pathophysiologic effects of, 558
    pregnancy considerations in, 562–563
    screening for, 561–562, 561t–562t
    treatment during pregnancy, 563–564
  cocaine in, 564–567
  heroin in, 567–569, 568b
  as high risk factor, 39
  intervention for positive screen, 574–575, 576t
  marijuana in, 569–570
  methamphetamines in, 570
  prevention and early detection of, 574, 575b
  tobacco in, 571–574
    fetal and neonatal complications in, 571–572
    maternal complications in, 571
    pathophysiologic effects of, 571
    treatment during pregnancy, 572–574, 573b
  traditional Chinese medicine for, 125
Drug therapy
  for asthma, 300t–301t
  for bacterial vaginosis, 520
  for candidiasis, 522
  for cardiac disease, 249–251
  for chlamydial infection, 523
  for gonorrhea, 525
  for group B streptococcal infection, 526, 527f
  for hepatitis C, 531
  for herpes simplex virus type2, 532
  for human immunodeficiency virus, 535–536
  for postpartum depression, 144–145
  for preeclampsia, 433–434
  for renal disease, 267
  for syphilis, 544
  for trichomoniasis, 545
  for urinary tract infection, 548–549, 548t
Drug withdrawal, 568b
Durable power of attorney, 177
Duty, 187
DVT; See Deep vein thrombosis
Dysfunctional labor, 610
  abnormal labor patterns in, 620t–621t
  cesarean birth and, 649–650
  diagnostic testing in, 619
  early detection and treatment of, 637–638

Dysfunctional labor *(Continued)*
  epidural or combined spinal/epidural in,
    646–648
  etiology of, 611
  external version in, 641–643
  fetal and neonatal effects of, 618–619
  fetal dystocia in, 612–617, 623,
    624t–626t
    breech presentation in, 615–617, 616f
    brow presentation in, 614, 615f
    compound presentation in, 614–615
    face presentation in, 613–614, 614f
    occiput posterior presentation in, 613,
      613f
    shoulder presentation in, 613–614,
      615f, 638–641, 639t, 640f–642f
  functional health patterns and, 627–637
    activity and position pattern in,
      629–634, 630f, 632f
    cognitive pattern in, 634–635
    coping and stress-tolerance pattern
      in, 637
    elimination pattern in, 629
    health-perception and health-
      management pattern in, 627
    nutritional and metabolic pattern in,
      627–628
    perceptual pattern in, 635–636
    rest and relaxation pattern in, 634
    role-relationship pattern in, 636–637
    self-perception and self-concept
      pattern in, 636
  incidence of, 610–611
  instrumental delivery with forceps or
    vacuum extractor in, 645–646
  labor management to decrease cesarean
    rate in, 619–623
  maternal effects of, 618
  normal physiology and, 612
  pelvic dystocia in, 617
  postpartum epidural analgesia in, 648
  prevention of, 627
  signs and symptoms of, 618
  uterine dystocia in, 612
  vaginal birth after cesarean and,
    643–644
Dyslipidemia
  in metabolic syndrome, 200
  preconception management of, 212
Dyspnea
  in respiratory distress, 292
  in venous thromboembolic disease, 283
Dysrhythmias, fetal, 64t
Dystocia, 595, 610; *See also* Dysfunctional
  labor

E
Early abortion, 311
Early decelerations of fetal heart rate,
  65t–67t, 69f
Echinacea, 522
Eclampsia, 417t, 425–426
  critical care in, 447–449
  disseminated intravascular coagulation
    and, 398
  hemodynamic changes in, 424–425
  signs and symptoms of, 429
Ecstasy, 570
Ectoderm, 6
Ectopic pregnancy, 331
  anticipatory grieving and, 348
  anxiety and, 347
  diagnostic testing in, 337–344,
    338t–341t, 343t
  etiology of, 331–333
  fetal and neonatal effects of, 337
  gestational trophoblastic neoplasia and,
    356
  incidence of, 331
  maternal effects of, 337
  medical management of, 347–348
  methotrexate for, 344–345
  normal physiology and, 333
  nursing assessment in, 346–347
  pathophysiology of, 333–336, 334t, 335f
  postoperative nursing interventions in,
    347
  prevention of, 346
  signs and symptoms of, 336–337
  surgical treatment of, 344–345
Edema
  hemodilution of plasma colloids and, 1
  in preeclampsia, 437t
  pulmonary
    acute, 307–308
    invasive hemodynamic monitoring
      and, 450
    maternal cardiac disease and, 247
    in preeclampsia, 424, 451t–452t
    preterm labor and, 481–482
  routine evaluation for, 36
  in venous thromboembolic disease, 283
Edinburgh Postnatal Depression Scale,
  141b–142b
Educational attainment as high risk factor,
  38
EFM; *See* Electronic fetal heart rate
  monitoring
Eggs, menu guidelines for, 17t
EIA test for anti-HCV, 530
Electrical stimulation, 110

Electroacupuncture, 110
Electrocardiogram changes during
    pregnancy, 2
Electrolyte imbalance
    in acute renal failure, 262
    in preeclampsia, 424
Electronic fetal heart rate monitoring,
    46–48
    acute asthma exacerbation and, 307
    after amniocentesis, 96
    cerebral palsy and, 47
    cesarean section and, 47–48
    during labor in prolonged pregnancy,
        667
    legal implications of, 48
    in preeclampsia, 452
Elimination pattern, 27b–33b
    diabetic mother and, 230
    dysfunctional labor and, 629
    in psychologic assessment for high-risk
        pregnancy, 135b–136b
Embolism
    in anaphylactoid syndrome of pregnancy
        critical care in, 308–309
        diagnostic testing in, 297
        disseminated intravascular
            coagulation and, 397
        fetal effects of, 294–295
        incidence of, 290
        signs of, 293
    maternal cardiac disease and, 247
    pulmonary, 282
        acute, 284–286, 285t
        anticoagulation therapy for, 286
        antiphospholipid syndrome and,
            274
        critical care in, 307–308
        diagnostic testing in, 283
        etiology of, 282
        fetal effects of, 283, 294–295
        incidence of, 282, 290
        intrapartum and postpartum
            management of heparin and,
            287
        maternal effects of, 283, 294
        normal physiology and, 283
        signs and symptoms of, 283
        thromboprophylaxis and, 284
        treatment of, 286
Embryo
    development of, 4, 313–314
    spontaneous abortion and, 315
Embryoblast, 313, 352–353
Emergency management in abruptio
    placentae, 372, 373t–375t

Emotional stress
    integrative therapies for, 119–120
    premature rupture of membranes and,
        497
    preterm labor and, 462b, 465
    prolonged pregnancy and, 663–664
    sporadic abortions and, 312
End-stage renal disease, 266–267
Endocervical culture for gonorrhea, 525
Endoderm, 6
Endometrial scarring, placenta previa and,
    377
Endothelial cell dysfunction in
    preeclampsia, 421, 422f
Endothelin, 421, 466t–467t
Energy therapies, 108, 115
    cranial sacral therapy in, 115
    polarity in, 115
Enoxaparin, 285t
Entrainment, 129
Environmental exposures, 38–39, 40t
Environmental factors in sporadic
    abortions, 312
Enzymes, nutritional therapy and, 113
Epidural analgesia
    in dysfunctional labor, 646–648
    instrumental delivery and, 645
    interventions to decrease risk for,
        627–637
    postpartum, 648
    risks of, 622
Episodic fetal heart patterns, 55
Erythromycin
    for chlamydial infection, 523
    for group B streptococcal infection, 526
    for premature rupture of membranes,
        494
Erythropoietin, 259, 261
Escherichia coli in urinary tract infection,
    259, 546
Essential fatty acids, 11
Estrogen, 585
    deficiency in prolonged pregnancy, 660
    fallopian tube and, 333
    preterm labor and, 463
    systemic vasodilation and, 244
Ethambutol, 302
Ethanol, 563
Ethical decision making, 170
    advance directive and, 177–178
    American Nurses Association code of
        ethics and, 177b
    clinical examples of, 178, 179b
    definitions of ethical principles and, 174t
    ethics committee and, 178

Ethical decision making *(Continued)*
  framework for ethics and, 173
  model for, 173–176
  moral judgment development and, 171–172
  Patient Self-Determination Act and, 176
  steps in, 176b
  values clarification and, 170–171
Ethical dilemma, 178, 179b
Ethical principles, 173, 174t
Ethics, 173
Ethics committee, 178
Ethnicity as high risk factor, 38
Evacuation of uterus in spontaneous abortion, 321
Evening primrose oil for induction of labor, 604
Evidence, legal term, 188t–189t
Evidence-based databases for integrative therapies, 126t
Exchange list for meal planning, 228, 228t–230t
Exercise, 6–8, 9b–10b
  for constipation, 119
  diabetic mother and, 219, 231
  for hypertensive disorders, 122
  for low back pain, 121
  during pregnancy, 629
Expectant management
  in abruptio placentae, 371–372
  in placenta previa, 379–380
  in preeclampsia, 431–432
  in premature rupture of membranes, 493–494
  in prolonged pregnancy, 667
Expert opinion, 188t–189t
Expert witness, 197
External contraction monitoring, 49–52, 51b, 51f
External fetal heart rate monitoring, 52, 52b
  after fetal intrauterine transfusion, 102
  after fetal kidney biopsy, 98
  after fetal muscle biopsy, 98
  after fetal skin biopsy, 97
  after fetal urine aspiration, 98
  after percutaneous umbilical blood sampling, 97
External version, 641–643
Extra-amniotic saline infusion for induction of labor, 591–592
Eye
  of diabetic mother, 224
  preeclampsia and, 424
  systemic lupus erythematosus and, 273t

Eye-to-eye contact in parent-infant attachment, 129

F
Face presentation, 613–614, 614f, 624t–626t
Facial anomalies in fetal alcohol syndrome, 559t
Facilitated diffusion, 5, 34
Factor V Leiden, 283
  recurrent abortions and, 313
Faintness
  after tubal rupture, 337
  in ectopic pregnancy, 347
Fallopian tube
  ectopic pregnancy and, 331, 332f
  normal physiology of, 333
Family planning, diabetic mother and, 225, 238
Family processes promotion in high risk pregnancy, 137
FAS; *See* Fetal alcohol syndrome
Fasting plasma glucose, 210
Father-infant attachment, 128
Fats
  daily food choices and, 16t
  diabetic mother and, 227
  exchange list for meal planning and, 229t–230t
  menu guidelines for, 17t
  needs during pregnancy, 11, 16t
Fear
  in ectopic pregnancy, 347
  in gestational trophoblastic disease, 361
  high risk pregnancy and, 134–136
  in placental abnormalities, 392
  in premature rupture of membranes, 497
Femstat 3; *See* Butoconazole
Ferguson reflex, 633
Ferrous gluconate, 11–12
Ferrous sulfate, 11–12
Fetal alcohol spectrum disorders, 559, 560t, 562
Fetal alcohol syndrome, 559, 559t–560t
Fetal anemia
  in hemolysis of fetal erythrocytes, 408
  placenta previa and, 379
Fetal aneuploidy tissue markers, 92b
Fetal arrhythmias, 59–62, 63f, 64t
Fetal biopsy
  kidney, 93t, 98
  muscle, 97–98
  skin, 97
Fetal bradycardia, 59t, 60f
Fetal dysrhythmias, 64t

Fetal dystocia, 612–617, 623, 624t–626t
  breech presentation in, 615–617, 616f
  brow presentation in, 614, 615f
  compound presentation in, 614–615
  face presentation in, 613–614, 614f
  occiput posterior presentation in, 613, 613f
  shoulder presentation in, 613–614, 615f, 638–641, 639t, 640f–642f
Fetal fibronectin, 469
Fetal gas exchange, premature rupture of membranes and, 497
Fetal heart
  capabilities for maintaining health, 45
  prolonged pregnancy and, 666
Fetal heart rate, 57
  in abruptio placentae, 371
  absence in hydatidiform mole, 353
  after amniocentesis, 96
  after chorionic villus sampling, 94
  amniotic fluid function and, 45
  baseline, 58–62, 58f, 59t
    variability of, 58–59, 60f, 61t, 62f
  central nervous system control of, 46
  in disseminated intravascular coagulation, 400
  electronic monitoring of, 46–48
    acute asthma exacerbation and, 307
    after amniocentesis, 96
    arrhythmia and artifact and, 59–62, 63f, 64t
    cerebral palsy and, 47
    cesarean section and, 47–48
    during labor in prolonged pregnancy, 667
    legal implications of, 48
    NICHD categories and, 56–57
    in preeclampsia, 452
  external monitoring of, 52, 52b
  in HELLP syndrome, 447
  in hemolytic incompatibility, 406, 408, 413
  induction of labor and, 599
  in maternal trauma, 514
  patient positioning and, 84
  patterns and periodic rate changes in, 63–65, 65t–67t, 68f–69f, 70t
  in placental abnormalities, 391
  in preeclampsia, 439
  in premature rupture of membranes, 493
  prostaglandin-initiated labor and, 587–589
  standardized definitions of, 48

Fetal hypoglycemia, 665
Fetal hypoxia, 294–295
  in abruptio placentae, 371
  in disseminated intravascular coagulation, 398
  dysfunctional labor and, 618
  prolonged pregnancy and, 665
Fetal intrauterine surgery, 102–103
Fetal intrauterine transfusion, 101–102
  in hemolytic incompatibility, 410
Fetal loss
  in abruptio placentae, 370–371
  after induction of labor, 597
  antiphospholipid syndrome and, 275
  in disseminated intravascular coagulation, 398
  in ectopic pregnancy, 337
  in end-stage renal disease, 266–267
  in fetal intrauterine transfusion, 101
  in maternal burn injury, 503
  maternal diabetes mellitus and, 208
  percutaneous umbilical blood sampling and, 96
  trauma-related, 500
  in vasa previa, 386
Fetal lung maturity
  amniocentesis in hemolytic incompatibility and, 411
  assessment in premature rupture of membranes, 492–493
  maternal diabetes mellitus and, 209
  placenta previa and, 380
  preeclampsia and, 434
Fetal malpresentation, 612–617, 623, 624t–626t
  breech presentation in, 615–617, 616f
  brow presentation in, 614, 615f
  compound presentation in, 614–615
  face presentation in, 613–614, 614f
  occiput posterior presentation in, 613, 613f
  in placenta previa, 378–379
  shoulder presentation in, 613–614, 615f, 638–641, 639t, 640f–642f
Fetal membranes, 489
  stripping of, 602
Fetal monitor, 49, 50f
Fetal movement, 37
Fetal movement counting, 75b
  in preeclampsia, 439
  in premature rupture of membranes, 493
Fetal muscle biopsy, 93t
Fetal oxygen saturation monitoring, 71–80
Fetal oxygenation, 43–44
  eclampsia and, 448

Fetal pulse oximetry, 71–80
Fetal skin biopsy, 93t
Fetal spiral electrode, 53f, 54
Fetal surveillance, 43
  in abruptio placentae, 372
  amniotic fluid volume evaluation in, 81b
  antepartum nursing assessment in,
    83–84
  baseline fetal heart rate and, 58–62, 58f,
    59t
    baseline variability and, 58–59, 60f,
      61t, 62f
    fetal arrhythmia and artifact and,
      59–62, 63f, 64t
  biophysical profile in, 81b–82b
  contraction stress test in, 76b–77b,
    78f–80f
  Doppler flow studies in, 83b
  electronic fetal heart rate monitoring in,
    46–48
    cerebral palsy and, 47
    cesarean section and, 47–48
    legal implications of, 48
  external contraction monitoring in,
    49–52, 51b, 51f
  external fetal heart rate monitoring in,
    52, 52b
  fetal heart rate and, 46, 57
  fetal heart rate patterns and periodic
    rate changes in, 63–65, 65t–67t,
    68f–69f, 70t
  fetal monitoring terms in, 55, 56b–57b
  fetal movement counting in, 75b
  fetal oxygen saturation monitoring with
    fetal pulse oximetry in, 71–80
  fetal oxygenation and, 43–44
  in hemolytic incompatibility, 410
  instrumentation in, 49–57, 50f
  intermittent auscultation in, 48–49
  internal monitoring in, 52–54, 53f
    advantages and limitations of, 54b
    fetal spiral electrode for, 53f, 54
    intrauterine pressure catheter for,
      52–54
  intrapartum nursing assessment in,
    83–84
  maternal diabetes mellitus and, 220,
    232–233
  modified biophysical profile in, 82b
  nonstress test in, 72b–73b, 73f
  nursing interventions in, 84
  perinatal screening and, 88
    amniocentesis in, 95–96
    chorionic villus sampling in, 93–94
    fetal kidney biopsy and, 98

Fetal surveillance (Continued)
    fetal muscle biopsy and, 97–98
    fetal skin biopsy and, 97
    fetal urine aspiration and, 99
    methods of, 89–91
    noninvasive prenatal diagnosis and,
      100
    nursing management in, 104
    percutaneous umbilical blood
      sampling in, 96–97
    preimplantation genetic diagnosis
      and, 99–100
    prenatal genetic screening and,
      88–89, 89t
    ultrasound evaluation for fetal
      abnormalities and, 91–92, 92b
  in placental abnormalities, 391
  in preeclampsia, 433, 439–440
  in prolonged pregnancy, 667
  uteroplacental-fetal exchange and,
    44–45
  vibroacoustic stimulation in, 74b
Fetal tachycardia, 59t, 60f
  maternal cocaine use and, 567
Fetal urine aspiration, 93t, 99
Fetopelvic disproportion, 617
Fetus
  abruptio placentae and, 370–371
  capabilities for maintaining health, 45
  coexisting hydatidiform mole with, 356
  development of, 6
  disseminated intravascular coagulation
    and, 398
  dysfunctional labor and, 618–619
  ectopic pregnancy and, 337
  effects of maternal conditions on
    autoimmune rheumatic diseases and,
      274–275
    cardiac disease and, 248
    diabetes mellitus and, 207–209
    pulmonary disease and, 294–295
    renal disease and, 263
    venous thromboembolic disease and,
      283
  hemolytic incompatibility and,
    407–408
  human parvovirus B19 and, 543
  maternal alcohol use during pregnancy
    and, 559–560, 559t–560t
  maternal cocaine use and, 565–566
  maternal establishment of relationship
    with, 130
  maternal heroin use and, 568
  maternal smoking and, 571–572
  maternal trauma and, 504–505, 516

Fetus *(Continued)*
  oxytocin for induction of labor and, 596–597
  placenta previa and, 379
  preeclampsia and, 427
  premature rupture of membranes and, 490–491
  preterm labor and, 465–468
  prolonged pregnancy and, 664–665
  secretion of oxytocin during labor, 593
  spontaneous abortion and, 311, 315, 317
  syphilis and, 544
  ultrasound evaluation for abnormalities of, 91–92, 92b
FFP; *See* Fresh frozen plasma
FHR; *See* Fetal heart rate
Fiber, diabetic mother and, 227–228
Fibrin, 396, 396f
Fibrinogen, 396, 396f
Fibrinoid layer of Nitabuch, 377, 381
Fibrinolysis, 396, 396f–397f
Fibrinolytic activity during pregnancy, 2–3
Fidelity, 174t
Fifth disease, 542
FIGO classification of gestational trophoblastic neoplasia, 357, 358t
Fimbriated tubal pregnancy, 331, 334t
Finality, 174t
First trimester
  diabetes mellitus and
    calculation guidelines for insulin in, 216t
    insulin needs and, 215t
    manifestations and consequences of, 205t
  screening during, 91
Fish, 17t
Flagyl; *See* Metronidazole
Fluid balance, 420
Fluid imbalance
  in acute renal failure, 262
  in preeclampsia, 424
Fluid intake
  in chronic kidney disease, 266
  needs during pregnancy, 13
  preeclampsia and, 434–435
  for prevention of urinary tract infection, 267
Fluid replacement
  in abruptio placentae, 372
  in acute renal failure, 265–266
  in disseminated intravascular coagulation, 400
Fluid shifts in pregnancy, 421
Fluid volume overload, 245

Focusing phase of pregnancy adjustment, 131
Folate
  needs during pregnancy, 12
  supplementation in multifetal pregnancy, 16
Folic acid
  maternal diabetes mellitus and, 219
  preeclampsia and, 432
Food
  dietary requirements for pregnancy and, 16t
  magnesium-rich, 20b
  menu guidelines and, 17t
  potassium-rich, 19b
Food groups, 15–16, 16t–17t
Food pyramid, 230
Forced expiratory volume at 1 second, 296t
Forced vital capacity, 296t
Forceps delivery, 645–646
Foreseeability, legal term, 188t–189t
Fracture
  clavicle, 646
  pelvic, 503
FRAMES acronym, 564
Frank breech, 615, 616f
Free beta subunit of human chorionic gonadotropin, 91
Free fetal DNA, 100
Freebase cocaine, 564
Fresh frozen plasma
  for abruptio placentae, 372
  for disseminated intravascular coagulation, 399
Fruits
  daily food choices and, 16t
  exchange list for meal planning and, 228t–230t
  menu guidelines for, 17t
Frustration in adaptation to high risk pregnancy, 132
Functional health patterns, 25–26, 27b–33b
  diabetic mother and, 225–234
  dysfunctional labor and, 627–637
    activity and position pattern in, 629–634, 630f, 632f
    cognitive pattern in, 634–635
    coping and stress-tolerance pattern in, 637
    elimination pattern in, 629
    health-perception and health-management pattern in, 627
    nutritional and metabolic pattern in, 627–628

Functional health patterns *(Continued)*
    perceptual pattern in, 635–636
    rest and relaxation pattern in, 634
    role-relationship pattern in, 636–637
    self-perception and self-concept
        pattern in, 636
    in psychologic assessment, 135b–136b
Functional residual capacity, 291
    changes during pregnancy, 2
Fundal growth, prolonged pregnancy and,
    666
Fundus height, 36
Fungal infections
    candidiasis in, 521–522
    sporadic abortions and, 312
Furosemide
    for acute renal failure, 265–266
    for maternal cardiac disease, 250

G
Gallbladder changes during pregnancy, 3
Gallstones during pregnancy, 3, 338t–341t
Gap junctions influence on uterine activity,
    466t–467t
Gastric aspiration in general anesthesia,
    628
Gastrointestinal system
    physiologic adaptations to pregnancy,
        3–4
    systemic lupus erythematosus and, 273t
Gastrulation, 6
Gene amplification molecular diagnostics,
    523
General anesthesia, gastric aspiration in,
    628
General damages, legal term, 187
Generality, 174t
Genetic risk, 37
Genetic screening
    prenatal, 88–89, 89t
    in recurrent spontaneous abortions, 328
Genetics
    blood type, 402–405, 403f–405f
    preeclampsia and, 426
Genital warts, 540
Genitalia of diabetic mother, 224
Genitourinary infections, 519
    bacterial vaginosis in, 519–521
    candidiasis in, 521–522
    chlamydial, 522–524
    gonorrhea in, 524–525
    group B streptococcus in, 525–527
    hepatitis B in, 527–530
    hepatitis C in, 530–531
    herpes simplex virus type 2 in, 531–533

Genitourinary infections *(Continued)*
    human immunodeficiency virus in,
        533–539
    human papillomavirus in, 539–541
    human parvovirus B19 in, 542–543
    prevention of, 549–551
    syphilis in, 543–545
    trichomoniasis in, 545–546
    urinary tract infection in, 546–549, 548t
Gentamicin, 265, 548–549
Geographic location as high risk factor, 38
Geranium essential oil, 120
Gestational age, premature rupture of
    membranes and, 492
Gestational diabetes, 200
    diagnostic testing in, 210–211, 211t
    dietary guidelines for, 227
    glucose test for, 34
    insulin therapy in, 219
    pathophysiology of, 204
    postpartum nursing interventions for,
        222, 238, 239b
    signs and symptoms of, 204
Gestational hypertension, 416, 417t
Gestational length variables, 665
Gestational trophoblastic disease, 351
    anticipatory grieving and, 361
    early detection of, 361–362
    gestational trophoblastic neoplasia and,
        358t–359t, 361
    maternal fear and, 361
    nursing assessment in, 360
    postevacuation nursing interventions in,
        360–361
    uterine evacuation in, 360
Gestational trophoblastic neoplasia,
    358t–359t, 361
    early detection of, 361–362
    nursing assessment in, 360
    prophylactic chemotherapy for, 356
GFR; *See* Glomerular filtration rate
Ginger for hyperemesis gravidarum, 18
Glargine, 216
Glomerular filtration, 260, 420
Glomerular filtration rate, 3
Glomerulus, 260
Gluco Watch G2 Biographer, 214
Glucose
    renal reabsorption of, 260
    requirements for diabetic mother in
        labor, 236
Glucose challenge test, 210
Glucose tolerance test
    for gestational diabetes, 34
    postpartum, 239b

Glyburide, 219
Glycosylated hemoglobin, 211
Gonococcal ophthalmia, 525
Gonorrhea, 524–525
Gordon's functional health patterns,
    25–26, 27b–33b; *See also* Functional
    health patterns
Graduated compression stockings, 284
Grains
    daily food choices and, 16t
    exchange list for meal planning and,
        229t–230t
    menu guidelines for, 17t
Grief and loss
    anticipatory grieving and
        in ectopic pregnancy, 348
        in gestational trophoblastic disease,
            361
        in maternal cardiac disease, 253
        in spontaneous abortion, 327
    bereavement care and, 149
        after-death care in home and,
            164–165
        contact with infant's body and, 153,
            154b
        continuing development of, 151–152
        grieving process and, 151–152
        historical background of, 149–150
        palliative care for dying infant and,
            164
        perinatal hospice care after diagnosis
            of life-limiting condition and,
            163–164
        Pregnancy Loss and Infant Death
            Alliance guidelines in,
            155b–162b, 165
        support during subsequent pregnancy
            and, 153–163
Grieving process, 151–152
Group B streptococcus infection, 525–527
    prophylaxis in premature rupture of
        membranes, 495
Group B streptococcus screening, 35
GTN; *See* Gestational trophoblastic
    disease
Gua sha, 110
Gunshot wound, 504
Gyne-Lotrimin; *See* Clotrimazole

H
hCG; *See* Human chorionic gonadotropin
Head injury, 502
Head-to-toe evaluation in trauma, 506,
    507f
Headache in preeclampsia, 424

Health care, effect of litigation on,
    186
Health care workers, human
    immunodeficiency virus and, 539
Health-perception and health-
    management pattern, 27b–33b
    diabetic mother and, 225–226
    dysfunctional labor and, 627
    in psychologic assessment for high-risk
        pregnancy, 135b–136b
Heart
    fetal, 45
    maternal, 2, 245
        normal physiology of, 244–245
        preeclampsia and, 437–438, 437t
Heart disease, 243
    anticipatory grieving and, 253
    critical care nursing interventions in,
        253–255
    diabetic mother and, 224
    diagnostic testing in, 248
    drug therapy for, 249–251
    early detection of preterm labor in,
        253
    etiology of, 243–244
    fetal and neonatal effects of, 248
    general management of, 248–249
    hemodynamic pressure readings in,
        255t
    incidence of, 243
    maternal effects of, 247–248
    maternal risk subgroups in, 247b
    normal antepartal cardiac physiology
        and, 244–245
    postpartum nursing interventions in,
        256
    prevention of cardiac decompensation
        in, 252–253
    signs and symptoms of, 246
    tertiary prevention in, 251–252
Heart rate
    abruptio placentae and, 369
    changes during pregnancy, 244
HELLP syndrome
    critical care in, 445–447
    diagnostic testing in, 431t
    eclampsia and, 449
    hypertension and, 416
    preeclampsia and, 425, 445–447
    renal disease and, 268
    signs of, 428
    systemic lupus erythematosus and,
        274
Hemabate; *See* Carboprost
Hematocrit, prenatal assessment of, 26

Hematologic system
  physiologic adaptations to pregnancy, 2–3
  preeclampsia and, 439
  systemic lupus erythematosus and, 273t
Hematoma in abruptio placentae, 367
Hemodilution during pregnancy, 1
Hemodynamic changes
  in preeclampsia, 424–425
  during pregnancy, 1
Hemodynamic monitoring
  in hypovolemic shock in placental abnormalities, 390
  in preeclampsia, 434, 450, 451t–452t
  pressure readings in cardiac disease, 255t
Hemoglobin
  fetal, 45
  prenatal assessment of, 27
Hemolytic incompatibility, 402
  ABO blood group system and, 405
  antepartum nursing interventions for, 413–414
  blood type genetics and, 402–405, 403f–405f
  CDE (Rh) blood group system and, 405
  diagnostic testing in, 408–409
  etiology of, 402
  fetal and neonatal effects of, 407–408
  incidence of, 402
  intrapartum nursing interventions for, 414
  maternal effects of, 407
  pathophysiology of, 406
  placental transport of fetal blood cells and, 405–406
  prevention of, 409–410, 412
  RhD$_O$ immune globulin for, 412–413
  signs and symptoms of, 406, 407f
  treatment for, 410–412
Heparin
  for acute venous thromboembolism, 284–286
  for antiphospholipid syndrome, 277
  intrapartum and postpartum management of, 287
  for maternal cardiac disease, 250
  for preeclampsia, 435
Hepatic alterations in preeclampsia, 439
Hepatitis B, 527–530
Hepatitis B immunoglobulin, 529
Hepatitis B virus screen, 34
Hepatitis C, 530–531

Herbal therapy, 112
  for analgesia in labor, 124
  Chinese, 109
  for constipation, 119
  contraindications during pregnancy, 113b
  for hyperemesis, 117
  for hypertensive disorders, 122
  for induction of labor, 123, 604
  for low back pain, 121
  for mental and emotional problems, 120
  for postpartum bleeding, 125
Herbicide exposure as high risk factor, 40t
Heroin, 567–569, 568b
Herpes simplex virus type2, 531–533
High-alert medication, oxytocin as, 597
High risk adaptation, 133–134
High risk factors, 37–41
  behavioral characteristics and, 39–41
  demographic characteristics and, 38–39
  genetic risk in, 37
  vaccination risk in, 37
High risk metastatic gestational trophoblastic neoplasia, 359, 359t
High risk pregnancy
  hormonal response to, 133
  psychologic adaptations to, 128
    allaying fear and facilitating coping and, 134–136
    anxiety and, 132
    attachment and, 128–129
    conflict in, 133
    crisis in, 133
    diversional activity interventions in, 137–138
    enhancing self-esteem and, 137
    frustration in, 132
    high risk adaptation and, 133–134
    high risk stressors and, 131–132
    maternal tasks in, 130
    paternal tasks in, 130
    postpartum depression and, 138–140; See also Postpartum depression
    prenatal depression and, 138
    promotion of family processes and, 137
    psychologic assessment in, 134, 135b–136b
    self-blaming in, 132
    threat to self-esteem in, 132
High risk stressors, 131–132
HMG-CoA reductase inhibitors, 212
Homans sign, 283
Home management
  of preeclampsia, 436–437
  of preterm labor, 482

Homeopathy, 110
  for analgesia in labor, 124–125
  for breech presentation, 118
  for induction of labor, 123
  for mental and emotional problems, 120
Homicide, 504, 509
Hormones
  cervical incompetence and, 315
  ectopic pregnancy and, 332
  influence on cardiovascular system, 244
  placental, 5
  recurrent spontaneous abortions and,
    324
  response to high risk pregnancy, 133
Hospice, perinatal, 163–164
Hospitalization
  in placental abnormalities, 392
  in preterm labor, 476–480
  stressors in, 132
Humalog, 215
Human chorionic gonadotropin
  free beta subunit of, 91
  role in embryo development, 313–314
  triple marker screening and, 90
Human immunodeficiency virus infection,
  533–539
Human immunodeficiency virus screening,
  34
Human insulin, 215, 216t
Human menopausal gonadotropin, 332
Human papillomavirus, 539–541
Human papillomavirus vaccine, 540
Human parvovirus B19, 542–543
Human wart viruses, 539
Humoral rheumatic diseases, 271
  etiology of, 272
  fetal and neonatal effects of, 274–275
  general management of, 276–277
  incidence of, 271
  maternal effects of, 274
  medical diagnosis of, 275–276
  pathophysiology of, 272
  secondary and tertiary prevention in,
    277–278
  signs and symptoms of, 272–273, 273t
Humulin, 215
Hydatidiform mole
  gestational trophoblastic neoplasia and,
    356
  prevention of, 360
  uterine evacuation of, 360
Hydralazine
  for hypertensive crisis during pregnancy,
    446b
  for preeclampsia, 433

Hydrocephalic disorders, fetal intrauterine
  surgery for, 103
Hydrops fetalis, 408
Hydrotherapy, 635
  for analgesia in labor, 124
Hydroxychloroquine, 277
Hyperbilirubinemia
  in HELLP syndrome, 425
  maternal diabetes mellitus and, 209
Hypercoagulation
  during pregnancy, 2–3, 283
  recurrent abortions and, 313
Hyperdynamic state during pregnancy, 2
Hyperemesis, 116–117
Hyperemesis gravidarum, 18–21, 19b–20b,
  20t
Hyperglycemia
  early morning, 217t
  effect on fetus, 208–209
Hyperinsulinemia, 4, 202
Hyperphenylalaninemia, 18
Hyperplasia, 10
Hyperreflexia, 503
  maternal cocaine use and, 565
Hypertension
  abruptio placentae and, 366
  in chronic kidney disease, 266
  in diabetes mellitus, 212–213
  in metabolic syndrome, 200
  in preeclampsia, 427
  stages of, 418t
Hypertensive crisis in preeclampsia,
  451t–452t
Hypertensive disorders of pregnancy, 416
  chronic hypertension in, 418–420
    antihypertensive medications for, 419t
    stages of, 418t
  classification of, 417t
  incidence of, 417–418
  integrative therapies for, 122
  preeclampsia in, 420–431
    activity restriction in, 432
    anticonvulsants for, 442–445,
      442b–443b, 444t, 446b
    cardiovascular alterations in,
      437–438, 437t
    central nervous system alterations in,
      438–439, 438t
    delivery and, 434
    diagnostic testing in, 429–431,
      430t–431t
    diet and, 432–433
    drug therapy for, 433–434
    early and appropriate prenatal care in,
      435–436

Hypertensive disorders of pregnancy
    (*Continued*)
    eclampsia and, 447–449
    expectant management in, 431–432
    fetal and neonatal effects of, 427
    fetal surveillance in, 433, 439–440
    HELLP syndrome and, 445–447
    hematologic alterations in, 439
    hepatic alterations in, 439
    home health care in, 436–437
    intensive hemodynamic monitoring
        in, 434, 450, 451t–452t
    intrapartum interventions for,
        450–453
    maternal effects of, 427
    mild *versus* severe, 429t
    normal physiology and, 420–421
    nursing interventions for, 440–441,
        441b
    pathophysiology of, 421–423, 422f
    postpartum interventions for,
        453–454
    prevention of, 434–435
    pulmonary alterations in, 439
    renal alterations in, 438, 438t
    reproductive system status and, 439
    signs and symptoms of, 427–429
Hypertrophy, 10
Hyperventilation during pregnancy, 2
Hypervolemia during pregnancy, 1, 3
Hypnotherapy, 111
    for addictions, 125
    for breech presentation, 118
    for hyperemesis, 117
    for mental and emotional problems,
        120
    for preterm labor, 123
Hypoglycemia
    diabetes mellitus and, 207
    effect on fetus, 207–208
    fetal, prolonged pregnancy and, 665
    management of, 233
    neonatal, maternal diabetes mellitus
        and, 209
    patient education in, 233
    postexercise, 231
Hypotension, regional analgesia and, 646
Hypothalamic-pituitary-adrenal axis, 133
Hypothenar refilling, spontaneous
    abortion and, 319b–320b
Hypovolemia
    in abruptio placentae, 365t
    in acute renal failure, 265–266
    disseminated intravascular coagulation
        and, 398

Hypovolemic shock
    in abruptio placentae, 369
    in placenta previa, 378
    in placental abnormalities, 389–390
Hypoxemia, fetal, 294–295
Hypoxia, fetal, 294–295
    in abruptio placentae, 371
    in disseminated intravascular
        coagulation, 398
    prolonged pregnancy and, 665
Hysterectomy
    in hydatidiform mole, 355
    in placenta cretas, 385
Hysterotomy in fetal intrauterine surgery,
    103

I

Iatrogenic prematurity, 596
Ideal body weight, diabetic mother and,
    226
Ignatia, 116–117
Immune system
    human immunodeficiency virus and, 533
    maladaptation in preeclampsia, 426
Immunoassay test in premature rupture of
    membranes, 492
Immunosuppression, placenta and, 314
Immunotolerance, placenta and, 314
Impaired fasting glucose, 200
Impaired glucose tolerance, 200
Incident report, 188t–189t
Incompetent cervix
    diagnostic testing in, 318
    medical management of, 324
    pathophysiology of, 315
    recurrent abortions and, 313
    signs and symptoms of, 316
Incomplete abortion, 316f, 317t
    medical management of, 321–322, 323f
    nursing interventions in, 326
Indirect Coombs test for RhD
    alloimmunization, 406, 408
Indirect monitoring of fetal heart rate, 52,
    52b
Indomethacin for preterm labor,
    477b–480b
Induction of labor, 582
    amniotomy for, 600–602
    balloon catheters and extra-amniotic
        saline infusion for, 591–592
    breast stimulation for, 602–604
    complementary therapies for, 604–605
    contraindications for, 585
    criteria for, 583–584
    dinoprostone for, 586–590, 588t

Induction of labor *(Continued)*
  incidence of, 582
  indications for, 583, 583b
  integrative therapies for, 123
  Laminaria and synthetic dilators for, 590–591
  misoprostol for, 590
  oxytocin for, 593–600
    dosages of, 594–595, 594t
    fetal and neonatal effects of, 596–597
    maternal side effects of, 595–596
    nursing interventions in, 597–600
    pharmacologic characteristics of, 593–594
    physiology of, 593
  physiology of uterotropins and uterotonins and, 585–586
  predictors of success in, 584, 584t
  prolonged pregnancy and, 666
  risks in, 585
  stripping of fetal membranes for, 602
Inevitable abortion, 316f, 317t
  medical management of, 321–322, 323f
  nursing interventions in, 326
Infant death, 149
  after-death care in home and, 164–165
  contact with infant's body and, 153, 154b
  continuing development of bereavement care and, 151–152
  electronic fetal heart rate monitoring and, 47
  grieving process and, 151–152
  historical background of perinatal bereavement care and, 149–150
  palliative care for dying infant and, 164
  perinatal hospice care after diagnosis of life-limiting condition and, 163–164
  Pregnancy Loss and Infant Death Alliance guidelines in, 155b–162b, 165
  support during subsequent pregnancy and, 153–163
Infection
  diabetes mellitus and, 206–207
  genitourinary, 519
    bacterial vaginosis in, 519–521
    candidiasis in, 521–522
    chlamydial, 522–524
    gonorrhea in, 524–525
    group B streptococcus in, 525–527
    hepatitis B in, 527–530
    hepatitis C in, 530–531

Infection *(Continued)*
    herpes simplex virus type 2 in, 531–533
    human immunodeficiency virus in, 533–539
    human papillomavirus in, 539–541
    human parvovirus B19 in, 542–543
    prevention of, 549–551
    syphilis in, 543–545
    trichomoniasis in, 545–546
    urinary tract infection in, 546–549, 548t
  Laminaria dilator-related, 591
  premature rupture of membranes and, 488
  preterm labor and, 461, 464
  respiratory
    etiology of, 290–291
    incidence of, 290
    maternal effects of, 294
    medical management of, 298–303
    nursing interventions for, 303–304
    pathophysiology of, 292
  risk for
    after abruptio placentae, 369
    after premature rupture of membranes, 496–497
  sporadic abortions and, 312
  urinary tract, 546–549, 548t
    diabetes mellitus and, 206, 230
    diagnostic testing in, 263–264
    drug therapy for, 267
    etiology of, 259
    general management of, 265–267
    incidence of, 258
    maternal effects of, 263
    prevention of, 267–268
    signs and symptoms of, 261–262
Inferior vena cava changes during pregnancy, 245
Inferior vena caval filter, 284
Infertility
  heroin use and, 568
  marijuana and, 569
Inflammatory response
  preeclampsia and, 426
  preterm labor and, 462b
Influenza, diabetes mellitus and, 207
Influenza vaccination, 302
Informed consent, 174t
  for epidural analgesia, 646
  for induction of labor, 597
INH; *See* Isoniazid
Inhaled corticosteroids, 300t–301t
Inhibin A, quad-screen and, 90

Injury during pregnancy; *See* Trauma
Instrumental delivery with forceps or
    vacuum extractor, 645–646
  interventions to decrease risk for,
    627–637
Instrumentation in fetal surveillance,
    49–57, 50f
Insulin
  breastfeeding effects on, 233
  diabetes mellitus and, 205t
  hyperinsulinemia and, 202
  increased tissue resistance to during
    pregnancy, 202
  needs during pregnancy, 215–218, 215t
Insulin pump, 218
Insulin resistance, 200
  during pregnancy, 4
  tumor necrosis factor-alpha and, 202
Insulin therapy in diabetes mellitus,
    215–218, 215t–216t
  calculation guidelines for, 216–217, 216t
  diabetic ketoacidosis and, 234
  dosage adjustments in, 218
  dosage distribution in, 217–218
  early morning hyperglycemia and, 217t
  gestational diabetes and, 219
  gestational diabetes mellitus and, 219
  insulin classifications in, 215–216, 216t
  insulin pump and, 218
  labor and, 221–222, 236, 236t
  postpartum, 237–238
  types of insulin in, 215
Insulinase, 202
Insurance, malpractice, 181–182
Intact fetal cells, 100
Intake and output in preeclampsia, 438,
    444
Integrative medicine, 107
Integrative therapies, 107
  for addictions, 125
  alternative medical systems in, 108–110
    homeopathy in, 110
    traditional Chinese medicine in,
      108–110
  for analgesia in labor, 123–125
  biologic-based therapies in, 112–113
    herbal medicine in, 112, 113b
    nutritional therapy in, 112–113
  for breech presentation, 117–118
  for constipation, 118–119
  energy therapies in, 115
    cranial sacral therapy in, 115
    polarity in, 115
  evidence-based databases for, 126t
  for hyperemesis, 116–117

Integrative therapies *(Continued)*
  for hypertensive disorders, 122
  for induction of labor, 123
  for low back pain, 121–122
  manipulative and body-based methods
    in, 113–115
    chiropractic in, 113–114
    massage therapy in, 114
    osteopathy in, 114–115
  for mental and emotional problems,
    119–120
  mind-body interventions in, 110–112
    aromatherapy in, 110–111, 111b
    hypnotherapy in, 111
    spiritual healing and prayer in, 111
    yoga in, 112
  for postpartum bleeding, 125
  for preterm labor, 122–123
Interferons for hepatitis C, 531
Intermediate-acting insulins, 215, 216t
Intermittent auscultation in fetal
    surveillance, 48–49
  NICHD categories of fetal heart rate
    and, 56–57, 56b
Intermittent pneumatic compression
    device, 284
Intermittent subcutaneous insulin during
    labor and delivery, 222, 236
Internal monitoring of fetus, 52–54, 53f,
    54b
  advantages and limitations of, 54b
  fetal spiral electrode for, 53f, 54
  intrauterine pressure catheter for,
    52–54
International bibliographic information on
    dietary supplements, 126t
International Federation of Gynecologists
    and Obstetricians classification of
    gestational trophoblastic neoplasia,
    357, 358t
Interstitial tubal pregnancy, 331, 334t
Intimate partner violence, 509–510,
    511b
Intraamniotic infection, 490, 493
  amniotomy and, 601
Intrapartum fetal surveillance, 65–80,
    83–84
Intrapartum period
  diabetic mother and, 221–222
  human immunodeficiency virus
    infection and, 536–538
  management of heparin during, 287
  nursing interventions in
    for alloimmunization, 414
    for asthma, 305

Intrapartum period *(Continued)*
  for premature rupture of membranes, 498
  nutritional and metabolic pattern and, 628
  position changes during, 629, 630f
  preeclampsia and, 450–453
  prolonged pregnancy and, 668
  vaginal birth after cesarean and, 644–645
Intraperitoneal transfusion in hemolytic incompatibility, 411
Intrathecal narcotics, 635
Intrauterine device, ectopic pregnancy and, 332, 346
Intrauterine growth restriction
  abruptio placentae and, 371
  antiphospholipid syndrome and, 275
  diabetes mellitus and, 208
  fetal alcohol syndrome and, 559t
  gonorrhea and, 525
  maternal heroin use and, 568
  placenta previa and, 379
  renal disease and, 263
  systemic lupus erythematosus and, 274
Intrauterine pressure catheter, 52–54
Intrauterine transfusion, 101–102
  in hemolytic incompatibility, 410
Intravascular transfusion in hemolytic incompatibility, 411
Intravenous therapy, 20t, 21
Intrinsic renal failure, 259
Invasive hemodynamic monitoring in preeclampsia, 434, 450, 451t–452t
Invasive placenta, 378, 381–385
Ipecac, 116–117
Iron
  need during pregnancy, 11–12
  supplementation of, 11–12
    in multifetal pregnancy, 15
    in placenta previa, 380
Iron deficiency anemia, 11
Isometric exercises, 8, 9b–10b
Isoniazid, 302
Isthmic tubal pregnancy, 331, 334t
IUD; *See* Intrauterine device

J
Jarisch-Herxheimer reaction, 544
Jasmine oil, 124
Jaundice in HELLP syndrome, 425
Joint Commission, 192t
Justice, 174t

K
Kali carbonicum, 124–125
Kegel exercises, 9b–10b
Ketoacidosis, diabetic, 207
  critical care interventions for, 234–235
  fetal mortality and, 209
  management of, 220–221
  signs and symptoms of, 204
Ketone bodies, diabetic ketoacidosis and, 207
Ketones, urine, 214
Ketonuria, 214
Kidney
  changes during pregnancy, 3, 420
  normal physiology of, 259–261
  preeclampsia and, 423–424, 438, 438t
Kidney biopsy, 264
Kidney disease, 258
  critical care for acute renal failure and, 269
  diagnostic testing in, 263–265, 264t
  drug therapy for, 267
  etiology of, 259
  fetal and neonatal effects of, 263
  general management of, 265–267
  incidence of, 258
  maternal effects of, 263
  normal renal physiology and, 259–261
  nursing interventions for, 268–269
  prevention of, 267–268
  signs and symptoms of, 261–262
Kidney stones
  diagnostic testing in, 264
  etiology of, 259
  general management of, 265
  incidence of, 258
  signs and symptoms of, 261
Klebsiella pneumoniae in urinary tract infection, 546
Kleihauer-Betke blood test
  in hemolytic incompatibility, 408
  in maternal trauma, 514
Kneeling position in occiput posterior presentation, 631
Kohlberg's moral judgment development, 171–172
Kussmaul respirations in diabetic ketoacidosis, 220–221

L
Labetalol
  for chronic hypertension during pregnancy, 418–419, 419t
  for hypertensive crisis during pregnancy, 446b

Labetalol *(Continued)*
  for maternal cardiac disease, 251
  for preeclampsia, 433
Labor
  diabetes mellitus and
    insulin needs and, 215t
    manifestations and consequences of,
      205t
  dysfunctional, 610
    abnormal labor patterns in, 620t–621t
    activity and position pattern and,
      629–634, 630f, 632f
    breech presentation in, 615–617, 616f
    brow presentation in, 614, 615f
    cesarean birth and, 649–650
    cognitive pattern and, 634–635
    compound presentation in, 614–615
    coping and stress-tolerance pattern
      and, 637
    diagnostic testing in, 619
    early detection and treatment of,
      637–638
    elimination pattern and, 629
    epidural or combined spinal/epidural
      in, 646–648
    etiology of, 611
    external version in, 641–643
    face presentation in, 613–614, 614f
    fetal and neonatal effects of, 618–619
    fetal dystocia in, 612–617, 623,
      624t–626t
    health-perception and health-
      management pattern and, 627
    incidence of, 610–611
    instrumental delivery with forceps or
      vacuum extractor in, 645–646
    labor management to decrease
      cesarean rate in, 619–623
    maternal effects of, 618
    normal physiology and, 612
    nutritional and metabolic pattern and,
      627–628
    occiput posterior presentation in, 613,
      613f
    pelvic dystocia in, 617
    perceptual pattern and, 635–636
    postpartum epidural analgesia in, 648
    prevention of, 627
    rest and relaxation pattern and, 634
    role-relationship pattern and,
      636–637
    self-perception and self-concept
      pattern and, 636
    shoulder presentation in, 613–614,
      615f, 638–641, 639t, 640f–642f

Labor *(Continued)*
    signs and symptoms of, 618
    uterine dystocia in, 612
    vaginal birth after cesarean and,
      643–644
  fetal oxygen saturation monitoring with
    fetal pulse oximetry during, 71–80
  hemodynamic responses to, 245
  induction of, 582
    amniotomy for, 600–602
    balloon catheters and extra-amniotic
      saline infusion for, 591–592
    breast stimulation for, 602–604
    complementary therapies for,
      604–605
    contraindications for, 585
    criteria for, 583–584
    dinoprostone for, 586–590, 588t
    incidence of, 582
    indications for, 583, 583b
    integrative therapies for, 123
    Laminaria and synthetic dilators for,
      590–591
    misoprostol for, 590
    oxytocin for, 593–600, 594t; *See also*
      Oxytocin
    physiology of uterotropins and
      uterotonins and, 585–586
    predictors of success in, 584, 584t
    prolonged pregnancy and, 666
    risks in, 585
    stripping of fetal membranes for, 602
  integrative therapies for analgesia in,
    123–125
  preterm, 460
    abdominal surgery management of,
      473
    cocaine use and, 565
    contraindications to halting, 472
    diabetes mellitus and, 206, 221, 235
    diagnostic testing in, 468–470
    estrogen and, 463
    etiology of, 461, 462b
    fetal and neonatal effects of, 465–468
    gonorrhea and, 525
    hepatitis B and, 529
    home management of, 482
    hospitalization in, 476–480
    incidence of, 460–461
    integrative therapies for, 122–123
    marijuana and, 569
    maternal cardiac disease and, 248, 253
    maternal effects of, 465
    maternal urinary tract infection and,
      263

Labor (Continued)
  multiple gestation and, 460
  national effects of, 468
  nontreatable cause, 472–473
  normal anatomy of cervix and, 461
  nursing management of, 474–482
  oxytocin and, 464
  pathophysiology of, 464–465,
    466t–467t
  physiology of labor contractions and,
    461–463
  premature rupture of membranes and,
    493
  primary prevention of, 470–471
  progesterone and, 464
  prostaglandins and, 463–464
  pulmonary edema in, 481–482
  secondary prevention of, 471–474
  systemic lupus erythematosus and,
    274
  tocolytic therapy for, 477b–480b,
    480–481
  urinary tract infection and, 549
  prolonged pregnancy and, 663, 667
Laboratory studies
  for diabetic mother, 219, 224–225
  prenatal, 26–35
Laboring down, 633–634
Lactated Ringer's solution
  for abruptio placentae, 372
  for hemorrhage
    in placental abnormalities, 389
    in uterine evacuation in spontaneous
      abortion, 322
Lactation, use of antidepressants during,
  144–145
Lactobacillus acidophilus, 522
Lamicel, 322, 590
Laminaria dilators, 322, 323f, 590–591
Lantus, 216
Lanugo, 6
Laparotomy salpingectomy, 345
Lasix; See Furosemide
Late abortion, 311
Late decelerations of fetal heart rate,
  65t–67t, 69f
  in RhD alloimmunization, 406, 407f
Late preterm birth, 460
  etiology of, 461
  prevention of, 474
Latency period in premature rupture of
  membranes, 488
Latent syphilis, 543
Lateral recumbent position, 629, 630f
Lavender essential oil, 120

Law, systems of, 186–187
LCR; See Ligase chain reaction
Lead exposure as high risk factor, 40t
Leaning-forward position in occiput
  posterior presentation, 631
LEAP assessment, 213
Learning disabilities, maternal diabetes
  mellitus and, 209
Leg pain in venous thromboembolic
  disease, 283
Leg sliding exercise, 9b–10b
Legal issues, 181
  clinical examples in, 197b
  commonly used legal terms, 188t–189t
  documentation and, 196b
  effect of litigation on health care, 186
  in electronic fetal heart rate monitoring,
    48
  expert witness and, 197
  litigation risk and, 183–185
  litigation sequence and, 187–190
  malpractice insurance and, 181–182
  mid-level providers and, 185–186
  nurse's deposition and, 190–191
  perinatal safety nurse and, 196–197
  policy and procedure writing and, 193b
  reasons parents sue and, 182–183
  risk management and, 194b–195b
  standards of care and, 192–195, 192t
  systems of law and, 186–187
  trial procedure and, 191–195
Leopold maneuver, 624t–626t
Leukocytosis
  during pregnancy, 3
  in respiratory distress, 292
Leukotriene mediators, 300t–301t
Levemir, 216
Liability
  professional, 181
  sources of, 194b–195b
Lifestyle modifications, gestational
  diabetes mellitus and, 238
Ligase chain reaction, 523
Linoleic acid, 11
Lispro, 215
Lithotomy position during labor,
  629–631
Litigation
  commonly used legal terms in,
    188t–189t
  effect on health care, 186
  reasons parents sue, 182–183
  risk for, 183–185
  sequence of, 187–190

Liver
    hepatitis B and, 527–530
    hepatitis C and, 530–531
    preeclampsia and, 425, 439
Living will, 177
Long-lever manipulation, 114–115
Long-term variability of fetal heart rate,
        46
Loop of Henle, 260
Loss and grief, 149
    after-death care in home and, 164–165
    contact with infant's body and, 153,
        154b
    continuing development of, 151–152
    grieving process and, 151–152
    historical background of, 149–150
    palliative care for dying infant and, 164
    perinatal hospice care after diagnosis
        of life-limiting condition and,
        163–164
    Pregnancy Loss and Infant Death
        Alliance guidelines in, 155b–162b,
        165
    support during subsequent pregnancy
        and, 153–163
Low back pain, 121–122
Low-molecular-weight heparins
    for acute venous thromboembolism, 285
    for antiphospholipid syndrome, 285t,
        324
    intrapartum and postpartum
        management of, 287
    for maternal cardiac disease, 250
    for prevention of valve thrombosis,
        247–248
    for thromboprophylaxis, 284
Low risk metastatic gestational
        trophoblastic neoplasia, 359, 359t
Lung
    preeclampsia and, 424, 439
    pulmonary edema and
        acute, 307–308
        invasive hemodynamic monitoring
            and, 450
        maternal cardiac disease and, 247
        in preeclampsia, 424, 451t–452t
        preterm labor and, 481–482
    pulmonary embolism and, 282
        acute, 284–286, 285t
        anticoagulation therapy for, 286
        antiphospholipid syndrome and, 274
        critical care in, 307–308
        diagnostic testing in, 283
        etiology of, 282
        fetal effects of, 283, 294–295

Lung (Continued)
        incidence of, 282, 290
        intrapartum and postpartum
            management of heparin and, 287
        maternal effects of, 283, 294
        normal physiology and, 283
        signs and symptoms of, 283
        thromboprophylaxis and, 284
        treatment of, 286
    respiratory disease and, 289
        diagnostic testing in, 295–297,
            295t–296t
        etiology of, 290–291
        fetal effects of, 294–295
        incidence of, 289–290
        maternal effects of, 293–294
        medical management of, 297–303,
            299t
        normal physiology and, 291
        nursing management of, 303–309
        pathophysiology of, 292
        signs and symptoms of, 292–293
    respiratory distress and
        in anaphylactoid syndrome of
            pregnancy, 292–293
        signs and symptoms of, 292–293
Lupus-like disease, 275
Luteal phase defect, 324

M
Macrobid; See Nitrofurantoin
Macrosomia, 664
    maternal diabetes mellitus and, 208
    obese mother and, 15
Magnesium rich foods, 20b
Magnesium sulfate
    for abruptio placentae, 372
    for maternal cardiac disease, 251
    for preeclampsia, 433, 442–445,
        442b–443b, 444t
    for preterm labor, 477b–480b
    for seizure control in eclampsia,
        448–449
    signs of toxicity, 444–445
Mainlining of heroin, 567
Major depressive syndrome, 143b
Malpractice, 188t–189t
Malpractice insurance, 181–182
Manipulative and body-based methods,
        108, 113–115
    chiropractic in, 113–114
    massage therapy in, 114
    osteopathy in, 114–115
Marfan syndrome, 247
Marginal abruptio placentae, 364, 366f

Marginal placenta previa, 370t, 376
Marijuana, 569–570
Marital status as high risk factor, 38
Martial law, 186
Massage therapy, 114
  for constipation, 119
  for hypertensive disorders, 122
  during labor, 125, 635
  for low back pain, 121
Mast-cell stabilizers, 300t–301t
Maternal age
  breech presentation and, 616
  as high risk factor, 38
  hydatidiform mole and, 352
  recurrent abortions and, 312
Maternal attachment, 128
Maternal death
  in abruptio placentae, 369
  diabetic ketoacidosis and, 207
  in disseminated intravascular
    coagulation, 398
  ectopic pregnancy and, 335, 337
  gestational trophoblastic neoplasia and,
    357
  maternal risk subgroups and, 247b
  in placenta cretas, 385
  in placenta previa, 378
  pneumonia and, 294
  preeclampsia and, 427
  premature rupture of membranes and,
    490
  pulmonary embolism and, 283, 294
  spontaneous abortion and, 316
  trauma-related, 500, 504
Maternal-fetal unit, 4–6
  amniotic fluid and, 5–6
  embryo and, 4
  fetus and, 6
  placenta and, 4–5
Maternal health disorders
  associated with fetal compromise, 71
  autoimmune rheumatic diseases in, 271
    etiology of, 272
    fetal and neonatal effects of,
      274–275
    general management of, 276–277
    incidence of, 271
    maternal effects of, 274
    medical diagnosis of, 275–276
    pathophysiology of, 272
    secondary and tertiary prevention in,
      277–278
    signs and symptoms of, 272–273, 273t
  cardiac disease in, 243
    anticipatory grieving and, 253

Maternal health disorders (Continued)
    critical care nursing interventions in,
      253–255
    diagnostic testing in, 248
    drug therapy for, 249–251
    early detection of preterm labor in,
      253
    etiology of, 243–244
    fetal and neonatal effects of, 248
    general management of, 248–249
    hemodynamic pressure readings in,
      255t
    incidence of, 243
    maternal effects of, 247–248
    maternal risk subgroups in, 247b
    normal antepartal cardiac physiology
      and, 244–245
    postpartum nursing interventions in,
      256
    prevention of cardiac decompensation
      in, 252–253
    signs and symptoms of, 246
    tertiary prevention in, 251–252
  diabetes mellitus in, 200
    blood glucose monitoring in, 214, 233
    causes of, 202
    coping with, 232
    diabetic ketoacidosis and, 234–235
    diagnostic testing in, 210–211, 211t
    diet and, 219, 226–230, 228t–230t
    early morning hyperglycemia and,
      217t
    exercise and, 219, 231
    fetal and neonatal effects of, 207–209
    fetal surveillance and, 220, 232–233
    hypoglycemia management and, 233
    incidence of, 201
    insulin management in, 215–218,
      215t–216t
    intrapartum management of, 221–
      222, 235–237, 236t
    ketoacidosis management and,
      220–221
    maternal effects of, 204–207
    maternal surveillance and, 219–220
    normal pregnancy physiology and,
      202
    pathophysiology of, 203–204, 203t
    postpartum management of, 222,
      237–238
    preconception management of,
      212–213, 223–225
    preterm labor management and, 221
    Revised White's Classification of
      perinatal diabetes and, 201t

Maternal health disorders *(Continued)*
    sick-day rule in, 234
    signs and symptoms of, 204, 205t
    urine testing in, 214
  genitourinary infections in, 519
    bacterial vaginosis in, 519–521
    candidiasis in, 521–522
    chlamydial, 522–524
    gonorrhea in, 524–525
    group B streptococcus in, 525–527
    hepatitis B in, 527–530
    hepatitis C in, 530–531
    herpes simplex virus type 2 in,
        531–533
    human immunodeficiency virus in,
        533–539
    human papillomavirus in, 539–541
    human parvovirus B19 in, 542–543
    prevention of, 549–551
    syphilis in, 543–545
    trichomoniasis in, 545–546
    urinary tract infection in, 546–549,
        548t
  pulmonary disease in, 289
    diagnostic testing in, 295–297,
        295t–296t
    etiology of, 290–291
    fetal effects of, 294–295
    incidence of, 289–290
    maternal effects of, 293–294
    medical management of, 297–303,
        299t
    normal physiology and, 291
    nursing management of, 303–309
    pathophysiology of, 292
    signs and symptoms of, 292–293
  renal disease in, 258
    critical care for acute renal failure
        and, 269
    diagnostic testing in, 263–265, 264t
    drug therapy for, 267
    etiology of, 259
    fetal and neonatal effects of, 263
    general management of, 265–267
    incidence of, 258
    maternal effects of, 263
    normal renal physiology and, 259–261
    nursing interventions for, 268–269
    prevention of, 267–268
    signs and symptoms of, 261–262
  venous thromboembolic disease in, 282
    acute, 284–286, 285t
    anticoagulation therapy for, 286
    diagnostic testing in, 283
    etiology of, 282

Maternal health disorders *(Continued)*
    fetal and neonatal effects of, 283
    incidence of, 282
    intrapartum and postpartum
        management of heparin and, 287
    maternal effects of, 283
    normal physiology and, 283
    signs and symptoms of, 283
    thromboprophylaxis and, 284
Maternal risk subgroups, 247b
Maternal serum alpha-fetoprotein, 90
    diabetic mother and, 220
Maternal serum markers screen, 35
Maternal surveillance in diabetes mellitus,
    219–220
Maternal tasks, 130
    establishing relationship with fetus in,
        130
    pregnancy acceptance in, 130
    role transition in, 130
Maturational stressors, 131–132
MCA Doppler velocity in hemolytic
    incompatibility, 409
McRobert's maneuver, 639t, 640f
Meal planning, diabetic mother and, 228t
Meats
    exchange list for meal planning and,
        228t–230t
    menu guidelines for, 17t
Mechanical methods for cervical ripening,
    590–591
Meconium, 45
Meconium aspiration syndrome, 665
Meconium contamination, 662–663
Meiosis, 313
Menstrual cycle
    fallopian tube and, 333
    prolonged pregnancy and, 666
Menstrual history in spontaneous
    abortion, 319b–320b
Menstruation, fallopian tube and, 333
Mental problems, integrative therapies for,
    119–120
Mental retardation, maternal alcohol use
    and, 559, 561
Mentum, 613–614, 614f, 624t–626t
Menu guidelines, 17t
Mercury exposure as high risk factor, 40t
Meridians, 109
Mesoderm, 6
Mesotrophoblast, 4–5
Metabolic acidosis, 297
    in acute renal failure, 262
Metabolic adaptations to pregnancy, 4
Metabolic alkalosis, 297

Metabolic syndrome, 200
Metabolites of cocaine, 565
Metaethics, 173
Metformin, 219
Methadone, 568–569
Methamphetamines, 570
Methergine; See Methylergonovine
    maleate
Methotrexate for ectopic pregnancy, 344
Methyldopa
    for chronic hypertension during
        pregnancy, 418–419, 419t
    for diabetes mellitus-related
        hypertension, 212
Methylergonovine maleate, 389
Metronidazole
    for bacterial vaginosis, 519
    for trichomoniasis, 545
Miconazole, 522
Microscopic examination in premature
    rupture of membranes, 492
Mid-level provider, legal issues and,
    185–186
Middle cerebral artery Doppler velocity in
    hemolytic incompatibility, 409
Midtrimester abortion, 311
Mild abruptio placentae, 368
Mild gestational hypertension, 416
Military law, 186
Milk, exchange list for meal planning and,
    228t–230t
Mind-body interventions, 108, 110–112
    aromatherapy in, 110–111, 111b
    hypnotherapy in, 111
    spiritual healing and prayer in, 111
    yoga in, 112
Minerals
    diabetic mother and, 227
    nutritional therapy and, 113
Minimal variability of fetal heart rate, 61t,
    62f
Minor injury management, 505, 514
Minute ventilation, 296t
Miscarriage, 311; See also Spontaneous
    abortion
Misoprostol for induction of labor, 588t,
    590
Missed abortion, 316f, 317t
    medical management of, 322
    nursing interventions in, 326
Mixed abruptio placentae, 364, 366f
Mixed metabolic and respiratory acidosis,
    297
Mixed respiratory and metabolic alkalosis,
    297

Mixed variability of fetal heart rate, 61t,
    62f
Moderate abruptio placentae, 368
Modified biophysical profile in fetal
    surveillance, 82b
Modified leg raises, 9b–10b
Molecular diagnostics
    for chlamydial infection, 523
    for gonorrhea, 525
Monistat; See Miconazole
Monitoring
    in diabetic ketoacidosis, 235
    electronic fetal heart rate, 46–48
        acute asthma exacerbation and, 307
        after amniocentesis, 96
        cerebral palsy and, 47
        cesarean section and, 47–48
        during labor in prolonged pregnancy,
            667
        legal implications of, 48
        in preeclampsia, 452
    hemodynamic
        in hypovolemic shock in placental
            abnormalities, 390
        in preeclampsia, 434, 450, 451t–452t
        pressure readings in cardiac disease,
            255t
    of trauma victim, 508
Monozygotic multiple fetus, 460
Montelukast, 300t–301t
Moral judgment development, 171–172
Moral relativism, 175
Moratorium phase of pregnancy
    adjustment, 130–131
Morning-after pill, ectopic pregnancy and,
    332
Morning sickness, 19b
Moro reflex, 640
Morphine, postpartum, 648
Morula, 4, 313, 352–353
Mother-infant attachment, 128
Motor vehicle collision prevention,
    508–509
Moxibustion, 109, 642
MSAFP; See Maternal serum
    alpha-fetoprotein
Mugwort plant, 109
Multifetal pregnancy, 460
    breech presentation and, 616
    electronic fetal monitor for, 55
    as high risk factor, 41
    normal physiologic adaptation to, 464
    preterm labor and, 460
        abdominal surgery management of,
            473

Multifetal pregnancy *(Continued)*
    contraindications to halting, 472
    diabetes mellitus and, 206, 221, 235
    diagnostic testing in, 468–470
    estrogen and, 463
    etiology of, 461, 462b
    fetal and neonatal effects of, 465–468
    home management of, 482
    hospitalization in, 476–480
    incidence of, 460–461
    integrative therapies for, 122–123
    maternal cardiac disease and, 248,
        253
    maternal effects of, 465
    maternal urinary tract infection and,
        263
    multiple gestation and, 460
    national effects of, 468
    nontreatable cause, 472–473
    normal anatomy of cervix and, 461
    nursing management of, 474–482
    oxytocin and, 464
    pathophysiology of, 464–465,
        466t–467t
    physiology of labor contractions and,
        461–463
    primary prevention of, 470–471
    progesterone and, 464
    prostaglandins and, 463–464
    pulmonary edema in, 481–482
    secondary prevention of, 471–474
    tocolytic therapy for, 477b–480b,
        480–481
    weight gain in, 15, 16t
Multifetal pregnancy reduction, 103–104

N
Nägele rule, 665
Naloxone, 648
Narcan; *See* Naloxone
Nasal congestion, 298
National Institute of Child Health and
        Human Development
    categorization of fetal heart rate
        tracings, 55, 56b
    on goals of fetal heart monitoring, 48
    terminology for communication and
        documentation, 193
National Practitioner Data Bank, 181
Natural food supplements, 113
Nausea in hyperemesis gravidarum, 18
Nebulizer, 303–304
Negligence, 187, 188t–189t
Neisseria gonorrhoeae, 524, 546
Neonatal lupus syndrome, 274

Neonate
    abruptio placentae and, 370–371
    chlamydial conjunctivitis in, 524
    ectopic pregnancy and, 337
    effects of dysfunctional labor on,
        618–619
    effects of maternal conditions on
        autoimmune rheumatic diseases and,
            274–275
        cardiac disease and, 248
        diabetes mellitus and, 207–209
        disseminated intravascular
            coagulation and, 398
        hepatitis B and, 529
        postpartum depression and, 140
        renal disease and, 263
        venous thromboembolic disease and,
            283
    fetal alcohol syndrome and, 559,
        559t–560t
    gonococcal ophthalmia in, 525
    group B streptococcal infection in, 526
    hemolytic incompatibility and,
        407–408
    herpes simplex virus type 2 and, 533
    human immunodeficiency virus and,
        536–537, 539
    maternal cocaine use and, 565–566
    maternal heroin use and, 568, 568b
    oxytocin for induction of labor and,
        596–597
    placenta previa and, 379
    preeclampsia and, 427
    premature rupture of membranes and,
        490–491
    preterm labor and, 465–468
    prolonged pregnancy and,
        664–665
Nephropathy in diabetes mellitus, 213
Neroli oil, 120, 124
Neural tube defects
    folic acid deficiency and, 12
    maternal diabetes mellitus and, 208
    maternal serum alpha-fetoprotein screen
        and, 90
Neurologic defects
    abruptio placentae and, 371
    in fetal alcohol syndrome, 559t
Neurologic injury, 502–503
Neurologic system of diabetic mother, 224
Neurotransmitters, cocaine and, 564
Neutral protamine Hagedorn, 215
New York Heart Association classification
        of cardiac disease, 246
Newborn; *See* Neonate

NICHD; *See* National Institute of Child
    Health and Human Development
Nicotine gum, 574
Nifedipine
    for chronic hypertension during
        pregnancy, 418–419, 419t
    for diabetes mellitus-related
        hypertension, 212
    for preeclampsia, 433
Nipple stimulation for induction of labor,
    76b–77b, 78f–79f, 602–604
Nitrazine test in premature rupture of
    membranes, 491–492
Nitric oxide, 421
Nitrofurantoin, 265, 548t
Nitrogenous waste buildup in acute renal
    failure, 262
Noncompliance with physician order, 185
Noninvasive prenatal diagnosis, 100
Nonmaleficence, 174t
Nonmetastatic gestational trophoblastic
    neoplasia, 357, 359t
Nonrecurring genetic abnormality in
    spontaneous abortion, 311
Nonstress test, 72b–73b, 73f, 380
    maternal chronic kidney disease and,
        266
    in premature rupture of membranes,
        493
Nontreatable cause preterm labor,
    472–473
Nonuniform accelerations of fetal heart
    rate, 65t–67t, 68f
Norepinephrine, cocaine and, 564
Normal saline for hemorrhage, in placental
    abnormalities, 389
Normative ethics, 173
NovoLog, 215
NST; *See* Nonstress test
Nuchal translucency ultrasound, 91
Nurse
    deposition in legal proceeding, 190–191
    inadequate communication with
        physician, 184
    role of, 25
Nurse anesthetist, 185
Nurse practitioner, 185
Nursing assessment, 25
    in ectopic pregnancy, 346–347
    in fetal surveillance, 83–84
    in gestational trophoblastic disease, 360
    Gordon's functional health patterns in,
        25–26, 27b–33b
    high risk factors and, 37–41, 40t
    laboratory studies and, 26–35

Nursing assessment *(Continued)*
    in perinatal screening, diagnoses, and
        fetal therapies, 104
    physical assessment and, 36–37
    in postpartum depression, 145
    in preeclampsia, 437–440, 437t
    ultrasound and, 35–36
Nutrient needs, 10–13
Nutrition
    alcohol use and, 563
    maternal cardiac disease and, 251
    preeclampsia and, 434–435
Nutritional and metabolic pattern,
        27b–33b
    diabetic mother and, 226–230
    dysfunctional labor and, 627–628
    in psychologic assessment for high-risk
        pregnancy, 135b–136b
Nutritional assessment, 10–21
    food groups and, 15–16, 16t–17t
    hyperemesis gravidarum and, 18–21,
        19b–20b, 20t
    hyperphenylalanemia and, 18
    nutrient needs and, 10–13
    prepregnancy weight status and, 13–14
    referrals and, 16–18
    weight gain and
        in multifetal pregnancy, 15, 16t
        in singleton pregnancy, 14–15, 14t
Nutritional status as high risk factor, 39
Nutritional therapy, 112–113
    Chinese, 109
    for constipation, 119
    for hyperemesis, 117
    for hypertensive disorders, 122
    for low back pain, 121
    for mental and emotional problems, 120
Nuts, 17t
Nux Vomica, 116–117

O
Obesity
    childhood, maternal diabetes mellitus
        and, 209
    metabolic syndrome and, 200
    preeclampsia and, 427
    prepregnancy weight status and, 14,
        14t, 39
    sporadic abortions and, 312
Occiput posterior presentation, 613, 613f,
        624t–626t
    maternal positioning in, 631
Occupational hazards, 38–39, 40t
    in sporadic abortions, 312
Oils, 17t

Oligohydramnios
  in chronic abruption, 368
  oral fluids and, 13
  premature rupture of membranes and,
    491
  prolonged pregnancy and, 662, 664
Oliguria in preeclampsia, 424–425, 450,
    451t–452t
Omega 3 fatty acids, 11
Omega 6 fatty acids, 11
Opiate analgesics during labor, 628
Oral corticosteroids, 300t–301t
Oral examination of diabetic mother, 224
Oral glucose-lowering agents, 219
Oral glucose tolerance test, 210, 211t
  postpartum, 239b
Orcytotrophoblast, 4–5
Ordering, 174t
Organization of Teratology Information
    Specialists, 39
Orgasm for induction of labor, 604
Osteopathy, 114–115
  for low back pain, 122
Ovarian cyst, 338t–341t
Ovary
  ectopic pregnancy and, 331, 334t
  enlargement in hydatidiform mole, 353
Overweight, prepregnancy weight status
    and, 13–14, 14t
Ovum, transmigration of, 333
Oxidative stress, preeclampsia and, 423,
    426
Oxygen consumption changes during
    pregnancy, 2
Oxygen partial pressure, fetal, 45
Oxygen therapy
  in eclampsia, 428
  in hypovolemic shock in placental
    abnormalities, 390
  during labor in cardiac disease, 249
  for pneumonia, 302
Oxygenation, fetal, 43–44
Oxytocin
  after uterine evacuation, 355
  for bleeding
    in placental abnormalities, 389
    in uterine evacuation, 322
  in contraction stress test, 76b–77b
  for induction of labor, 593–600
  influence on uterine activity,
    466t–467t
  preterm labor and, 464
  secretion during labor, 586
  for spontaneous abortion, 325–326
  stripping of fetal membranes and, 602

P

Pain
  abdominal
    in abruptio placentae, 367
    after tubal rupture, 337
    in ectopic pregnancy, 336–337, 346
    in spontaneous abortion, 315
  low back, 121–122
  pelvic, 338t–341t
  in venous thromboembolic disease, 283
Palliative care for dying infant, 164
PAMG-1 test, 492
Pancreas, diabetes mellitus and, 202
Papanicolaou test
  during first prenatal visit, 35
  in spontaneous abortion, 318
Parasitic infection, sporadic abortions and,
    312
Parasympathetic nervous system in control
    of fetal heart rate, 46
Parent-infant attachment, 128–129
Paroxysmal atrial tachycardia, fetal, 64t
Partial fetal alcohol syndrome, 560t
Partial hydatidiform mole, 351, 354
Partial placenta previa, 370t, 376
Partial pressure of carbon dioxide, 295t
Partial pressure of oxygen, 295t
Partial thromboplastin time in
    disseminated intravascular
    coagulation, 390–391
Passageway, 611
Passenger, 611
Passive diffusion, 44
Passive smoking as high risk factor, 40t
Paternal attachment, 128
Paternal cocaine use, 566
Paternal tasks, 130
Patient Self-Determination Act, 176
PCOS; *See* Polycystic ovary syndrome
PCR; *See* Polymerase chain reaction
PCWP; *See* Pulmonary capillary wedge
    pressure
Peak expiratory flow rate, 296t
Pelvic dystocia, 617
Pelvic examination in pelvic pain,
    338t–341t, 342
Pelvic fracture, 503
Pelvic infection, ectopic pregnancy and,
    331
Pelvic inflammatory disease
  Chlamydia in, 523–524
  ectopic pregnancy and, 346
  gonorrhea and, 525
  pelvic pain in, 338t–341t
Pelvic pain, 338t–341t

Pelvic surgery, ectopic pregnancy and, 331
Penicillin G
  for group B streptococcal infection, 526
  for syphilis, 544
Perceptual pattern, dysfunctional labor
    and, 635–636
Percutaneous umbilical blood sampling,
    93t, 96–97
Perimortem cesarean delivery, 506–507
Perinatal death, 149
  in abruptio placentae, 370
  after-death care in home and, 164–165
  contact with infant's body and, 153,
    154b
  continuing development of bereavement
    care and, 151–152
  ectopic pregnancy and, 337
  electronic fetal heart rate monitoring
    and, 47
  in end-stage renal disease, 266–267
  grieving process and, 151–152
  historical background of perinatal
    bereavement care and, 149–150
  maternal diabetes mellitus and, 208
  palliative care for dying infant and, 164
  perinatal hospice care after diagnosis
    of life-limiting condition and,
    163–164
  in placenta previa, 379
  in preeclampsia, 427
  Pregnancy Loss and Infant Death
    Alliance guidelines in, 155b–162b,
    165
  support during subsequent pregnancy
    and, 153–163
  in vasa previa, 386
Perinatal hospice care, 163–164
Perinatal nurse, 25
Perinatal safety nurse, 196–197
Perinatal screening, 88
  fetal biopsy and
    kidney, 98
    muscle, 97–98
    skin, 97
  fetal urine aspiration and, 99
  methods of, 89–91
  noninvasive prenatal diagnosis and, 100
  nursing management in, 104
  preimplantation genetic diagnosis and,
    99–100
  prenatal diagnostic tests and, 92–97, 93t
    amniocentesis in, 95–96
    chorionic villus sampling in, 93–94
    percutaneous umbilical blood
      sampling in, 96–97

Perinatal screening (Continued)
  prenatal genetic screening and, 88–89,
    89t
  ultrasound evaluation for fetal
    abnormalities and, 91–92, 92b
Periodic fetal heart patterns, 55
Peripheral sensory neuropathy in diabetes
    mellitus, 213
Peripheral vascular disease, 224
Pest control and garbage disposal
    assessment, 27b–33b
Pesticide exposure as high risk factor,
    40t
pH, 295t
Pharmacologic labor induction with
    oxytocin, 593–600
  dosages of, 594–595, 594t
  fetal and neonatal effects of,
    596–597
  maternal side effects of, 595–596
  nursing interventions in, 597–600
  pharmacologic characteristics of,
    593–594
  physiology of, 593
Pharmacologic methods for cervical
    ripening, 588t
  dinoprostone in, 586–590
  misoprostol in, 590
Phenylketonuria, 18
Phenytoin for preeclampsia, 433,
    442b–443b
Phosphorus for hyperemesis, 116–117
Physical abuse during pregnancy, 41
Physical examination
  of diabetic mother, 224
  in pelvic pain, 338t–341t
Physician-nurse communication, 184
Physiologic adaptations to pregnancy, 1
  cardiovascular, 1–4
  gastrointestinal, 3–4
  hematologic, 2–3
  metabolic, 4
  renal, 3
  respiratory, 2
Physiologic methods of labor induction
  amniotomy in, 600–602
  breast stimulation in,
    602–604
  stripping of fetal membranes in, 602
PID; See Pelvic inflammatory disease
Pindolol, 418–419, 419t
Pitocin, 593
Pituitary necrosis in abruptio placentae,
    369
PKU; See Phenylketonuria

Placenta
  development of, 4–5, 313–314
  immunology of, 314
  marijuana and, 569
  multiple gestation and, 464
  normal physiology of, 661
  preterm labor and, 462b, 465
  prolonged pregnancy and, 662
  spontaneous abortion and, 315, 321
  transport of fetal blood cells and,
      405–406
  tubal rupture and, 335
  uteroplacental-fetal exchange and,
      44–45
Placenta accreta, 381
Placenta cretas, 381–385
Placenta increta, 381
Placenta percreta, 381
Placenta previa, 376–381
  abruptio placentae *versus,* 382t–384t
  classifications of, 376, 376f
  delivery in, 380–381, 382t–384t
  diagnostic testing in, 379
  etiology of, 376–377
  expectant management in, 379–380
  fetal and neonatal effects of, 379
  maternal effects of, 378
  pathophysiology of, 377
  signs and symptoms of, 378
Placental abnormalities, 364
  abruptio placentae in, 364–376
    classifications of, 365t, 366f
    complications of, 368–369, 370t
    delivery in, 372–376
    diagnostic testing in, 371
    emergency management in, 372,
        373t–375t
    etiology of, 366
    expectant management in, 371–372
    fetal and neonatal effects of, 370–371
    incidence of, 364
    maternal effects of, 369
    normal physiology and, 366
    pathophysiology of, 366
    signs and symptoms of, 367–368
  antepartum fetal surveillance in, 391
  assessment of blood loss in, 387
  bedrest in, 392–393
  disseminated intravascular coagulation
      in, 390–391
  fear and, 392
  hospitalization in, 392
  hypovolemic shock in, 389–390
  invasive placenta in, 381–385
  mild bleeding in, 388

Placental abnormalities *(Continued)*
  moderate to severe bleeding in, 388–389
  placenta previa in, 376–381
    classifications of, 376, 376f
    delivery in, 380–381, 382t–384t
    diagnostic testing in, 379
    etiology of, 376–377
    expectant management in, 379–380
    fetal and neonatal effects of, 379
    maternal effects of, 378
    pathophysiology of, 377
    signs and symptoms of, 378
  prevention of, 386–387
  RhD alloimmunization and, 393
  vasa previa in, 385–386, 385f
Placental membrane, 5, 405–406
Plaintiff, 188t–189t
Plasma fibrinogen, 2–3
Plasma protein-A, 91
Plasma volume changes during pregnancy,
    1
Plasmin, 396–397, 397f
Plasminogen, 396–397, 397f
Plate method, 230
Platelet aggregation, diabetes mellitus and,
    212
Platelet transfusion
  in abruptio placentae, 372
  in disseminated intravascular
      coagulation, 399
PLIDA; *See* Pregnancy Loss and Infant
    Death Alliance
Plum blossom needling, 110
PMI; *See* Point of maximal impulse
Pneumococcal vaccine, 302
Pneumonia
  incidence of, 290
  maternal effects of, 294
  medical management of, 298–302
Pneumonitis, neonatal, 524
Point of maximal impulse, 2
Polarity therapy, 115
  for hyperemesis, 117
  for mental and emotional problems, 120
Policy and procedure writing, 193b
Policy revision, 194b–195b
Polycystic ovary syndrome, 324
Polycythemia
  fetal, 665
  neonatal, 209
Polydipsia in diabetes mellitus, 210
Polyhydramnios, diabetes mellitus and, 206
Polymerase chain reaction
  for chlamydial infection, 523
  for herpes simplex virus type2, 532

Polyuria in diabetes mellitus, 210
Population groups at high risk for genetic conditions, 89t
Positioning
    changes during intrapartum period, 629, 630f
    fetal heart rate and, 84
Post-term pregnancy, 660
    diagnostic testing in, 665–666
    etiology of, 660–661
    fetal and neonatal effects of, 664–665
    incidence of, 660
    maternal effects of, 663–664
    medical management of, 666–667
    normal physiology of amniotic fluid and placenta and, 661
    nursing management of, 667–669
    pathophysiology of, 662
    signs and symptoms of, 662–663
Postconventional level of moral judgment development, 172
Posteriorly implanted abruptio placentae, 368
Postexercise hypoglycemia, 231
Postmaturity, 660
Postmaturity syndrome, 664
Postmortem cesarean delivery, 506–507
Postnasal discharge, 298
Postoperative care
    in cesarean birth, 649–650
    in ectopic pregnancy, 347
Postpartum anemia
    in abruptio placentae, 369
    in placenta previa, 378
Postpartum bleeding
    integrative therapies for, 125
    in placental abnormalities, 389
    premature rupture of membranes and, 490
    risk after abruptio placentae, 369
Postpartum depression, 138–140
    criteria for major depressive syndrome and, 143b
    diagnosis of, 140–143
    differential diagnosis of, 139
    Edinburgh Postnatal Depression Scale and, 141b–142b
    neonatal effects of, 140
    screening for, 140
    treatment of, 143–145
Postpartum epidural analgesia, 648
Postpartum period
    asthma and, 306
    cardiac disease and, 256
    diabetes mellitus and

Postpartum period (Continued)
    calculation guidelines for insulin in, 216t
    insulin needs and, 215t
    management of, 222, 237–238
    manifestations and consequences of, 205t
    eclampsia and, 449
    HELLP syndrome and, 447, 453
    human immunodeficiency virus infection and, 538–539
    management of heparin during, 287
    preeclampsia and, 441, 453–454
Postpartum psychosis, 139
Postprandial glucose, 210
Postprocedural care
    in amniocentesis, 96
    in chorionic villus sampling, 94
    in fetal intrauterine transfusion, 102
    in fetal kidney biopsy, 98
    in fetal muscle biopsy, 98
    in fetal skin biopsy, 97
    in fetal urine aspiration for, 99
    in percutaneous umbilical blood sampling, 97
    in spontaneous abortion, 326–327
    in uterine evacuation of hydatidiform mole, 360–361
Postrenal failure, 259
Potassium
    diabetic ketoacidosis and, 234–235
    excess in acute renal failure, 262
    foods rich in, 19b
Poultry, menu guidelines for, 17t
Power, essential labor force, 611
Practice statement, 193b
Prayer and spiritual healing, 111
Precipitous labor, 620t–621t
Preconception health status as high risk factor, 39
Preconception management
    of diabetes mellitus, 212–213, 223–225
    Preconventional level of moral judgment development, 171
Preeclampsia, 417t, 420–431
    activity restriction in, 432
    anticonvulsants for, 442–445, 442b–443b, 444t, 446b
    aspirin and, 212
    cardiovascular alterations in, 437–438, 437t
    central nervous system alterations in, 438–439, 438t
    chronic hypertension and, 212

Preeclampsia *(Continued)*
  chronic kidney disease and, 262
  delivery and, 434
  diabetes mellitus and, 206
  diagnostic testing in, 429–431,
      430t–431t
  diet and, 432–433
  disseminated intravascular coagulation
      and, 398
  drug therapy for, 433–434
  early and appropriate prenatal care in,
      435–436
  eclampsia and, 447–449
  expectant management in, 431–432
  fetal and neonatal effects of, 427
  fetal surveillance in, 433, 439–440
  HELLP syndrome and, 445–447
  hematologic alterations in, 439
  hepatic alterations in, 439
  home health care in, 436–437
  intensive hemodynamic monitoring in,
      434, 450, 451t–452t
  intrapartum interventions for, 450–453
  low dose aspirin for prevention of, 266
  maternal effects of, 427
  mild *versus* severe, 428, 429t
  normal physiology and, 420–421
  nursing interventions for, 440–441, 441b
  pathophysiology of, 421–423, 422f
  postpartum interventions for, 453–454
  prevention of, 434–435
  pulmonary alterations in, 439
  renal alterations in, 438, 438t
  reproductive system status and, 439
  signs and symptoms of, 427–429
  supplemental calcium and, 12–13
  systemic lupus erythematosus and, 274
Pregestational diabetes, 204, 205t
Pregnancy
  acceptance of, 130
  antepartum nutrition and, 10–21
      assessment of, 13–16
      food groups and, 15–16, 16t–17t
      hyperemesis gravidarum and, 18–21,
          19b–20b, 20t
      hyperphenylalanemia and, 18
      nutrient needs in, 10–13
      prepregnancy weight status and,
          13–14
      weight gain in multifetal pregnancy
          and, 15, 16t
      weight gain in singleton pregnancy
          and, 14–15, 14t
  development of maternal-fetal unit in,
      4–6

Pregnancy *(Continued)*
  amniotic fluid and, 5–6
  embryo and, 4
  fetus and, 6
  placenta and, 4–5
  dietary requirements for, 16t
  ectopic; *See* Ectopic pregnancy
  exercise and bedrest in, 6–8, 9b–10b
  integrative therapies in, 107
      for addictions, 125
      alternative medical systems in,
          108–110
      for analgesia in labor, 123–125
      biologic-based therapies in, 112–113
      for breech presentation, 117–118
      for constipation, 118–119
      energy therapies in, 115
      evidence-based databases for, 126t
      for hyperemesis, 116–117
      for hypertensive disorders, 122
      for induction of labor, 123
      for low back pain, 121–122
      manipulative and body-based
          methods in, 113–115
      for mental and emotional problems,
          119–120
      mind-body interventions in, 110–112
      for postpartum bleeding, 125
      for preterm labor, 122–123
  physiologic adaptations to, 1
      cardiovascular, 1–4
      cervical changes and, 314
      gastrointestinal, 3–4
      hematologic, 2–3
      metabolic, 4
      renal, 3
      respiratory, 2
  prolonged, 660
      diagnostic testing in, 665–666
      etiology of, 660–661
      fetal and neonatal effects of,
          664–665
      incidence of, 660
      maternal effects of, 663–664
      medical management of, 666–667
      normal physiology of amniotic fluid
          and placenta and, 661
      nursing management of, 667–669
      pathophysiology of, 662
      signs and symptoms of, 662–663
  substance abuse during, 558
      alcohol in, 558–564, 559t–560t
      cocaine in, 564–567
      heroin in, 567–569, 568b
      as high risk factor, 39

Pregnancy *(Continued)*
  intervention for positive screen,
    574–575, 576t
  marijuana in, 569–570
  methamphetamines in, 570
  prevention and early detection of, 574,
    575b
  tobacco in, 571–574, 573b
  traditional Chinese medicine for, 125
  use of antidepressants during, 144–145
Pregnancy complications
  chronic hypertension in, 418–420
    antihypertensive medications for, 419t
    stages of, 418t
  disseminated intravascular coagulation
    in, 395
    anticoagulants for, 400
    blood replacement in, 399–400
    diagnostic testing in, 399
    etiology of, 395–396
    fetal and neonatal effects of, 398
    incidence of, 395
    maternal effects of, 398
    normal process of clot formation and,
      396–397, 396f–397f
    nursing management in, 400–401
    pathophysiology of, 397–398
    signs and symptoms of, 398
  ectopic pregnancy in, 331
    anticipatory grieving and, 348
    anxiety and, 347
    diagnostic testing in, 337–344,
      338t–341t, 343t
    etiology of, 331–333
    fetal and neonatal effects of, 337
    incidence of, 331
    maternal effects of, 337
    medical management of, 347–348
    methotrexate for, 344–345
    normal physiology and, 333
    nursing assessment in, 346–347
    pathophysiology of, 333–336, 334t,
      335f
    postoperative nursing interventions
      in, 347
    prevention of, 346
    signs and symptoms of, 336–337
    surgical treatment of, 344–345
  gestational trophoblastic disease in, 351
    anticipatory grieving and, 361
    early detection of, 361–362
    gestational trophoblastic neoplasia
      and, 358t–359t, 361
    maternal fear and, 361
    nursing assessment in, 360

Pregnancy complications *(Continued)*
    postevacuation nursing interventions
      in, 360–361
    uterine evacuation in, 360
  hemolytic incompatibility in, 402
    ABO blood group system and, 405
    antepartum nursing interventions for,
      413–414
    blood type genetics and, 402–405,
      403f–405f
    CDE (Rh) blood group system and,
      405
    diagnostic testing in, 408–409
    etiology of, 402
    fetal and neonatal effects of, 407–408
    incidence of, 402
    intrapartum nursing interventions
      for, 414
    maternal effects of, 407
    pathophysiology of, 406
    placental transport of fetal blood cells
      and, 405–406
    prevention of, 409–410, 412
    Rh_o D immune globulin for,
      412–413
    signs and symptoms of, 406, 407f
    treatment for, 410–412
  placental abnormalities in, 364
    abruptio placentae in, 364–376; *See
      also* Abruptio placentae
    antepartum fetal surveillance in, 391
    assessment of blood loss in, 387
    bedrest in, 392–393
    disseminated intravascular
      coagulation in, 390–391
    fear and, 392
    hospitalization in, 392
    hypovolemic shock in, 389–390
    invasive placenta in, 381–385
    mild bleeding in, 388
    moderate to severe bleeding in,
      388–389
    placenta previa in, 376–381; *See also*
      Placenta previa
    prevention of, 386–387
    RhD alloimmunization and, 393
    vasa previa in, 385–386, 385f
  preeclampsia in, 420–431
    activity restriction in, 432
    anticonvulsants for, 442–445,
      442b–443b, 444t, 446b
    cardiovascular alterations in,
      437–438, 437t
    central nervous system alterations in,
      438–439, 438t

Pregnancy complications *(Continued)*
  delivery and, 434
  diagnostic testing in, 429–431,
    430t–431t
  diet and, 432–433
  drug therapy for, 433–434
  early and appropriate prenatal care in,
    435–436
  eclampsia and, 447–449
  expectant management in, 431–432
  fetal and neonatal effects of, 427
  fetal surveillance in, 433, 439–440
  HELLP syndrome and, 445–447
  hematologic alterations in, 439
  hepatic alterations in, 439
  home health care in, 436–437
  intensive hemodynamic monitoring
    in, 434, 450, 451t–452t
  intrapartum interventions for,
    450–453
  maternal effects of, 427
  mild *versus* severe, 429t
  normal physiology and, 420–421
  nursing interventions for, 440–441,
    441b
  pathophysiology of, 421–423, 422f
  postpartum interventions for,
    453–454
  prevention of, 434–435
  pulmonary alterations in, 439
  renal alterations in, 438, 438t
  reproductive system status and, 439
  signs and symptoms of, 427–429
  premature rupture of membranes in, 488
    abruptio placentae and, 366
    antepartum complications in, 498
    bedrest in, 497–498
    diagnostic testing in, 491–492
    etiology of, 488–489
    fear and stress in, 497
    fetal and neonatal effects of, 490–491
    impaired fetal gas exchange in, 497
    incidence of, 488–489
    intrapartum nursing interventions
      in, 498
    maternal effects of, 490
    medical management of, 492–495
    normal physiology and, 489
    pathophysiology of, 489–490
    prevention of, 495–496
    risk for infection in, 496–497
  preterm labor in, 460
    abdominal surgery management of,
      473
    contraindications to halting, 472

Pregnancy complications *(Continued)*
    diabetes mellitus and, 206, 221, 235
    diagnostic testing in, 468–470
    estrogen and, 463
    etiology of, 461, 462b
    fetal and neonatal effects of, 465–468
    home management of, 482
    hospitalization in, 476–480
    incidence of, 460–461
    integrative therapies for, 122–123
    maternal cardiac disease and, 248,
      253
    maternal effects of, 465
    maternal urinary tract infection and,
      263
    multiple gestation and, 460
    national effects of, 468
    nontreatable cause, 472–473
    normal anatomy of cervix and, 461
    nursing management of, 474–482
    oxytocin and, 464
    pathophysiology of, 464–465,
      466t–467t
    physiology of labor contractions and,
      461–463
    primary prevention of, 470–471
    progesterone and, 464
    prostaglandins and, 463–464
    pulmonary edema in, 481–482
    secondary prevention of, 471–474
    tocolytic therapy for, 477b–480b,
      480–481
  spontaneous abortion in, 311
    anticipatory grieving and, 327
    antiphospholipid syndrome and, 275
    classification of, 316, 316f, 317t
    diabetes mellitus and, 206
    diagnostic testing in, 317–318
    in end-stage renal disease, 266–267
    etiology of, 311–313
    fetal effects of, 317
    hemorrhage management in, 325–326
    incidence of, 311
    inevitable, complete, or incomplete
      abortion and, 321–322
    interventions to decrease risk for
      recurrence, 328
    maternal cardiac disease and, 248
    maternal effects of, 316
    medical management of, 318–325
    missed abortion and, 322, 323f
    normal physiology and, 313–314
    nurse practitioner workup summary
      for, 319b–320b
    pathophysiology of, 315

Pregnancy complications *(Continued)*
  pelvic pain in, 338t–341t
  postsurgical nursing interventions in,
    326–327
  prevention of, 325
  recurrent, 323–325
  signs and symptoms of, 315–316
  systemic lupus erythematosus and,
    274
  threatened abortion and, 320–321
  tubal pregnancy and, 334
  trauma in, 500
    abruptio placentae and, 366
    burn in, 503
    cardiopulmonary resuscitation in,
      506–507
    chest injury in, 503
    continued monitoring in, 508
    critical care in, 514–516
    etiology of, 500–501
    fetal effects of, 504–505
    gunshot and stab wounds in, 504
    hemorrhage in, 501–504
    homicide in, 504
    incidence of, 500
    intimate partner violence and,
      509–510, 511b
    maternal effects of, 504
    minor injury management in, 505, 514
    motor vehicle collision prevention
      and, 508–509
    neurologic injury in, 502–503
    pathophysiology of, 501
    pelvic fracture in, 503
    primary survey in, 505–506
    recovery and rehabilitation in, 516
    secondary physical assessment in,
      506, 507f
    tertiary assessment in, 507–508
Pregnancy Loss and Infant Death
  Alliance, 155b–162b, 165
Prehypertension, 418t
Preimplantation genetic diagnosis, 99–100
Preimplantation genetic screening, 93t
Preload, 246
Premature atrial contractions, fetal, 64t
Premature rupture of membranes, 488
  abruptio placentae and, 366
  antepartum complications in, 498
  bedrest in, 497–498
  cocaine use and, 565
  diagnostic testing in, 491–492
  etiology of, 488–489
  fear and stress in, 497
  fetal and neonatal effects of, 490–491

Premature rupture of membranes
  (Continued)
  gonorrhea and, 525
  impaired fetal gas exchange in, 497
  incidence of, 488–489
  intrapartum nursing interventions in,
    498
  Laminaria dilator-related, 591
  maternal effects of, 490
  medical management of, 492–495
  normal physiology and, 489
  pathophysiology of, 489–490
  prevention of, 495–496
  risk for infection in, 496–497
Premature ventricular contractions, fetal,
  64t
Prematurity
  abruptio placentae and, 371
  breech presentation and, 616
  heroin use and, 568
  maternal cocaine use and, 565
  multiple gestation and, 468
  oxytocin-induced labor and, 596
  placenta previa and, 379
  premature rupture of membranes and,
    490
Prenatal assessment guide, 26, 27b–33b
Prenatal care
  high risk factors and, 39
  preeclampsia and, 435–436
Prenatal depression, 138, 143–145
Prenatal diagnostic tests, 92–97, 93t
  amniocentesis in, 95–96
  chorionic villus sampling in, 93–94
  percutaneous umbilical blood sampling
    in, 96–97
Prenatal genetic screening, 88–89, 89t
Prenatal therapy, 101–104
  fetal intrauterine surgery in, 102–103
  fetal intrauterine transfusion in, 101–102
  multifetal pregnancy reduction in,
    103–104
  nursing management in, 104
Preoperative management of cesarean
  birth, 649
Prepidil; *See* Dinoprostone
Prerenal failure, 259, 264t
Preterm labor, 460
  abdominal surgery management of, 473
  cocaine use and, 565
  contraindications to halting, 472
  diabetes mellitus and, 206, 221, 235
  diagnostic testing in, 468–470
  estrogen and, 463
  etiology of, 461, 462b

Preterm labor *(Continued)*
 fetal and neonatal effects of, 465–468
 gonorrhea and, 525
 hepatitis B and, 529
 heroin use and, 568
 home management of, 482
 hospitalization in, 476–480
 incidence of, 460–461
 integrative therapies for, 122–123
 marijuana and, 569
 maternal cardiac disease and, 248, 253
 maternal effects of, 465
 maternal urinary tract infection and,
  263
 multiple gestation and, 460
 national effects of, 468
 nontreatable cause, 472–473
 normal anatomy of cervix and, 461
 nursing management of, 474–482
 oxytocin and, 464
 pathophysiology of, 464–465, 466t–467t
 physiology of labor contractions and,
  461–463
 premature rupture of membranes and,
  493
 primary prevention of, 470–471
 progesterone and, 464
 prostaglandins and, 463–464
 pulmonary edema in, 481–482
 secondary prevention of, 471–474
 systemic lupus erythematosus and, 274
 tocolytic therapy for, 477b–480b,
  480–481
 urinary tract infection and, 549
Preterm premature rupture of membranes,
 488
Prevention
 of autoimmune rheumatic diseases,
  277–278
 of cardiac decompensation in cardiac
  disease, 252–253
 of disseminated intravascular
  coagulation, 400
 of dysfunctional labor, 627
 of ectopic pregnancy, 346
 of genitourinary infection, 549–551
 of hemolytic incompatibility, 409–410,
  412
 of human papillomavirus infection, 540
 of hydatidiform mole, 360
 of intimate partner violence, 510–511
 of maternal trauma, 508–511
 of motor vehicle collisions, 508–509
 of placental abnormalities, 386–387
 of preeclampsia, 434–435

Prevention *(Continued)*
 of premature rupture of membranes,
  495–496
 of preterm labor, 470–471
 of renal disease, 267–268
 of sexually transmitted infections,
  549–550
 of spontaneous abortion, 325
 of substance abuse during pregnancy,
  574, 575b
 of vaginal infection, 551
Primary survey in trauma, 505–506
Primary syphilis, 543
Prizing, process of valuing and, 170–171
Procardia; *See* Nifedipine
Process of valuing, 170–171
Professional liability, 181
Professional negligence, 188t–189t
Progesterone, 585
 aldosterone and, 261
 embryo development and, 4
 influence on uterine activity, 466t–467t
 preterm labor and, 464, 471
 role in embryo development, 313–314
 spontaneous abortion and, 318
Progestin-only contraceptives, ectopic
  pregnancy and, 332
Prolactin, myocardial contractility and,
  244
Prolonged decelerations of fetal heart rate,
  65t–67t, 69f
Prolonged pregnancy, 660
 diagnostic testing in, 665–666
 etiology of, 660–661
 fetal and neonatal effects of, 664–665
 incidence of, 660
 maternal effects of, 663–664
 medical management of, 666–667
 normal physiology of amniotic fluid and
  placenta and, 661
 nursing management of, 667–669
 pathophysiology of, 662
 signs and symptoms of, 662–663
PROM; *See* Premature rupture of
  membranes
Prophylactic antibiotic therapy
 for group B streptococcus, 526
 in premature rupture of membranes, 494
Prophylactic cerclage, 324
Prophylactic chemotherapy in
  hydatidiform mole, 356
Propranolol, 251
Prostacyclin, 421, 585
Prostaglandin inhibitors for preterm labor,
  477b–480b

Prostaglandins, 585
  cervical ripening and, 587
  influence on uterine activity, 466t–467t
  preterm labor and, 463–464
  prolonged pregnancy and, 660
  stripping of fetal membranes and, 602
Protein
  daily food choices and, 16t
  deficiency in hyperemesis gravidarum,
    18
  diabetic mother and, 227
  needs during pregnancy, 10–11, 16t
  nutritional therapy and, 113
Protein C deficiency, 283, 313
Protein S deficiency, 283, 313
Proteinuria in preeclampsia, 427–428, 438t
Prothrombin activator, 396, 396f
Prothrombin gene mutation G20210A,
    283
Prothrombin time in disseminated
  intravascular coagulation, 390–391
Proventil; See Albuterol
Proximate cause, 187
Psychologic adaptations, 128
  anxiety and, 132
  attachment and, 128–129
  conflict in, 133
  crisis in, 133
  frustration in, 132
  high risk adaptation and, 133–134
  high risk stressors and, 131–132
  hormonal response to high risk
    pregnancy and, 133
  maternal tasks in, 130
  nursing management during high risk
    pregnancy and, 134–138
    diversional activity interventions in,
      137–138
    interventions to allay fear and
      facilitate coping in, 134–136
    interventions to enhance self-esteem
      in, 137
    interventions to promote family
      processes in, 137
    psychologic assessment in, 134,
      135b–136b
  paternal tasks in, 130
  postpartum depression and, 138–140
    criteria for major depressive syndrome
      and, 143b
    diagnosis of, 140–143
    differential diagnosis of, 139
    Edinburgh Postnatal Depression
      Scale and, 141b–142b
    neonatal effects of, 140

Psychologic adaptations (Continued)
    screening for, 140
    treatment of, 143–145
  prenatal depression and, 138
  self-blaming in, 132
  threat to self-esteem in, 132
Psychosocial assessment of diabetic
    mother, 224
Psychosocial effects
  of bedrest, 8
  of intimate partner violence, 512
Psychotherapy for postpartum depression,
    143
Publicity, 174t
PUBS; See Percutaneous umbilical blood
    sampling
Pulmicort; See Budesonide
Pulmonary arterial carbon dioxide, 295t
Pulmonary artery catheter
  in hypovolemic shock in placental
    abnormalities, 390
  in preeclampsia, 450
Pulmonary artery wedge pressure, 255t
Pulmonary capillary wedge pressure, 1
Pulmonary disease, 289
  diagnostic testing in, 295–297,
    295t–296t
  etiology of, 290–291
  fetal effects of, 294–295
  incidence of, 289–290
  maternal effects of, 293–294
  medical management of, 297–303, 299t
  normal physiology and, 291
  nursing management of, 303–309
  pathophysiology of, 292
  signs and symptoms of, 292–293
Pulmonary edema
  acute, 307–308
  invasive hemodynamic monitoring and,
    450
  maternal cardiac disease and, 247
  in preeclampsia, 424, 451t–452t
  preterm labor and, 481–482
Pulmonary embolism, 282
  acute, 284–286, 285t
  anticoagulation therapy for, 286
  antiphospholipid syndrome and, 274
  critical care in, 307–308
  diagnostic testing in, 283
  etiology of, 282
  fetal effects of, 283, 294–295
  incidence of, 282, 290
  intrapartum and postpartum
    management of heparin and, 287
  maternal effects of, 283, 294

Pulmonary embolism *(Continued)*
  normal physiology and, 283
  signs and symptoms of, 283
  thromboprophylaxis and, 284
  treatment of, 286
Pulmonary hypoplasia, premature rupture
  of membranes and, 491
Pulmonary wedge pressure, 249
Pulsatile oxytocin management, 595
Pulsatilla
  for analgesia in labor, 124–125
  for breech presentation, 118
  for hyperemesis, 116–117
  for induction of labor, 123
Pulse oximetry, fetal, 71–80
Pulse pressure
  blood loss and, 370t
  spontaneous abortion and, 319b–320b
Punitive exemplary damages, legal term,
  187
Purified protein derivative, 35
Pushing methods, 633
Pyelonephritis, 258
  diabetes mellitus and, 206
  diagnostic testing in, 263–264
  signs and symptoms of, 261
Pyridoxine
  for hyperemesis gravidarum, 19
  isoniazid with, 302
  multifetal pregnancy and, 15

Q
Qi, 108
Quadruple marker screen, 35, 90
Quality assurance, 194b–195b
Quickening, prolonged pregnancy and,
  666
Quinidine, 251

R
Race as high risk factor, 38
Radiation therapy as high risk factor, 40t
Rapid-acting insulins, 215, 216t
Rapid plasma reagin test, 34
Raspberry leaf tea, 124, 604
Reactive oxygen species, premature
  rupture of membranes and, 490
Recombinant human activated protein
  C for disseminated intravascular
  coagulation, 399
Recombinant immunoblot assay, 530
Recovery and rehabilitation in trauma,
  508, 516
Recumbent position during labor,
  629–631

Recurrent spontaneous abortions, 317t
  etiology of, 312–313
  medical management of, 323–325
  nursing interventions to decrease risk
    of, 325
Red blood cell transfusion in disseminated
  intravascular coagulation, 399
Referral, diabetic mother and, 230, 232
Referred pain after tubal rupture, 337
Refusal to follow order, 185
Regional analgesia for labor, 633, 635,
  646–648
Rehabilitation in trauma, 516
Relationship-based care, 150
Relaxin
  cervical incompetence and, 315
  fetal membranes and, 489
  influence on uterine activity, 466t–467t
Renal artery, 260
Renal biopsy, 264
Renal calculi
  diagnostic testing in, 264
  etiology of, 259
  general management of, 265
  incidence of, 258
  signs and symptoms of, 261
Renal disease, 258
  critical care for acute renal failure and,
    269
  diagnostic testing in, 263–265, 264t
  drug therapy for, 267
  etiology of, 259
  fetal and neonatal effects of, 263
  general management of, 265–267
  incidence of, 258
  maternal effects of, 263
  normal renal physiology and, 259–261
  nursing interventions for, 268–269
  prevention of, 267–268
  signs and symptoms of, 261–262
Renal failure
  in abruptio placentae, 369
  in placenta previa, 378
Renal function studies, 264, 264t
Renal plasma flow, multiple gestation and,
  464
Renal system
  changes during pregnancy, 3, 420
  normal physiology of, 259–261
  systemic lupus erythematosus and,
    273t
Renal tubule, 260
Renin, 261
Reparation, 174t
Replacement child syndrome, 153–162

Reproductive system status, preeclampsia and, 439
Rescue cerclage, 325
Residual volume, 296t
Respiratory acidosis, 297
Respiratory alkalosis, 297
    chest injury and, 503
    compensatory, 2
Respiratory compromise, 295–296
Respiratory disease, 289
    diagnostic testing in, 295–297, 295t–296t
    etiology of, 290–291
    fetal effects of, 294–295
    incidence of, 289–290
    maternal effects of, 293–294
    medical management of, 297–303, 299t
    normal physiology and, 291
    nursing management of, 303–309
    pathophysiology of, 292
    signs and symptoms of, 292–293
Respiratory distress
    in anaphylactoid syndrome of pregnancy, 292–293
    signs and symptoms of, 292–293
Respiratory emergencies
    critical care in, 307
    fetal effects of, 294–295
    incidence of, 290
    maternal effects of, 294
Respiratory infections
    etiology of, 290–291
    incidence of, 290
    maternal effects of, 294
    medical management of, 298–303
    nursing interventions for, 303–304
    pathophysiology of, 292
Respiratory rate, 296t
    abruptio placentae and, 369
    in disseminated intravascular coagulation, 398
    in preeclampsia, 439
Respiratory system
    normal physiology of, 291
    physiologic adaptations to pregnancy, 2
    systemic lupus erythematosus and, 273t
Respondent superior, legal term, 188t–189t
Rest and relaxation pattern, dysfunctional labor and, 634
Retinopathy, diabetic, 207, 213
Reverse Woods screw maneuver, 639t
Revised White's classification of perinatal diabetes, 201t

RhD alloimmunization, 402
    ABO blood group system and, 405
    antepartum nursing interventions for, 413–414
    blood type genetics and, 402–405, 403f–405f
    CDE (Rh) blood group system and, 405
    diagnostic testing in, 408–409
    etiology of, 402
    fetal and neonatal effects of, 407–408
    incidence of, 402
    intrapartum nursing interventions for, 414
    maternal effects of, 407
    pathophysiology of, 406
    placental abnormalities and, 378, 393
    placental transport of fetal blood cells and, 405–406
    prevention of, 409–410, 412
    Rh_o D immune globulin for, 412–413
    signs and symptoms of, 406, 407f
    treatment for, 410–412
RhD antigen, 405
Rh_o D immune globulin
    after ectopic pregnancy, 347
    after maternal trauma, 514
    after spontaneous abortion procedures, 327
    after uterine evacuation of hydatidiform mole, 355
    for hemolytic incompatibility, 409, 412–413
Rheumatic fever, 249
Rh_o(D) blood typing, 33
Ribavirin, 531
Rifampin, 302
Right action, 172
Risk assessment for preterm labor, 468–469
Risk drinking, 563
Risk management, 188t–189t, 194b–195b
Rocephin; See Ceftriaxone
Rodenticide exposure as high risk factor, 40t
Role-relationship pattern, 27b–33b
    diabetic mother and, 231
    dysfunctional labor and, 636–637
    in psychologic assessment for high-risk pregnancy, 135b–136b
Role transition in pregnancy, 130
Rose oil, 124
Rubella/rubeola/varicella screen, 34
Rubin rotational maneuver, 639t, 642f

Rupture
    tubal, 334, 335f, 345
    uterine
        small birth canal and, 618
        trauma-related, 509

S
Safety issues in intimate partner violence,
    512–513
Saint John's wort, 124
Saline wet mount
    in bacterial vaginosis, 520
    in candidiasis, 521
Salpingo-oophorectomy in tubal rupture,
    345
Screening
    for alcohol use, 561–562, 561t–562t
    antepartum diagnostic assessment and,
        26–36
    for cocaine use, 566
    for depression
        postpartum, 140
        prenatal, 138
    for genitourinary infections
        bacterial vaginosis and, 520
        candidiasis and, 521
        chlamydial infection and, 523
        gonorrhea and, 524–525
        group B streptococcus and, 526
        hepatitis B and, 528
        hepatitis C and, 530
        herpes simplex virus type 2 and, 532
        human immunodeficiency virus and,
            534–535
        human papillomavirus and, 540
        syphilis and, 544
        trichomoniasis and, 545
        urinary tract infection and, 547
    for iron deficiency anemia, 11
    for marijuana use, 570
    perinatal, 88
        amniocentesis in, 95–96
        chorionic villus sampling in, 93–94
        fetal kidney biopsy and, 98
        fetal muscle biopsy and, 97–98
        fetal skin biopsy and, 97
        fetal urine aspiration and, 99
        methods of, 89–91
        noninvasive prenatal diagnosis and,
            100
        nursing management in, 104
        percutaneous umbilical blood
            sampling in, 96–97
        preimplantation genetic diagnosis
            and, 99–100

Screening (Continued)
        prenatal diagnostic tests and, 92–97,
            93t
        prenatal genetic screening and,
            88–89, 89t
        ultrasound evaluation for fetal
            abnormalities and, 91–92, 92b
    for substance abuse, 575b
    for thrombophilia, 283
Second stage of labor, 631–633, 632f
Second trimester
    diabetes mellitus and
        calculation guidelines for insulin in,
            216t
        insulin needs and, 215t
        manifestations and consequences of,
            205t
    screening in, 90–91
Secondary physical assessment in trauma,
    506, 507f
Secondary prevention
    of disseminated intravascular
        coagulation, 400
    of preterm labor, 471–474
    of sexually transmitted infections,
        550
Secondary syphilis, 543
Seizure in eclampsia, 425–426, 447–448
Selective transfer, 5, 34
Self-blaming in high risk pregnancy, 132
Self-esteem
    interventions to enhance, 137
    sexually transmitted infections and,
        550–551
    threat in high-risk pregnancy, 132
Self-management education, diabetic
    mother and, 225
Self-monitoring of blood glucose, 214
    after delivery, 222
    patient education in, 233
Self-perception and self-concept pattern,
    27b–33b
    diabetic mother and, 27b–33b, 231
    dysfunctional labor and, 636
    in psychologic assessment for high-risk
        pregnancy, 135b–136b
Sensitization to fetal blood cells, 406
Sepia, 116–117
Septic abortion, 317t
Septicemia in placenta previa, 378
Serial clot observation testing in
    disseminated intravascular
    coagulation, 391
Serotonin, cocaine and, 564
Serum albumin, preeclampsia and, 424

Serum beta-human chorionic gonadotropin
in ectopic pregnancy, 342, 343t
in hydatidiform mole, 351
in metastatic gestational trophoblastic neoplasia, 359
in spontaneous abortion, 318
Serum blood glucose, oral glucose tolerance test and, 211t
Serum creatinine changes during pregnancy, 3
Serum ferritin, iron deficiency anemia and, 11
Serum progesterone in ectopic pregnancy, 343t, 344
Severe abruptio placentae, 368
Severe gestational hypertension, 416
Severe preeclampsia, 440–441
Sexual intercourse for induction of labor, 604
Sexuality and reproductive pattern, 27b–33b
diabetic mother and, 232
in psychologic assessment for high-risk pregnancy, 135b–136b
Sexually transmitted infections, 519
chlamydial, 522–524
ectopic pregnancy and, 331
gonorrhea in, 524–525
hepatitis B in, 527–530
herpes simplex virus type 2 in, 531–533
human immunodeficiency virus in, 533–539
human papillomavirus in, 539–541
primary prevention of, 549–550
screening for, 34
secondary prevention of, 550
self-esteem and, 550–551
syphilis in, 543–545
tertiary prevention for, 550
trichomoniasis in, 545–546
Sheehan syndrome
in abruptio placentae, 369
hypovolemic shock in, 390
Shepherd's purse, 125
Shock
in abruptio placentae, 368–369
after tubal rupture, 337
disseminated intravascular coagulation and, 398
trauma-related, 504
Short-acting beta$_2$-agonists, 300t–301t
Short-acting insulins, 215, 216t
Short-term variability of fetal heart rate, 46

Shoulder pain after tubal rupture, 337
Shoulder presentation, 614, 615f, 624t–626t
management of, 638–641, 639t, 640f–642f
Sick-day rule in diabetes mellitus, 234
Sidelines support group, 8, 136
Simple diffusion, 44
Sim's lateral position
in occiput posterior presentation, 631
second stage of labor and, 633
Single footling breech, 616f
Singulair; See Montelukast
Sinoatrial arrest, fetal, 64t
Sinusoidal pattern of fetal heart rate, 70f, 70t
in hemolytic incompatibility, 407f, 408
Situational stressors, 131–132
Sitz bath for candidiasis, 522
Skin
of diabetic mother, 224
disseminated intravascular coagulation and, 398
systemic lupus erythematosus and, 273t
SLE; See Systemic lupus erythematosus
Sleep and rest pattern, 27b–33b
diabetic mother and, 231
in psychologic assessment for high-risk pregnancy, 135b–136b
Smoking, 571–574
abruptio placentae and, 366
ectopic pregnancy and, 332
fetal and neonatal complications in, 571–572
maternal complications in, 571
pathophysiologic effects of, 571
premature rupture of membranes and, 496
treatment during pregnancy, 572–574, 573b
Smoking cessation program, 572, 573b, 576t
Snack foods, 229t–230t
Sniffing cocaine, 564
Social drinking, 563
Socioeconomic status as high risk factor, 38
Sodium
diabetic mother and, 228
excess in acute renal failure, 262
glomerular filtration and, 260
needs during pregnancy, 12
preeclampsia and, 432–433
restriction in maternal cardiac disease, 251

Somogyi effect, 217t
Special damages, legal term, 187
Spectinomycin for gonorrhea, 525
Speculum examination
    in placenta previa, 379
    in premature rupture of membranes,
        491
    in spontaneous abortion, 318,
        319b–320b
Spinal cord injury, 502
Spiritual healing and prayer, 111
    for mental and emotional problems, 120
Spontaneous abortion, 311
    anticipatory grieving and, 327
    antiphospholipid syndrome and, 275
    classification of, 316, 316f, 317t
    cocaine use and, 565
    diabetes mellitus and, 206
    diagnostic testing in, 317–318
    in end-stage renal disease, 266–267
    etiology of, 311–313
    fetal effects of, 317
    gestational trophoblastic neoplasia and,
        356
    hemorrhage management in, 325–326
    incidence of, 311
    inevitable, complete, or incomplete
        abortion and, 321–322
    interventions to decrease risk for
        recurrence, 328
    maternal cardiac disease and, 248
    maternal effects of, 316
    medical management of, 318–325
    missed abortion and, 322, 323f
    normal physiology and, 313–314
    nurse practitioner workup summary for,
        319b–320b
    pathophysiology of, 315
    pelvic pain in, 338t–341t
    postsurgical nursing interventions in,
        326–327
    prevention of, 325
    recurrent, 323–325
    signs and symptoms of, 315–316
    systemic lupus erythematosus and,
        274
    threatened abortion and, 320–321
    tubal pregnancy and, 334
Sporadic abortions, 311–312
Squatting position, 631, 632f
Stab wound, 504
Standard Advanced Cardiac Life Support,
    506
Standards of care, 188t–189t
    legal issues in, 192–195, 192t

Starch, exchange list for meal planning
    and, 228t–230t
Starvation ketosis, 204–206
Statins for preconception management of
    dyslipidemia, 212
Statute of limitations, 188t–189t
Statutory law, 188t–189t
Stillbirth
    cocaine use and, 565
    diabetes mellitus and, 208
    systemic lupus erythematosus and, 274
Streptococcus agalactiae, 525
Stress, 131
    integrative therapies for, 119–120
    premature rupture of membranes and,
        497
    preterm labor and, 462b, 465
    prolonged pregnancy and, 663–664
    sporadic abortions and, 312
Stripping of fetal membranes for induction
    of labor, 602
Stroke, antiphospholipid syndrome and,
    274
Stroke volume, 245
    uterine contractions and, 245
Substance abuse, 558
    alcohol in, 558–564
        childhood effects of, 561
        fetal complications in, 559–560,
            559t–560t
        maternal complications in, 559
        pathophysiologic effects of, 558
        pregnancy considerations in, 562–563
        screening for, 561–562, 561t–562t
        treatment during pregnancy, 563–564
    cocaine in, 564–567
    heroin in, 567–569, 568b
    as high risk factor, 39
    intervention for positive screen,
        574–575, 576t
    marijuana in, 569–570
    methamphetamines in, 570
    prevention and early detection of, 574,
        575b
    tobacco in, 571–574
        fetal and neonatal complications in,
            571–572
        maternal complications in, 571
        pathophysiologic effects of, 571
        treatment during pregnancy, 572–574,
            573b
    traditional Chinese medicine for, 125
Sulfonamides for urinary tract infection,
    548t
Supervision, litigation risk and, 183–184

Supine position
  avoidance during labor, 629, 631
  exercise performed in, 7
  fetal oxygenation and, 43
Support group for spontaneous abortion, 327
Suprapubic pressure, 639t, 640f–641f
Supraventricular tachycardia, fetal, 62, 64t
Surfactant protein A, labor contractions and, 461–463
Surgery
  bariatric, 14
  in ectopic pregnancy, 345
  fetal intrauterine, 102–103
  in preterm labor, 473
Sustained-release theophylline, 300t–301t
Sweets
  daily food choices and, 16t
  exchange list for meal planning and, 229t–230t
Swimming for low back pain, 121
Sympathetic nervous system in control of fetal heart rate, 46
Symptom-relief drinking, 563
Synchrony in parent-infant attachment, 129
Syncope
  blood loss and, 370t
  in ectopic pregnancy, 347
Syncytiotrophoblast, 4–5, 314
Syndrome X, 200
Synthetic dilators for induction of labor, 590–591
Syphilis, 543–545
Systemic corticosteroids, 300t–301t
Systemic disease, sporadic abortions and, 312
Systemic lupus erythematosus, 271
  critical care interventions for, 280
  drug therapy for, 277
  etiology of, 272
  fetal and neonatal effects of, 274–275
  general management of, 276
  incidence of, 271
  intrapartum nursing interventions for, 279
  maternal effects of, 274
  medical diagnosis of, 275
  pathophysiology of, 272
  postpartum nursing interventions for, 279
  prenatal nursing interventions for, 278
  secondary and tertiary prevention in, 277–278
  signs and symptoms of, 272, 273t

Systemic vascular resistance, 246
  changes during pregnancy, 2, 244
Systems of law, 186–187

T
T-ACE questionnaire for at-risk drinking patterns, 561, 561t
Tachycardia
  fetal, 59t, 60f
  in venous thromboembolic disease, 283
Tachypnea
  blood loss and, 370t
  in venous thromboembolic disease, 283
Tactile contact in parent-infant attachment, 129
Tai ji, 108
Teleology, 175
Telephone advice, 184
Tenormin; See Atenolol
Teratogen
  alcohol as, 563
  marijuana as, 569
  in sporadic abortions, 311–312, 325
Terazol; See Terconazole
Terbutaline
  for acute exacerbation of asthma, 306
  for maternal cardiac disease, 251
  for preterm labor, 477b–480b
Terconazole for candidiasis, 522
Term gestation, ACOG confirmation of, 583b
Tertiary assessment in trauma, 507–508
Tertiary prevention
  in cardiac disease, 251–252
  of disseminated intravascular coagulation, 400
  of sexually transmitted infections, 550
Tertiary syphilis, 544
Tetracycline contraindication in pregnancy, 267
Theca lutein cyst, 353
Theophylline, 300t–301t
Therapeutic cerclage, 324–325
Therapeutic massage, 114
Thermal trauma, 503
Third trimester
  diabetes mellitus and
    calculation guidelines for insulin in, 216t
    insulin needs and, 215t
    manifestations and consequences of, 205t
  placental abnormalities and, 364
    abruptio placentae in, 364–376
    antepartum fetal surveillance in, 391

Third trimester *(Continued)*
  assessment of blood loss in, 387
  bedrest in, 392–393
  disseminated intravascular
      coagulation in, 390–391
  fear and, 392
  hospitalization in, 392
  hypovolemic shock in, 389–390
  invasive placenta in, 381–385
  mild bleeding in, 388
  moderate to severe bleeding in,
      388–389
  placenta previa in, 376–381
  prevention of, 386–387
  RhD alloimmunization and, 393
  vasa previa in, 385–386, 385f
Thoracic breathing during pregnancy, 2
Threatened abortion, 316f, 317t, 320–321
Three-hour glucose tolerance test, 210–211
Thrombin, 396, 396f
Thrombocytopenia, preeclampsia-related,
    452–453
Thrombophilia, 282
  abruptio placentae and, 366
  preeclampsia and, 427
  recurrent abortions and, 313
Thromboprophylaxis, 284
Thrombosis in placenta previa, 378
Thromboxane, 421, 463
Thyroid palpation in diabetic mother, 224
Tidal volume, 291, 296t
  changes during pregnancy, 2
Tinzaparin, 285t
Tissue culture for *Chlamydia*, 523
Tobacco use, 571–574; *See also* Smoking
Tocolytic therapy
  for abruptio placentae, 372
  for maternal cardiac disease, 251
  for placenta previa, 380
  for premature rupture of membranes,
      495
  for preterm labor, 477b–480b, 480–481
Tocotransducer, 49, 51f
Tort, 187
Total body surface area, 503
Total placenta previa, 370t, 376
Traditional Chinese medicine, 108–110
  for addictions, 125
  for analgesia in labor, 123–124
  for breech presentation, 117–118
  for constipation, 118
  for hyperemesis, 116
  for hypertensive disorders, 122
  for induction of labor, 123
  for low back pain, 121–122

Traditional Chinese medicine *(Continued)*
  for mental and emotional problems,
      119–120
  for postpartum bleeding, 125
  for preterm labor, 122–123
Trandate; *See* Labetalol
Transabdominal chorionic villus sampling,
    94
Transcervical chorionic villus sampling, 94
Transcutaneous electrical nerve
      stimulation for induction of labor, 604
Transfusion
  in abruptio placentae, 372, 373t–375t
  in disseminated intravascular
      coagulation, 399–400
  fetal, 101–102
  in hemolytic incompatibility, 410
  in placenta previa, 380
  in preeclampsia-related
      thrombocytopenia, 452–453
  in spontaneous abortion, 321–322,
      325–326
Transmigration of ovum, 333
Transvaginal Foley catheter for labor
      induction, 591
Transvaginal ultrasound
  in ectopic pregnancy, 342, 343t
  in hydatidiform mole, 351, 360
  in placenta previa, 379
  as predictor of success in labor
      induction, 584
  in risk assessment for preterm labor, 469
Trauma, 500
  abruptio placentae and, 366
  birth, 618
  burn in, 503
  cardiopulmonary resuscitation in,
      506–507
  chest injury in, 503
  continued monitoring in, 508
  critical care in, 514–516
  etiology of, 500–501
  fetal effects of, 504–505
  gunshot and stab wounds in, 504
  hemorrhage in, 501–504
  homicide in, 504
  incidence of, 500
  intimate partner violence and, 509–510,
      511b
  Laminaria dilator-related, 591
  maternal effects of, 504
  minor injury management in, 505, 514
  motor vehicle collision prevention and,
      508–509
  neurologic injury in, 502–503

Trauma *(Continued)*
  pathophysiology of, 501
  pelvic fracture in, 503
  primary survey in, 505–506
  recovery and rehabilitation in, 516
  secondary physical assessment in, 506, 507f
  tertiary assessment in, 507–508
Treponema pallidum, 543
Trial of labor, 644–645
Trial procedure, 191–195
Trichomoniasis, 545–546
Trimethoprim-sulfamethoxazole
  for acute pyelonephritis, 547
  for urinary tract infection, 265
Tripelennamine, 298
Triple marker screening, 90
Trophoblast, 4, 313, 352–353
  hydatidiform mole and, 351, 352f
Tubal abortion, 334, 335f
Tubal ectopic pregnancy, 333–335
  medical management of, 344–345
  tubal rupture in, 345
Tubal infection, 331
Tubal ligation, 332
Tubal rupture, 334, 335f
Tubal surgery, ectopic pregnancy and, 331
Tuberculosis
  incidence of, 290
  medical management of, 302–303
  purified protein derivative test for, 35
Tuboabdominal pregnancy, 331, 335
Tuboovarian pregnancy, 331, 335
Tuina, 109
Tumor necrosis factor-alpha, hyperinsulinemia and, 202
TWEAK questionnaire for at-risk drinking patterns, 561, 562t
Twin pregnancy, 460
  breech presentation and, 616
  electronic fetal monitor for, 55
  as high risk factor, 41
  normal physiologic adaptation to, 464
  preterm labor and, 460
    abdominal surgery management of, 473
    contraindications to halting, 472
    diabetes mellitus and, 206, 221, 235
    diagnostic testing in, 468–470
    estrogen and, 463
    etiology of, 461, 462b
    fetal and neonatal effects of, 465–468
    home management of, 482
    hospitalization in, 476–480
    incidence of, 460–461

Twin pregnancy *(Continued)*
    integrative therapies for, 122–123
    maternal cardiac disease and, 248, 253
    maternal effects of, 465
    maternal urinary tract infection and, 263
    national effects of, 468
    nontreatable cause, 472–473
    normal anatomy of cervix and, 461
    nursing management of, 474–482
    oxytocin and, 464
    pathophysiology of, 464–465, 466t–467t
    physiology of labor contractions and, 461–463
    primary prevention of, 470–471
    progesterone and, 464
    prostaglandins and, 463–464
    pulmonary edema in, 481–482
    secondary prevention of, 471–474
    tocolytic therapy for, 477b–480b, 480–481
  weight gain in, 15, 16t
Twin-twin transfusion syndrome, 103
Two-hour glucose tolerance test, 210–211
Two-hour postprandial glucose, 210
Type 1 diabetes mellitus, 200, 202, 210
Type 2 diabetes mellitus, 200, 202
  development due to maternal diabetes mellitus, 209
  diagnostic testing in, 210
TYVU acronym, 318

U
Ultrasound, 35–36
  in cardiac disease, 249
  in chronic kidney disease, 266
  diabetic mother and, 220
  in ectopic pregnancy, 342, 343t
  for fetal abnormalities, 91–92, 92b
  in hemolytic incompatibility, 409
  in hydatidiform mole, 351, 360
  in placenta cretas, 381
  in placenta previa, 379
  as predictor of success in labor induction, 584
  in prolonged pregnancy, 666
  in risk assessment for preterm labor, 469
  in spontaneous abortion, 318
  in vasa previa, 386
Ultrasound transducer, 49, 51f
Umbilical artery, 5

Umbilical cord
  prolonged pregnancy and, 662
  velamentous inserted, 385, 385f
Umbilical vein, 5
Unconjugated estriol, triple marker
    screening and, 90
Underweight, prepregnancy weight status
    and, 13–14, 14t
Unfractionated heparin
  for acute venous thromboembolism,
    285
  for antiphospholipid syndrome, 285t,
    324
  intrapartum and postpartum
    management of, 287
  for maternal cardiac disease, 250
  for prevention of valve thrombosis,
    247–248
  for thromboprophylaxis, 284
Uniform accelerations of fetal heart rate,
    65t–67t, 68f
Universality, 174t
Unproductive uterine activity, 596
Upper respiratory infection, 298
Upright position during labor,
    629, 630f
Urea, 260
Urethral calculi
  diagnostic testing in, 264
  etiology of, 259
  general management of, 265
  incidence of, 258
  signs and symptoms of, 261
Urinary output
  in abruptio placentae, 372
  in chronic kidney disease, 266
  in disseminated intravascular
    coagulation, 398
  in placental abnormalities, 387, 390
Urinary stasis, 261
Urinary tract infection, 546–549, 548t
  diabetes mellitus and, 206, 230
  diagnostic testing in, 263–264
  drug therapy for, 267
  etiology of, 259
  general management of, 265–267
  incidence of, 258
  maternal effects of, 263
  prevention of, 267–268
  signs and symptoms of, 261–262
Urine culture, 26
Urine dipstick test, 36
Urine ketones, 214
Urine testing in diabetes mellitus, 214
Urine toxicology screening, 566

Uterine anomalies
  hydatidiform mole and, 353
  recurrent spontaneous abortions and,
    312, 323
Uterine contractions
  cardiac output and, 245
  cocaine use and, 565
  dysfunctional labor and, 611
  induction of labor and, 582
    amniotomy for, 600–602
    balloon catheters and extra-amniotic
      saline infusion for, 591–592
    breast stimulation for, 602–604
    complementary therapies for,
      604–605
    contraindications for, 585
    criteria for, 583–584
    dinoprostone for, 586–590, 588t
    incidence of, 582
    indications for, 583, 583b
    integrative therapies for, 123
    Laminaria and synthetic dilators for,
      590–591
    misoprostol for, 590
    oxytocin for, 593–600, 594t; See also
      Oxytocin
    physiology of uterotropins and
      uterotonins and, 585–586
    predictors of success in, 584, 584t
    risks in, 585
    stripping of fetal membranes for,
      602
  normal physiology of, 461–463, 612
Uterine dystocia, 612
Uterine evacuation
  of hydatidiform mole, 355, 360
  in spontaneous abortion, 321
Uterine rupture, 509
  small birth canal and, 618
Uterine tachysystole
  breast stimulation and, 603
  dinoprostone and, 587
  oxytocin and, 595–596
  vaginal birth after cesarean and, 644
Uteroplacental-fetal exchange,
    44–45
Uteroplacental insufficiency in
    preeclampsia, 423
Uterotonins, 585–586
Uterus
  factors influencing activity of,
    466t–467t
  preterm labor and, 464–465
  prolonged pregnancy and, 663
Utility, 174t

V

Vaccination risk, 37
Vacuum aspiration in spontaneous
　　abortion, 321
Vacuum extractor delivery, 645–646
Vaginal birth after cesarean, 623, 643–644
Vaginal bleeding
　　in ectopic pregnancy, 336, 346–347
　　in placenta previa, 378
　　in spontaneous abortion, 315, 317–318
Vaginal delivery
　　breech presentation and, 617
　　cardiac disease and, 249
　　HELLP syndrome and, 447
　　heparin therapy after, 287
　　human immunodeficiency virus
　　　　infection and, 538
　　preeclampsia and, 434
Vaginal infections
　　bacterial vaginosis in, 519–521
　　candidiasis in, 521–522
　　chlamydial, 522–524
　　diabetes mellitus and, 206
　　gonorrhea in, 524–525
　　primary prevention of, 551
Vaginal speculum examination
　　in placenta previa, 379
　　in premature rupture of membranes, 491
　　in spontaneous abortion, 318,
　　　　319b–320b
Vaginal ultrasound
　　in ectopic pregnancy, 342, 343t
　　in hydatidiform mole, 351, 360
　　in placenta previa, 379
　　in risk assessment for preterm labor, 469
　　in spontaneous abortion, 318
Valium; See Diazepam
Valsalva maneuver, 7
Value and belief pattern, 135b–136b
Values clarification, 170–171
Variability of fetal heart rate, 58–59, 60f,
　　61t, 62f
　　amniotomy and, 601
　　decelerations in, 65t–67t, 69f
　　in hemolytic incompatibility, 408
　　maternal cocaine use and, 567
　　prostaglandin-initiated labor and,
　　　　587–589
Varicella infection, 312
Vasa previa, 385–386, 385f
Vascular defect, preeclampsia and, 426
Vasopressin influence on uterine activity,
　　466t–467t
Vasopressors for hypovolemic shock in
　　placental abnormalities, 390

VBAC; See Vaginal birth after cesarean
VDRL; See Venereal Disease Research
　　Laboratory test
Vegetables
　　daily food choices and, 16t
　　exchange list for meal planning and,
　　　　228t–230t
　　menu guidelines for, 17t
Velamentous inserted umbilical cord, 385,
　　385f
Venereal Disease Research Laboratory
　　test, 34
Venous pressure changes during
　　pregnancy, 245
Venous thromboembolic disease, 282
　　acute, 284–286, 285t
　　anticoagulation therapy for, 286
　　antiphospholipid syndrome and, 274
　　diagnostic testing in, 283
　　etiology of, 282
　　fetal and neonatal effects of, 283
　　incidence of, 282
　　intrapartum and postpartum
　　　　management of heparin and, 287
　　maternal effects of, 283
　　normal physiology and, 283
　　signs and symptoms of, 283
　　thromboprophylaxis and, 284
Veracity, 174t
Verbal contact in parent-infant
　　attachment, 129
Verbal orders, legal issues in, 185
Vibroacoustic stimulation, 74b
Villi, placental, 4–5, 34
Violence as high risk factor, 41
Viral infections
　　bronchitis in, 298
　　hepatitis B in, 527–530
　　hepatitis C in, 530–531
　　herpes simplex virus type 2 in, 531–533
　　human immunodeficiency virus in,
　　　　533–539
　　human papillomavirus in, 539–541
　　human parvovirus B19 in, 542–543
　　pneumonia in, 302
　　sporadic abortions and, 312
Viremia, 312
Visken; See Pindolol
Visual changes in preeclampsia, 424
Visual contact in parent-infant attachment,
　　129
Vital capacity, 291
Vital signs
　　of diabetic mother, 224
　　in ectopic pregnancy, 347

Vitamin(s)
    diabetic mother and, 227
    renal excretion of, 261
    supplementation in hyperemesis
        gravidarum, 18
Vitamin A, 13
Vitamin B complex deficiency, 18
Vitamin B$_6$ supplementation
    for hyperemesis gravidarum, 19
    with isoniazid, 302
    in multifetal pregnancy, 15
Vitamin C supplementation in multifetal
        pregnancy, 16
Vitamin D
    needs during pregnancy, 13
    supplementation in multifetal
        pregnancy, 16
Volume overload in preeclampsia, 424
Vomiting
    in hyperemesis gravidarum, 18
    integrative therapies for, 116–117
Vulnerable child syndrome, 153–162

W
Waning insulin, 217t
Warfarin
    for prevention of valve thrombosis,
        247–248
    resumption after delivery, 287
    for thromboprophylaxis, 284
Warm compress breast stimulation, 603
Water
    diabetic mother and, 227, 231
    reabsorption of, 260
Water intoxication, 596
Water therapy in preeclampsia, 435
Weight, prepregnancy weight status and,
        13–14
Weight gain
    dietary requirements for pregnancy and,
        16t
    in multifetal pregnancy, 15, 16t
    in singleton pregnancy, 14–15, 14t

Weight loss
    in diabetes mellitus, 210
    in hyperemesis gravidarum, 18
    prolonged pregnancy and, 663
Wharton jelly, prolonged pregnancy and,
        662
Whiff test
    in bacterial vaginosis, 520
    in candidiasis, 521
Whirlpool bath, 635
White's classification of perinatal diabetes,
        201t
WIC; See Women, Infants, and Children
Wild yam cream, 117
Withdrawal, 568b
Women, Infants, and Children, 16–18
Woods screw maneuver, 639t, 641f

Y
Yarrow, 125
Yin and yang, 108
Yoga, 112
    for constipation, 119
    for hypertensive disorders, 122
    for low back pain, 121
    for mental and emotional problems, 120
Yolk sac, 5

Z
Zafirlukast, 300t–301t
Zidovudine, 535–536
Zinc
    needs during pregnancy, 12
    supplementation in multifetal
        pregnancy, 15
Zygote, 313, 352–353